W9-BKK-235

THEORETICAL BASIS *for Nursing*

THEORETICAL BASIS *for Nursing*

FOURTH EDITION

Melanie McEwen, PhD, RN, CNE, ANEF

Associate Professor
University of Texas Health Science Center at Houston
School of Nursing
Houston, Texas

Evelyn M. Wills, PhD, RN

Professor (Retired)
Department of Nursing
College of Nursing and Allied Health Professions
University of Louisiana at Lafayette
Lafayette, Louisiana

Wolters Kluwer Health | Lippincott Williams & Wilkins

Philadelphia • Baltimore • New York • London
Buenos Aires • Hong Kong • Sydney • Tokyo

Acquisitions Editor: Patrick Barbera
Product Development Editor: Helen Kogut
Editorial Assistant: Dan Reilly
Production Project Manager: Cynthia Rudy
Design Coordinator: Holly McLaughlin
Illustration Coordinator: Jennifer Clements
Manufacturing Coordinator: Karin Duffield
Prepress Vendor: Absolute Service, Inc.

4th edition

Copyright © 2014 Wolters Kluwer Health | Lippincott Williams & Wilkins.

Copyright © 2011 Wolters Kluwer Health | Lippincott Williams & Wilkins. Copyright © 2007, 2002 Lippincott Williams & Wilkins. All rights reserved. This book is protected by copyright. No part of this book may be reproduced or transmitted in any form or by any means, including as photocopies or scanned-in or other electronic copies, or utilized by any information storage and retrieval system without written permission from the copyright owner, except for brief quotations embodied in critical articles and reviews. Materials appearing in this book prepared by individuals as part of their official duties as U.S. government employees are not covered by the above-mentioned copyright. To request permission, please contact Lippincott Williams & Wilkins at Two Commerce Square, 2001 Market Street, Philadelphia, PA 19103, via email at permissions@lww.com, or via our website at lww.com (products and services).

9 8 7 6 5 4 3 2

Printed in China

Library of Congress Cataloging-in-Publication Data
McEwen, Melanie, author.
Theoretical basis for nursing / Melanie McEwen, Evelyn M. Wills.—Edition 4.
p. ; cm.
Includes bibliographical references and indexes.
ISBN 978-1-4511-9031-1
I. Wills, Evelyn M., author. II. Title.
[DNLM: 1. Nursing Theory. WY 86]
RT84.5
610.73--dc23

2013035526

Care has been taken to confirm the accuracy of the information presented and to describe generally accepted practices. However, the author(s), editors, and publisher are not responsible for errors or omissions or for any consequences from application of the information in this book and make no warranty, expressed or implied, with respect to the currency, completeness, or accuracy of the contents of the publication. Application of this information in a particular situation remains the professional responsibility of the practitioner; the clinical treatments described and recommended may not be considered absolute and universal recommendations.

The author(s), editors, and publisher have exerted every effort to ensure that drug selection and dosage set forth in this text are in accordance with the current recommendations and practice at the time of publication. However, in view of ongoing research, changes in government regulations, and the constant flow of information relating to drug therapy and drug reactions, the reader is urged to check the package insert for each drug for any change in indications and dosage and for added warnings and precautions. This is particularly important when the recommended agent is a new or infrequently employed drug.

Some drugs and medical devices presented in this publication have U.S. Food and Drug Administration (FDA) clearance for limited use in restricted research settings. It is the responsibility of the health care provider to ascertain the FDA status of each drug or device planned for use in his or her clinical practice.

LWW.com

CCS1214

DEDICATION

To Kaitlin and Grant—You have helped me broaden my thoughts and consider all kinds of possibilities; I hope I've done the same for you.

Also for Helen and Keith—Our children chose well. Besides, you have given us Madelyn, Logan, Brenna, Liam, Lucy, and Andrew; they are gifts beyond words.

Melanie McEwen

To Tom, Paul, and Vicki, who light up my life, and to Marian, who is my applause. To Teddy, Gwen, Merlyn, and Madelyn, who have been so patient and loving during this process. A thousand thank yous to Peggy, who has supported me through this writing process.

Evelyn M. Wills

CONTRIBUTORS

Grace Bielkiewicz, RN, PMHCNS-BC
Assistant Professor (Retired)
Department of Nursing
Southern University
Baton Rouge, Louisiana
Chapter 13: Theories From the Sociologic Sciences

Debra Brossett Garner, DNP, APRN, ACNS-BC, PMHNP-BC
Psychiatric Mental Health Nurse Practitioner
Delhi Rural Health Clinic
Delhi, Louisiana
Chapter 14: Theories From the Behavioral Sciences

Melinda Granger Oberleitner, DNS, RN
Associate Dean, College of Nursing and Allied Health Professions
Professor, Department of Nursing
SLEMCO/BORSF Endowed Professor of Nursing
University of Louisiana at Lafayette
Lafayette, Louisiana
Chapter 16: Theories, Models, and Frameworks From Administration and Management
Chapter 20: Application of Theory in Nursing Administration and Management

REVIEWERS

Kimamer Amer, PhD
Associate Professor
Department of Nursing
DePaul University
Chicago, Illinois

Margaret Barnes, MSN, RN
Assistant Professor
School of Nursing, RNBSN Post-Licensure Division
Indiana Wesleyan University
Florence, Kentucky

Shari Cherney, RN, BScN, MHSc
Professor
Department of Nursing
George Brown College
Toronto, Ontario, Canada

Cheryl Delgado, PhD
Associate Professor
Department of Nursing
Cleveland State University
Cleveland, Ohio

Dolores Furlong, PhD
Professor
Department of Nursing
University of New Brunswick
Fredericton, New Brunswick, Canada

Maryanne Garon, DNSc
Professor
Department of Nursing
California State University Fullerton
Fullerton, California

Carol Grantham, PhD, MSN, CPNP-PC
Faculty
Byrdine F. Lewis School of Nursing & Health Professions
Georgia State University
Atlanta, Georgia

Barbara Harris, PhD
Assistant Professor
School of Nursing
DePaul University
Chicago, Illinois

Seongkum Heo, PhD
Assistant Professor
Department of Nursing
University of Arkansas for Medical Sciences
Little Rock, Arkansas

Donna Murnaghan, PhD
Associate Professor
School of Nursing
University of Prince Edward Island
Charlottetown, Prince Edward Island, Canada

Pamela Reis, PhD, CNM
Assistant Professor
Department of Nursing
East Carolina University
Greenville, North Carolina

Sue Robertson, PhD
Assistant Professor
Department of Nursing
California State University, Fullerton
Fullerton, California

Denice Sheehan, PhD
Assistant Professor
Department of Nursing
Kent State University
Kent, Ohio

Ida Slusher, DSN
Professor & Nursing Education Coordinator
Department of Baccalaureate & Graduate Nursing
Eastern Kentucky University
Richmond, Kentucky

Sharon Van Sell, BSN, MEd, MS, EdD
Professor
Department of Nursing
Texas Woman's University
Dallas, Texas

PREFACE

Frequently, nursing students respond with a cringing expression or a resounding "ugh!" when faced with the requirement of taking a course on theory. Indeed, many fail to see theory's relevance to the real world of nursing practice and often have difficulty applying the information in later courses and in their research. This book is the result of the frustration felt by a group of nursing instructors who met a number of years ago to adopt a textbook for a theory course. Indeed, because of student complaints and faculty dissatisfaction, we were changing textbooks yet again. A fairly lengthy discussion arose in which we concluded that the available books did not meet the needs of our students or course faculty. Ultimately, we determined to "build a better mousetrap." Our intent was to write a book that was a general overview of theory per se, stressing how it is—and should be—used by nurses to improve practice, research, education, and management/leadership.

As in past editions, an ongoing review of trends in nursing theory and nursing science has shown an increasing emphasis on middle range theory, evidence-based practice, and situation-specific theories. To remain current and timely, in this fourth edition, we have added a new chapter discussing evidence-based practice, highlighting how it relates to theory in nursing, and presenting several evidence-based practice models commonly used by nurses. We have also included new middle range nursing theories and added a significant section discussing situation-specific nursing theories, describing how they relate to evidence-based practice. Updates and application examples have been added throughout the discussions on the various theories.

Organization of the Text

Theoretical Basis for Nursing is designed to be a basic nursing theory textbook that includes the essential information students need to understand and apply theory.

The book is divided into four units. **Unit I, Introduction to Theory,** provides the background needed to understand what theory is and how it is used in nursing. It outlines tools and techniques used to develop, analyze, and evaluate theory so that it can be used in nursing practice, research, administration and management, and education. In this unit, we have provided a balanced view of "hot" topics (e.g., philosophical world views and utilization of shared or borrowed theory). Also, rather than espousing one strategy for activities such as concept development and theory evaluation, we have included a variety of strategies.

Unit II, Nursing Theories, focuses largely on the grand nursing theories and begins with a chapter describing their historical development. This unit divides the grand nursing theories into three groups based on their focus (human needs, interactive process, and unitary process). The works of many of the grand theorists are briefly summarized in Chapters 7, 8, and 9. We acknowledge that these analyses are not comprehensive; rather, they are intended to provide the reader with enough information to understand the basis of the work and to whet the reader's appetite to select one or more for further study.

Chapters 10 and 11 cover the significant topic of middle range nursing theory. Chapter 10 presents a detailed overview of the origins and growth of middle range theory in nursing and gives numerous examples of how middle range theories have been developed by nurses. Chapter 11 provides an overview of some of the growing number of middle range nursing theories. The theories presented include some of the most commonly used middle range nursing theories (e.g., Pender's Health Promotion Model and Leininger's Culture Care Diversity and Universality Theory) as well as some that are less well known but have a growing body of research support (e.g., Meleis' Transitions Theory, the Theory of Unpleasant Symptoms, and the Uncertainty in Illness Theory). The intent is to provide a broad range of middle range theories to familiarize the reader with examples and to encourage them to search for others appropriate to their practice or research. Ultimately, it is hoped that readers will be challenged to develop new theories that can be used by nurses.

Chapter 12, which discusses evidence-based practice (EBP), is new to this edition. This chapter explains and defines the idea/process of EBP and describes how it relates to nursing theory and application of theory in nursing practice and research. The chapter concludes with a short presentation and review of five different EBP models that have been widely used by nurses and are well supported in the literature.

Unit III, Shared Theories Used by Nurses, is rather unique in nursing literature. Our book acknowledges that "shared" or "borrowed" theories are essential to nursing and negates the idea that the use of shared theory in practice or research is detrimental. In this unit, we have identified some of the most significant theories that have been developed outside of the discipline of nursing but are continually used in nursing. We have organized these theories based on broad disciplines: theories from the sociologic sciences, behavioral sciences, and biomedical sciences, as well as from administration and management and learning. Each of these chapters was written by a nurse with both educational and practical experience in her respective area. These theories are presented with sufficient information to allow the reader to understand the theories and to recognize those that might be appropriate for her or his own work. These chapters also provide original references and give examples of how the concepts, theories, and models described have been used by other nurses.

Finally, **Unit IV, Application of Theory in Nursing Practice,** explains how theories are applied in nursing. Separate chapters cover nursing practice, nursing research, nursing administration and management, and nursing education. These chapters include many specific examples for the application of theory and are intended to be a practical guide for theory use. The heightened development of practice theories and EBP guidelines are critical to theory application in nursing today, so these areas have been expanded. The unit concludes with a chapter that discusses some of the future issues in theory within the discipline.

Key Features

In addition to numerous tables and boxes that highlight and summarize important information, *Theoretical Basis for Nursing* contains case studies, learning activities, exemplars, and illustrations that help students visualize various concepts. New to this edition is a special feature called Link to Practice.

- **Link to Practice**: All chapters include at least one "Link to Practice" box, which presents useful information or clinically related examples related to the subject being discussed. The intent is to give additional tools or resources that can be used by nurses to apply the content in their own practice or research.
- **Case Studies:** At the end of Chapter 1 and the beginning of Chapters 2 to 22, case studies help the reader understand how the content in the chapter relates to the everyday experience of the nurse, whether in practice, research, or other aspects of nursing.
- **Learning Activities:** At the end of each chapter, learning activities pose critical thinking questions, propose individual and group projects related to topics covered in the chapter, and stimulate classroom discussion.
- **Exemplars:** In five chapters, an exemplar discusses a scholarly study from the perspectives of concept analysis (Chapter 3); theory development (Chapter 4); theory analysis and evaluation (Chapter 5); middle range theory development (Chapter 10); and theory generation via research, theory testing via research, and use of a theory as the conceptual framework for a research study (Chapter 19).
- **Illustrations:** Diagrams and models are included throughout the book to help the reader better understand the many different theories presented.

New To This Edition

- New Chapter 12, *Evidence-Based Practice and Nursing Theory*
- More detailed explanation of EBP and its relationship to theory in nursing
- Enhanced attention to situation-specific theories and how they relate to EBP
- Numerous recent examples of application of theories in nursing practice, nursing research, leadership/administration, and education
- NEW instructional support

Student Resources Available on thePoint

- **Literature Assessment Activity** provides an interactive tool featuring journal articles along with questions that will encourage students to think critically about the literature. Students can print or e-mail their responses to their instructor.
- **Case Studies** with applicable questions guide students in understanding how the various theories link to nursing practice.
- **Learning Objectives** for each chapter help focus the student.
- **Internet Resources** provide live web links to pertinent sites so that students can further their study and understanding of the various theories.
- **Journal Articles** for each chapter offer opportunities to gain more knowledge and understanding of the chapter content.

Instructor Resources Available on thePoint

- **Instructor's Guide** includes application-level discussion questions and classroom/online activities that Melanie McEwen uses in her own teaching!
- **Strategies for Effective Teaching of Nursing Theory** provide ideas for instructors to help make the nursing theory class come alive.
- **Test Generator Questions** provide multiple-choice questions that can be used for testing general content knowledge.
- **PowerPoints with audience response (Iclicker) questions**, based on the ones used by Melanie McEwen in her own classroom, help highlight important points to enhance the classroom, experience.
- **Case Studies** with questions, answers, and related activities offer opportunities for instructors to make the student case studies an exciting, fun, and rewarding classroom/online experience.
- **Image Bank** provides images from the text that instructors can use to enhance their own presentations.

In summary, the focus of this learning package is on the application of theory rather than on the study, analysis, and critique of grand theorists or a presentation of a specific aspect of theory (e.g., construction or evaluation). It is hoped that practicing nurses, nurse researchers, and nursing scholars, as well as graduate students and theory instructors, will use this book and its accompanying resources to gain a better understanding and appreciation of theory.

Melanie McEwen, PhD, RN, CNE, ANEF
Evelyn M. Wills, PhD, RN

ACKNOWLEDGMENTS

Our heartfelt thanks to Product Development Editor, Helen Kogut, for her assistance, patience, and persistence in helping us complete this project. She has made a difficult task seem easy! We also want to thank Acquisitions Editor, Christina Burns, for her wonderful support and assistance in getting this project started and Patrick Barbera for seeing it through to the end. Finally, a huge word of thanks to our contributors who have diligently worked to present the notion of theory in a manner that will engage nursing students and to look for new examples and applications to help make theory fresh and relevant.

CONTENTS

Unit I: Introduction to Theory 1

1. Philosophy, Science, and Nursing 2
Melanie McEwen
Nursing as a Profession 2
Nursing as an Academic Discipline 4
Introduction to Science and Philosophy 5
Science and Philosophical Schools of Thought 7
Nursing Philosophy, Nursing Science, and Philosophy of Science in Nursing 11
Knowledge Development and Nursing Science 12
Research Methodology and Nursing Science 16

2. Overview of Theory in Nursing 23
Melanie McEwen
Overview of Theory 24
The Importance of Theory in Nursing 25
Terminology of Theory 26
Historical Overview: Theory Development in Nursing 26
Classification of Theories in Nursing 36
Issues in Theory Development in Nursing 40

3. Concept Development: Clarifying Meaning of Terms 49
Evelyn M. Wills, Melanie McEwen
The Concept of "Concept" 50
Concept Analysis/Concept Development 54
Strategies for Concept Analysis and Concept Development 57

4. Theory Development: Structuring Conceptual Relationships in Nursing 72
Melanie McEwen
Overview of Theory Development 73
Categorizations of Theory 73
Components of a Theory 79
Theory Development 82

5. Theory Analysis and Evaluation 95
Melanie McEwen
Definition and Purpose of Theory Evaluation 96
Historical Overview of Theory Analysis and Evaluation 97
Comparisons of Methods 106
Synthesized Method of Theory Evaluation 106

Unit II: Nursing Theories 115

6. Overview of Grand Nursing Theories 116
Evelyn M. Wills
Categorization of Conceptual Frameworks and Grand Theories 118
Specific Categories of Models and Theories for This Unit 124
Analysis Criteria for Grand Nursing Theories 124
The Purpose of Critiquing Theories 127

7. Grand Nursing Theories Based on Human Needs 131
Evelyn M. Wills
Florence Nightingale: Nursing: What It Is and What It Is Not 132
Virginia Henderson: The Principles and Practice of Nursing 136
Faye G. Abdellah: Patient-Centered Approaches to Nursing 139
Dorothea E. Orem: The Self-Care Deficit Nursing Theory 142
Dorothy Johnson: The Behavioral System Model 146
Betty Neuman: The Neuman Systems Model 149

8. Grand Nursing Theories Based on Interactive Process 159
Evelyn M. Wills
Myra Estrin Levine: The Conservation Model 160
Barbara M. Artinian: The Intersystem Model 164
Helen C. Erickson, Evelyn M. Tomlin, and Mary Ann P. Swain: Modeling and Role-Modeling 169
Imogene M. King: King's Conceptual System and Theory of Goal Attainment and Transactional Process 173
Sister Callista Roy: The Roy Adaptation Model 177
Jean Watson: Caring Science as Sacred Science 182

9. Grand Nursing Theories Based on Unitary Process 192
Evelyn M. Wills
Martha Rogers: The Science of Unitary and Irreducible Human Beings 193
Margaret Newman: Health as Expanding Consciousness 198
Rosemarie Parse: The Humanbecoming Paradigm 202

10. Introduction to Middle Range Nursing Theories 213
Melanie McEwen
Purposes of Middle Range Theory 214
Characteristics of Middle Range Theory 215
Concepts and Relationships for Middle Range Theory 216
Categorizing Middle Range Theory 217
Development of Middle Range Theory 217
Analysis and Evaluation of Middle Range Theory 225

11. Overview of Selected Middle Range Nursing Theories 229
Melanie McEwen
High Middle Range Theories 230
Middle Middle Range Theories 241
Low Middle Range Theories 248

12. Evidence-Based Practice and Nursing Theory 258
Evelyn M. Wills, Melanie McEwen
Overview of Evidence-Based Practice 259
Definition and Characteristics of Evidence-Based Practice 259
Concerns Related to Evidence-Based Practice in Nursing 261
Evidence-Based Practice and Practice-Based Evidence 261

Promotion of Evidence-Based Practice in Nursing 263
Theory and Evidence-Based Practice 263
Theoretical Models of EBP 264

Unit III: Shared Theories Used by Nurses 277

13. Theories From the Sociologic Sciences 278
Grace Bielkiewicz
Exchange Theories 279
Interactionist Frameworks 284
Conflict Theories 289
Chaos Theory 295
Postmodern Social Theory 298

14. Theories From the Behavioral Sciences 305
Debra Brossett Garner
Psychodynamic Theories 306
Behavioral and Cognitive-Behavioral Theories 313
Humanistic Theories 315
Stress Theories 318
Social Psychology 321

15. Theories From the Biomedical Sciences 331
Melanie McEwen
Theories and Models of Disease Causation 332
Theories and Principles Related to Physiology and Physical Functioning 339

16. Theories, Models, and Frameworks From Leadership and Management 354
Melinda Granger Oberleitner
Overview of Concepts of Leadership and Management 355
Early Leadership Theories 355
Contemporary Leadership Theories 362
Organizational/Management Theories 365
Motivational Theories 366
Concepts of Power, Empowerment, and Change 368
Problem-Solving and Decision-Making Processes 372
Conflict Management 374
Quality Improvement 375
Evidence-Based Practice 380

17. Learning Theories 386
Evelyn M. Wills, Melanie McEwen
What Is Learning? 387
What Is Teaching? 388
Categorization of Learning Theories 388
Behavioral Learning Theories 389
Cognitive Learning Theories 392
Summary of Learning Theories 404
Learning Styles 405
Principles of Learning 406
Application of Learning Theories in Nursing 407

Unit IV: Application of Theory in Nursing 411

18. Application of Theory in Nursing Practice 412
Melanie McEwen
Relationship Between Theory and Practice 413
Theory-Based Nursing Practice 414
The Theory–Practice Gap 416
Situation-Specific/Practice Theories in Nursing 418
Application of Theory in Nursing Practice 422

19. Application of Theory in Nursing Research 430
Melanie McEwen
Historical Overview of Research and Theory in Nursing 431
Relationship Between Research and Theory 432
Types of Theory and Corresponding Research 434
How Theory Is Used in Research 437
Nursing and Non-Nursing Theories in Nursing Research 444
Other Issues in Nursing Theory and Nursing Research 445

20. Application of Theory in Nursing Administration and Management 452
Melinda Granger Oberleitner
Organizational Design 453
Shared Governance 456
Transformational Leadership in Nursing and in Health Care 458
Patient Care Delivery Models 459
Case Management 466
Disease/Chronic Illness Management 468
Quality Management 470

21. Application of Theory in Nursing Education 479
Evelyn M. Wills, Melanie McEwen
Theoretical Issues in Nursing Curricula 481
Theoretical Issues in Nursing Instruction 488

22. Future Issues in Nursing Theory 497
Melanie McEwen
Future Issues in Nursing Science 499
Future Issues in Nursing Theory 500
Theoretical Perspectives on Future Issues in Nursing Practice, Research, Administration and Management, and Education 502

Glossary 513
Author Index 523
Subject Index 554

UNIT I

Introduction to Theory

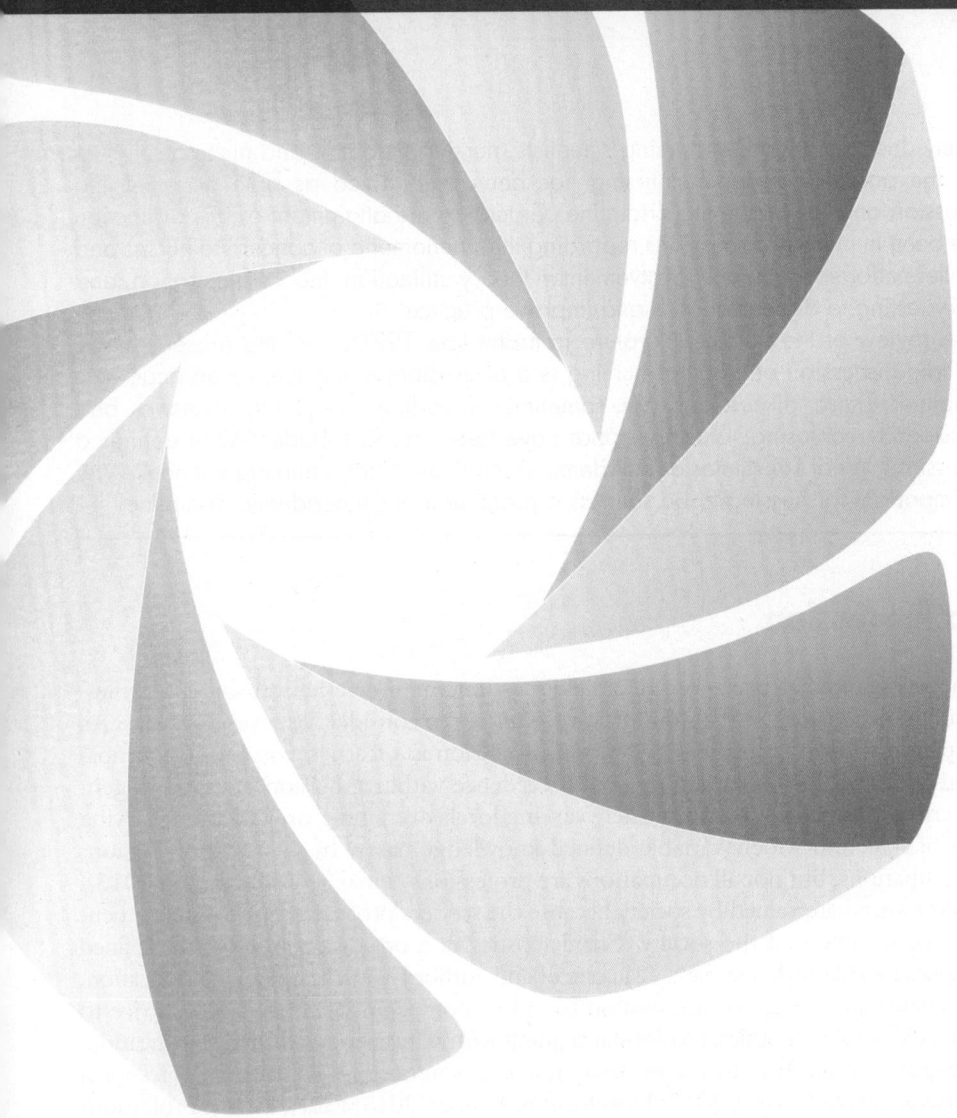

CHAPTER 1

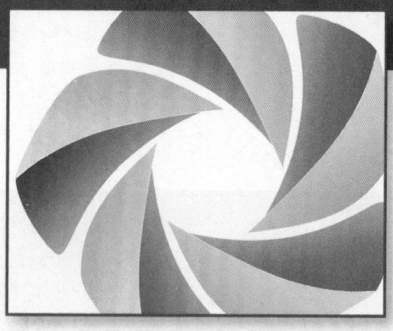

Philosophy, Science, and Nursing

Melanie McEwen

Largely due to the work of nursing scientists, nursing theorists, and nursing scholars over the past five decades, nursing has been recognized as both an emerging profession and an academic discipline. Crucial to the attainment of this distinction have been numerous discussions regarding the phenomena of concern to nurses and countless efforts to enhance involvement in theory utilization, theory generation, and theory testing to direct research and improve practice.

A review of the nursing literature from the late 1970s until the present shows sporadic discussion of whether nursing is a profession, a science, or an academic discipline. These discussions are sometimes pleading, frequently esoteric, and occasionally confusing. Questions that have been raised include: What defines a profession? What constitutes an academic discipline? What is nursing science? Why is it important for nursing to be seen as a profession or an academic discipline?

Nursing as a Profession

In the past, there has been considerable discussion about whether nursing is a profession or an occupation. This is important for nurses to consider for several reasons. An occupation is a job or a career, whereas a profession is a learned vocation or occupation that has a status of superiority and precedence within a division of work. In general terms, occupations require widely varying levels of training or education, varying levels of skill, and widely variable defined knowledge bases. In short, all professions are occupations, but not all occupations are professions (Finkelman & Kenner, 2013).

Professions are valued by society because the services professionals provide are beneficial for members of the society. Characteristics of a profession include (1) defined and specialized knowledge base, (2) control and authority over training and education, (3) credentialing system or registration to ensure competence, (4) altruistic service to society, (5) a code of ethics, (6) formal training within institutions of higher education, (7) lengthy socialization to the profession, and (8) autonomy (control of professional activities) (Ellis & Hartley, 2012; Finkelman & Kenner, 2013; Rutty, 1998). Professions must have a group of scholars, investigators, or researchers who work to continually advance the knowledge of the profession with the goal of improving practice (Schlotfeldt, 1989). Finally, professionals are responsible and accountable to the public for their work (Hood, 2010). Traditionally, professions have included the clergy, law, and medicine.

Until near the end of the 20th century, nursing was viewed as an occupation rather than a profession. Nursing has had difficulty being deemed a profession because many of the services provided by nurses have been perceived as an extension of those offered by wives and mothers. Additionally, historically, nursing has been seen as subservient to medicine, and nurses have delayed in identifying and organizing professional knowledge. Furthermore, education for nurses is not yet standardized, and the three-tier entry-level system (diploma, associate degree, and bachelor's degree) into practice that persists has hindered professionalization because a college education is not yet a requirement. Finally, autonomy in practice is incomplete because nursing is still dependent on medicine to direct much of its practice.

On the other hand, many of the characteristics of a profession can be observed in nursing. Indeed, nursing has a social mandate to provide health care for clients at different points in the health–illness continuum. There is a growing knowledge base, authority over education, altruistic service, a code of ethics, and registration requirements for practice. Although the debate is ongoing, it can be successfully argued that nursing is an aspiring, evolving profession (Finkelman & Kenner, 2013; Hood, 2010; Judd, Sitzman, & Davis, 2010). See Link to Practice 1-1 for more information on the future of nursing as a profession.

Link to Practice 1-1

The Future of Nursing

The Institute of Medicine (IOM, 2011) recently issued a series of sweeping recommendations directed to the nursing profession. The IOM explained their "vision" is to make quality, patient-centered care accessible for all Americans. Recommendations included a three-pronged approach to meeting the goal.

The first "message" was directed toward transformation of practice and precipitated the notion that nurses should be able to practice to the full extent of their education. Indeed, the IOM advocated for removal of regulatory, policy, and financial barriers to practice to ensure that "current and future generations of nurses can deliver safe, quality, patient-centered care across all settings, especially in such areas as primary care and community and public health" (p. 30).

A second key message related to the transformation of nursing education. In this regard, the IOM promotes "seamless academic progression" (p. 30), which includes a goal to increase the number and percentage of nurses who enter the workforce with a baccalaureate degree or who progress to the degree early in their career. Specifically, they recommend that 80% of RNs be BSN prepared by 2020. Last, the IOM advocated that nurses be full partners with physicians and other health professionals in the attempt to redesign health care in the United States.

These "messages" are critical to the future of nursing as a profession. Indeed, standardization of entry level into practice at the BSN level, coupled with promotion of advanced education and independent practice, and inclusion as "leaders" in the health care transformation process, will help solidify nursing as a true profession.

Nursing as an Academic Discipline

Disciplines are distinctions between bodies of knowledge found in academic settings. A *discipline* is "a branch of knowledge ordered through the theories and methods evolving from more than one worldview of the phenomenon of concern" (Parse, 1997, p. 74). It has also been termed a field of inquiry characterized by a unique perspective and a distinct way of viewing phenomena (Butts, Rich, & Fawcett, 2012; Parse, 1999).

Viewed another way, a discipline is a branch of educational instruction or a department of learning or knowledge. Institutions of higher education are organized around disciplines into colleges, schools, and departments (e.g., business administration, chemistry, history, and engineering).

Disciplines are organized by structure and tradition. The structure of the discipline provides organization and determines the amount, relationship, and ratio of each type of knowledge that comprises the discipline. The tradition of the discipline provides the content, which includes ethical, personal, esthetic, and scientific knowledge (Northrup et al., 2004; Risjord, 2010). Characteristics of disciplines include (1) a distinct perspective and syntax, (2) determination of what phenomena are of interest, (3) determination of the context in which the phenomena are viewed, (4) determination of what questions to ask, (5) determination of what methods of study are used, and (6) determination of what evidence is proof (Donaldson & Crowley, 1978).

Knowledge development within a discipline proceeds from several philosophical and scientific perspectives or worldviews (Litchfield & Jonsdottir, 2008; Newman, Sime, & Corcoran-Perry, 1991; Parse, 1999; Risjord, 2010). In some cases, these worldviews may serve to divide or segregate members of a discipline. For example, in psychology, practitioners might consider themselves behaviorists, Freudians, or any one of a number of other divisions.

Several ways of classifying academic disciplines have been proposed. For instance, they may be divided into the basic sciences (physics, biology, chemistry, sociology, anthropology) and the humanities (philosophy, ethics, history, fine arts). In this classification scheme, it is arguable that nursing has characteristics of both.

Distinctions may also be made between academic disciplines (e.g., physics, physiology, sociology, mathematics, history, philosophy) and professional disciplines (e.g., medicine, law, nursing, social work). In this classification scheme, the academic disciplines aim to "know," and their theories are descriptive in nature. Research in academic disciplines is both basic and applied. Conversely, the professional disciplines are practical in nature, and their research tends to be more prescriptive and descriptive (Donaldson & Crowley, 1978).

Nursing's knowledge base draws from many disciplines. In the past, nursing depended heavily on physiology, sociology, psychology, and medicine to provide academic standing and to inform practice. In recent decades, however, nursing has been seeking what is unique to nursing and developing those aspects into an academic discipline. Areas that identify nursing as a distinct discipline are as follows:

- An identifiable philosophy
- At least one conceptual framework (perspective) for delineation of what can be defined as nursing
- Acceptable methodologic approaches for the pursuit and development of knowledge (Oldnall, 1995)

To begin the quest to validate nursing as both a profession and an academic discipline, this chapter provides an overview of the concepts of science and philosophy.

It examines the schools of philosophical thought that have influenced nursing and explores the epistemology of nursing to explain why recognizing the multiple "ways of knowing" is critical in the quest for development and application of theory in nursing. Finally, this chapter presents issues related to how philosophical worldviews affect knowledge development through research. This chapter concludes with a case study that depicts how "the ways of knowing" in nursing are used on a day-to-day, even moment-by-moment, basis by all practicing nurses.

Introduction to Science and Philosophy

Science is concerned with causality (cause and effect). The scientific approach to understanding reality is characterized by observation, verifiability, and experience; hypothesis testing and experimentation are considered scientific methods. In contrast, *philosophy* is concerned with the purpose of human life, the nature of being and reality, and the theory and limits of knowledge. Intuition, introspection, and reasoning are examples of philosophical methodologies. Science and philosophy share the common goal of increasing knowledge (Butts et al., 2012; Fawcett, 1999; Silva, 1977). The science of any discipline is tied to its philosophy, which provides the basis for understanding and developing theories for science (Gustafsson, 2002; Silva & Rothbert, 1984).

Overview of Science

Science is both a process and a product. Parse (1997) defines science as the "theoretical explanation of the subject of inquiry and the methodological process of sustaining knowledge in a discipline" (p. 74). Science has also been described as a way of explaining observed phenomena as well as a system of gathering, verifying, and systematizing information about reality (Streubert & Carpenter, 2011). As a process, science is characterized by systematic inquiry that relies heavily on empirical observations of the natural world. As a product, it has been defined as empirical knowledge that is grounded and tested in experience and is the result of investigative efforts. Furthermore, science is conceived as being the consensual, informed opinion about the natural world, including human behavior and social action (Gortner & Schultz, 1988).

Science has come to represent knowledge, and it is generated by activites that combine advancement of knowledge (research) and explanation for knowledge (theory) (Powers & Knapp, 2011). Citing Van Laer, Silva (1977) lists six characteristics of science (Box 1-1).

Box 1-1 Characteristics of Science

1. Science must show a certain coherence.
2. Science is concerned with definite fields of knowledge.
3. Science is preferably expressed in universal statements.
4. The statements of science must be true or probably true.
5. The statements of science must be logically ordered.
6. Science must explain its investigations and arguments.

Source: Silva (1977).

Table 1-1 Classifications of Science

Classification	Examples
Natural sciences	Chemistry, physics, biology, physiology, geology, meteorology
Basic or pure sciences	Mathematics, logic, chemistry, physics, English (language)
Human or social sciences	Psychology, anthropology, sociology, economics, political science, history, religion
Practice or applied sciences	Architecture, engineering, medicine, pharmacology, law

Science has been classified in several ways. These include pure or basic science, natural science, human or social science, and applied or practice science. The classifications are not mutually exclusive and are open to interpretation based on philosophical orientation. Table 1-1 lists examples of a number of sciences by this manner of classification.

Some sciences defy classification. For example, computer science is arguably applied or perhaps pure. Law is certainly a practice science, but it is also a social science. Psychology might be a basic science, a human science, or an applied science, depending on what aspect of psychology one is referring to.

There are significant differences between the human and natural sciences. Human sciences refer to the fields of psychology, anthropology, and sociology and may even extend to economics and political science. These disciplines deal with various aspects of humans and human interactions. Natural sciences, on the other hand, are concentrated on elements found in nature that do not relate to the totality of the individual. There are inherent differences between the human and natural sciences that make the research techniques of the natural sciences (e.g., laboratory experimentation) improper or potentially problematic for human sciences (Gortner & Schultz, 1988).

It has been posited that although nursing draws on the basic and pure sciences (e.g., physiology and chemistry) and has many characteristics of social sciences, it is without question an applied or practice science. However, it is important to note that it is also synthesized, in that it draws on the knowledge of other established disciplines—including other practice disciplines (Dahnke & Dreher, 2011; Holzemer, 2007; Risjord, 2010).

Overview of Philosophy

Within any discipline, both scholars and students should be aware of the philosophical orientations that are the basis for developing theory and advancing knowledge (Dahnke & Dreher, 2011; DiBartolo, 1998; Northrup et al., 2004; Risjord, 2010). Rather than a focus on solving problems or answering questions related to that discipline (which are tasks of the discipline's science), the philosophy of a discipline studies the concepts that structure the thought processes of that discipline with the intent of recognizing and revealing foundations and presuppositions (Blackburn, 2008; Cronin & Rawlings-Anderson, 2004).

Philosophy has been defined as "a study of problems that are ultimate, abstract, and general. These problems are concerned with the nature of existence, knowledge, morality, reason, and human purpose" (Teichman & Evans, 1999, p. 1). Philosophy

Table 1-2 Branches of Philosophy

Branch	Pursuit
Metaphysics	Study of the fundamental nature of reality and existence—general theory of reality
Ontology	Study of theory of being (what is or what exists)
Cosmology	Study of the physical universe
Epistemology	Study of knowledge (ways of knowing, nature of truth, and relationship between knowledge and belief)
Logic	Study of principles and methods of reasoning (inference and argument)
Ethics (axiology)	Study of nature of values; right and wrong (moral philosophy)
Esthetics	Study of appreciation of the arts or things beautiful
Philosophy of science	Study of science and scientific practice
Political philosophy	Study of citizen and state

Sources: Blackburn (2008); Teichman & Evans (1999).

tries to discover knowledge and truth and attempts to identify what is valuable and important.

Modern philosophy is usually traced to Rene Descartes, Francis Bacon, Baruch Spinoza, and Immanuel Kant (ca. 1600–1800). Descartes (1596–1650) and Spinoza (1632–1677) were early rationalists. Rationalists believe that reason is superior to experience as a source of knowledge. Rationalists attempt to determine the nature of the world and reality by deduction and stress the importance of mathematical procedures.

Bacon (1561–1626) was an early empiricist. Like rationalists, he supported experimentation and scientific methods for solving problems.

The work of Kant (1724–1804) set the foundation for many later developments in philosophy. Kant believed that knowledge is relative and that the mind plays an active role in knowing. Other philosophers have also influenced nursing and the advance of nursing science. Several are discussed later in the chapter.

Although there is some variation, traditionally, the branches of philosophy include metaphysics (ontology and cosmology), epistemology, logic, esthetics, and ethics or axiology. Political philosophy and philosophy of science are added by some authors (Rutty, 1998; Teichman & Evans, 1999). Table 1-2 summarizes the major branches of philosophy.

Science and Philosophical Schools of Thought

The concept of science as understood in the 21st century is relatively new. In the period of modern science, three philosophies of science (paradigms or worldviews) dominate: rationalism, empiricism, and human science/phenomenology. Rationalism and empiricism are often termed *received view* and human science/phenomenology and related worldviews (i.e., historicism) are considered *perceived view* (Hickman, 2011; Meleis, 2012). These two worldviews dominated theoretical discussion in nursing through the 1990s. More recently, attention has focused on another dominant worldview: "postmodernism" (Meleis, 2012; Reed, 1995).

Received View (Empiricism, Positivism, Logical Positivism)

Empiricism has its roots in the writings of Francis Bacon, John Locke, and David Hume, who valued observation, perception by senses, and experience as sources of knowledge (Gortner & Schultz, 1988; Powers & Knapp, 2011). Empiricism is founded on the belief that what is experienced is what exists, and its knowledge base requires that these experiences be verified through scientific methodology (Dahnke & Dreher, 2011; Gustafsson, 2002). This knowledge is then passed on to others in the discipline and subsequently built on. The term *received view* or *received knowledge* denotes that individuals learn by being told or receiving knowledge.

Empiricism holds that truth corresponds to observable, reduction, verification, control, and bias-free science. It emphasizes mathematic formulas to explain phenomena and prefers simple dichotomies and classification of concepts. Additionally, everything can be reduced to a scientific formula with little room for interpretation (DiBartolo, 1998; Gortner & Schultz, 1988; Risjord, 2010).

Empiricism focuses on understanding the parts of the whole in an attempt to understand the whole. It strives to explain nature through testing of hypotheses and development of theories. Theories are made to describe, explain, and predict phenomena in nature and to provide understanding of relationships between phenomena. Concepts must be operationalized in the form of propositional statements, thereby making measurement possible. Instrumentation, reliability, and validity are stressed in empirical research methodologies. Once measurement is determined, it is possible to test theories through experimentation or observation, which results in verification or falsification (Cull-Wilby & Pepin, 1987; Suppe & Jacox, 1985).

Positivism is often equated with empiricism. Like empiricism, positivism supports mechanistic, reductionist principles, where the complex can be best understood in terms of its basic components. *Logical positivism* was the dominant empirical philosophy of science between the 1880s and 1950s. Logical positivists recognized only the logical and empirical bases of science and stressed that there is no room for metaphysics, understanding, or meaning within the realm of science (Polifroni & Welch, 1999; Risjord, 2010). Logical positivism maintained that science is value free, independent of the scientist, and obtained using objective methods. The goal of science is to explain, predict, and control. Theories are either true or false, subject to empirical observation, and capable of being reduced to existing scientific theories (Rutty, 1998).

Contemporary Empiricism/Postpositivism

Positivism came under criticism in the 1960s when positivistic logic was deemed faulty (Rutty, 1998). An overreliance on strictly controlled experimentation in artificial settings produced results that indicated that much significant knowledge or information was missed. In recent years, scholars have determined that the positivist view of science is outdated and misleading in that it contributes to overfragmentation in knowledge and theory development (DiBartolo, 1998). It has been observed that positivistic analysis of theories is fundamentally defective due to insistence on analyzing the logically ideal, which results in findings that have little to do with reality. It was maintained that the context of discovery was artificial and that theories and explanations can be understood only within their discovery contexts (Suppe & Jacox, 1985). Also, scientific inquiry is inherently value laden, as even choosing what to investigate and/or what techniques to employ will reflect the values of the researcher.

The current generation of postpositivists accept the subjective nature of inquiry but still support rigor and objective study through quantitative research methods. Indeed, it has been observed that modern empiricists or postpositivists are concerned with explanation and prediction of complex phenomena, recognizing contextual variables (Powers & Knapp, 2011; Reed, 2008).

Nursing and Empiricism

As an emerging discipline, nursing has followed established disciplines (e.g., physiology) and the medical model in stressing logical positivism. Early nurse scientists embraced the importance of objectivity, control, fact, and measurement of smaller and smaller parts. Based on this influence, acceptable methods for knowledge generation in nursing have stressed traditional, orthodox, and preferably experimental methods.

Although positivism continues to heavily influence nursing science, that viewpoint has been challenged in recent years (Risjord, 2010). Consequently, postpositivism has become one of the most accepted contemporary worldviews in nursing.

Perceived View (Human Science, Phenomenology, Constructivism, Historicism)

In the late 1960s and early 1970s, several philosophers, including Kuhn, Feyerbend, and Toulmin, challenged the positivist view by arguing that the influence of history on science should be emphasized (Dahnke & Dreher, 2011). The perceived view of science, which may also be referred to as the interpretive view, includes phenomenology, constructivism, and historicism. The interpretive view recognizes that the perceptions of both the subject being studied and the researcher tend to de-emphasize reliance on strict control and experimentation in laboratory settings (Monti & Tingen, 1999).

The perceived view of science centers on descriptions that are derived from collectively lived experiences, interrelatedness, human interpretation, and learned reality, as opposed to artificially invented (i.e., laboratory-based) reality (Rutty, 1998). It is argued that the pursuit of knowledge and truth is naturally historical, contextual, and value laden. Thus, there is no single truth. Rather, knowledge is deemed true if it withstands practical tests of utility and reason (DiBartolo, 1998).

Phenomenology is the study of phenomena and emphasizes the appearance of things as opposed to the things themselves. In phenomenology, *understanding* is the goal of science, with the objective of recognizing the connection between one's experience, values, and perspective. It maintains that each individual's experience is unique, and there are many interpretations of reality. Inquiry begins with individuals and their experiences with phenomena. Perceptions, feelings, values, and the meanings that have come to be attached to things and events are the focus.

For social scientists, the *constructivist* approaches of the perceived view focus on understanding the actions of, and meaning to, individuals. What exists depends on what individuals perceive to exist. Knowledge is subjective and created by individuals. Thus, research methodology entails the investigation of the individual's world (Wainwright, 1997). There is an emphasis on subjectivity, multiple truths, trends and patterns, discovery, description, and understanding.

Feminism and critical social theory may also be considered to be perceived view. These philosophical schools of thought recognize the influence of gender, culture, society, and shared history as being essential components of science (Riegel et al., 1992). Critical social theorists contend that reality is dynamic and shaped by social, political, cultural, economic, ethnic, and gender values (Streubert & Carpenter, 2011). Critical social theory and feminist theories will be described in more detail in Chapter 13.

Nursing and Phenomenology/Constructivism/Historicism

Because they examine phenomena within context, phenomenology, as well as other perceived views of philosophy, are conducive to discovery and knowledge development inherent to nursing. Phenomenology is open, variable, and relativistic and based on human experience and personal interpretations. As such, it is an important, guiding paradigm for nursing practice theory and education (DiBartolo, 1998).

In nursing science, the dichotomy of philosophic thought between the received, empirical view of science and the perceived, interpretative view of science has persisted. This may have resulted, in part, because nursing draws heavily both from natural sciences (physiology, biology) and social sciences (psychology, sociology).

Postmodernism (Poststructuralism, Postcolonialism)

Postmodernism began in Europe in the 1960s as a social movement centered on a philosophy that rejects the notion of a single "truth." Although it recognizes the value of science and scientific methods, postmodernism allows for multiple meanings of reality and multiple ways of knowing and interpreting reality (Hood, 2010; Reed, 1995). In postmodernism, knowledge is viewed as uncertain, contextual, and relative. Knowledge development moves from emphasis on identifying a truth or fact in research to discovering practical significance and relevance of research findings (Reed, 1995).

Similar or related constructs and worldviews found in the nursing literature include "deconstruction," "postcolonialism," and at times, feminist philosophies. In nursing, the postcolonial worldview can be connected to both feminism and critical theory, particularly when considering nursing's historical reliance on medicine (Holmes, Roy, & Perron, 2008; Mackay, 2009; Racine, 2009).

Postmodernism has loosened the notions of what counts as knowledge development that have persisted among supporters of qualitative and quantitative research methods. Rather than focusing on a single research methodology, postmodernism promotes use of multiple methods for development of scientific understanding and incorporation of different ways to improve understanding of human nature (Hood, 2010; Meleis, 2012; Reed, 1995). Increasingly, in postmodernism, there is a consensus that synthesis of both research methods can be used at different times to serve different purposes (Hood, 2010; Meleis, 2012; Risjord, Dunbar, & Moloney, 2002).

Criticisms of postmodernism have been made and frequently relate to the perceived reluctance to address error in research. Taken to the extreme as Paley (2005) pointed out, when there is absence of strict control over methodology and interpretation of research, "nobody can ever be wrong about anything" (p. 107). Chinn and Kramer (2011) echoed the concerns by acknowledging that knowledge development should never be "sloppy." Indeed, although application of various methods in research is legitimate and may be advantageous, research must still be carried out carefully and rigorously.

Nursing and Postmodernism

Postmodernism has been described as a dominant scientific theoretical paradigm in nursing in the late 20th century (Meleis, 2012). As the discipline matures, there has been recognition of the pluralistic nature of nursing and an enhanced understanding that the goal of research is to provide an integrative basis for nursing care (Walker & Avant, 2011).

In terms of scientific methodology, the attention is increasingly on combining multiple methods within a single research project (Chinn & Kramer, 2011). Postmodernism has helped dislodged the authority of a single research paradigm in nursing science by emphasizing the blending or integration of qualitative and quantitative research into a holistic, dynamic model to improve nursing practice. Table 1-3 compares the dominant philosophical views of science in nursing.

Table 1-3 Comparison of the Received, Perceived, and Postmodern Views of Science

Received View of Science—Hard Sciences	Perceived View of Science—Soft Sciences	Postmodernism, Poststructuralism, and Postcolonialism
Empiricism/positivism/ logical positivism	Historicism/phenomenology	Macroanalysis
Reality/truth/facts considered acontextual (objective)	Reality/truth/facts considered in context (subjective)	Contextual meaning; narration
Deductive	Inductive	Contextual, political, and structural analysis
Reality/truth/facts considered ahistorical	Reality/truth/facts considered with regard to history	Reality/truth/facts considered with regard to history
Prediction and control	Description and understanding	Metanarrative analysis
One truth	Multiple truths	Different views
Validation and replication	Trends and patterns	Uncovering opposing views
Reductionism	Constructivism/holism	Macrorelationship; microstructures
Quantitative research methods	Qualitative research methods	Methodologic pluralism

Sources: Meleis (2012); Moody (1990).

Nursing Philosophy, Nursing Science, and Philosophy of Science in Nursing

The terms *nursing philosophy, nursing science,* and *philosophy of science in nursing* are sometimes used interchangeably. The differences, however, in the general meaning of these concepts are important to recognize.

Nursing Philosophy

Nursing philosophy has been described as "a statement of foundational and universal assumptions, beliefs and principles about the nature of knowledge and thought (epistemology) and about the nature of the entities represented in the metaparadigm (i.e., nursing practice and human health processes [ontology])" (Reed, 1995, p. 76). Nursing philosophy, then, refers to the belief system or worldview of the profession and provides perspectives for practice, scholarship, and research (Gortner, 1990).

No single dominant philosophy has prevailed in the discipline of nursing. Many nursing scholars and nursing theorists have written extensively in an attempt to identify the overriding belief system, but to date, none has been universally successful. Most would agree then that nursing is increasingly recognized as a "multiparadigm discipline" (Powers & Knapp, 2011, p. 129), in which using multiple perspectives or worldviews in a "unified" way is valuable and even necessary for knowledge development (Giuliano, Tyer-Viola, & Lopez, 2005).

Nursing Science

Barrett (2002) defined nursing science as "the substantive, discipline-specific knowledge that focuses on the human-universe-health process articulated in the nursing frameworks and theories" (p. 57). To develop and apply the discipline-specific knowledge, nursing science recognizes the relationships of human responses in health and illness and addresses biologic, behavioral, social, and cultural domains. The goal of nursing science is to represent the nature of nursing—to understand it, to explain it, and to use it for the benefit of humankind. It is nursing science that gives direction to the future generation of substantive nursing knowledge, and it is nursing science that provides the knowledge for all aspects of nursing (Barrett, 2002; Holzemer, 2007).

Philosophy of Science in Nursing

Philosophy of science in nursing helps to establish the meaning of science through an understanding and examination of nursing concepts, theories, laws, and aims as they relate to nursing practice. It seeks to understand truth; to describe nursing; to examine prediction and causality; to critically relate theories, models, and scientific systems; and to explore determinism and free will (Nyatanga, 2005; Polifroni & Welch, 1999).

Knowledge Development and Nursing Science

Development of nursing knowledge reflects the interface between nursing science and research. The ultimate purpose of knowledge development is to improve nursing practice. Approaches to knowledge development have three facets: ontology, epistemology, and methodology. Ontology refers to the study of being: what is or what exists. Epistemology refers to the study of knowledge or ways of knowing. Methodology is the means of acquiring knowledge (Powers & Knapp, 2011). The following sections discuss nursing epistemology and issues related to methods of acquiring knowledge.

Epistemology

Epistemology is the study of the theory of knowledge. Epistemologic questions include: What do we know? What is the extent of our knowledge? How do we decide whether we know? and What are the criteria of knowledge? (Schultz & Meleis, 1988).

According to Streubert and Carpenter (2011), it is important to understand the way in which nursing knowledge develops to provide a context in which to judge the appropriateness of nursing knowledge and methods that nurses use to develop that knowledge. This in turn will refocus methods for gaining knowledge as well as establishing the legitimacy or quality of the knowledge gained.

Ways of Knowing

In epistemology, there are several basic types of knowledge. These include the following:

- Empirics—the scientific form of knowing. Empirical knowledge comes from observation, testing, and replication.
- Personal knowledge—a priori knowledge. Personal knowledge pertains to knowledge gained from thought alone.

- Intuitive knowledge—includes feelings and hunches. Intuitive knowledge is not guessing but relies on nonconscious pattern recognition and experience.
- Somatic knowledge—knowledge of the body in relation to physical movement. Somatic knowledge includes experiential use of muscles and balance to perform a physical task.
- Metaphysical (spiritual) knowledge—seeking the presence of a higher power. Aspects of spiritual knowing include magic, miracles, psychokinesis, extrasensory perception, and near-death experiences.
- Esthetics—knowledge related to beauty, harmony, and expression. Esthetic knowledge incorporates art, creativity, and values.
- Moral or ethical knowledge—knowledge of what is right and wrong. Values and social and cultural norms of behavior are components of ethical knowledge.

Nursing Epistemology

Nursing epistemology has been defined as "the study of the origins of nursing knowledge, its structure and methods, the patterns of knowing of its members, and the criteria for validating its knowledge claims" (Schultz & Meleis, 1988, p. 21). Like most disciplines, nursing has both scientific knowledge and knowledge that can be termed conventional wisdom (knowledge that has not been empirically tested).

Traditionally, only what stands the test of repeated measures constitutes truth or knowledge. Classical scientific processes (i.e., experimentation), however, are not suitable for creating and describing all types of knowledge. Social sciences, behavioral sciences, and the arts rely on other methods to establish knowledge. Because it has characteristics of social and behavioral sciences, as well as biologic sciences, nursing must rely on multiple ways of knowing.

In a classic work, Carper (1978) identified four fundamental patterns for nursing knowledge: (1) empirics—the science of nursing, (2) esthetics—the art of nursing, (3) personal knowledge in nursing, and (4) ethics—moral knowledge in nursing.

Empirical knowledge is objective, abstract, generally quantifiable, exemplary, discursively formulated, and verifiable. When verified through repeated testing over time, it is formulated into scientific generalizations, laws, theories, and principles that explain and predict (Carper, 1978, 1992). It draws on traditional ideas that can be verified through observation and proved by hypothesis testing.

Empirical knowledge tends to be the most emphasized way of knowing in nursing because there is a need to know how knowledge can be organized into laws and theories for the purpose of describing, explaining, and predicting phenomena of concern to nurses. Most theory development and research efforts are engaged in seeking and generating explanations that are systematic and controllable by factual evidence (Carper, 1978, 1992).

Esthetic knowledge is expressive, subjective, unique, and experiential rather than formal or descriptive. Esthetics includes sensing the meaning of a moment. It is evident through actions, conduct, attitudes, and interactions of the nurse in response to another. It is not expressed in language (Carper, 1978).

Esthetic knowledge relies on perception. It is creative and incorporates empathy and understanding. It is interpretive, contextual, intuitive, and subjective and requires synthesis rather than analysis. Furthermore, esthetics goes beyond what is explained by principles and creates values and meaning to account for variables that cannot be quantitatively formulated (Carper, 1978, 1992).

Personal knowledge refers to the way in which nurses view themselves and the client. Personal knowledge is subjective and promotes wholeness and integrity in personal encounters. Engagement, rather than detachment, is a component of personal knowledge.

Personal knowledge incorporates experience, knowing, encountering, and actualizing the self within the practice. Personal maturity and freedom are components of personal knowledge, which may include spiritual and metaphysical forms of knowing. Because personal knowledge is difficult to express linguistically, it is largely expressed in personality (Carper, 1978, 1992).

Ethics refers to the moral code for nursing and is based on obligation to service and respect for human life. Ethical knowledge occurs as moral dilemmas arise in situations of ambiguity and uncertainty and when consequences are difficult to predict. Ethical knowledge requires rational and deliberate examination and evaluation of what is good, valuable, and desirable as goals, motives, or characteristics (Carper, 1978, 1992). Ethics must address conflicting norms, interests, and principles and provide insight into areas that cannot be tested.

Fawcett, Watson, Neuman, Walkers, and Fitzpatrick (2001) stress that integration of all patterns of knowing is essential for professional nursing practice and that no one pattern should be used in isolation from others. Indeed, they are interrelated and interdependent because there are multiple points of contact between and among them (Carper, 1992). Thus, nurses should view nursing practice from a broadened perspective that places value on ways of knowing beyond the empirical (Silva, Sorrell, & Sorrell, 1995). Table 1-4 summarizes selected characteristics of Carper's patterns of knowing in nursing.

Table 1-4 Characteristics of Carper's Patterns of Knowing in Nursing

Pattern of Knowing	Relationship to Nursing	Source or Creation	Source of Validation	Method of Expression	Purpose or Outcome
Empirics	Science of nursing	Direct or indirect observation and measurement	Replication	Facts, models, scientific principles, laws statements, theories, descriptions	Description, explanation, prediction
Esthetics	Art of nursing	Creation of value and meaning, synthesis of abstract and concrete	Appreciation; experience; inspiration; perception of balance, rhythm, proportion, and unity	Appreciation; empathy; esthetic criticism; engaging, intuiting, and envisioning	Move beyond what can be explained, quantitatively formulated, understanding, balance
Personal knowledge	Therapeutic use of self	Engagement, opening, centering, actualizing self	Response, reflection, experience	Empathy, active participation	Therapeutic use of self
Ethics	Moral component of nursing	Values clarification, rational and deliberate reasoning, obligation, advocating	Dialogue, justification, universal generalizability	Principles, codes, ethical theories	Evaluation of what is good, valuable, and desirable

Sources: Carper (1978); Carper (1992); Chinn & Kramer (2011).

Other Views of Patterns of Knowledge in Nursing

Although Carper's work is considered classic, it is not without critics. Schultz and Meleis (1988) observed that Carper's work did not incorporate practical knowledge into the ways of knowing in nursing. Because of this and other concerns, they described three patterns of knowledge in nursing: clinical, conceptual, and empirical.

Clinical knowledge refers to the individual nurse's personal knowledge. It results from using multiple ways of knowing while solving problems during client care provision. Clinical knowledge is manifested in the acts of practicing nurses and results from combining personal knowledge and empirical knowledge. It may also involve intuitive and subjective knowing. Clinical knowledge is communicated retrospectively through publication in journals (Schultz & Meleis, 1988).

Conceptual knowledge is abstracted and generalized beyond personal experience. It explicates patterns revealed in multiple client experiences, which occur in multiple situations, and articulates them as models or theories. In conceptual knowledge, concepts are drafted and relational statements are formulated. Propositional statements are supported by empirical or anecdotal evidence or defended by logical reasoning.

Conceptual knowledge uses knowledge from nursing and other disciplines. It incorporates curiosity, imagination, persistence, and commitment in the accumulation of facts and reliable generalizations that pertain to the discipline of nursing. Conceptual knowledge is communicated in propositional statements (Schultz & Meleis, 1988).

Empirical knowledge results from experimental, historical, or phenomenologic research and is used to justify actions and procedures in practice. The credibility of empirical knowledge rests on the degree to which the researcher has followed procedures accepted by the community of researchers and on the logical, unbiased derivation of conclusions from the evidence. Empirical knowledge is evaluated through systematic review and critique of published research and conference presentations (Schultz & Meleis, 1988).

Chinn and Kramer (2011) also expanded on Carper's patterns of knowing to include "emancipatory knowing"—what they designate as the "praxis of nursing." In their view, emancipatory knowing refers to human's ability to critically examine the current status quo and to determine why it currently exists. This, in turn, supports identification of inequities in social and political institutions and clarification of cultural values and beliefs to improve conditions for all. In this view, emancipatory knowledge is expressed in actions that are directed toward changing existing social structures and establishing practices that are more equitable and favorable to human health and well-being.

Summary of Ways of Knowing in Nursing

For decades, the importance of the multiple ways of knowing has been recognized in the discipline of nursing. If nursing is to achieve a true integration between theory, research, and practice, theory development and research must integrate different sources of knowledge. Kidd and Morrison (1988) state that in nursing, synthesis of theories derived from different sources of knowledge will

1. Encourage the use of different types of knowledge in practice, education, theory development, and research
2. Encourage the use of different methodologies in practice and research
3. Make nursing education more relevant for nurses with different educational backgrounds
4. Accommodate nurses at different levels of clinical competence
5. Ultimately promote high-quality client care and client satisfaction

Research Methodology and Nursing Science

Being heavily influenced by logical empiricism, as nursing began developing as a scientific discipline in the mid-1900s, quantitative methods were used almost exclusively in research. In the 1960s and 1970s, schools of nursing aligned nursing inquiry with scientific inquiry in a desire to bring respect to the academic environment, and nurse researchers and nurse educators valued quantitative research methods over other forms.

A debate over methodology began in the 1980s, however, when some nurse scholars asserted that nursing's ontology (what nursing is) was not being adequately and sufficiently explored using quantitative methods in isolation. Subsequently, qualitative research methods began to be put into use. The assumptions were that qualitative methods showed the phenomena of nursing in ways that were naturalistic and unstructured and not misrepresented (Holzemer, 2007; Rutty, 1998).

The manner in which nursing science is conceptualized determines the priorities for nursing research and provides measures for determining the relevance of various scientific research questions. Therefore, the way in which nursing science is conceptualized also has implications for nursing practice. The philosophical issues regarding methods of research relate back to the debate over the worldviews of received versus perceived views of science versus postmodernism and whether nursing is a practice or applied science, a human science, or some combination. The notion of evidence-based practice has emerged over the last few years, largely in response to these and related concerns. Evidence-based practice as it relates to the theoretical basis of nursing will be examined in Chapter 13.

Nursing as a Practice Science

In early years, the debate focused on whether nursing was a basic science or an applied science. The goal of basic science is the attainment of knowledge. In basic research, the investigator is interested in understanding the problem and produces knowledge for knowledge's sake. It is analytical and the ultimate function is to analyze a conclusion backward to its proper principles.

Conversely, an applied science is one that uses the knowledge of basic sciences for some practical end. Engineering, architecture, and pharmacology are examples. In applied research, the investigator works toward solving problems and producing solutions for the problem. In practice sciences, research is largely clinical and action oriented (Moody, 1990). Thus, as an applied or practical science, nursing requires research that is applied and clinical and that generates and tests theories related to health of human beings within their environments as well as the actions and processes used by nurses in practice.

Nursing as a Human Science

The term *human science* is traced to philosopher Wilhelm Dilthey (1833–1911). Dilthey proposed that the human sciences require concepts, methods, and theories that are fundamentally different from those of the natural sciences. Human sciences study human life by valuing the lived experience of persons and seek to understand life in its matrix of patterns of meaning and values. Some scholars believe that there is a need to approach human sciences differently from conventional empiricism and contend that human experience must be understood in context (Cody & Mitchell, 2002; Mitchell & Cody, 1992).

In human sciences, scientists hope to create new knowledge to provide understanding and interpretation of phenomena. In human sciences, knowledge takes the form of descriptive theories regarding the structures, processes, relationships, and traditions that underlie psychological, social, and cultural aspects of reality. Data are interpreted within context to derive meaning and understanding. Humanistic scientists value the subjective component of knowledge. They recognize that humans are not capable of total objectivity and embrace the idea of subjectivity (Streubert & Carpenter, 2011). The purpose of research in human science is to produce descriptions and interpretations to help understand the nature of human experience.

Nursing is sometimes referred to as a human science (Cody & Mitchell, 2002; Mitchell & Cody, 1992). Indeed, the discipline has examined issues related to behavior and culture, as well as biology and physiology, and sought to recognize associations among factors that suggest explanatory variables for human health and illness. Thus, it fits the pattern of other humanistic sciences (i.e., anthropology, sociology).

Quantitative Versus Qualitative Methodology Debate

Nursing scholars accept the premise that scientific knowledge is generated from systematic study. The research methodologies and criteria used to justify the acceptance of statements or conclusions as true within the discipline result in conclusions and statements that are appropriate, valid, and reliable for the purpose of the discipline.

The two dominant forms of scientific inquiry have been identified in nursing: (1) empiricism, which objectifies and attempts to quantify experience and may test propositions or hypotheses in controlled experimentation; and (2) phenomenology and other forms of qualitative research (i.e., grounded theory, hermeneutics, historical research, ethnography), which study lived experiences and meanings of events (Gortner & Schultz, 1988; Monti & Tingen, 1999; Risjord, 2010). Reviews of the scientific status of nursing knowledge usually contrast the positivist–deductive–quantitative approach with the interpretive–inductive–qualitative alternative.

Although nursing theorists and nursing scientists emphasize the importance of sociohistorical contexts and person–environment interactions, they tend to focus on "hard science" and the research process. It has been argued that there is an overvaluation of the empirical/quantitative view because it is seen as "true science" (Tinkle & Beaton, 1983). Indeed, the experimental method is held in the highest regard. A viewpoint has persisted into the 21st century in which scholars assume that descriptive or qualitative research should be performed only where there is little information available or when the science is young. Correlational research may follow, and then experimental methods can be used when the two lower ("less rigid" or "less scientific") levels have been explored.

Quantitative Methods

Traditionally, within the "received" or positivistic worldview, science has been uniquely quantitative. The quantitative approach has been justified by its success in measuring, analyzing, replicating, and applying the knowledge gained (Streubert & Carpenter, 2011). According to Wolfer (1993), science should incorporate methodologic principles of objective observation/description, accurate measurement, quantification of variables, mathematical and statistical analysis, experimental methods, and verification through replication whenever possible.

Kidd and Morrison (1988) state that in their haste to prove the credibility of nursing as a profession, nursing scholars have emphasized reductionism and empirical validation through quantitative methodologies, emphasizing hypothesis testing. In this framework, the scientist develops a hypothesis about a phenomenon and seeks to prove or disprove it.

Qualitative Methods

The tradition of using qualitative methods to study human phenomena is grounded in the social sciences. Phenomenology and other methods of qualitative research arose because aspects of human values, culture, and relationships were unable to be described fully using quantitative research methods. It is generally accepted that qualitative research findings answer questions centered on social experience and give meaning to human life. Beginning in the 1970s, nursing scientists were challenged to explain phenomena that defy quantitative measurement, and qualitative approaches, which emphasize the importance of the client's perspective, began to be used in nursing research (Kidd & Morrison, 1988).

Repeatedly, scholars state that nursing research should incorporate means for determining interpretation of the phenomena of concern from the perspective of the client or care recipient. Contrary to the assertions of early scientists, many later nurse scientists believe that qualitative inquiry contains features of good science including theory and observation, logic, precision, clarity, and reproducibility (Monti & Tingen, 1999).

Methodologic Pluralism

In many respects, nursing is still undecided about which methodologic approach (qualitative or quantitative) best demonstrates the essence and uniqueness of nursing because both methods have strengths and limitations. Munhall (2007), Risjord (2010), and Sandelowski (2000), among others, believe that the two approaches may be considered complementary and appropriate for nursing as a research-based discipline. Indeed, it is repeatedly argued that both approaches are equally important and even essential for nursing science development (Foss & Ellefsen, 2002; Risjord et al., 2002; Thurmond, 2001; Young, Taylor, & Renpenning, 2001).

Although basic philosophical viewpoints have guided and directed research strategies in the past, recently, scholars have called for theoretical and methodologic pluralism in nursing philosophy and nursing science as presented in the discussion on postmodernism. Pluralism of research designs is essential for reflecting the uniqueness of nursing, and multiple approaches to theory development and testing should be encouraged. Because there is no one best method of developing knowledge, it is important to recognize that valuing one standard as exclusive or superior restricts the ability to progress.

Summary

Nursing is an evolving profession, an academic discipline, and a science. As nursing progresses and grows as a profession, some controversy remains on whether to emphasize a humanistic, holistic focus or an objective, scientifically derived means of comprehending reality. What is needed, and is increasingly more evident as nursing matures as a profession, is an open philosophy that ties empirical concepts that are capable of being validated through the senses with theoretical concepts of meaning and value.

It is important that future nursing leaders and novice nurse scientists possess an understanding of nursing's philosophical foundations. The legacy of philosophical positivism continues to drive beliefs in the scientific method and research strategies, but it is time to move forward to face the challenges of the increasingly complex and volatile health care environment.

Key Points

- Nursing can be considered an aspiring or evolving profession.
- Nursing is a professional discipline that draws much of its knowledge base from other disciplines, including psychology, sociology, physiology, and medicine.
- Nursing is an applied or practice science that has been influenced by several philosophical schools of thought or worldviews, including the received view (empiricism, positivism, logical positivism), the perceived view (humanism, phenomenology, constructivism), and postmodernism.
- *Nursing philosophy* refers to the worldview(s) of the profession and provides perspective for practice, scholarship, and research. *Nursing science* is the discipline-specific knowledge that focuses on the human-environment-health process and is articulated in nursing theories and generated through nursing research. *Philosophy of science in nursing* establishes the meaning of science through examination of nursing concepts, theories, and laws as they relate to nursing practice.
- Nursing epistemology (ways of knowing in nursing) has focused on four predominant or "fundamental" ways of knowledge: empirical knowledge, esthetic knowledge, personal knowledge, and ethical knowledge.
- As nursing science has developed, there has been a debate over what research methods to use (i.e., quantitative methods vs. qualitative methods). Increasingly, there has been a call for "methodologic pluralism" to better ensure that research findings are applicable in nursing practice.

Case Study

The following is adapted from a paper written by a graduate student describing an encounter in nursing practice that highlights Carper's (1978) ways of knowing in nursing.

In her work, Carper (1978) identified four patterns of knowing in nursing: empirical knowledge (science of nursing), esthetic knowledge (art of nursing), personal knowledge, and ethical knowledge. Each is essential and depends on the others to make the whole of nursing practice, and it is impossible to state which of the patterns of knowing is most important. If nurses focus exclusively on empirical knowledge, for example, nursing care would become more like medical care. But without an empirical base, the art of nursing is just tradition. Personal knowledge is gained from experience and requires a scientific basis, understanding, and empathy. Finally, the moral component is necessary to determine what is valuable, ethical, and compulsory. Each of these ways of knowing is illustrated in the following scenario.

Mrs. Smith was a 24-year-old primigravida who presented to our unit in early labor. Her husband, and father of her unborn child, had abandoned her 2 months prior to delivery, and she lacked close family support.

I cared for Mrs. Smith throughout her labor and assisted during her delivery. During this process, I taught breathing techniques to ease pain and improve coping. Position changes were encouraged periodically, and assistance was provided as needed.

Mrs. Smith's care included continuous fetal monitoring, intravenous hydration, analgesic administration, back rubs, coaching and encouragement, assistance while getting an epidural, straight catheterization as needed, vital sign monitoring per policy, oxytocin administration after delivery, newborn care, and breastfeeding assistance, among many others. All care was explained in detail prior to rendering.

***Empirical knowledge** was clearly utilized in Mrs. Smith's care. Examples would be those practices based on the Association of Women's Health, Obstetric and Neonatal Nurses (AWHONN) evidence-based standards. These include guidelines for fetal heart rate monitoring and interpretation, assessment and management of Mrs. Smith while receiving her epidural analgesia, the assessment and management of side effects secondary to her regional analgesia, and even frequency for monitoring vital signs. Other examples would be assisting Mrs. Smith to an upright position during her second stage of labor to facilitate delivery and delaying nondirected pushing once she was completely dilated.*

***Esthetic knowledge,** or the art of nursing, is displayed in obstetrical nursing daily. Rather than just responding to biologic developments or spoken requests, the whole person was valued and cues were perceived and responded to for the good of the patient. The care I gave Mrs. Smith was holistic; her social, spiritual, psychological, and physical needs were all addressed in a comprehensive and seamless fashion. The empathy conveyed to the patient took into account her unique self and situation, and the care provided was reflexively tailored to her needs. I recognized the profound experience of which I was a part and adapted my actions and attitude to honor the patient and value the larger experience.*

*Many aspects of **personal knowledge** seem intertwined with esthetics, though more emphasis seems to be on the meaningful interaction between the patient and nurse. As above, the patient was cared for as a unique individual. Though secondary to the awesome nature of birth, much of the experience revolved around the powerful interpersonal relationship established. Mrs. Smith was accepted as herself. Though efforts were made by me to manage certain aspects of the experience, Mrs. Smith was allowed control and freedom of expression and reaction. She and I were both committed to the mutual though brief relationship. This knowledge stems from my own personality and ability to accept others, willingness to connect to others, and desire to collaborate with the patient regarding her care and ultimate experience.*

*The **ethical knowledge** of nursing is continuously utilized in nursing care to promote the health and well-being of the patient; and in this circumstance, the unborn child as well. Every decision made must be weighed against desired goals and values, and nurses must strive to act as advocates for each patient. When caring for a patient and an unborn child, there is a constant attempt to do no harm to either, while balancing the care of both. A very common example is the administration of medications for the mother's comfort that can cause sedation and respiratory depression in the neonate. This case involved fewer ethical considerations than many others in obstetrics. These include instances in which physicians do not respond when the nurse feels there is imminent danger and the chain of command must be utilized, or when assistance is required for the care of abortion patients or in other situations that may be in conflict with the nurses moral or religious convictions.*

A close bond was formed while I cared for Mrs. Smith and her baby. Soon after admission, she was holding my hand during contractions and had shared very intimate details of her life, separation, and fears. Though she had shared her financial concerns and had a new baby to provide for, a few weeks after her delivery I received a beautiful gift basket and card. In her note she shared that I had touched her in a way she had never expected and she vowed never to forget me; I've not forgotten her either.

Contributed by Shelli Carter, RN, MSN

Learning Activities

1. Reflect on the previous case study. Think of a situation from personal practice in which multiple ways of knowing were used. Write down the anecdote and share it with classmates.
2. With classmates, discuss whether nursing is a profession or an occupation. What can current and future nurses do to enhance nursing's standing as a profession?
3. Debate with classmates the dominant philosophical schools of thought in nursing (received view, perceived view, postmodernism). Which worldview best encompasses the profession of nursing? Why?

REFERENCES

Barrett, E. A. M. (2002). What is nursing science? *Nursing Science Quarterly, 15*(1), 51–60.

Blackburn, S. (2008). *Oxford dictionary of philosophy* (2nd ed., rev.). New York: Oxford University Press.

Butts, J. B., Rich, K. L., & Fawcett, J. (2012). The future of nursing: How important is discipline-specific knowledge? A conversation with Jacqueline Fawcett. *Nursing Science Quarterly, 25*(2), 151–154.

Carper, B. A. (1978). Fundamental patterns of knowing in nursing. *Advances in Nursing Science, 1*(1), 13–24.

Carper, B. A. (1992). Philosophical inquiry in nursing: An application. In J. F. Kikuchi & H. Simmons (Eds.), *Philosophic inquiry in nursing* (pp. 71–80). Newbury Park, CA: Sage.

Chinn, P. L., & Kramer, M. K. (2011). *Theory and nursing: Integrated knowledge development* (7th ed.). St. Louis: Mosby.

Cody, W. K., & Mitchell, G. J. (2002). Nursing knowledge and human science revisited: Practical and political considerations. *Nursing Science Quarterly, 15*(1), 4–13.

Cronin, P., & Rawlings-Anderson, K. (2004). *Knowledge for contemporary nursing practice.* London, United Kingdom: Mosby.

Cull-Wilby, B. L., & Pepin, J. I. (1987). Towards a coexistence of paradigms in nursing knowledge development. *Journal of Advanced Nursing, 12*(4), 515–522.

Dahnke, M. D., & Dreher, H. M. (2011). *Philosophy of science for nursing practice: Concepts and application.* New York: Springer.

DiBartolo, M. C. (1998). Philosophy of science in doctoral nursing education revisited. *Journal of Professional Nursing, 14*(6), 350–360.

Donaldson, S. K., & Crowley, D. M. (1978). The discipline of nursing. *Nursing Outlook, 26*(2), 113–120.

Ellis, J. R., & Hartley, C. L. (2012). *Nursing in today's world: Trends, issues, and management* (10th ed.). Philadelphia: Lippincott Williams & Wilkins.

Fawcett, J. (1999). The state of nursing science: Hallmarks of the 20th and 21st centuries. *Nursing Science Quarterly, 12*(4), 311–318.

Fawcett, J., Watson, J., Neuman, B., Walkers, P. H., & Fitzpatrick, J. (2001). On nursing theories and evidence. *Journal of Nursing Scholarship, 3*(2), 115–119.

Finkelman, A., & Kenner, C. (2013). *Professional nursing concepts: Competencies for quality leadership* (2nd ed.). Burlington, MA: Jones & Bartlett.

Foss, C., & Ellefsen, B. (2002). The value of combining qualitative and quantitative approaches in nursing research by means of method triangulation. *Journal of Advanced Nursing, 40*(2), 242–248.

Giuliano, K. K., Tyer-Viola, L., & Lopez, R. P. (2005). Unity of knowledge in the advancement of nursing knowledge. *Nursing Science Quarterly, 18*(3), 243–248.

Gortner, S. R. (1990). Nursing values and science: Toward a science philosophy. *Image: Journal of Nursing Scholarship, 22*(2), 101–105.

Gortner, S. R., & Schultz, P. R. (1988). Approaches to nursing science methods. *Image: Journal of Nursing Scholarship, 20*(1), 22–24.

Gustafsson, B. (2002). The philosophy of science from a nursing-scientific perspective. *Theoria: Journal of Nursing Theory, 11* (2), 3–13.

Hickman, J. S. (2011). An introduction to nursing theory. In J. B. George (Ed.), *Nursing theories: The base for professional nursing practice* (6th ed., pp. 1–22). Upper Saddle River, NJ: Pearson Education.

Holmes, D., Roy, B., & Perron, A. (2008). The use of postcolonialism in the nursing domain: Colonial patronage, conversion, and resistance. *Advances in Nursing Science, 31*(1), 42–51.

Holzemer, W. L. (2007). Towards understanding nursing science. *Japan Journal of Nursing Science, 4*(1), 57–59.

Hood, L. J. (2010). *Leddy & Pepper's conceptual bases of professional nursing.* Philadelphia: Lippincott Williams & Wilkins.

Institute of Medicine. (2011). The future of nursing: Leading change, advancing health. Washington, DC: National Academies Press.

Judd, D., Sitzman, K., & Davis, G. M. (2010). *A history of American nursing: Trends and eras.* Sudbury, MA: Jones and Bartlett Publishers.

Kidd, P., & Morrison, E. F. (1988). The progression of knowledge in nursing research: A search for meaning. *Image: Journal of Nursing Scholarship, 20*(4), 222–224.

Litchfield, M. C., & Jonsdottir, H. (2008). A practice discipline that's here and now. *Advances in Nursing Science, 31*(1), 79–91.

Mackay, M. (2009). Why nursing has not embraced the clinician-scientist role. *Nursing Philosophy, 10*(4), 287–296.

Meleis, A. I. (2012). *Theoretical nursing: Development and progress* (5th ed.). Philadelphia: Lippincott Williams & Wilkins.

Mitchell, G. J., & Cody, W. K. (1992). Nursing knowledge and human science: Ontological and epistemological considerations. *Nursing Science Quarterly, 5*(2), 54–61.

Monti, E. J., & Tingen, M. S. (1999). Multiple paradigms of nursing science. *Advances in Nursing Science, 21*(4), 64–80.

Moody, L. E. (1990). *Advancing nursing science through research.* Newbury Park, CA: Sage.

Munhall, P. L. (2007). *Nursing research: A qualitative perspective* (4th ed.). Boston: Jones & Bartlett Publishers.

Newman, M. A., Sime, A. M., & Corcoran-Perry, S. A. (1991). The focus of the discipline of nursing. *Advances in Nursing Science, 14*(1), 1–6.

Northrup, D. T., Tschanz, C. L., Olynyk, V. G., Makaroff, K. L. S., Szabo, J., & Biasio, H. A. (2004). Nursing: Whose discipline is it anyway? *Nursing Science Quarterly, 17*(1), 55–62.

Nyatanga, L. (2005). Nursing and the philosophy of science. *Nurse Education Today, 25*, 670–674.

Oldnall, A. S. (1995). Nursing as an emerging academic discipline. *Journal of Advanced Nursing, 21*, 605–612.

Paley, J. (2005). Phenomenology as rhetoric. *Nursing Inquiry, 12*(2), 106–116.

Parse, R. R. (1997). The language of nursing knowledge: Saying what we mean. In I. M. King & J. Fawcett (Eds.), *The language of nursing theory and metatheory* (pp. 73–77). Indianapolis: Center Nursing Press.

Parse, R. R. (1999). Nursing: The discipline and the profession. *Nursing Science Quarterly, 12*(4), 275–276.

Polifroni, E. C., & Welch, M. (1999). *Perspectives on philosophy of science in nursing.* Philadelphia: Lippincott Williams & Wilkins.

Powers, B. A., & Knapp, T. R. (2011). *Dictionary of nursing theory and research* (4th ed.). New York: Springer.

Racine, L. (2009). Applying Antonio Gramsci's philosophy to postcolonial feminist social and political activism in nursing. *Nursing Philosophy, 10*(2), 180–190.

Reed, P. G. (1995). A treatise on nursing knowledge development in the 21st century: Beyond postmodernism. *Advances in Nursing Science, 17*(3), 70–84.

Reed, P. G. (2008). Adversity and advancing nursing knowledge. *Nursing Science Quarterly, 21*(2), 133–139.

Riegel, B., Omery, A., Calvillo, E., Elsayed, N. G., Lee, P., Shuler, P., & Siegal, B. E. (1992). Moving beyond: A generative philosophy of science. *Image: Journal of Nursing Scholarship, 24*(2), 115–119.

Risjord, M. (2010). *Nursing knowledge: Science, practice, and philosophy.* West Sussex, United Kingdom: Wiley-Blackwell.

Risjord, M. W., Dunbar, S. B., & Moloney, M. F. (2002). A new foundation for methodological triangulation. *Journal of Nursing Scholarship, 34*(3), 269–275.

Rutty, J. E. (1998). The nature of philosophy of science, theory and knowledge relating to nursing and professionalism. *Journal of Advanced Nursing, 28*(2), 243–250.

Sandelowski, M. (2000). Combining qualitative and quantitative sampling, data collection, and analysis techniques in mixed-method studies. *Research in Nursing & Health, 23*(3), 246–255.

Schlotfeldt, R. M. (1989). Structuring nursing knowledge: A priority for creating nursing's future. *Nursing Science Quarterly, 1*(1), 35–38.

Schultz, P. R., & Meleis, A. I. (1988). Nursing epistemology: Traditions, insights, questions. *Image: Journal of Nursing Scholarship, 20*(4), 217–221.

Silva, M. C. (1977). Philosophy, science, theory: Interrelationships and implications for nursing research. *Image: Journal of Nursing Scholarship, 9*(3), 59–63.

Silva, M. C., & Rothbert, D. (1984). An analysis of changing trends of philosophies of science on nursing theory development and testing. *Advances in Nursing Science, 6*(2), 1–13.

Silva, M. C., Sorrell, J. M., & Sorrell, C. D. (1995). From Carper's patterns of knowing to ways of being: An ontological philosophical shift in nursing. *Advances in Nursing Science, 18*(1), 1–13.

Streubert, H. J., & Carpenter, D. R. (2011). *Qualitative research in nursing: Advancing the humanistic imperative* (5th ed.). Philadelphia: Lippincott Williams & Wilkins.

Suppe, F., & Jacox, A. (1985). Philosophy of science and development of nursing theory. In H. H. Werley & J. J. Fitzpatrick (Eds.), *Annual review of nursing research.* New York: Springer.

Teichman, J., & Evans, K. C. (1999). *Philosophy: A beginner's guide* (3rd ed.). Cambridge, MA: Blackwell.

Thurmond, V. A. (2001). The point of triangulation. *Journal of Nursing Scholarship, 33*(3), 253–258.

Tinkle, M. B., & Beaton, J. L. (1983). Toward a new view of science: Implications for nursing research. *Advances in Nursing Science, 5*(2), 27–36.

Wainwright, S. P. (1997). A new paradigm for nursing: The potential of realism. *Journal of Advanced Nursing, 26*(6), 1262–1271.

Walker, L. O., & Avant, K. (2011). *Strategies for theory construction in nursing* (5th ed.). Upper Saddle River, NJ: Pearson Health Sciences.

Wolfer, J. (1993). Aspects of reality and ways of knowing in nursing: In search of an integrating paradigm. *Image: Journal of Nursing Scholarship, 25*(2), 141–146.

Young, A., Taylor, S. G., & Renpenning, K. M. (2001). *Connections: Nursing research, theory, and practice.* St. Louis: Mosby.

CHAPTER 2

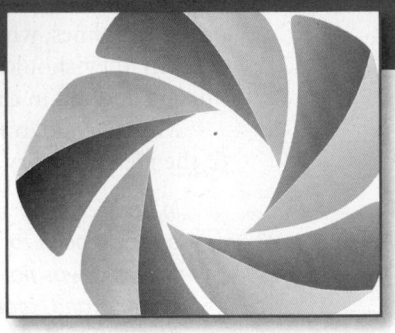

Overview of Theory in Nursing

Melanie McEwen

Matt Ng has been an emergency room nurse for almost 6 years and recently decided to enroll in a master's degree program to become an acute care nurse practitioner. As he read over the degree requirements, Matt was somewhat bewildered. One of the first courses required by his program was entitled Application of Theory in Nursing. He was interested in the courses in advanced pharmacology, advanced physical assessment, and pathophysiology and was excited about the advanced practice clinical courses, but a course that focused on nursing theory did not appear congruent with his goals.

Looking over the syllabus for the theory application course did little to reassure Matt, but he was determined to make the best of the situation and went to the first class with an open mind. The first few class periods were increasingly interesting as the students and instructor discussed the historical evolution of the discipline of nursing and the stages of nursing theory development. As the course progressed, the topics became more relevant to Matt. He learned ways to analyze and evaluate theories, examined a number of different types of theories used by nurses, and completed several assignments, including a concept analysis, an analysis of a middle range nursing theory, and a synthesis paper that examined the use of non-nursing theories in nursing research.

By the end of the semester, Matt was able to recognize the importance of the study of theory. He understood how theoretical principles and concepts affected his current practice and how they would be essential to consider as he continued his studies to become an advanced practice nurse.

When asked about theory, many nurses and nursing students, and often even nursing faculty will respond with a furrowed brow, a pained expression, and a resounding "ugh." When questioned about their negative response, most will admit that the idea of studying theory is confusing, that they see no practical value, and that theory is, in essence, too theoretical.

Likewise, some nursing scholars believe that nursing theory is practically nonexistent, whereas others recognize that many practitioners have not heard of nursing theory. Some nurses lament that nurse researchers use theories and frameworks from other disciplines, whereas others believe the notion of nursing theory is outdated and ask why they should bother with theory. Questions and debates about "theory" in nursing abound in the nursing literature.

Myra Levine, one of the pioneer nursing theorists, wrote that "the introduction of the idea of theory in nursing was sadly inept" (Levine, 1995, p. 11). She stated,

> *In traditional nursing fashion, early efforts were directed at creating a procedure—a recipe book for prospective theorists—which then could be used to decide what was and was not a theory. And there was always the thread of expectation that the great, grand, global theory would appear and end all speculation. Most of the early theorists really believed they were achieving that.*

Levine went on to explain that every new theory posited new central concepts, definitions, relational statements, and goals for nursing, and then attracted a chorus of critics. This resulted in nurses finding themselves confused about the substance and intention of the theories. Indeed, "in early days, theory was expected to be obscure. If it was clearly understandable, it wasn't considered a very good theory" (Levine, 1995, p. 11).

The drive to develop nursing theory has been marked by nursing theory conferences, the proliferation of theoretical and conceptual frameworks for nursing, and the formal teaching of theory development in graduate nursing education. It has resulted in the development of many systems, techniques or processes for theory analysis and evaluation, a fascination with the philosophy of science, and confusion about theory development strategies and division of choice of research methodologies.

There is debate over the types of theories that should be used by nurses. Should they be only nursing theories or can nurses use theories "borrowed" from other disciplines? There is debate over terminology such as *conceptual framework, conceptual model,* and *theory.* There have been heated discussions concerning the appropriate level of theory for nurses to develop, as well as how, why, where, and when to test, measure, analyze, and evaluate these theories/models/conceptual frameworks. The question has been repeatedly asked: Should nurses adopt a single theory, or do multiple theories serve them best? It is no wonder, then, that nursing students display consternation, bewilderment, and even anxiety when presented with the prospect of studying theory. One premise, however, can be agreed upon: To be useful, a theory must be meaningful and relevant, but above all, it must be understandable. This chapter discusses many of the issues described previously. It presents the rationale for studying and using theory in nursing practice, research, management/administration, and education; gives definitions of key terms; provides an overview of the history of development of theory utilization in nursing; describes the scope of theory and levels of theory; and, finally, introduces the widely accepted nursing metaparadigm.

Overview of Theory

Most scholars agree that it is the unique theories and perspectives used by a discipline that distinguish it from other disciplines. The theories used by members of a profession clarify basic assumptions and values shared by its members and define the nature, outcome, and purpose of practice (Alligood, 2010; Butts, Rich, & Fawcett, 2012; Rutty, 1998).

Definitions of the term *theory* abound in the nursing literature. At a basic level, theory has been described as a systematic explanation of an event in which constructs and concepts are identified and relationships are proposed and predictions made (Streubert & Carpenter, 2011). Theory has also been defined as a "creative and rigorous structuring of ideas that project a tentative, purposeful and systematic view of phenomena" (Chinn & Kramer, 2011, p. 257). Finally, theory has been called a set of interpretative assumptions, principles, or propositions that help explain or guide action (Young, Taylor, & Renpenning, 2001).

In their classic work, Dickoff and James (1968) state that theory is invented, rather than found in or discovered from reality. Furthermore, theories vary according to the number of elements, the characteristics and complexity of the elements, and the kind of relationships between or among the elements.

The Importance of Theory in Nursing

Before the advent of development of nursing theories, nursing was largely subsumed under medicine. Nursing practice was generally prescribed by others and highlighted by traditional, ritualistic tasks with little regard to rationale. The initial work of nursing theorists was aimed at clarifying the complex intellectual and interactional domains that distinguish expert nursing practice from the mere doing of tasks (Omrey, Kasper, & Page, 1995). It was believed that conceptual models and theories could create mechanisms by which nurses would communicate their professional convictions, provide a moral/ethical structure to guide actions, and foster a means of systematic thinking about nursing and its practice (Chinn & Kramer, 2011; Peterson, 2013; Sitzman & Eichelberger, 2011; Ziegler, 2005). The idea that a single, unified model of nursing—a worldview of the discipline—might emerge was encouraged by some (Levine, 1995; Tierney, 1998).

It is widely believed that use of theory offers structure and organization to nursing knowledge and provides a systematic means of collecting data to describe, explain, and predict nursing practice. Use of theory also promotes rational and systematic practice by challenging and validating intuition. Theories make nursing practice more overtly purposeful by stating not only the focus of practice but also specific goals and outcomes. Theories define and clarify nursing and the purpose of nursing practice to distinguish it from other caring professions by setting professional boundaries. Finally, use of a theory in nursing leads to coordinated and less fragmented care (Alligood, 2010; Chinn & Kramer, 2011; Ziegler, 2005).

Ways in which theories and conceptual models developed by nurses have influenced nursing practice are described by Fawcett (1992), who stated that in nursing they:

- Identify certain standards for nursing practice
- Identify settings in which nursing practice should occur and the characteristics of what the model's author considers recipients of nursing care
- Identify distinctive nursing processes and technologies to be used, including parameters for client assessment, labels for client problems, a strategy for planning, a typology of intervention, and criteria for evaluation of intervention outcomes
- Direct the delivery of nursing services
- Serve as the basis for clinical information systems, including the admission database, nursing orders, care plan, progress notes, and discharge summary
- Guide the development of client classification systems
- Direct quality assurance programs

Terminology of Theory

Young and colleagues (2001) wrote that in nursing, conceptual models or frameworks detail a network of concepts and describe their relationships, thereby explaining broad nursing phenomena. Theories, they noted, are the narrative that accompanies the conceptual model. These theories typically provide a detailed description of all of the components of the model and outline relationships in the form of propositions. Critical components of the theory or narrative include definitions of the central concepts or constructs; propositions or relational statements, the assumptions on which the framework is based; and the purpose, indications for use, or application. Many conceptual frameworks and theories will also include a schematic drawing or model depicting the overall structure of or interactivity of the components (Chinn & Kramer, 2011).

Some terms may be new to students of theory and others need clarification. Table 2-1 lists definitions for a number of terms that are frequently encountered in writings on theory. Many of these terms will be described in more detail later in the chapter and in subsequent chapters.

Historical Overview: Theory Development in Nursing

Most nursing scholars credit Florence Nightingale with being the first modern nursing theorist. Nightingale was the first to delineate what she considered nursing's goal and practice domain, and she postulated that "to nurse" meant having charge of the personal health of someone. She believed the role of the nurse was seen as placing the client "in the best condition for nature to act upon him" (Hilton, 1997, p. 1211).

Florence Nightingale

Nightingale received her formal training in nursing in Kaiserswerth, Germany, in 1851. Following her renowned service for the British army during the Crimean War, she returned to London and established a school for nurses. According to Nightingale, formal training for nurses was necessary to "teach not only what is to be done, but how to do it." She was the first to advocate the teaching of symptoms and what they indicate. Further, she taught the importance of rationale for actions and stressed the significance of "trained powers of observation and reflection" (Kalisch & Kalisch, 2004, p. 36).

In *Notes on Nursing,* published in 1859, Nightingale proposed basic premises for nursing practice. In her view, nurses were to make astute observations of the sick and their environment, record observations, and develop knowledge about factors that promoted healing. Her framework for nursing emphasized the utility of empirical knowledge, and she believed that knowledge developed and used by nurses should be distinct from medical knowledge. She insisted that trained nurses control and staff nursing schools and manage nursing practice in homes and hospitals (Chinn & Kramer, 2011; Kalisch & Kalisch, 2004).

Stages of Theory Development in Nursing

Subsequent to Nightingale, almost a century passed before other nursing scholars attempted the development of philosophical and theoretical works to describe and define nursing and to guide nursing practice. Kidd and Morrison (1988) described five stages in the development of nursing theory and philosophy: (1) silent knowledge,

Table 2-1 Definitions and Characteristics of Theory Terms and Concepts

Term	Definition and Characteristics
Assumptions	Assumptions are beliefs about phenomena one must accept as true to accept a theory about the phenomena as true. Assumptions may be based on accepted knowledge or personal beliefs and values. Although assumptions may not be susceptible to testing, they can be argued philosophically.
Borrowed or shared theory	A borrowed theory is a theory developed in another discipline that is not adapted to the worldview and practice of nursing.
Concept	Concepts are the elements or components of a phenomenon necessary to understand the phenomenon. They are abstract and derived from impressions the human mind receives about phenomena through sensing the environment.
Conceptual model/ conceptual framework	A conceptual model is a set of interrelated concepts that symbolically represents and conveys a mental image of a phenomenon. Conceptual models of nursing identify concepts and describe their relationships to the phenomena of central concern to the discipline.
Construct	Constructs are the most complex type of concept. They comprise more than one concept and are typically built or constructed by the theorist or philosopher to fit a purpose. The terms *concept* and *construct are* often used interchangeably, but some authors use concept as the more general term—all constructs are concepts, but not all concepts are constructs.
Empirical indicator	Empirical indicators are very specific and concrete identifiers of concepts. They are actual instructions, experimental conditions, and procedures used to observe or measure the concept(s) of a theory.
Epistemology	Epistemology refers to theories of knowledge or how people come to have knowledge; in nursing, it is the study of the origins of nursing knowledge.
Hypotheses	Hypotheses are tentative suggestions that a specific relationship exists between two concepts or propositions. As the hypothesis is repeatedly confirmed, it progresses to an empirical generalization and ultimately to a law.
Knowledge	Knowledge refers to the awareness or perception of reality acquired through insight, learning, or investigation. In a discipline, knowledge is what is collectively seen to be a reasonably accurate understanding of the world as seen by members of the discipline.
Laws	A law is a proposition about the relationship between concepts in a theory that has been repeatedly validated. Laws are highly generalizable. Laws are found primarily in disciplines that deal with observable and measurable phenomena, such as chemistry and physics. Conversely, social and human sciences have few laws.
Metaparadigm	A metaparadigm represents the worldview of a discipline—the global perspective that subsumes more specific views and approaches to the central concepts with which the discipline is concerned. The metaparadigm is the ideology within which the theories, knowledge, and processes for knowing find meaning and coherence. Nursing's metaparadigm is generally thought to consist of the concepts of person, environment, health, and nursing.
Middle range theory	Middle range theory refers to a part of a discipline's concerns related to particular topics. The scope is narrower than that of broad-range or grand theories.
Model	Models are graphic or symbolic representations of phenomena that objectify and present certain perspectives or points of view about nature or function or both. Models may be theoretical (something not directly observable—expressed in language or mathematics symbols) or empirical (replicas of observable reality—model of an eye, for example).
Ontology	Ontology is concerned with the study of existence and the nature of reality.

(continued)

331-3083060

Table 2-1 Definitions and Characteristics of Theory Terms and Concepts *(continued)*

Term	Definition and Characteristics
Paradigm	A paradigm is an organizing framework that contains concepts, theories, assumptions, beliefs, values, and principles that form the way a discipline interprets the subject matter with which it is concerned. It describes work to be done and frames an orientation within which the work will be accomplished. A discipline may have a number of paradigms. The term *paradigm* is associated with Kuhn's *Structure of Scientific Revolutions.*
Phenomena	Phenomena are the designation of an aspect of reality; the phenomena of interest become the subject matter particular to the primary concerns of a discipline.
Philosophy	A philosophy is a statement of beliefs and values about human beings and their world.
Practice or situation-specific theory	A practice or situation-specific theory deals with a limited range of discrete phenomena that are specifically defined and are not expanded to include their link with the broad concerns of a discipline.
Praxis	Praxis is the application of a theory to cases encountered in experience.
Relationship statements	Relationship statements indicate specific relationships between two or more concepts. They may be classified as propositions, hypotheses, laws, axioms, or theorems.
Taxonomy	A taxonomy is a classification scheme for defining or gathering together various phenomena. Taxonomies range in complexity from simple dichotomies to complicated hierarchical structures.
Theory	Theory refers to a set of logically interrelated concepts, statements, propositions, and definitions, which have been derived from philosophical beliefs of scientific data and from which questions or hypotheses can be deduced, tested, and verified. A theory purports to account for or characterize some phenomenon.
Worldview	Worldview is the philosophical frame of reference used by a social or cultural group to describe that group's outlook on and beliefs about reality.

Sources: Alligood & Tomey (2010); Blackburn (2008); Chinn & Kramer (2011); Powers & Knapp (2011).

(2) received knowledge, (3) subjective knowledge, (4) procedural knowledge, and (5) constructed knowledge. Table 2-2 gives an overview of characteristics of each of these stages in the development of nursing theory, and each stage is described in the following sections. To contemporize Kidd and Morrison's work, attention will be given to the current decade and a new stage—that of "integrated knowledge."

Silent Knowledge Stage

Recognizing the impact of the poorly trained nurses on the health of soldiers during the Civil War, in 1868, the American Medical Association advocated the formal training of nurses and suggested that schools of nursing be attached to hospitals with instruction being provided by medical staff and resident physicians. The first training school for nurses in the United States was opened in 1872 at the New England Hospital. Three more schools, located in New York, New Haven, and Boston, opened shortly thereafter (Kalisch & Kalisch, 2004). Most schools were under the control of hospitals and superintended by hospital administrators and physicians. Education and practice were based on rules, principles, and traditions that were passed along through an apprenticeship form of education.

There followed rapid growth in the number of hospital-based training programs for nurses, and by 1909, there were more than 1,000 such programs (Kalisch & Kalisch, 2004). In these early schools, a meager amount of theory was taught by

Table 2-2 Stages in the Development of Nursing Theory

Stage	Source of Knowledge	Impact on Theory and Research
Silent knowledge	Blind obedience to medical authority	Little attempt to develop theory. Research was limited to collection of epidemiologic data.
Received knowledge	Learning through listening to others	Theories were borrowed from other disciplines. As nurses acquired non-nursing doctoral degrees, they relied on the authority of educators, sociologists, psychologists, physiologists, and anthropologists to provide answers to nursing problems. Research was primarily educational research or sociologic research.
Subjective knowledge	Authority was internalized to foster a new sense of self.	A negative attitude toward borrowed theories and science emerged. Nurse scholars focused on defining nursing and on developing theories about and for nursing. Nursing research focused on the nurse rather than on clients and clinical situations.
Procedural knowledge	Includes both separate and connected knowledge	Proliferation of approaches to theory development. Application of theory in practice was frequently underemphasized. Emphasis was placed on the procedures used to acquire knowledge, with focused attention to the appropriateness of methodology, the criteria for evolution, and statistical procedures for data analysis.
Constructed knowledge	Combination of different types of knowledge (intuition, reason, and self-knowledge)	Recognition that nursing theory should be based on prior empirical studies, theoretical literature, client reports of clinical experiences and feelings, and the nurse scholar's intuition or related knowledge about the phenomenon of concern.
Integrated knowledge	Assimilation and application of "evidence" from nursing and other health care disciplines	Nursing theory will increasingly incorporate information from published literature with enhanced emphasis on clinical application as situation-specific/practice theories and middle range theories.

Source: Kidd & Morrison (1988).

physicians, and practice was taught by experienced nurses. The curricula contained some anatomy and physiology and occasional lectures on special diseases. Few nursing books were available, and the emphasis was on carrying out physicians' orders. Nursing education and practice focused on the performance of technical skills and application of a few basic principles, such as aseptic technique and principles of mobility. Nurses depended on physicians' diagnosis and orders and as a result largely adhered to the medical model, which views body and mind separately and focuses on cure and treatment of pathologic problems (Donahue, 2011). Hospital administrators saw nurses as inexpensive labor. Nurses were exploited both as students and as experienced workers. They were taught to be submissive and obedient, and they learned to fulfill their responsibilities to physicians without question (Chinn & Kramer, 2011).

Unfortunately, with a few exceptions, this model of nursing education persisted for more than 80 years. One exception was Yale University, which started the first autonomous school of nursing in 1924. At Yale, and in other later collegiate programs, professional training was strengthened by in-depth exposure to the underlying theory of disease as well as the social, psychological, and physical aspects of client welfare. The growth of collegiate programs lagged, however, due to opposition from many physicians who argued that university-educated nurses were overtrained. Hospital schools continued to insist that nursing education meant acquisition of technical skills and that knowledge of theory was unnecessary and might actually handicap the nurse (Andrist, 2006; Donahue, 2011; Kalisch & Kalisch, 2004).

Received Knowledge Stage

It was not until after World War II that substantive changes were made in nursing education. During the late 1940s and into the 1950s, serious nursing shortages were fueled by a decline in nursing school enrollments. A 1948 report, *Nursing for the Future,* by Esther Brown, PhD, compared nursing with teaching. Brown noted that the current model of nursing education was central to the problems of the profession and recommended that efforts be made to provide nursing education in universities as opposed to the apprenticeship system that existed in most hospital programs (Donahue, 2011; Kalisch & Kalisch, 2004).

Other factors during this time challenged the tradition of hospital-based training for nurses. One of these factors was a dramatic increase in the number of hospitals resulting from the Hill-Burton Act, which worsened the ongoing and sometimes critical nursing shortage. In addition, professional organizations for nurses were restructured and began to grow. It was also during this time that state licensure testing for registration took effect, and by 1949, 41 states required testing. The registration requirement necessitated that education programs review the content matter they were teaching to determine minimum criteria and some degree of uniformity. In addition, the techniques and processes used in instruction were also reviewed and evaluated (Kalisch & Kalisch, 2004).

Over the next decade, a number of other events occurred that altered nursing education and nursing practice. In 1950, the journal *Nursing Research* was first published. The American Nurses Association (ANA) began a program to encourage nurses to pursue graduate education to study nursing functions and practice. Books on research methods and explicit theories of nursing began to appear. In 1956, the Health Amendments Act authorized funds for financial aid to promote graduate education for full-time study to prepare nurses for administration, supervision, and teaching. These events resulted in a slow but steady increase in graduate nursing education programs.

The first doctoral programs in nursing originated within schools of education at Teachers College of Columbia University (1933) and New York University (1934). But it would be 20 more years before the first doctoral program in nursing began at the University of Pittsburgh (1954) (Kalisch & Kalisch, 2004).

Subjective Knowledge Stage

Until the 1950s, nursing practice was principally derived from social, biologic, and medical theories. With the exceptions of Nightingale's work in the 1850s, nursing theory had its beginnings with the publication of Hildegard Peplau's book in 1952. Peplau described the interpersonal process between the nurse and the client. This started a revolution in nursing, and in the late 1950s and 1960s, a number of nurse theorists emerged seeking to provide an independent conceptual framework for nursing education and practice (Donahue, 2011). The nurse's role came under scrutiny during this decade as nurse leaders debated the nature of nursing practice and theory development.

During the 1960s, the development of nursing theory was heavily influenced by three philosophers, James Dickoff, Patricia James, and Ernestine Weidenbach, who, in a series of articles, described theory development and the nature of theory for a practice discipline. Other approaches to theory development combined direct observations of practice, insights derived from existing theories and other literature sources, and insights derived from explicit philosophical perspectives about nursing and the nature of health and human experience. Early theories were characterized by a functional view of nursing and health. They attempted to define what nursing is, describe the social purposes nursing serves, explain how nurses function to realize these purposes, and identify parameters and variables that influence illness and health (Chinn & Kramer, 2011).

In the 1960s, a number of nurse leaders (Abdellah, Orlando, Widenbach, Hall, Henderson, Levine, and Rogers) developed and published their views of nursing. Their descriptions of nursing and nursing models evolved from their personal, professional, and educational experiences, and reflected their perception of ideal nursing practice.

Procedural Knowledge Stage

By the 1970s, the nursing profession viewed itself as a scientific discipline evolving toward a theoretically based practice focusing on the client. In the late 1960s and early 1970s, several nursing theory conferences were held. Also, significantly, in 1972, the National League for Nursing implemented a requirement that the curricula for nursing educational programs be based on conceptual frameworks. During these years, many nursing theorists published their beliefs and ideas about nursing and some developed conceptual models.

During the 1970s, a consensus developed among nursing leaders regarding common elements of nursing. These were the nature of nursing (roles/actions/interventions), the individual recipient of care (client), the context of nurse–client interactions (environment), and health. Nurses debated whether there should be one conceptual model for nursing or several models to describe the relationships among the nurse, client, environment, and health. Books were written for nurses on how to critique, develop, and apply nursing theories. Graduate schools developed courses on analysis and application of theory, and researchers identified nursing theories as conceptual frameworks for their studies. Through the late 1970s and early 1980s, theories moved to characterizing nursing's role from "what nurses do" to "what nursing is." This changed nursing from a context-dependent, reactive position to a context-independent, proactive arena (Chinn & Kramer, 2011).

Although master's programs were growing steadily, doctoral programs grew more slowly, but by 1970, there were 20 such programs. This growth in graduate nursing education allowed nurse scholars to debate ideas, viewpoints, and research methods in the nursing literature. As a result, nurses began to question the ideas that were taken for granted in nursing and the traditional basis in which nursing was practiced.

Constructed Knowledge Stage

During the late 1980s, scholars began to concentrate on theories that provide meaningful foundation for nursing practice. There was a call to develop substance in theory and to focus on nursing concepts grounded in practice and linked to research. The 1990s into the early 21st century saw an increasing emphasis on philosophy and philosophy of science in nursing. Attention shifted from grand theories to middle range theories, as well as application of theory in research and practice.

In the 1990s, the idea of evidence-based practice (EBP) was introduced into nursing to address the widespread recognition of the need to move beyond attention given to research per se, in order to address the gap in research and practice. The "evidence" is research that has been completed and published (LoBiondo-Wood & Haber, 2010). Ostensibly, EBP promotes employment of theory-based, research-derived evidence to guide nursing practice.

During this period, graduate education in nursing continued to grow rapidly, particularly among programs that produced advanced practice nurses (APNs). A seminal event during this time was the introduction of the doctor of nursing practice (DNP). The DNP was initially proposed by the American Association of Colleges of Nursing (AACN) in 2004 to be the terminal degree for APNs. The impetus for the DNP was based on recognition of the need for expanded competencies due to the increasing complexity of clinical practice, enhanced knowledge to improve nursing practice and outcomes, and promotion of leadership skills (American Association of Colleges of Nursing [AACN], 2004).

Integrated Knowledge Stage

More recently, development of nursing knowledge shifted to a trend that blends and uses a variety of processes to achieve a given research aim as opposed to adherence to strict, accepted methodologies (Chinn & Kramer, 2011). In the second decade of the 21st century, there has been significant attention to the need to direct nursing knowledge development toward clinical relevance, to address what Risjord (2010) terms the "relevance gap." Indeed, as Risjord states, and virtually all nursing scholars would agree, "the primary goal . . . of nursing research is to produce knowledge that supports practice" (p. 4). But he continues to note that in reality, a significant portion of research supports practice imperfectly, infrequently, and often insignificantly.

In the current stage of knowledge development, considerable focus in nursing science has been on integration of knowledge into practice, largely with increased attention on EBP and translational research (Chinn & Kramer, 2011). Indeed, it is widely accepted that systematic review of research from a variety of health disciplines, often in the form of meta-analyses, should be undertaken to inform practice and policy making in nursing (Schmidt & Brown, 2012; Melnyk & Fineout-Overholt, 2011). Further, this involves or includes application of evidence from across all health-related sciences (i.e., translational research).

Translational research was designated a priority initiative by the National Institute of Health in 2005 (Powers & Knapp, 2011). The idea of translational research is to close the gap between scientific discovery and translation of research into practice; the intent is to validate evidence in the practice setting (Chinn & Kramer, 2011). Translational research shifts focus to interdisciplinary efforts and integration of the perspectives of different disciplines to "a contemporary movement aimed at producing a concerted multidisciplinary effort to address recognized health disparities and care delivery inadequacies" (Powers & Knapp, 2011, p. 191).

Into the second decade of the 21st century, the number of doctoral programs in the United States continued to grow steadily, and by 2013, there were 128 doctoral programs granting a PhD in nursing (AACN, 2013b). Further, after a sometimes contentious debate, the DNP gained widespread acceptance, and by 2013, there were 123 programs granting the DNP, with more being planned (AACN, 2013a).

In this current stage of theory development in nursing, it is anticipated that there will be ongoing interest in EBP and growth of translational research. In this regard, development and application of middle range and practice theories will continue to be stressed, with attention increasing on practical/clinical application and relevance of both research and theory.

Summary of Stages of Nursing Theory Development

A number of events and individuals have had an impact on the development and utilization of theory in nursing practice, research, and education. Table 2-3 provides a summary of significant events.

Beginning in the early 1950s, efforts to represent nursing theoretically produced broad conceptualizations of nursing practice. These conceptual models or frameworks proliferated during the 1960s and 1970s. Although the conceptual models were not developed using traditional scientific research processes, they did provide direction for nursing by focusing on a general ideal of practice that served as a guide for research and education. Table 2-4 lists the works of many of the nursing theorists and the titles and

(text continues on page 36)

Table 2-3 Significant Events in Theory Development in Nursing

Event	Year
Nightingale publishes *Notes on Nursing*	1859
American Medical Association advocates formal training for nurses	1868
Teacher's College—Columbia University—Doctorate in Education degree for nursing	1920
Yale University begins the first collegiate school of nursing	1924
Report by Dr. Esther Brown—"Nursing for the Future"	1948
State licensure for registration becomes standard	1949
Nursing Research first published	1950
H. Peplau publishes *Interpersonal Relations in Nursing*	1952
University of Pittsburgh begins the first PhD program in nursing	1954
Health Amendments Act passes—funds graduate nursing education	1956
Process of theory development discussed among nursing scholars (works published by Abdellah, Henderson, Orlando, Wiedenbach, and others)	1960–1966
First symposium on Theory Development in Nursing (published in *Nursing Research* in 1968)	1967
Symposium Theory Development in Nursing	1968
Dickoff, James, and Weidenbach—"Theory in a Practice Discipline"	
First Nursing Theory Conference	1969
Second Nursing Theory Conference	1970
Third Nursing Theory Conference	1971
National League for Nursing adopts Requirement for Conceptual Framework for Nursing Curricula	1972
Key articles publish in *Nursing Research* (Hardy—Theories: Components, Development, and Evaluation; Jacox—Theory Construction in Nursing; and Johnson—Development of Theory)	1974
Nurse educator conferences on nursing theory	1975, 1978
Advances in Nursing Science first published	1979
Books written for nurses on how to critique theory, develop theory, and apply nursing theory	1980s
Graduate schools of nursing develop courses on how to analyze and apply theory in nursing	1980s
Research studies in nursing identify nursing theories as frameworks for study	1980s
Publication of numerous books on analysis, application, evaluation, and development of nursing theories	1980s
Philosophy and philosophy of science courses offered in doctoral programs	1990s
Increasing emphasis on middle range and practice theories for nursing	1990s
Nursing literature describes the need to establish interconnections among central nursing concepts	1990s
Introduction of evidence-based practice into nursing	1990s
Philosophy of Nursing first published	1999
Books published describing, analyzing, and discussing application of middle range theory and evidence-based practice	2000s
Introduction of the Doctor of Nursing Practice (DNP)	2004
Growing emphasis on development of situation-specific and middle range theories in nursing	2010+

Sources: Bishop & Hardin (2010); Donahue, 2011; Kalisch & Kalisch (2004); Meleis (2012); Moody (1990).

Table 2-4 Chronology of Publications of Selected Nursing Theorists

Theorist	Year	Title of Theoretical Writings
Florence Nightingale	1859	*Notes on Nursing*
Hildegard Peplau	1952	*Interpersonal Relations in Nursing*
Virginia Henderson	1955	*Principles and Practice of Nursing*, 5th edition
	1966	*The Nature of Nursing: A Definition and Its Implications for Practice, Research, and Education*
	1991	*The Nature of Nursing: Reflections After 25 Years*
Dorothy Johnson	1959	*A Philosophy of Nursing*
	1980	*The Behavioral System Model for Nursing*
Faye Abdellah	1960	*Patient-Centered Approaches to Nursing*
	1968	2nd edition
Ida Jean Orlando	1961	*The Dynamic Nurse–Patient Relationship*
Ernestine Wiedenbach	1964	*Clinical Nursing: A Helping Art*
Lydia E. Hall	1964	*Nursing: What Is It?*
Joyce Travelbee	1966	*Interpersonal Aspects of Nursing*
	1971	2nd edition
Myra E. Levine	1967	*The Four Conservation Principles of Nursing*
	1973	*Introduction to Clinical Nursing*
	1989	*The Conservation Principles: Twenty Years Later*
Martha Rogers	1970	*An Introduction to the Theoretical Basis of Nursing*
	1980	*Nursing: A Science of Unitary Man*
	1983	*Science of Unitary Human Being: A Paradigm for Nursing*
	1989	*Nursing: A Science of Unitary Human Beings*
Dorothea E. Orem	1971	*Nursing: Concepts of Practice*
	1980	2nd edition
	1985	3rd edition
	1991	4th edition
	1995	5th edition
	2001	6th edition
	2011	*Self-Care Science, Nursing Theory and Evidence-Based Practice* (Taylor & Renpenning)
Imogene M. King	1971	*Toward a Theory for Nursing: General Concepts of Human Behavior*
	1981	*A Theory for Nursing: Systems, Concepts, Process*
	1989	*King's General Systems Framework and Theory*

Table 2-4 Chronology of Publications of Selected Nursing Theorists *(continued)*

Theorist	Year	Title of Theoretical Writings
Betty Neuman	1974	*The Betty Neuman Health-Care Systems Model: A Total Person Approach to Patient Problems*
	1982	*The Neuman Systems Model*
	1989	2nd edition
	1995	3rd edition
	2002	4th edition
	2011	5th edition
Evelyn Adam	1975	*A Conceptual Model for Nursing*
	1980	*To Be a Nurse*
	1991	2nd edition
Callista Roy	1976	*Introduction to Nursing: An Adaptation Model*
	1980	*The Roy Adaptation Model*
	1984	*Introduction to Nursing: An Adaptation Model,* 2nd edition
	1991	*The Roy Adaptation Model*
	1999	2nd edition
	2009	3rd edition
Josephine Paterson and Loretta Zderad	1976	*Humanistic Nursing*
Jean Watson	1979	*Nursing: The Philosophy and Science of Caring*
	1985	*Nursing: Human Science and Human Care*
	1989	*Watson's Philosophy and Theory of Human Caring in Nursing*
	1999	*Human Science and Human Care*
	2012	2nd edition
Margaret A. Newman	1979	*Theory Development in Nursing*
	1983	*Newman's Health Theory*
	1986	*Health as Expanding Consciousness*
	2000	2nd edition
Madeleine Leininger	1980	*Caring: A Central Focus of Nursing and Health Care Services*
	1988	*Leininger's Theory of Nursing: Cultural Care Diversity and Universality*
	2001	*Culture Care Diversity and Universality*
	2006	2nd edition
Joan Riehl Sisca	1980	*The Riehl Interaction Model*
	1989	2nd edition

(continued)

Table 2-4 Chronology of Publications of Selected Nursing Theorists *(continued)*

Theorist	Year	Title of Theoretical Writings
Rosemary Parse	1981	*Man-Living-Health: A Theory for Nursing*
	1985	*Man-Living-Health: A Man-Environment Simultaneity Paradigm*
	1987	*Nursing Science: Major Paradigms, Theories, Critiques*
	1989	*Man-Living-Health: A Theory of Nursing*
	1999	*Illuminations: The Human Becoming Theory in Practice and Research*
Joyce Fitzpatrick	1983	*A Life Perspective Rhythm Model*
	1989	2nd edition
Helen Erickson et al.	1983	*Modeling and Role Modeling*
Nancy Roper, Winifred Logan, and Alison Tierney	1983	*A Model for Nursing*
	1983	*The Roper/Logan/Tierney Model for Nursing*
	1996	*The Elements of Nursing: A Model for Nursing Based on a Model of Living*
	2000	*The Roper/Logan/Tierney Model for Nursing*
Patricia Benner and Judith Wrubel	1984	*From Novice to Expert: Excellence and Power in Clinical Nursing Practice*
	1989	*The Primacy of Caring: Stress and Coping in Health and Illness*
Anne Boykin and Savina Schoenhofer	1993	*Nursing as Caring*
	2001	2nd edition
Barbara Artinian	1997	*The Intersystem Model: Integrating Theory and Practice*
	2011	2nd edition
Brendan McCormack and Tanya McCance	2010	*Person-Centred Nursing: Theory and Practice*

Sources: Chinn & Kramer (2011); Hickman (2011); Hilton (1997).

year of key theoretical publications. The works of a number of the major theorists are discussed in Chapters 7 through 9. Reference lists and bibliographies outlining application of their work to research, education, and practice are described in those chapters.

Classification of Theories in Nursing

Over the last 40 years, a number of methods for classifying theory in nursing have been described. These include classification based on range/scope or abstractness (grand or macrotheory to practice or situation-specific theory) and type or purpose of the theory (descriptive, predictive, or prescriptive theory). Both of these classification schemes are discussed in the following sections.

Scope of Theory

One method for classification of theories in nursing that has become common is to differentiate theories based on scope, which refers to complexity and degree of abstraction. The scope of a theory includes its level of specificity and the concreteness of its concepts

Theory	Level of Abstraction
Metatheory	Most abstract
Grand theories	↓
Middle range theories	
Practice theories	Least abstract

FIGURE 2-1 Comparison of the scope of nursing theories.

and propositions. This classification scheme typically uses the terms *metatheory, philosophy,* or *worldview* to describe the philosophical basis of the discipline; *grand theory* or *macrotheory* to describe the comprehensive conceptual frameworks; *middle range* or *midrange* theory to describe frameworks that are relatively more focused than the grand theories; and *situation-specific theory, practice theory,* or *microtheory* to describe those smallest in scope (Higgins & Moore, 2000; Peterson, 2013). Theories differ in complexity and scope along a continuum from practice or situation-specific theories to grand theories. Figure 2-1 compares the scope of nursing theory by level of abstractness.

Metatheory

Metatheory refers to a theory about theory. In nursing, metatheory focuses on broad issues such as the processes of generating knowledge and theory development, and it is a forum for debate within the discipline (Chinn & Kramer, 2011; Powers & Knapp, 2011). Philosophical and methodologic issues at the metatheory or worldview level include identifying the purposes and kinds of theory needed for nursing, developing and analyzing methods for creating nursing theory, and proposing criteria for evaluating theory (Hickman, 2011; Walker & Avant, 2011).

Walker and Avant (2011) presented an overview of historical trends in nursing metatheory. Beginning in the 1960s, metatheory discussions involved nursing as an academic discipline and the relationship of nursing to basic sciences. Later discussions addressed the predominant philosophical worldviews (received view versus perceived view) and methodologic issues related to research (see Chapter 1). Recent metatheoretical issues relate to the philosophy of nursing and address what levels of theory development are needed for nursing practice, research, and education (i.e., grand theory versus middle range and practice theory) and the increasing focus on the philosophical perspectives of critical theory, postmodernism, and feminism.

Grand Theories

Grand theories are the most complex and broadest in scope. They attempt to explain broad areas within a discipline and may incorporate numerous other theories. The term *macrotheory* is used by some authors to describe a theory that is broadly conceptualized and is usually applied to a general area of a specific discipline (Higgins & Moore, 2000; Peterson, 2013).

Grand theories are nonspecific and are composed of relatively abstract concepts that lack operational definitions. Their propositions are also abstract and are not generally amenable to testing. Grand theories are developed through thoughtful and insightful appraisal of existing ideas as opposed to empirical research (Fawcett & DeSanto-Madeya, 2013). The majority of the nursing conceptual frameworks (e.g., Orem, Roy, and Rogers) are considered to be grand theories. Chapters 6 through 9 discuss many of the grand nursing theories.

Middle Range Theories

Middle range theory lies between the grand nursing models and more circumscribed, concrete ideas (practice or situation-specific theories). Middle range theories are substantively specific and encompass a limited number of concepts and a limited aspect of the real world. They are composed of relatively concrete concepts that can be operationally defined and relatively concrete propositions that may be empirically tested (Higgins & Moore, 2000; Peterson, 2013; Whall, 2005).

A middle range theory may be (1) a description of a particular phenomenon, (2) an explanation of the relationship between phenomena, or (3) a prediction of the effects of one phenomenon or another (Fawcett & DeSanto-Madeya, 2013). Many investigators favor working with propositions and theories characterized as middle range rather than with conceptual frameworks because they provide the basis for generating testable hypotheses related to particular nursing phenomena and to particular client populations (Chinn & Kramer, 2011; Ketefian & Redman, 1997). The number of middle range theories developed and used by nurses has grown significantly over the past two decades. Examples include social support, quality of life, and health promotion. Chapters 10 and 11 describe middle range theory in more detail.

Practice Theories

Practice theories are also called *situation-specific theories, prescriptive theories*, or *microtheories* and are the least complex. Practice theories are more specific than middle range theories and produce specific directions for practice (Higgins & Moore, 2000; Peterson, 2013; Whall, 2005). They contain the fewest concepts and refer to specific, easily defined phenomena. They are narrow in scope, explain a small aspect of reality, and are intended to be prescriptive. They are usually limited to specific populations or fields of practice and often use knowledge from other disciplines (McKenna, 1993). Examples of practice theories developed and used by nurses are theories of postpartum depression, infant bonding, and oncology pain management. Chapters 12 and 18 present additional information on practice theories.

Type or Purpose of Theory

In their seminal work, Dickoff and James (1968) defined theories as intellectual inventions designed to describe, explain, predict, or prescribe phenomena. They described four kinds of theory, each of which builds on the other. These are:

- Factor-isolating theories (descriptive theories)
- Factor-relating theories (explanatory theories)
- Situation-relating theories (predictive theories or promoting or inhibiting theories)
- Situation-producing theories (prescriptive theories)

Dickoff and James (1968) stated that nursing as a profession should go beyond the level of descriptive or explanatory theories and attempt to attain the highest levels—that of situation-relating/predictive and situation-producing/prescriptive theories.

Descriptive (Factor-Isolating) Theories

Descriptive theories are those that describe, observe, and name concepts, properties, and dimensions. Descriptive theory identifies and describes the major concepts of phenomena but does not explain how or why the concepts are related. The purpose of descriptive theory is to provide observation and meaning regarding the phenomena. It is generated and tested by descriptive research techniques including concept analysis, case studies, literature review phenomenology, ethnography, and grounded theory (Young et al., 2001).

Examples of descriptive theories are readily found in the nursing literature. Dombrowsky and Gray (2012), for example, used the process of concept analysis to develop a conceptual model describing the experiences and contributing factors of urinary continence and incontinence. In other works, using grounded theory methodology, Kanacki, Roth, Georges, and Herring (2012) developed a theoretical model describing the experience of caring for a dying spouse, and Busby and Witucki-Brown (2011) constructed a theory describing situational awareness among emergency response providers. Lastly, Robles-Silva (2008) used ethnography to construct a conceptual model explaining the multiple phases that caregivers experience while working with poor, chronically ill adults in Mexico.

Explanatory (Factor-Relating) Theories

Factor-relating theories, or explanatory theories, are those that relate concepts to one another, describe the interrelationships among concepts or propositions, and specify the associations or relationships among some concepts. They attempt to tell *how* or *why* the concepts are related and may deal with cause and effect and correlations or rules that regulate interactions. They are developed by correlational research and increasingly through comprehensive literature review and synthesis. An example of an explanatory theory is the theory of spirituality-based nursing practice (Nardi & Rooda, 2011). This theory was developed from a mixed-method research study that surveyed senior nursing students on several aspects of awareness and application of spirituality in their practice. In other works, comprehensive literature review and synthesis were used by Reimer and Moore (2010) to develop a middle range theory explaining flight nursing expertise and by Murrock and Higgins (2009) to develop a middle range theory explaining the effects of music on improved health outcomes.

Predictive (Situation-Relating) Theories

Situation-relating theories are achieved when the conditions under which concepts are related are stated and the relational statements are able to describe future outcomes consistently. Situation-relating theories move to prediction of precise relationships between concepts. Experimental research is used to generate and test them in most cases.

Predictive theories are relatively difficult to find in the nursing literature. In one example, Cobb (2012) used a quasi-experimental, model building approach to predict the relationship between spirituality and health status among adults living with HIV. In another example, Chang, Wung, and Crogan (2008) used a quasi-experimental research design to create a theoretical model supporting an intervention designed to improve elderly nursing home resident's ability to provide self-care. Their research validated the premise that the theory-based intervention improved performance of activities of daily living among residents in the study group compared with a control group.

Another example of a predictive theory in nursing can be found in the Caregiving Effectiveness Model. The process outlining development of this theory was described by Smith and colleagues (2002) and combined numerous steps in theory construction and empirical testing and validation. In the model, caregiving effectiveness is dependent on the interface of a number of factors including the characteristics of the caregiver, interpersonal interactions between the patient and caregiver, and the educational preparedness of the caregiver, combined with adaptive factors, such as economic stability, and the caregiver's own health status and family adaptation and coping mechanisms. The model itself graphically details the interaction of these factors and depicts how they collectively work to impact caregiving effectiveness.

Prescriptive (Situation-Producing) Theories

Situation-producing theories are those that prescribe activities necessary to reach defined goals. Prescriptive theories address nursing therapeutics and consequences of interventions. They include propositions that call for change and predict consequences of nursing interventions. They should describe the prescription, the consequence(s), the type of client, and the conditions (Meleis, 2012).

Prescriptive theories are among the most difficult to identify in the nursing literature. One example is a work by Walling (2006) that presented a "prescriptive theory explaining medical acupuncture" for nurse practitioners. The model describes how acupuncture can be used to reduce stress and enhance well-being. In another example, Auvil-Novak (1997) described the development of a middle range theory of chronotherapeutic intervention for postsurgical pain based on three experimental studies of pain relief among postsurgical clients. The theory uses a time-dependent approach to pain assessment and provides directed nursing interventions to address postoperative pain.

Issues in Theory Development in Nursing

A number of issues related to use of theory in nursing have received significant attention in the literature. The first is the issue of borrowed versus unique theory in nursing. A second issue is nursing's metaparadigm, and a third is the importance of the concept of caring in nursing.

Borrowed Versus Unique Theory in Nursing

Since the 1960s, the question of borrowing—or sharing—theory from other disciplines has been raised in the discussion of nursing theory. The debate over borrowed/shared theory centers in the perceived need for theory unique to nursing discussed by many nursing theorists.

The main premise held by those opposed to borrowed theory is that only theories that are grounded in nursing should guide the actions of the discipline. A second premise that supports the need for unique theory is that any theory that evolves out of the practice arena of nursing is substantially nursing. Although one might "borrow" theory and apply it to the realm of nursing actions, it is transformed into nursing theory because it addresses phenomena within the arena of nursing practice.

Opponents of using borrowed theory believe that nursing knowledge should not be tainted by using theory from physiology, psychology, sociology, and education. Furthermore, they believe "borrowing" requires returning and that the theory is not in essence nursing if concepts are borrowed (Levine, 1995; Risjord, 2010).

Proponents of using borrowed theory in nursing believe that knowledge belongs to the scientific community and to society at large, and it is not the property of individuals or disciplines (Powers & Knapp, 2011). Indeed, these individuals feel that knowledge is not the private domain of one discipline, and the use of knowledge generated by any discipline is not borrowed but shared. Further, shared theory does not lessen nursing scholarship but enhances it (Levine, 1995).

Furthermore, advocates of borrowed or shared theory believe that, like other applied sciences, nursing depends on the theories from other disciplines for its theoretical foundations. For example, general systems theory is used in nursing, biology, sociology, and engineering. Different theories of stress and adaptation are valuable to nurses, psychologists, and physicians.

In reality, all nursing theories incorporate concepts and theories shared with other disciplines to guide theory development, research, and practice. However, simply adopting concepts or theories from another discipline does not convert them into nursing concepts or theories. It is important, therefore, for theorists, researchers, and practitioners to use concepts from other disciplines appropriately. Emphasis should be placed on redefining and synthesizing the concepts and theories according to a nursing perspective (Fawcett & DeSanto-Madeya, 2013; Levine, 1995).

Nursing's Metaparadigm

The most abstract and general component of the structural hierarchy of nursing knowledge is what Kuhn (1977) called the *metaparadigm*. A metaparadigm refers "globally to the subject matter of greatest interest to member of a discipline" (Powers & Knapp, 2011, p. 107). The metaparadigm includes major philosophical orientations or worldviews of a discipline, the conceptual models and theories that guide research and other scholarly activities, and the empirical indicators that operationalize theoretical concepts (Fawcett & Malinski, 1996). The purpose or function of the metaparadigm is to summarize the intellectual and social missions of the discipline and place boundaries on the subject matter of that discipline (Kim, 1989). Fawcett and DeSanto-Madeya (2013) identified four requirements for a metaparadigm. These are summarized in Box 2-1.

According to Fawcett and DeSanto-Madeya (2013), in the 1970s and early 1980s, a number of nursing scholars identified a growing consensus that the dominant phenomena within the science of nursing revolved around the concepts of man (person), health, environment, and nursing. Fawcett first wrote on the central concepts of nursing in 1978 and formalized them as the metaparadigm of nursing in 1984. This articulation of four metaparadigm concepts (person, health, environment, and nursing) served as an organizing framework around which conceptual development proceeded.

Wagner (1986) examined the nursing metaparadigm in depth. Her sample of 160 doctorally prepared chairpersons, deans, or directors of programs for bachelor's of science in nursing revealed that between 94% and 98% of the respondents agreed that the concepts that comprise the nursing metaparadigm are person, health, nursing, and environment. She concluded that these findings indicated a consensus within the discipline of nursing that these are the dominant phenomena within the science. A summary of definitions for each term is presented here.

Person refers to a being composed of physical, intellectual, biochemical, and psychosocial needs; a human energy field; a holistic being in the world; an open system;

Box 2-1 Requirements for a Metaparadigm

1. A metaparadigm must identify a domain that is distinctive from the domains of other disciplines . . . the concepts and propositions represent a unique perspective for inquiry and practice.
2. A metaparadigm must encompass all phenomena of interest to the discipline in a parsimonious manner . . . the concepts and propositions are global and there are no redundancies.
3. A metaparadigm must be perspective-neutral . . . the concepts and propositions do not represent a specific perspective (i.e., a specific paradigm or conceptual model or combination of perspectives).
4. A metaparadigm must be global in scope and substance . . . the concepts and propositions do not reflect particular national, cultural, or ethnic beliefs and values.

Adapted from: Fawcett & DeSanto-Madeya, 2013

an integrated whole; an adaptive system; and a being who is greater than the sum of his or her parts (Wagner, 1986). Nursing theories are often most distinguishable from each other by the various ways in which they conceptualize the person or recipient of nursing care. Most nursing models organize data about the individual person as a focus of the nurse's attention, although some nursing theorists have expanded to include family or community as the focus (Thorne et al., 1998). *Health* is the ability to function independently; successful adaptation to life's stressors; achievement of one's full life potential; and unity of mind, body, and soul (Wagner, 1986). Health has been a phenomenon of central interest to nursing since its inception. Nursing literature indicates great diversity in the explication of health and quality of life (Thorne et al., 1998). Indeed, in a recent work, following a critical appraisal of the works of several nurse-theorists, Plummer and Molzahn (2012) suggested replacing the term "health" with "quality of life." They posited that quality of life is a more inclusive notion, as health is often understood in terms of physical status. Alternatively, quality of life better encompasses a holistic perspective, involving physical, psychological, and social well-being, as well as the spiritual and environmental aspects of the human experience.

Environment typically refers to the external elements that affect the person; internal and external conditions that influence the organism; significant others with whom the person interacts; and an open system with boundaries that permit the exchange of matter, energy, and information with human beings (Wagner, 1986). Many nursing theories have a narrow conceptualization of the environment as the immediate surroundings or circumstances of the individual. This view limits understanding by making the environment rigid, static, and natural. A multilayered view of the environment encourages understanding of an individual's perspective and immediate context and incorporates the sociopolitical and economic structures and underlying ideologies that influence reality (Thorne et al., 1998).

Nursing is a science, an art, and a practice discipline and involves caring. Goals of nursing include care of the well, care of the sick, assisting with self-care activities, helping individuals attain their human potential, and discovering and using nature's laws of health. The purposes of nursing care include placing the client in the best condition for nature to restore health, promoting the adaptation of the individual, facilitating the development of an interaction between the nurse and the client in which jointly set goals are met, and promoting harmony between the individual and the environment (Wagner, 1986). Furthermore, nursing practice facilitates, supports, and assists individuals, families, communities, and societies to enhance, maintain, and recover health and to reduce and ameliorate the effects of illness (Thorne et al., 1998).

In addition to these definitions, many grand nursing theorists, and virtually all of the theoretical commentators, incorporate these four terms into their conceptual or theoretical frameworks. Table 2-5 presents theoretical definitions of the metaparadigm concepts from selected nursing conceptual frameworks and other writings.

Relationships Among the Metaparadigm Concepts

The concepts of nursing's metaparadigm have been linked in four propositions identified in the writings of Donaldson and Crowley (1978) and Gortner (1980). These are as follows:

1. Person and health: Nursing is concerned with the principles and laws that govern human processes of living and dying.
2. Person and environment: Nursing is concerned with the patterning of human health experiences within the context of the environment.
3. Health and nursing: Nursing is concerned with the nursing actions or processes that are beneficial to human beings.

Table 2-5 Selected Theoretical Definitions of the Concepts of Nursing's Metaparadigm

Metaparadigm Concept	Author/Source of Definition	Definition
Person/human being/client	D. Johnson	A behavioral system with patterned, repetitive, and purposeful ways of behaving that link person to the environment.
	B. Neuman	A dynamic composite of the interrelationships between physiologic, psychological, sociocultural, developmental, spiritual, and basic structure variables. May be an individual, group, community, or social system.
	D. Orem	Are distinguished from other living things by their capacity (1) to reflect upon themselves and their environment, (2) to symbolize what they experience, and (3) to use symbolic creations (ideas, words) in thinking, in communicating, and in guiding efforts to do and to make things that are beneficial for themselves or others.
	M. Rogers	An irreducible, indivisible, pan-dimensional energy field identified by pattern and manifesting characteristics that are specific to the whole and that cannot be predicted from knowledge of the parts.
Nursing	M. Leininger	A learned humanistic and scientific profession and discipline that is focused on human care phenomena and activities to assist, support, facilitate, or enable individuals or groups to maintain or regain their well-being (or health) in culturally meaningful and beneficial ways, or to help people face handicaps or death.
	M. Newman	Caring in the human health experience.
	D. Orem	A specific type of human service required whenever the maintenance of continuous self-care requires the use of special techniques and the application of scientific knowledge in providing care or in designing it.
	J. Watson	A human science of persons and human health–illness experiences that are mediated by professional, personal, scientific, esthetic, and ethical human care transactions.
Health	M. Leininger	A state of well-being that is culturally defined, valued, and practiced, and that reflects the ability of individuals (or groups) to perform their daily role activities in culturally expressed, beneficial, and patterned lifeways.
	M. Newman	A pattern of evolving, expanding consciousness regardless of the form or direction it takes.
	C. Roy	A state and process of being and becoming an integrated and whole person. It is a reflection of adaptation, that is, the interaction of the person and the environment.
	J. Watson	Unity and harmony within the mind, body, and soul. Health is also associated with the degree of congruence between the self as perceived and the self as experienced.
Environment	M. Leininger	The totality of an event, situation, or particular experience that gives meaning to human expressions, interpretations, and social interactions in particular physical, ecologic, sociopolitical, and cultural settings.
	B. Neuman	All internal and external factors of influences that surround the client or client system.
	M. Rogers	An irreducible, pan-dimensional energy field identified by pattern and integral with the human field.
	C. Roy	All conditions, circumstances, and influences that surround and affect the development and behavior of human adaptive systems with particular consideration of person and earth resources.

Sources: Johnson (1980); Leininger (1991); Neuman (1995); Newman (1990); Orem (2001); Rogers (1990); Roy & Andrews (1999); Watson (1985).

4. Person, environment, and health: Nursing is concerned with the human processes of living and dying, recognizing that human beings are in a continuous relationship with their environments (Fawcett & DeSanto-Madeya, 2013, p. 6).

In addressing how the four concepts meet the requirements for a metaparadigm, Fawcett and DeSanto-Madeya (2013) explain that the first three propositions represent recurrent themes identified in the writings of Nightingale and other nursing scholars. Furthermore, the four concepts and propositions identify the unique focus of the discipline of nursing and encompass all relevant phenomena in a parsimonious manner. Finally, the concepts and propositions are perspective-neutral because they do not reflect a specific paradigm or conceptual model and they do not reflect the beliefs and values of any one country or culture.

Other Viewpoints on Nursing's Metaparadigm

There is some dissension in the acceptance of person/health/environment/nursing as nursing's metaparadigm. Kim (1987, 1989, 2010) identified four domains (client, client–nurse, practice, and environment) as an organizing framework or typology of nursing. In this framework, the most significant difference appears to be in placing health issues (i.e., health care experiences and health care environment) within the client domain and differentiating the nursing practice domain from the client–nurse domain. The latter focuses specifically on interactions between the nurse and the client.

Meleis (2012) maintained that nursing encompasses seven central concepts: interaction, nursing client, transitions, nursing process, environment, nursing therapeutics, and health. Addition of the concepts of interaction, transitions, and nursing process denotes the greatest difference between this framework and the more commonly described person/health/environment/nursing framework. (See Link to Practice 2-1 for another thought on expanding the metaparadigm to include social justice.)

Link to Practice 2-1

Should Social Justice Be Part of Nursing's Metaparadigm?

Schim, Benkert, Bell, Walker, and Danford (2006) proposed that the construct of "social justice" be added to nursing's metaparadigm. They argued that social justice is interconnected with the four acknowledged metaparadigm concepts of nursing, person, health, and environment. In their model, social justice actually acts as the central, organizational foundation that links the other four concepts, particularly within the context of public health nursing, and more specifically in urban settings.

Using this macroperspecitve, the goal of nursing is to ensure adequate distribution of resources to benefit those who are marginalized. Suggested strategies to enhance attention to social justice in nursing include shifting to a population health and health promotion/disease prevention perspective; diversifying nursing by recruiting and educating underrepresented minorities into the profession; and engaging in political action at local, state, national and international levels. They concluded that as a caring profession, nursing should expand efforts with a social justice orientation to help ensure equal access to benefits and protections of society for all.

Caring as a Central Construct in the Discipline of Nursing

A final debate that will be discussed in this chapter centers on the place of the concept of caring within the discipline and science of nursing. This debate has been escalating over the last decade and has been motivated by the perceived urgency of identifying nursing's unique contribution to the health care disciplines and revolves around the defining attributes and roles within the practice of nursing (Thorne et al., 1998).

The concept of caring has occupied a prominent position in nursing literature and has been touted as the essence of nursing by renowned nursing scholars, including Leininger, Watson, and Erikkson. Indeed, it has been proposed that nursing be defined as the study of caring in the human health experience (Newman, Sime, & Corcoran-Perry, 1991).

Although some theorists (i.e., Watson, Leininger, and Boykin) have gone so far as to identify caring as the essence of nursing, there is little if any rejection of caring as *a* central concept for nursing, although not necessarily *the* most significant concept. Thorne and colleagues (1998) cited three major areas of contention in the debate about caring in nursing. The first is the diverse views on the nature of caring. These range from caring as a human trait to caring as a therapeutic intervention and differ according to whether the act of caring is conceptualized as being client centered, nurse centered, or both.

A second major issue in the caring debate concerns the use of caring terminology to conceptualize a specialized role. It has been asked whether there is a compelling reason to lay claim to caring as nursing's unique domain when so many professions describe their function as involving caring, and the concept of caring is prominent in the work of many other disciplines (e.g., medicine, social work, and psychology) (Thorne et al., 1998).

A third issue centers on the implications for the future development of the profession that nursing should espouse caring as its unique mandate. It has been observed that nurses should ask themselves if it is politically astute to be the primary interpreters of a construct that is both gendered and devalued (Meadows, 2007; Thorne et al., 1998).

Thus, it is argued by Fawcett and Malinski (1996) that although caring is included in several conceptualizations of the discipline of nursing, it is not a dominant term in every conceptualization and therefore does not represent a discipline-wide viewpoint. Furthermore, caring is not uniquely a nursing phenomenon, and caring behaviors may not be generalizable across national and cultural boundaries.

Summary

Like Matt Ng, the graduate nursing student described in the opening case study, nurses who are in a position to learn more about theory, and to recognize how and when to apply it, must often be convinced of the relevance of such study to understand the benefits. The study of theory requires exposure to many new concepts, principles, thoughts, and ideas, as well as a student who is willing to see how theory plays an important role in nursing practice, research, education, and administration.

Although study and use of theoretical concepts in nursing dates back to Nightingale, little progress in theory development was made until the 1960s. The past five decades, however, have produced significant advancement in theory development for nursing. This chapter has presented an overview of this evolutionary process. In addition, the basic types of theory and purposes of theory were described. Subsequent chapters will explain many of the ideas introduced here to assist professional nurses to understand the relationship among theory, practice, and research and to further develop the discipline, the science, and the profession of nursing.

Key Points

- "Theory" refers to the systematic explanation of events in which constructs and concepts are identified, relationships are proposed, and predictions are made.
- Theory offers structure and organization to nursing knowledge and provides a systematic means of collecting data to describe, explain, and predict nursing practice.
- Florence Nightingale was the first modern nursing theorist; she described what she considered nurses' goals and practice domain to be.
- There has been an evolution of stages of theory development in nursing. Nursing is currently in the "integrated knowledge" stage, which emphasizes EBP and translational research. Theory development increasingly sources meta-analyses, as well as nursing research, and is largely directed toward middle range and situation-specific/practice theories.
- Theories can be classified by scope of level of abstraction (e.g., metatheory, grand theory, middle range theory, and situation-specific theory) or by type or purpose of the theory (e.g., description, explanation, prediction, and prescription).
- Nursing "borrows" or "shares" theories and concepts from other disciplines to guide theory development, research, and practice. It is critical that nurses redefine and synthesize these shared concept and theories according to a nursing perspective.
- The concepts of nursing, person, environment, and health are widely accepted as the dominant phenomena in nursing; they have been identified as nursing's metaparadigm.

Learning Activities

1. Examine early issues of *Nursing Research* (1950s and 1960s) and determine whether theories or theoretical frameworks were used as a basis for research. What types of theories were used? Review current issues to analyze how this has changed.
2. Examine early issues of *American Journal of Nursing* (1900–1950). Determine if and how theories were used in nursing practice. What types of theories were used? Review current issues to analyze how this has changed.
3. Find reports that present middle range or practice theories in the nursing literature. Identify if these theories are descriptive, explanatory, predictive, or prescriptive in nature.

REFERENCES

Alligood, M. R. (2010). Introduction to nursing theory: Its history, significance, and analysis. In M. R. Alligood & A. M. Tomey (Eds.), *Nursing theorists and their work* (7th ed., pp. 3–15). Maryland Heights, MO: Mosby.

Alligood, M. R., & Tomey, A. M. (2010). *Nursing theorists and their work* (7th ed.). Maryland Heights, MO: Mosby.

American Association of Colleges of Nursing. (2004). *AACN position statement on the practice doctorate in nursing.* Retrieved from http://www.aacn.nche.edu/dnp/position-statement

American Association of Colleges of Nursing (2013a). *CCNE-Accredited Doctor of Nursing Practice (DNP) Programs.* Retrieved from http://apps.aacn.nche.edu/CCNE/reports/rptAccredited Programs_New.asp?sort=state&sProgramType=3

American Association of Colleges of Nursing. (2013b). *PhD nursing programs in the U.S.* Retrieved from http://www.aacn.nche.edu/membership/nursing-program-search?search=&name=&state=&category_id=9&x=19&y=8

Andrist, L. C. (2006). The history of the relationship between feminism and nursing. In L. C. Andrist, P. K. Nicholas, & K. A. Wolfe (Eds.), *A history of nursing ideas.* Boston: Jones & Bartlett Publishers.

Auvil-Novak, S. E. (1997). A middle range theory of chronotherapeutic intervention for postsurgical pain. *Nursing Research, 46*(2), 66–71.

Bishop, S. M., & Hardin, S. R. (2010). History and philosophy of science. In M. R. Alligood & A. M. Tomey (Eds.), *Nursing theorists and their work* (7th ed., pp. 16–24). St. Louis: Mosby.

Blackburn, S. (2008). *Oxford dictionary of philosophy.* New York: Oxford University Press.

Busby, S., & Witucki-Brown, J. (2011). Theory development for situational awareness in multi-casualty incidents. *Journal of Emergency Nursing, 37*(5), 444–452.

Butts, J. B., Rich, K. L., & Fawcett, J. (2012). The future of nursing: How important is discipline-specific knowledge? A conversation with Jacqueline Fawcett. *Nursing Science Quarterly, 25*(2), 151–154.

Chang, S. H., Wung, S. F., & Crogan, N. L. (2008). Improving activities of daily living for nursing home elder persons in Taiwan. *Nursing Research, 57*(3), 191–198.

Chinn, P. L., & Kramer, M. K. (2011). *Integrated theory and knowledge development in nursing* (8th ed.). St. Louis: Elsevier/Mosby.

Cobb, R. K. (2012). How well does spirituality predict health status in adults living with HIV-disease: A Neuman systems model study. *Nursing Science Quarterly, 25*(4), 347–355.

Dickoff, J., & James, P. (1968). A theory of theories: A position paper. *Nursing Research, 17*(3), 197–203.

Dombrowsky, T. A., & Gray, J. (2012). Continence and incontinence: A concept analysis. *The Journal of Theory Construction & Testing, 16*(2), 31–41.

Donahue, M. P. (2011). *Nursing the finest art: An illustrated history* (3rd ed.). St. Louis: Mosby.

Donaldson, S. K., & Crowley, D. M. (1978). The discipline of nursing. *Nursing Outlook, 26*(2), 113–120.

Fawcett, J. (1992). Contemporary conceptualizations of nursing: Philosophy or science? In J. F. Kikuchi & H. Simmons (Eds.), *Philosophic inquiry in nursing* (pp. 64–70). Newbury Park, CA: Sage.

Fawcett, J., & DeSanto-Madeya, S. (2013). *Contemporary nursing knowledge: Analysis and evaluation of nursing models and theories* (3rd ed.). Philadelphia: F. A. Davis.

Fawcett, J., & Malinski, V. M. (1996). On the requirements for a metaparadigm: An invitation to dialogue. *Nursing Science Quarterly, 9*(3), 94–97, 100–101.

Gortner, S. R. (1980). Nursing science in transition. *Nursing Research, 29*(3), 180–183.

Hickman, J. S. (2011). An introduction to nursing theory. In J. George (Ed.), *Nursing theories: The base for professional nursing practice* (6th ed., pp. 1–22). Upper Saddle River, NJ: Pearson Education.

Higgins, P. A., & Moore, S. M. (2000). Levels of theoretical thinking in nursing. *Nursing Outlook, 48*(4), 179–183.

Hilton, P. A. (1997). Theoretical perspective of nursing: A review of the literature. *Journal of Advanced Nursing, 26*(6), 1211–1220.

Johnson, D. E. (1980). The behavioral system model for nursing. In J. P. Riehl & C. Roy (Eds.), *Conceptual models for nursing practice* (2nd ed., pp. 209–216). New York: Appleton-Century-Crofts.

Kalisch, P. A., & Kalisch, B. J. (2004). *The advance of American nursing* (4th ed.). Philadelphia: Lippincott Williams & Wilkins.

Kanacki, L. S., Roth, P., Georges, J. M., & Herring, P. (2012). Shared presence: Caring for a dying spouse. *Journal of Hospice & Palliative Care Nursing, 14*(6), 414–425.

Ketefian, S., & Redman, R. W. (1997). Nursing science in the global community. *Image: Journal of Nursing Scholarship, 29*(1), 11–16.

Kidd, P., & Morrison, E. F. (1988). The progression of knowledge in nursing research: A search for meaning. *Image: Journal of Nursing Scholarship, 20*(4), 222–224.

Kim, H. S. (1987). Structuring the nursing knowledge system: A typology of four domains. *Scholarly Inquiry for Nursing Practice, 1*(2), 99–110.

Kim, H. S. (1989). Theoretical thinking in nursing: Problems and prospects. *Recent Advances in Nursing, 24,* 106–122.

Kim, H. S. (2010). *The nature of theoretical thinking in nursing* (3rd ed.). New York: Springer.

Kuhn, T. S. (1977). Second thought on paradigms. In F. Suppe (Ed.), *The structure of scientific theory* (pp. 459–482). Urbana, IL: University of Illinois Press.

Leininger, M. (1991). *Culture care diversity and universality: A theory of nursing.* New York: National League for Nursing.

Levine, M. E. (1995). The rhetoric of nursing theory. *Image: Journal of Nursing Scholarship, 27*(1), 11–14.

LoBiondo-Wood, G., & Haber, J. (2010). *Nursing research: Methods and critical appraisal for evidence based practice* (7th ed.). St. Louis: Mosby.

McKenna, G. (1993). Unique theory—Is it essential in the development of a science of nursing? *Nurse Education Today, 15,* 121–127.

Meadows, R. (2007). Beyond caring. *Nursing Administration Quarterly, 31*(2), 158–161.

Meleis, A. I. (2012). *Theoretical nursing: Development and progress* (5th ed.). Philadelphia: Lippincott Williams & Wilkins.

Melnyk, B. M., & Fineout-Overholt, E. (2011). *Evidence-based practice in nursing and healthcare: A guide to practice* (2nd ed.). Philadelphia: Lippincott Williams and Wilkins.

Moody, L. E. (1990). *Advancing nursing science through research.* Newbury Park, CA: Sage.

Murrock, C. J., & Higgins, P. A. (2009). The theory of music, mood and movement to improve health outcomes. *Journal of Advanced Nursing, 65*(10), 2249–2257.

Nardi, D., & Rooda, L. (2011). Spirituality-based nursing practice by nursing students: An exploratory study. *Journal of Professional Nursing, 27*(4), 255–263.

Neuman, B. (1995). *The Neuman systems model* (3rd ed.). Norwalk, CT: Appleton & Lange.

Newman, M. A. (1990). Newman's theory of health as praxis. *Nursing Science Quarterly, 3*(1), 37–41.

Newman, M. A., Sime, A. M., & Corcoran-Perry, S. A. (1991). The focus of the discipline of nursing. *Advances in Nursing Science, 14*(1), 1–6.

Omrey, A., Kasper, C. E., & Page, G. G. (1995). *In search of nursing science.* Thousand Oaks, CA: Sage.

Orem, D. E. (2001). *Nursing: Concepts of practice* (6th ed.). St. Louis: Mosby.

Peplau, H. (1952). *Interpersonal relations in nursing.* New York: Putnam's Sons.

Peterson, S. J. (2013). Introduction to the nature of nursing knowledge. In S. J. Peterson & T. S. Bredow (Eds.), *Middle range theories: Application to nursing research* (3rd ed., pp. 1–37). Philadelphia: Lippincott Williams & Wilkins.

Plummer, M., & Molzahn, A. E. (2012). Quality of life in contemporary nursing theory: A concept analysis. *Nursing Science Quarterly, 22*(2), 123–140.

Powers, B. A., & Knapp, T. R. (2011). *A dictionary of nursing theory and research* (4th ed.). New York: Springer.

Reimer, A. P., & Moore, S. M. (2010). Flight nursing expertise: Towards a middle-range theory. *Journal of Advanced Nursing, 66*(5), 1183–1192.

Risjord, M. (2010). *Nursing knowledge: Science, practice, and philosophy.* West Sussex, UK: Wiley-Blackwell.

Robles-Silva, L. (2008). The caregiving trajectory among poor and chronically ill people. *Qualitative Health Research, 18*(3), 358–368.

Rogers, M. E. (1990). Nursing: Science of unitary, irreducible, human beings: Update 1990. In E. A. M. Barrett (Ed.), *Visions of Rogers' science-based nursing* (pp. 5–11). New York: National League for Nursing.

Roy, C., & Andrews, H. A. (1999). *The Roy adaptation model* (2nd ed.). Norwalk, CT: Appleton & Lange.

Rutty, J. E. (1998). The nature of philosophy of science, theory and knowledge relating to nursing and professionalism. *Journal of Advanced Nursing, 28*(2), 243–250.

Schim, S. M., Benkert, R., Bell, S. E., Walker, D. S., & Danford, C. A. (2012). Social justice: Added metaparadigm concept for urban health nursing. *Public Health Nursing, 24*(1), 73–80.

Schmidt, N. A., & Brown, J. M. (2012). *Evidence-based practice for nursing: Appraisal and application of research.* New York: Jones & Bartlett Learning.

Sitzman, K., & Eichelberger, L. W. (2011). *Understanding the work of nurse theorists: A creative beginning* (2nd ed.). New York: Jones & Bartlett Learning.

Smith, C. E., Pace, K., Kochinda, C., Kleinbeck, S. V. M., Loehler, J., & Popkess-Vawter, S. (2002). Caregiving effectiveness model evolution to a midrange theory of home care: A process for critique and replication. *Advances in Nursing Science, 25*(1), 50–64.

Streubert, H. J., & Carpenter, D. R. (2011). *Qualitative research in nursing: Advancing the humanistic imperative* (5th ed.). Philadelphia: Lippincott Williams & Wilkins.

Thorne, S., Canam, C., Dahinten, S., Hall, W., Henderson, A., & Kirkham, S. R. (1998). Nursing's metaparadigm concepts: Disimpacting the debates. *Journal of Advanced Nursing, 27*(6), 1257–1268.

Tierney, A. F. (1998). Nursing models: Extant or extinct? *Journal of Advanced Nursing, 28*(1), 77–85.

Wagner, J. (1986). *Nurse scholar's perceptions of nursing's metaparadigm* (Doctoral dissertation, Ohio State University).

Walker, L. O., & Avant, K. C. (2011). *Strategies for theory construction in nursing* (5th ed.). Upper Saddle River, NJ: Prentice-Hall.

Walling, A. (2006). Therapeutic modulation of the psychoneuroimmune system by medical acupuncture creates enhanced feelings of well-being. *Journal of the American Academy of Nurse Practitioners, 18*(4), 135–143.

Watson, J. (1985). *Nursing: Human science and human care.* Norwalk, CT: Appleton-Century-Crofts.

Whall, A. L. (2005). The structure of nursing knowledge: Analysis and evaluation of practice, middle range, and grand theory. In J. J. Fitzpatrick & A. L. Whall (Eds.), *Conceptual models of nursing: Analysis and application* (4th ed., pp. 5–20). Upper Saddle River, NJ: Prentice-Hall.

Young, A., Taylor, S. G., & Renpenning, K. M. (2001). *Connections: Nursing research, theory and practice.* St. Louis: Mosby.

Ziegler, S. M. (2005). *Theory-directed nursing practice* (2nd ed.). New York: Springer.

CHAPTER 3

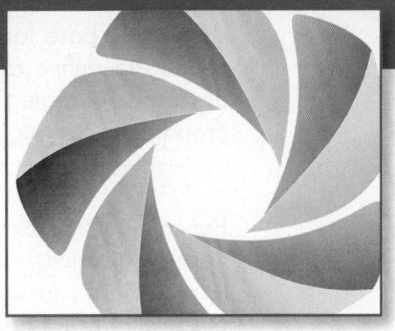

Concept Development

Clarifying Meaning of Terms

Evelyn M. Wills and Melanie McEwen

Mary Talbot is a home health nurse with several years of experience. Recently, Mary was assigned to care for Mrs. Janet Benson, who had had a mastectomy. The pathology report revealed a slow-growing, noninvasive carcinoma in situ; there were no involved nodes, and further tests showed no metastasis. Mrs. Benson was thankful that she was most likely free of the disease.

In the hospital, Mrs. Benson progressed well. But after she was discharged and began chemotherapy, she would frequently weep over things that seemed trivial. Her husband called Mary because he was concerned as this was not Mrs. Benson's usual behavior. Typically, she was self-contained, stoic, and accepting of life's circumstances, seldom demonstrating excessive emotion. To try to better understand Mrs. Benson's response, and to plan care accordingly, Mary consulted Rebecca Wallis, a certified oncology nurse specialist (ONS). After discussing the case with Mary, Rebecca set up an appointment with the Bensons. To gather data from both Mr. and Mrs. Benson's viewpoints, Rebecca asked each of them to explain how they felt about Mrs. Benson's cancer. Mr. Benson replied that the loss of his wife's breast was a small matter to him; he loved her for herself, and he was grateful that she was getting well.

Mrs. Benson seemed relieved by his pronouncement. In response to Rebecca's questioning, she focused on her sadness and inquired if this was normal in women who had undergone mastectomy. Rebecca explained that the reaction was quite common and that oncology nurses in the region used the term postmastectomy grief (PMG) reaction to describe it. The ONSs had worked out a protocol of nursing therapy for PMG, but it had not been formally tested. In the protocol, they requested that the physician oncologist refer the patient to a psychiatric home health nurse for an assessment. The psychiatric home health nurse would confer with the oncologist and the nurse practitioner and, if needed, would request a referral to a licensed therapist. Additionally, a group called "Breast Cancer Support" had been organized in the area by women who had undergone a mastectomy. In this group, problems, such as sadness, were discussed by women who had experienced them, and support was given to those who were going through recovery from breast cancer surgery. Rebecca recommended that the Bensons attend a meeting.

Mrs. Benson's case, and the problem of PMG in general, prompted Rebecca to seek more information about this reaction of breast cancer patients. Her review of the literature suggested that the phenomena needed further study to develop the knowledge base for practice. Because of her education, she realized that she first needed to define and name the problem. To this end, she chose to use concept development strategies she had learned in her graduate nursing program to initiate preparation for a formal research study.

Experienced nurses who are focused on the practical application of evidence-based nursing knowledge demonstrate an inclination toward generalizing what they have learned from a group of clients to other clients with similar problems. This is obvious in the professional discussions of clinical nurses, particularly those educated for advanced practice, who might state, "We see certain phenomenon frequently enough in practice that we have developed clinical protocols or interventions."

These observed phenomena are considered by nurses to be reliable, enduring, and stable features of practical experience, whether or not they have acquired a name and whether or not they have been studied in research (Kim, 2010). Expert practice and enhanced education lead advanced practice nurses to recognize commonalities in phenomena that suggest the need for inquiry. This, in turn, may guide development of clinical hypotheses and testing of interventions. With the current focus on evidence-based practice, clear delineation of the concepts under study in research requires that the linkages among phenomena, concepts, and practice be clarified (Hupcey & Penrod, 2008).

For the nurse who desires to discriminately, formally, and concretely examine a phenomenon in depth, such as described earlier, the most logical place to start is by defining the phenomenon or concept for further study. This is not an easy task, however, and significant time, research, and effort must be made to adequately define nursing concepts. To simplify the process, a number of strategies and methods for concept analysis, concept development, and concept clarification have been proposed and used by nursing scholars for many years.

The rationale for concept development and several methods commonly used by nurses are discussed in this chapter. This will allow expert nurse clinicians and advanced practice nurses to develop or clarify meanings for the phenomena encountered in practice. The outcome can then serve as the basis for further development of theory for research and practice.

The Concept of "Concept"

Concepts are terms that refer to phenomena that occur in nature or in thought. *Concept* has been defined as an abstract term derived from particular attributes (Kerlinger, 1986) and "a symbolic statement describing a phenomenon or a class of phenomena" (Kim, 2010, p. 22). Concepts may be abstract (e.g., hope, love, desire) or relatively concrete (e.g., airplane, body temperature, pain). Concepts are formulated in words that enable people to communicate their meanings about realities in the world (Cutcliffe & McKenna, 2005; Kim, 2010; Penrod & Hupcey, 2005) and give meaning to phenomena that can directly or indirectly be seen, heard, tasted, smelled, or touched (Fawcett, 1999). A concept may be a word (e.g., grief, empathy, power, pain), two words (e.g., job satisfaction, need fulfillment, role strain), or a phrase (e.g., maternal role attachment, biomarkers of preterm labor, health-promoting behaviors). Finally, when they are operationalized, concepts become variables used in hypotheses to be tested in research.

Concepts have been compared to bricks in a wall that lend structure to science (Hardy, 1973). Chinn and Kramer (2011) believe that concepts are more than terms, and constructing conceptual meaning is a vital approach to theory building in which mental constructions or ideas are used to represent experiences. Similarly, Parse (2006) agrees that formal study of concepts enhances knowledge development for nursing through naming, creating, and confirming the phenomena of interest.

Although it was once thought that concepts could be defined once and for all, that idea has been disputed (Penrod & Hupcey, 2005; Rodgers & Knafl, 2000). Theorists now understand that conceptual meaning is created by scholars to assist in imparting the meaning to their readers and, ultimately, to benefit the discipline. Conceptual fluidity and dependence on the context is common in writings on concept analysis in current literature (Duncan, Cloutier, & Bailey, 2007; Penrod & Hupcey, 2005). This makes it imperative that scholars and researchers define concepts clearly and distinctly so that their readers may thoroughly and accurately comprehend their work. Because conceptual meanings are dynamic, they should be defined for each specific use the writer or researcher makes of the term. Indeed, concepts are defined and their meanings are understood only within the framework of the theory of which they are a part (Hardy, 1973).

Types of Concepts

Concepts explicate the subject matter of the theories of a discipline. For example, concepts from psychology include personality, intelligence, and cognition; concepts from biology include cell, species, and protoplasm (Jacox, 1974). Dubin (1978) explained the differences between various types of concepts, characterizing them as enumerative, associative, relational, statistical, and summative. Table 3-1 shows characteristics and examples of each of these types of concepts.

Table 3-1 Types of Concepts

Concept	Characteristics	Examples
Enumerative concepts	Are always present and universal	Age, height, weight
Associative concepts	Exist only in some conditions within a phenomenon; may have a zero value	Income, presence of disease, anxiety
Relational concepts	Can be understood only through the combination or interaction of two or more enumerative or associative concepts	Elderly (must combine concepts of age and longevity), mother (must combine man, woman, and birth)
Statistical concepts	Relate the property of one thing in terms of its distribution in the population rate	Average blood pressure, HIV/AIDS prevalence rate
Summative concepts	Represent an entire complex entity of a phenomenon; are complex and not measurable	Nursing, health, and environment

Source: Dubin (1978).

In nursing, concepts have been borrowed or derived from other disciplines (e.g., adaptation, culture, homeostasis) as well as developed directly from nursing practice and research (e.g., maternal–infant bonding, health-promoting behaviors, breastfeeding attrition). In nursing literature, concepts have been categorized in several ways. For example, they have been described as concrete or abstract, variable or nonvariable (Hardy, 1973), and as operationally or theoretically defined.

Abstract Versus Concrete Concepts

Concepts may be viewed on a continuum from concrete (specific) to abstract (general). At one end of the continuum are concrete concepts, which have simple, directly observable empirical referents that can be seen, felt, or heard (e.g., a chair, the color red, jazz music). Concrete concepts are limited by time and space and are observable in reality.

At the other end of the continuum are abstract concepts (e.g., art, social support, personality, role). These are not clearly observable directly or indirectly and must be defined in terms of observable concepts (Jacox, 1974). Abstract concepts are independent of time and space. The more abstract a concept is, the more it transcends time and geography (Meleis, 2012).

Some concepts are formed from direct experiences with reality, whereas others are formed from indirect experiences. Relatively concrete or "empirical" concepts are formed from direct observations of objects, properties, or events. Concepts describing objects (e.g., desk or dog) or properties (e.g., cold, hard) are more empirical because the object or property that represents the idea (the empirical indicator) can be directly observed. Slightly more abstract properties, such as height, weight, and gender, can also be observed or measured.

As concepts become more abstract, their empirical indicators become less concrete and less directly measurable, and assessment of abstract concepts increasingly depends on indirect measures. For example, cardiovascular fitness, social support, and self-esteem are not directly observable properties or objects. To study these and similar concepts, their empirical referents must be defined and means must be identified or developed to measure them.

Variable (Continuous) Versus Nonvariable (Discrete) Concepts

Concepts may be categorized as variable or nonvariable (Hardy, 1973). Concepts that describe phenomena according to some dimensions of the phenomena are termed *variables.* A discrete (noninterval level) concept identifies categories or classes of characteristics. Discrete concepts include gender, ethnic background, religion, and marital status. Discrete variables can be single variable categories that may be answered as "yes" or "no" (e.g., either one is pregnant or not pregnant; one is a nurse or is not a nurse) or fits into a predefined category (e.g., religion, marital status, educational attainment).

Continuous (variable) concepts permit classification of dimension or graduation of phenomena on a continuum (e.g., blood pressure, pain) (Hardin & Bishop, 2010). Variable concepts include quality of life, health-promoting behaviors, and cultural identity. An examination of recent nursing research led to numerous examples of continuous or variable concepts that were being studied. These included the concepts of hope, quality of life, resilience, and grief. In each case, the concept was defined operationally and measured by tools, scales, or some other indicator to show where the respondent's level of the variable fell relative to others or relative to a predefined norm.

Theoretically Versus Operationally Defined Concepts

Concepts may be theoretically or operationally defined. A theoretical definition gives meaning to a term in context of a theory and permits any reader to assess the validity of the definition. The operational definition tells how the concept is linked to concrete situations and describes a set of procedures that will be performed to assign a value for the concept. Operational definitions permit the concept to be measured and allow hypotheses to be tested. Thus, operational definitions form the bridge between the theory and the empirical world (Hardy, 1973). Examples of theoretically and operationally defined concepts are shown in Table 3-2.

Sources of Concepts

When beginning a review of concepts found in nursing practice, research, education, and administration, one may look to several places or sources for relevant concepts. Indeed, the source of nursing concepts may be from the natural world, from research, or derived from other disciplines.

Table 3-2 Examples of Theoretically and Operationally Defined Concepts

Concept	Theoretical Definition	Operational Definition	Source
Health risk behaviors	Unhealthy lifestyle choices, such as smoking cigarettes, drug abuse, alcohol abuse, exposure to violence, and unhealthy dietary behaviors	Score on the Youth Risk Behaviors surveillance questionnaire	Dowdell, E. B. (2012). Urban seventh grade students: A report of health risk behaviors and exposure to violence. *Journal of School Nursing, 28*(2), 130–137.
Health-related quality of life	"value given to the duration of life as altered by one's functioning ability and disability, perceptions and social opportunities as a result of body changes, illness, injury, treatment or policy" (p. E63).	Scores on the SF-12 Health Survey summary scales—physical (HRQoL-physical) and mental (HRQoL-mental)	Emmanuel, E., St. John, W., & Sun, J. (2012). Social support and quality of life in the perinatal period. *Journal of Obstetric, Gynecologic and Neonatal Nursing, 41*(6), E62–E70.
Spiritual care	Frequency of assessment and interventions related to spiritual practice and barriers to providing spiritual care	Score on the Spiritual Care Practice Questionnaire	Ronaldson, S., Hayes, L., Aggar, C., Green, J., & Carey, M. (2012). Spirituality and spiritual caring: Nurses' perspectives and practice in palliative and acute care environments. *Journal of Clinical Nursing, 21*(19), 2126–2135.

Naturalistic concepts are concepts seen in nature or in nursing practice such as body weight, thermoregulation, hematologic complications, depression, pain, and spirituality. These may be on a continuum from concrete to abstract, and some may be measurable in fact (e.g., body weight and temperature) and others (e.g., pain or spirituality) measurable only indirectly and only in principle.

Research-based concepts are the result of conceptual development that is grounded in research processes. The theorist/researcher studies the realm of interest and identifies themes. Through qualitative, phenomenologic, or grounded theory approaches, the researcher may uncover meanings of the phenomena of interest and their theoretical relationships (Parse, 1999; Rodgers, 2000). Examples include help-seeking behavior (Cornally & McCarthy, 2011), care transitions (Geary & Schumacher, 2012), compassion fatigue (Jenkins & Warren, 2012), and shared presence (Kanacki, Roth, & Georges, 2012).

Existing concepts are the final type of concept. The nursing literature is filled with adapted concepts, more or less well synthesized through derivation from other disciplines. Such concepts include human needs from Maslow's (1954) hierarchy of needs and stress from Selye's (1956) physiologic theory of the stress of life. Theories of bodily function come from the study of physiology (Guyton & Hall, 1996). Borrowed concepts from medicine are clearly seen in clinical practice, especially in critical care areas of institutions. Other existing concepts commonly used in nursing research, administration, and practice are empathy, suffering, abuse, hope, and burnout. Table 3-3 summarizes the three sources of concepts for nursing.

Concept Analysis/Concept Development

Concept analysis, concept development, concept synthesis, and other terms refer to the rigorous process of bringing clarity to the definition of the concepts used in

Table 3-3 Sources of Concepts

Concept	Source	Characteristics	Examples From Nursing Literature
Naturalistic concepts	Present in nursing practice	May be defined and developed for use in research and theory development Often have medical implications as well as nursing use	Body weight, pain, thermoregulation, depression, hematologic complications, circadian dysregulation
Research-based concepts	Developed through qualitative research processes (e.g., grounded theory or existential phenomenology)	Often relate to a nursing specialty	Hope, grief, cultural competence, chronic pain
Existing concepts	Borrowed from other disciplines	Developed for nursing practice but are useful in research and theory	Job satisfaction, quality of life, abuse, adaptation, stress

Sources: Cowles & Rogers (1993); Parse (1999); Verhulst & Schwartz-Barcott (1993); Wang (2000).

science. Concept analysis and concept development are the terms used most commonly in nursing and are generally applied to the process of inquiry that examines concepts for their level of development as revealed by their internal structure, use, representativeness, and relationship to other concepts. Thus, concept analysis/concept development explores the meaning of concepts to promote understanding.

Purposes of Concept Development

Clarifying, recognizing, and defining concepts that describe phenomena is the purpose of concept development or concept analysis. These processes serve as the basis for development of conceptual frameworks, theories, and research studies.

Because a considerable portion of the conceptual basis of nursing theory, research, and practice has been constructed using concepts adopted from other disciplines, reexamination of these concepts for relevance and fit is important. The process of applying "borrowed" or "shared" concepts may have altered their meaning, and it is important to review them for appropriateness of application (Hupcey, Morse, Lenz, & Tason, 1996). Also, as knowledge is continually developing, new concepts are being introduced and accepted, and concepts are continually being investigated and refined. Furthermore, some concepts are poorly defined with characteristics that have not been described, whereas other concepts that have been defined may present with inconsistency between the definition and its use in research (Morse, Hupcey, Mitcham, & Lenz, 1996).

In summary, concept analysis can be used to evaluate the level of maturity or development of nursing concepts by:

- Identifying gaps in nursing knowledge
- Determining the need to refine or clarify a concept when it appears to have multiple meanings
- Evaluating the adequacy of competing concepts in their relation to other phenomena
- Examining the congruence between the definition of the concept and the way it has been operationalized
- Determining the fit between the definition of the concept and its clinical application (Morse et al., 1996)

Link to Practice 3-1 gives examples of a number of different concepts that have been suggested for development by graduate nursing students. Some of the examples (e.g., "first time parentitis in the ED" and "normal birth experience reconciliation") were derived from clinical practice and others (e.g., chemo brain and hoarding) were derived from non-nursing sources. A few (e.g., chemo brain, wholeness, and successful aging) may have already been presented in the nursing literature and even been a component of nursing research, but most have not.

Context for Concept Development

In the course of nursing practice, multiple instances of a problem will be seen as shown in the opening case study. When talking among peers, nurses may clarify a problem so that colleagues can understand the situation. Eventually, the nurse will develop a term, a word, or a phrase as a name for the problem. Thus begins the most elemental method for identifying a theoretical phenomenon—concept naming.

In refining the phenomenon so that the phenomenon can be studied, the steps of the concept development process are instituted. In this process, instances of the

Link to Practice 3-1

Student-Generated Examples of Concepts of Interest to Nurses

Like Rebecca, the ONS in the opening case study, nurses routinely encounter ideas, concepts, and phenomena in practice. Here are some concepts suggested by graduate students in the past that might be amenable to concept analysis or concept development and ultimately to theory development and research.

Concepts from the literature and other disciplines:

- Chemo brain
- Chronic fatigue
- Denial
- Forgiveness
- Functional status
- Healing
- Hoarding
- Inner strength
- Postdeployment reassimilation
- Second victim
- Successful aging
- Thermoregulation
- Waiting
- Wholeness
- Genetic health promotion

Phenomena from observation in clinical settings:

- First-time parentitis in the ED
- Males are nurturing caregivers
- Normal birth experience reconciliation
- Palliative care in the NICU
- Rally at the end-of-life

phenomenon are collected, the similarities and differences between the concept being studied and other concepts are reviewed, and those that are material to the use of the concept are extracted and the concept is defined from its existence in nature. Isolating specific information from all the surrounding information (the context) is important, but nurses must see the concept emerging and take note of the context in which the concept occurs.

In the case study at the beginning of the chapter, the nurses recognized the problem of women with breast cancer and their periodic sadness and noted the context in which the phenomenon occurred. It was important to focus on those situations that are relevant. Questions that might be asked to assess the context include: Did the women have unsupportive husbands? Were their lives threatened by nodal involvement and metastasis? What were the previous experiences of the women with disease or injury? What is the history of cancer in the women's families?

Concept Development and Conceptual Frameworks

Once concepts have been identified, named, and developed, the nurse can test them in descriptive studies, particularly qualitative studies to further develop the concept and make explicit its use in real situations. The concept can be analyzed for its relation to many facets of the nursing discipline and the meaning made explicit for the nurse's use in daily work or scholarly endeavors.

Conceptual frameworks are structures that relate concepts together in a meaningful way. Although relationships are posited in conceptual frameworks, frequently neither the direction nor the strength of the relationships is made explicit for use in practice or for testing in a research project. Chapter 4 provides a detailed discussion of the processes used in the development of theories and conceptual frameworks.

Concept Development and Research

A common language is necessary for communicating the meanings of concepts that comprise theories. Theory, research, and practice are linked, and most scholars recognize that they cannot be separated. Researchers relate concepts together into structures that are called models and theories and derive from them testable relationships called hypotheses (Kerlinger, 1986).

Hickman (2011) points out that nursing research, theory, and practice form a cycle and that entry into this cycle may be at any point. Research both precedes theory and is guided by theory. Both theory and research direct practice, and conversely, research and theory are derived from practice situations. Thus, theory, while guiding research, is simultaneously being tested in the research process. The conceptual elements of the theory that guide the research or are being tested by the research are named and defined during concept analysis.

Difficulties with studying a problem in nursing may be related to the exactness with which the terms in use are developed and defined. Poorly defined concepts may lead to faulty construction of research instruments and methods (Morse, 1995). Frequently, a nursing problem does not lend itself precisely to existing terminology. In this situation, the nurse should engage in the effort of concept development. Furthermore, if one cannot successfully define the problem so that other professionals can understand it, concept development is necessary.

Strategies for Concept Analysis and Concept Development

There are multiple methods of constructing meaning for concepts. This can be accomplished through review of research literature, scholarly critique, and thoughtful definition. When a formal or detailed meaning is warranted, however, a more structured method for concept development will need to be used.

In the early 1960s, John Wilson (1963), a social scientist, developed a process for defining concepts to improve communication and comprehension of the meanings of terms in scientific use. Wilson used 11 steps, or techniques, to guide the concept analysis process. A few recent examples, which used Wilson's method of concept development, were discovered in the nursing literature. Buettner-Schmidt and Lobo (2011) used Wilson's method to review the concept of social justice, and Saiki and Lobo (2011) used Wilson's method to review the concept of disclosure. In a third example, Matutina (2010) used Wilson's method to examine the concept of therapeutic misconception.

Building on the process presented by Wilson, nurses have published several techniques, methods, and strategies for concept development. Strategies devised by several nurse scholars will be presented briefly in the following sections, and examples of published works using these methods will be provided where available.

Walker and Avant

Walker and Avant first explicated the process of concept analysis for nurses in 1986. Their procedures were based on Wilson's method and clarified his methods so that graduate students could apply them to examine phenomena of interest to nurses. Three different processes were described by Walker and Avant (2011): concept analysis, concept synthesis, and concept derivation.

Concept Analysis

Concept analysis is an approach espoused by Walker and Avant (2011) to clarify the meanings of terms and to define terms (concepts) so that writers and readers share a common language. Concept analysis should be conducted when concepts require clarification or further development to define them for a nurse scholar's purposes, whether that is research, theory development, or practice. This method for concept analysis requires an eight-step approach, as listed in Box 3-1.

Concept Synthesis

Concept synthesis is used when concepts require development based on observation or other forms of evidence. The individual must develop a way to group or order the information about the phenomenon from his or her own viewpoint or theoretical requirement. Methods of synthesizing concepts follow:

1. Qualitative synthesis—relies on sensory data and looking for similarities, differences, and patterns among the data to identify the new concept
2. Quantitative synthesis—requires numerical data to delineate those attributes that belong to the concept and those that do not
3. Literary synthesis—involves reviewing a wide range of the literature to acquire new insights about the concept or to find new concepts
4. Mixed methods—use of any of the three methods described together, either sequentially or combined (Walker & Avant, 2011)

Box 3-1 Steps in Concept Analysis

1. Select a concept.
2. Determine the aims or purposes of analysis.
3. Identify all the uses of the concept possible.
4. Determine the defining attributes.
5. Identify model case.
6. Identify borderline, related, contrary, invented, and illegitimate cases.
7. Identify antecedents and consequences.
8. Define empirical referents.

Source: Walker & Avant (2011, p. 160).

Box 3-2 Steps in Concept Derivation

1. Become thoroughly familiar with the existing literature related to the topic of interest.
2. Search other fields for new ways of looking at the topic of interest.
3. Select a parent concept or set of concepts from another field to use in the derivation process.
4. Redefine the concept(s) from the parent field in terms of the topic of interest.

Source: Walker & Avant (2011, p. 76).

Concept Derivation

Concept derivation from Walker and Avant's (2011) perspective is often necessary when there are few concepts currently available to a nurse that explain a problem area. It is applicable when a comparison or analogy can be made between one field or area that is conceptually defined and another that is not. Concept derivation can be helpful in generating new ways of thinking about a phenomenon of interest. A four-step plan for the work of moving likely concepts from disciplines outside nursing into the nursing lexicon has been developed (Box 3-2).

Examples of Concept Analysis Using Walker and Avant's Techniques

Walker and Avant's techniques have been taught for three decades in graduate nursing programs, and their method of concept analysis is the most commonly used in nursing. Table 3-4 lists several examples from recent nursing literature. In their most recent edition, Walker and Avant (2011) outline the processes for each of the methods described in depth and provide a number of examples for clarification. The reader is referred to their work, as well as to the examples listed, for more information.

Rodgers

Rodgers first published her evolutionary method for concept analysis in 1989. According to Rodgers (2000), concept analysis is necessary because concepts are dynamic, "fuzzy," and context dependent and possess some pragmatic utility or purpose. Furthermore, because phenomena, needs, and goals change, concepts must be continually refined and variations introduced to achieve a clearer and more useful meaning.

Rodgers (2000) examined two viewpoints or schools of thought regarding concept development and showed that the methods of each differ significantly. She termed these methods "essentialism" and "evolutionary" viewpoints. In her work, she contrasted the essentialist method of concept development as exemplified by Wilson (1963) and Walker and Avant (1995) with concept development using the evolutionary method.

The evolutionary method of concept development is a concurrent task approach. In it, the tasks may be going on all at the same time, rather than a sequence of specific steps that are completed before going to the next step. The activities involved in the evolutionary method are listed in Box 3-3.

Rodgers (2000) defined many terms and explained the process of concept analysis using the evolutionary view. The goal of the concept analysis will, to an extent, determine how the researcher *identifies the concept of interest* and terms

Table 3-4 Examples of Concept Analyses Using Walker and Avant's Methods

Concept	Reference
Compassion fatigue	Jenkins, B., & Warrant, N. A. (2012). Concept analysis: Compassion fatigue and effects upon critical care nurses. *Critical Care Nursing Quarterly, 35*(4), 388–395.
Compliance	Ingram, T. L. (2009). Compliance: A concept analysis. *Nursing Forum, 44*(3), 189–194.
Confidence/ self-confidence	Perry, P. (2011). Concept analysis: Confidence/self-confidence. *Nursing Forum, 46*(4), 218–230.
Managerial coaching	Batson, V. D., & Yoder, L. H. (2012). Managerial coaching: A concept analysis. *Journal of Advanced Nursing, 67*(8), 1658–1669.
Migration	Freeman, M., Baumann, A., Blythe, J., Fisher, A., & Akhtar-Danesh, N. (2011). Migration: A concept analysis from a nursing perspective. *Journal of Advanced Nursing, 68*(5), 1176–1186.
Nursing care	DalPezzo, N. K. (2009). Nursing care: A concept analysis. *Nursing Forum, 44*(4), 256–264.
Shame	McFall, L., & Johnson, V. A. (2009). Shame: A concept analysis. *Journal of Testing and Theory Construction, 13*(2), 57–62.
Suicidal behavior	Sun, F. K. (2011). A concept analysis of suicidal behavior. *Public Health Nursing, 28*(5), 458–468.
Tolerance	Moore, H. K., & Walker, C. A. (2011). Tolerance: A concept analysis. *The Journal of Theory Construction & Testing, 15*(2), 48–52.

and expressions selected. The incorporation of a new term into a nurse's way of viewing a client situation is often a circumstance warranting analysis of a new concept.

The goal of the analysis will also influence *selection of the setting and sample* for data collection. For instance, the setting may be a library and the sample might be literature. The sampling might be time-oriented, say literature from the previous 5 years. In any case, the researcher's goal is to develop a rigorous design consistent with the purpose of the analysis. The selection of literature from related disciplines might include those that typically use the concept. An exhaustive review includes all

Box 3-3 Steps in Rodgers' Process of Concept Analysis

1. Identify the concept and associated terms.
2. Select an appropriate realm (a setting or a sample) for data collection.
3. Collect data to identify the attributes of the concept and the contextual basis of the concept (i.e., interdisciplinary, sociocultural, and temporal variations).
4. Analyze the data regarding the characteristics of the concept.
5. Identify an exemplar of the concept, if appropriate.
6. Identify hypotheses and implications for further development.

Source: Rodgers (2000, p. 85).

the indexed literature using the concept and may be limited by a time frame such as several years.

A randomization process is then used to select the sample across each discipline over time. In *collecting and managing the data,* a discovery approach is preferred. The focus of the data analysis is on identifying the attributes, antecedents, and consequences and related concepts or surrogate terms. The attributes located by this means constitute a "real definition as opposed to a nominal or dictionary definition" (Rodgers, 2000, p. 91).

Rodgers defines *surrogate terms* as ways of expressing the concept other than by the term of interest. She distinguishes between surrogate terms and *related concepts* by showing that surrogate terms are different words that express the concept, whereas "related concepts are part of a network that provide a background" and "lend significance to the concept of interest" (Rodgers, 2000, p. 92).

Analyzing the data can go on simultaneously with its collection according to Rodgers (2000), or it can be delayed until all the data are collected. The latter is allowed in concept analysis using the evolutionary process because data are currently available, rather than being constantly created by the subjects as in qualitative research study. The researcher must beware of considering the data "saturated," that is, redundant, too early.

Identifying an exemplar from the literature, field observation, or interview is important and will provide a clear example of the concept. Examples of actual cases are preferred over constructed cases (in contrast to Wilson's [1963] method). The goal is to illustrate the characteristics of the concept in relevant contexts to enhance the clarity and effective application of the concept.

Interpreting the results involves gaining insight on the current status of the concept and generating implications for inquiry based on this status and identified gaps. Interpreting the results may involve interdisciplinary comparison, temporal comparison, and assessment of the social context within which the concept analysis was conducted.

Identifying implications for further development and formal inquiry may be the result. The results of the analysis may direct further inquiry rather than giving the final answer on the meaning of the concept. The implications of this form of research-based concept analysis may yield questions for further research, or hypotheses may be extracted from the findings. The major outcome of the evolutionary method of concept analysis is the generation of further questions for research rather than the static definition of the concept. Table 3-5 lists a number of references for concept analyses using this method. For more information, the reader is referred to Rodgers (2000).

Schwartz-Barcott and Kim

A hybrid model of concept development was initially presented by Schwartz-Barcott and Kim in 1986 and expanded and revised in 1993 and 2000. This method for concept development involves a three-phase process, which is summarized in Table 3-6.

Theoretical Phase

In the theoretical phase, a borrowed concept, an underdeveloped nursing concept, or a concept from clinical practice may be selected. The main consideration is that the concept has relevance for nursing. A clinical encounter may be described in detail to arrive at the concept through analysis. *The literature is searched* broadly and systematically across disciplines that may use the concept. A set of questions that provides

Cancer Survivorship – Doyle, N. (2008) Cancer Survivorship. Evolutionary concept analysis. Journal of Advanced Nursing 62(4) -498-509

Table 3-5 Examples of Concept Analyses Using Rodgers' Methods

Concept	Reference
Chronic fatigue	Jorgenson, R. (2008). Chronic fatigue: An evolutionary concept analysis. *Journal of Advanced Nursing, 63*(2), 199–207.
Community health	Baisch, M. J. (2009). Community health: An evolutionary concept analysis. *Journal of Advanced Nursing, 65*(11), 2464–2476.
Death anxiety	Lehto, R. H., & Stein, K. F. (2009). Death anxiety: An analysis of an evolving concept. *Research and Theory for Nursing Practice: An International Journal, 23*(1), 23–33.
Interdisciplinary collaboration	Petri, L. (2010). Concept analysis of interdisciplinary collaboration. *Nursing Forum, 45*(2), 73–82.
Knowing in nursing	Bonis, S. A. (2009). Knowing in nursing: A concept analysis. *Journal of Advanced Nursing, 65*(6), 1328–1341.
Moral distress	Russell, A. C. (2012). Moral distress in neuroscience nursing: An evolutionary concept analysis. *Journal of Neuroscience Nursing, 44*(1), 15–26.
Nurse–physician communication	Cypress, B. S. (2011). Exploring the concept of nurse-physician communication within the context of health care outcomes using the evolutionary method of concept analysis. *Dimensions of Critical Care Nursing, 30*(1), 28–38.
School violence	Jones, S. N., Waite, R., & Thomas-Clements, P. (2012). An evolutionary concept analysis of school violence: From bullying to death. *Journal of Forensic Nursing, 8*(1), 4–12.
awareness	Eckroth-Bucher, M. (2010). Self-awareness: A review and analysis of a basic nursing concept. *Advances in Nursing Science, 33*(4), 297–309.

Cancer Survivorship Doyle N (2008) Cancer survivorship evolutionary concept analysis

inquiry into the essential nature of the concept, the means of clear definition, and ways to enhance its measurability focuses on questions of measurement and definition. *Meaning and measurement* are dealt with. This requires thought for comparing and contrasting the data. *A working definition* is chosen to be used in the final phase. The definition should maintain a nursing perspective.

Table 3-6 Phases of Schwartz-Barcott and Kim's Hybrid Model of Concept Development

Phase	Activities
Theoretical phase	Select a concept. Review the literature. Determine meaning and measurement. Choose a working definition.
Fieldwork phase	Set the stage. Negotiate entry into a setting. Select cases. Collect and analyze data.
Final analytical phase	Weigh findings. Write report.

Source: Schwartz-Barcott & Kim (2000).

Fieldwork Phase

In the *fieldwork* phase, the concept is corroborated and refined. The fieldwork phase integrates with the literature phase and expands into a modified qualitative research approach (e.g., participant observation). The steps of this phase are setting the stage, negotiating entry, selecting cases, and collecting and analyzing the data.

Analytical Phase

The final analytical phase includes examination of the details in the light of the literature review. The researcher reviews the findings with the original purpose in view. Three questions guide the final analysis:

1. How much is the concept applicable and important to nursing?
2. Does the initial selection of the concept seem justified?
3. To what extent do the review of literature, theoretical analysis, and empirical findings support the presence and frequency of the concept within the population selected for empirical study? (Schwartz-Barcott & Kim, 2000, p. 147)

The final step of the process is to *write up the findings*. The work may be reported as either fieldwork or as a concept analysis. Elements the researcher must consider when writing the findings are length of the study, the intended audience, timing, pacing of the authorship process, anticipated length of the manuscript, how much detail of the process to include, and ethics of the interpretation of the analysis (Schwartz-Barcott & Kim, 2000).

Several results can be realized by this type of analysis:

1. The current meaning of the concept can be supported or refined.
2. A different definition than previously used may stand out.
3. The concept may be completely redefined.
4. A new or refined way of measuring the concept may be the result (Schwartz-Barcott & Kim, 1993).

Examples of published reports using this model are listed in Table 3-7.

Meleis

Meleis (2012) described three strategies to develop conceptual meaning for use in nursing theory, research, and practice. These are concept exploration, concept clarification, and concept analysis.

Concept Exploration

Concept exploration is used when concepts are new and ambiguous in a discipline, when concepts are camouflaged by being embedded in the daily nursing discussion, or when a concept from another discipline is being redesigned for use in nursing. Concept exploration may awaken nurses to a new concept or revitalize the meanings of an overused concept to make it explicit for practice, research, and theory building. The steps Meleis (2012) suggests for this endeavor follow:

1. Identifying the major components and dimensions of the concept
2. Raising appropriate questions about the concept
3. Proposing triggers for continuing the exploration
4. Identifying and defining the advantages to the discipline of continuing the exploration of this concept (p. 373)

Table 3-7 Examples of Concept Analyses Using Schwartz-Barcott and Kim's Hybrid Method

Concept	Reference
Being sensitive	Sayers, K. L., & de Vries, K. (2008). A concept development of "being sensitive" in nursing. *Nursing Ethics, 15*(3), 289–303.
Pain identification in demented patients	Chang, S. O., Oh, Y., Park, E. Y., Kim, G. M., & Ki, K. Y. (2011). Concept analysis of nurses' identification of pain in demented patients in a nursing home: Development of a hybrid model. *Pain Management Nursing, 12*(2), 61–69.
Service awareness	Crist, J. D., Michaels, C., Gelfand, D. E., & Phillips, L. R. (2007). Defining and measuring service awareness among elders and caregivers of Mexican descent. *Research and Theory for Nursing Practice: An International Journal, 21*(2), 119–129.
Situation awareness	Sitterding, M. C., Broome, M. E., Everett, L. Q., & Ebright, P. (2012). Understanding situation awareness in nursing work: A hybrid concept analysis. *Advances in Nursing Science, 35*(1), 77–92.
Transition to motherhood	Shin, H., & White-Traut, R. (2007). The conceptual structure of transition to motherhood in the neonatal intensive care unit. *Journal of Advanced Nursing, 58*(1), 90–98.

Concept Clarification

Concept clarification is used to "refine concepts that have been used in nursing without a clear, shared, and conscious agreement on the properties of meanings attributed to them" (Meleis, 2012, p. 374). Concept clarification is a way to refine existing concepts when they lack clarity for a specific nursing endeavor. The processes involved in concept clarification allow for reduction of ambiguities while critically reviewing the properties. The processes are presented in Box 3-4.

Concept Analysis

Concept analysis, according to Meleis (2012), assumes that the concept has been introduced into nursing literature but is ready to move to the level of development for research. This process implies that the concept will be broken down to its essentials and then reconstructed for its contribution to the nursing lexicon. The goal of

Box 3-4 Process of Concept Clarification

1. Clarify the boundaries of the concept, including what attributes should be included and what should be excluded.
2. Critically review the properties of the concept.
3. Bring to light new dimensions that had not been considered.
4. Compare, contrast, delineate, and differentiate these properties and provide exemplars of the concept.
5. Identify assumptions and philosophical bases about the events that trigger the phenomena and propose questions from a nursing perspective.

Source: Meleis (2012, p. 374).

Table 3-8 Meleis' Processes for Concept Development

Process	Task or Activity
Defining	Creating theoretical and operational definitions that clarify ambiguities, enhance precision, and relate concepts to empirical referents
Differentiating	Sorting in and out similarities and differences between the concept being developed and other like concepts
Delineating antecedents	Defining the contextual conditions under which the concept is perceived and expected to occur
Delineating consequences	Defining events, situations, or conditions that may result from the concept
Modeling	Defining and identifying exemplars (i.e., clinical referents or research referents) to illustrate some aspect of the concept. Models may be same or like models, or contrary models
Analogizing	Describing the concept through another concept or phenomenon that is similar and has been studied more extensively
Synthesizing	Bringing together findings, meanings, and properties that have been discovered and describing future steps in theorizing

Source: Meleis (2012, pp. 384–386).

the analysis is to bring the concept close to use in research or clinical practice and to ultimately contribute to instrument development and theory testing.

Meleis (2012) focused on an integrated approach to concept development, which includes defining, differentiating, delineating antecedents and consequences, modeling, analogizing, and synthesizing. Table 3-8 lists each of these components and presents related activities or tasks to be accomplished for each phase. A few examples using Meleis' strategies were located in the literature. For example, Olsen & Harder (2010) combined Meleis' strategies with Schwartz-Barcott and Kim's to describe "network-focused nursing." Clark and Robinson (2000) used Meleis' earlier work to describe the concept of multiculturalism, and Felten and Hall (2001) used Meleis' strategies to describe the concept of resilience in elderly women.

Morse

In response to concerns that some concepts in the nursing lexicon had been derived and not developed adequately for nursing, or had become overused by those who did not clarify them, Morse (1995) developed a method of concept development to enhance clarity and distinctiveness of nursing concepts. In this method, she used the term "advanced techniques of concept analysis" and described the processes of concept delineation, concept comparison, and concept clarification.

Concept Delineation

Concept delineation is a strategy that requires an extensive literature search and assists in separating two terms that seem closely linked. The concepts are then compared and contrasted to identify commonalities, similarities, and differences such that distinctions may be drawn between the terms (Morse, 1995).

Concept Comparison

Concept comparison clarifies competing concepts, again using an extensive literature review and keeping the literature for each concept separate. Three phases are used in the comparison:

1. Preconditions—the status of the concept in nursing and its use in teaching or clinical practice
2. Process—the type of nursing response to the concept, at what level of consciousness it occurs, and, if it is identified with the client, at what level
3. Outcomes—whether the concept was used to identify process or product, its accuracy in prediction, the client's condition, and the client's experience with the concept (Morse, 1995, pp. 39–41).

Concept Clarification

For Morse (1995), *concept clarification* is used with concepts that are "mature" and have a large body of literature identifying and using them. The concept clarification process requires a "literature review to identify the underlying values and to identify, describe and compare and contrast the attributes of each" (p. 41).

Published reports using Morse's methods for concept development can be found in the nursing literature. For example, Weaver, Morse, and Mitcham (2008) used Morse's process to analyze the concept of ethical sensitivity, and Olson and Morse (2005) used it to delineate the concept of fatigue. In other works, Whitehead (2004) used Morse's method to analyze health promotion and health education; Fasnacht (2003) used Morse's methods to "refine" the concept of creativity; and McCormack and colleagues (2002) used it to analyze "context."

Penrod and Hupcey

Penrod and Hupcey (2005) built on Morse's method and termed their method "principle-based concept analysis." Explaining their intent to "determine and evaluate the state of the science surrounding the concept" (p. 405) and "produce evidence that reveals scholars' best estimate of 'probable truth' in the scientific literature" (p. 406), they outlined four principles for their method: epistemologic, pragmatic, linguistic, and logical (Box 3-5).

Penrod and Hupcey (2005) explain that in their method of concept analysis, the findings "are summarized as a theoretical definition that integrates an evaluative summary of each of the criteria posed by the four over-arching principles." To do this, the researcher must consider three issues: (1) selection of appropriate disciplinary literature for review, (2) assurance of the adequacy and appropriateness of the sample derived from the literature, and (3) employment of "within- and across-discipline analytic techniques." They have elucidated that this advanced level of concept development seems to be more relevant to the research endeavor, as it is a research-based concept analysis.

Despite being developed relatively recently, examples of published works using Penrod and Hupcey's (2005) method for concept analysis can be found. For example, Bell, Lucas, and White-Traut (2008) used the principle-based method to clarify the term "neonatal neurobehavioral organization," Steis, Penrod, Adkins, and Hupcey (2009) examined the concept of recognition within the context of nurse–patient interactions, and Griffith, Hall, and Fields (2011) used the process to describe "crying that heals." Lastly, Mikkelsen and Frederiksen (2011) analyzed the concept of "family-centered care" using the Penrod and Hupcey method.

Box 3-5 Four Principles of Concept Analysis

Epistemologic principle is based on the question "Is the concept clearly defined and well differentiated from other concepts?" (p. 405).

Pragmatic principle, in which the question to be answered is "Is the concept applicable and useful within the scientific realm or inquiry? Has it been operationalized?" In this principle, they believe that an operationalized concept has achieved a level of maturity (p. 405).

Linguistic principle asks "Is the concept used consistently and appropriately within context?" (p. 406). Similarly to Morse and to Rodgers, they find that context or lack of context is a factor important in this type of analysis (p. 406).

Logical principle applies the question "Does the concept hold its boundaries through theoretical integration with other concepts?" (p. 406). The authors require that the concept not be blurred with respect to other concepts but that it remains logically clear and distinct.

Source: Penrod & Hupcey (2005, pp. 405–406).

Comparison of Models for Concept Development

The nursing literature contains several comparisons and critiques of the various models and methods for concept development/concept analysis. Indeed, Hupcey and colleagues (1996) and Morse and colleagues (1996) provided a detailed and well-researched comparison of the techniques presented by Walker and Avant (1986), Schwartz-Barcott and Kim (1993), and Rodgers (1989). Strengths and weaknesses of each method were described in their papers. More recently, Duncan and colleagues (2007) and Weaver and Mitcham (2008) reviewed the history of concept analysis comparing the major methods in common use. Finally, Risjord (2009) reexamined the philosophical basis and intent of concept analysis and concluded that rather than *preceding* theory development, it must be a *part of* theory development. Table 3-9 compares the various formats for concept development/concept analysis described earlier.

Summary

Rebecca Wallis, one of the nurses from the opening case study, identified what she thought was a new phenomenon that was pertinent to her practice of oncology nursing and decided to develop the concept more fully. By applying techniques of concept analysis to the PMG reaction, she began the process of formulating information on this concept that could ultimately be used by other nurses in practice or research.

The process of developing concepts includes reviewing the nurse's area of interest, examining the phenomena closely, pondering the terms that are relevant and that fit together with reality, and operationalizing the concept for practice, research, or educational use. Whether advanced practice nurses or nursing scholars elect to use the methods proposed by Wilson (1963), Walker and Avant (2011), Morse (1995), Rodgers (2000), Schwartz-Barcott and Kim (2000), Meleis (2012), Penrod and Hupcey (2005), or a combination, it is clear that the process of developing, clarifying, comparing and contrasting, and integrating well-derived and defined concepts is necessary for theory development and to guide research studies. This will, in turn, ultimately benefit practice. Chapter 4 builds on the process of concept development by describing the processes used to link concepts to form relationship statements and to construct conceptual models, frameworks, and theories.

Table 3-9 Comparison of Selected Methods of Concept Development

Author(s)	Method	Purpose	No. of Steps	Constructed Cases	Other Factors/Steps
Walker & Avant	Concept analysis	Clarify meaning of terms	8	Model, borderline, related, contrary	Identify empirical referents and defining attributes; delineate antecedents and consequences
Rodgers	Evolutionary concept analysis	Refine and clarify concepts for use in research and practice	5	Model only (identified—not constructed)	Identify appropriate realm (setting and sample); analyze data about characteristics, conduct interdisciplinary or temporal comparisons; identify hypotheses and implications for further study
Schwartz-Barcott & Kim	Hybrid model of concept development	Support or refine the meaning of a concept and/or develop a new or refined way to measure a concept	3 phases	Model case, contrary case	Develop working definitions, search literature, participant observation, collect and analyze data, write findings
Meleis	Concept development	Define concepts theoretically and operationally, clarify ambiguities, relate concepts to empirical referents	7	Same or like models; contrary models	Define concept, use an analogy to describe a similar concept, synthesize findings; differentiate similarities and differences between like concepts; delineate antecedents and consequences
Morse	Concept comparison	Clarifies the meaning of competing concepts	3 phases	Not specified	Uses extensive literature review to examine and describe preconditions (status of use of the concepts in teaching or practice), process, and outcomes of use of the concept
Penrod & Hupcey	Principle-based concept analysis	Concept analysis	4 phases based on principles	Not specified	Sampling within bodies of large multidisciplinary literature yields a theoretically based scientific definition

Key Points

- A concept is a symbolic statement that describes a phenomenon or a class of phenomena.
- There are many different ways to explain or classify concepts (e.g., abstract vs. concrete and variable vs. discrete).
- Concepts used in nursing practice, research, education, and administration can come from the natural world (e.g., biology and environment), from research, or from other disciplines.
- Concept analysis/concept development refers to the rigorous process of bringing clarity to the definition of the concepts used in nursing science.

- When theoretically and operationally defined, the concepts can be readily applied in nursing practice, research, education, and administration.
- Several methods for concept analysis/concept development have been described in the nursing literature.

CONCEPT ANALYSIS EXEMPLAR

The following is an outline delineating the steps of a concept analysis using Rodgers' (2000) evolutionary method.

Ballard, J. (2010). Forgetfulness and older adults: Concept analysis. *Journal of Advanced Nursing, 66*(6), 1409–1419.

1. *Identify the concept and associated terms.*

Concept: Forgetfulness
Associated terms: memory loss, dementia, memory test, age-acquired memory impairment

2. *Select an appropriate realm (setting) for data collection.*

The realm for the study was a search of the Cumulative Index to Nursing and Allied Health Literature (CINAHL), Excerpta Medica Database (EMBASE), and Internurse databases and included papers published in English between 1962 and 2009. Educational references and references related to health care staff were omitted.

3. *Identify the attributes of the concept and the contextual basis of the concept.*

Attributes of forgetfulness:
Increased episodes of prospective memory loss with delayed processing and response time in aging adults characterized by the following:
   a. Retrieval-induced forgetting
   b. Decline in prospective and working memory
   c. Delayed recall and processing time

4. *Specify the characteristics of the concept.*

Antecedents: Neurobiologic changes in aging (changes in the hippocampus, dementia, stroke), stress and tension, sensory input impairment, medication side effects, depression, delirium, vitamin B deficiency, and thyroid dysfunction

Consequences: Two themes were presented.
   a. Perception of social impact/emotions—fear, embarrassment, anger, and low self-esteem
   b. Coping mechanism—adherence to routines, reminders/lists, humor

5. *Identify an exemplar of the concept.*

Definition of forgetfulness—increased incidence of episodic prospective memory loss, slower processing time, and delayed recall associated with aging

Two case studies from practice were presented:

Forgetfulness with no deficits on testing—Case study of a 76-year-old woman with transient inability to recall information while visiting her son. Follow-up evaluation and cognitive assessment yielded normal results. The lapse in memory was attributed to fatigue and stress.

Forgetfulness with deficits on testing—Case study of a 72-year-old experiencing sudden withdrawal and depression. Initial examination revealed depression and significant impairment of short-term and procedural memory. A follow-up CT scan revealed a large, inoperable brain mass.

6. *Identify hypotheses and implications for development.*

For further study and application, the author suggested:

Research to investigate the benefits of nurse-led population screening for memory deficits in older adults.

Require nurse education in the assessment of memory and promotion of enhanced access to adequate referral pathways when abnormal results are uncovered.

Learning Activities

1. Collect and review several of the concept analyses mentioned in the chapter. How are they operationalized? Can they readily be used for research?
2. Review the different methods for concept development presented. How are the methods alike? How are they different? Which method appears to be the easiest to use?
3. Consider a phenomenon you have observed in your practice that might be appropriate for further development. Discuss the phenomenon with colleagues and try to name it and determine how you might develop it further.

REFERENCES

Bell, A. F., Lucas, R., & White-Traut, R. C. (2008). Concept clarification of neonatal neurobehavioral organization. *Journal of Advanced Nursing, 61*(5), 570–581.

Buettner-Schmidt, K., & Lobo, M. L. (2011). Social justice: A concept analysis. *Journal of Advanced Nursing, 68*(4), 948–958.

Chinn, P. L., & Kramer, M. K. (2011). *Theory and nursing: Integrated knowledge development* (8th ed.). St. Louis: Elsevier/Mosby.

Clark, C., & Robinson, T. (2000). Multiculturalism as a concept in nursing. *Journal of National Black Nurses' Association, 11*(2), 39–43.

Cornally, N., & McCarthy, G. (2011). Help-seeking behavior: A concept analysis. *International Journal of Nursing Practice, 17*(3), 280–288,

Cowles, K. V., & Rogers, B. L. (1993). The concept of grief: An evolutionary perspective. In B. L. Rogers & K. A. Knafl (Eds.), *Concept development in nursing: Foundations, techniques, and applications.* Philadelphia: Saunders.

Cutcliffe, J. R., & McKenna, H. P. (2005). *The essential concepts of nursing: Building blocks for practice.* New York: Elsevier.

Dubin, R. (1978). *Theory building.* New York: Free Press.

Duncan, C., Cloutier, J. D., & Bailey, P. H. (2007). Concept analysis: The importance of differentiating the ontological focus. *Journal of Advanced Nursing, 58*(3), 293–300.

Fasnacht, P. H. (2003). Creativity: A refinement of the concept for nursing practice. *Journal of Advanced Nursing, 41*(2), 195–202.

Fawcett, J. (1999). *The relationship of theory and research* (3rd ed.). Philadelphia: F. A. Davis.

Felten, B. S., & Hall, J. M. (2001). Conceptualizing resilience in women older than 85: Overcoming adversity from illness or loss. *Journal of Gerontological Nursing, 27*(11), 46–53.

Geary, C. R., & Schumacher, K. L. (2012). Care transitions: Integrating transition theory and complexity science concepts. *Advances in Nursing Science, 35*(3), 236–248.

Griffith, M. B., Hall, J. M., & Fields, B. (2011). Crying that heals: Concept evaluation. *Journal of Holistic Nursing, 29*(3), 167–179.

Guyton, A. C., & Hall, J. E. (1996). *Textbook of medical physiology* (9th ed.). Philadelphia: Saunders.

Hardin, S. R., & Bishop, S. M. (2010). Theory development process. In M. R. Alligood & A. M. Tomey (Eds.), *Nursing theorists and their work* (7th ed., pp. 36–49). St. Louis: Mosby.

Hardy, M. (1973). Theories: Components, development, evaluation. *Theoretical foundations for nursing.* New York: MSS Information Systems.

Hickman, J. S. (2011). An introduction to nursing theory. In J. George (Ed.), *Nursing theories: The base for professional nursing practice* (6th ed., pp. 1–22). Upper Saddle River, NJ: Pearson Education.

Hupcey, J. E., Morse, J. M., Lenz, E. R., & Tason, M. C. (1996). Wilsonian methods of concept analysis: A critique. *Scholarly Inquiry for Nursing Practice, 10*(3), 185–210.

Hupcey, J. E., & Penrod, J. (2008). Enhancing methodological clarity: Principle-based concept analysis. *Journal of Advanced Nursing, 50*(4), 403–409.

Jacox, A. K. (1974). Theory construction in nursing: An overview. *Nursing Research, 23*(1), 4–13.

Jenkins, B., & Warren, N. A. (2012). Concept analysis: Compassion fatigue and effects upon critical care nurses. *Critical Care Nursing Quarterly, 35*(4), 388–395.

Kanacki, L. S., Roth, P., & Georges, J. M. (2012). Shared presence: Caring for a dying spouse. *Journal of Hospice and Palliative Nursing, 14*(6), 414–425.

Kerlinger, F. N. (1986). *Foundations of behavioral research* (3rd ed.). New York: Holt, Rinehart & Winston.

Kim, H. S. (2010). *The nature of theoretical thinking in nursing* (3rd ed.). New York: Springer.

Maslow, A. H. (1954). *Motivation and personality.* New York: Harper.

Matutina, R. E. (2010). The concept analysis of therapeutic misconception. *Nurse Researcher, 17*(4), 83–93.

McCormack, B., Kitson, A., Harvey, G., Rycroft-Malone, J., Tichen, A., & Seers, K. (2002). Getting evidence into practice: The meaning of "context." *Journal of Advanced Nursing, 38*(1), 94–104.

Meleis, A. I. (2012). *Theoretical nursing: Development and progress* (4th ed.). Philadelphia: Lippincott Williams & Wilkins.

Mikkelsen, G., & Frederiksen, K. (2011). Family-centred care of children in hospital—A concept analysis. *Journal of Advanced Nursing, 67*(5), 1152–1162.

Morse, J. M. (1995). Exploring the theoretical basis of nursing using advanced techniques of concept analysis. *Advances in Nursing Science, 17*(3), 31–46.

Morse, J. M., Hupcey, J. E., Mitcham, C., & Lenz, E. R. (1996). Concept analysis in nursing research: A critical appraisal. *Scholarly Inquiry for Nursing Practice, 10*(3), 253–277.

Olsen, P. R., & Harder, I. (2010). Network-focused nursing development of a new concept. *Advances in Nursing Science, 33*(4), 272–284.

Olson, K., & Morse, J. M. (2005). Delineating the concept of fatigue using a pragmatic utility approach. In J. R. Cutcliffe & H. P. McKenna (Eds.), *The essential concepts of nursing.* New York: Elsevier.

Parse, R. R. (1999). *Hope: An international human becoming perspective.* Sudbury, MA: Jones & Bartlett and National League for Nursing.

Parse, R. R. (2006). Concept inventing: Continuing clarification. *Nursing Science Quarterly, 19*(4), 289.

Penrod, J., & Hupcey, J. E. (2005). Enhancing methodological clarity: Principle-based concept analysis. *Journal of Advanced Nursing, 50*(4), 403–409.

Risjord, M. (2009). Rethinking concept analysis. *Journal of Advanced Nursing, 65*(3), 684–691.

Rodgers, B. L. (1989). Concept analysis and the development of nursing knowledge: The evolutionary cycle. *Journal of Advanced Nursing, 14*(4), 330–335.

Rodgers, B. L. (2000). Concept analysis: An evolutionary view. In B. L. Rodgers & K. A. Knafl (Eds.), *Concept development in nursing: Foundations, techniques, and applications* (2nd ed., pp. 77–102). Philadelphia: Saunders.

Rodgers, B. L., & Knafl, K. A. (2000). *Concept development in nursing: Foundations, techniques, and applications* (2nd ed.). Philadelphia: Saunders.

Saiki, L. S., & Lobo, M. L. (2011). Disclosure: A concept analysis. *Journal of Advanced Nursing, 67*(12), 2713–2722.

Schwartz-Barcott, D., & Kim, H. S. (1986). A hybrid model for concept development. In P. L. Chinn (Ed.), *Nursing research methodology: Issues and implementation.* Rockville, MD: Aspen.

Schwartz-Barcott, D., & Kim, H. S. (1993). An expansion and elaboration of the hybrid model of concept development. In B. L. Rodgers & K. A. Knafl (Eds.), *Concept development in nursing* (pp. 107–133). Philadelphia: Saunders.

Schwartz-Barcott, D., & Kim, H. S. (2000). An expansion and elaboration of the hybrid model of concept development. In B. L. Rodgers & K A. Knafl (Eds.), *Concept development in nursing* (2nd ed., pp. 129–160). Philadelphia: Saunders.

Selye, H. (1956). *The stress of life.* New York: McGraw-Hill.

Shin, H., & White-Traut, R. (2007). The conceptual structure of transition to motherhood in the neonatal intensive care unit. *Journal of Advanced Nursing, 58*(1), 90–98.

Steis, M. R., Penrod, J., Adkins, C. S., & Hupcey, J. E. (2009). Principle-based concept analysis: Recognition in the context of nurse-patient interactions. *Journal of Advanced Nursing, 65*(0), 1964–1975.

Verhulst, G., & Swartz-Barcott, D. (1993). A concept analysis of withdrawal: Application of the hybrid model of concept development. In B. L. Rogers & K. A. Knafl (Eds.), *Concept development in nursing: Foundations, techniques, and applications* (pp. 135–158). Philadelphia: Saunders.

Walker, L. O., & Avant, K. (1986). *Strategies for theory construction in nursing* (1st ed.). Norwalk, CT: Appleton & Lange.

Walker, L. O., & Avant, K. (1995). *Strategies for theory construction in nursing* (3rd ed.). Norwalk, CT: Appleton & Lange.

Walker, L. O., & Avant, K. (2011). *Strategies for theory construction in nursing* (5th ed.). Upper Saddle River, NJ: Pearson Education.

Wang, C. H. (2000). Developing a concept of hope from a human science perspective. *Nursing Science Quarterly, 13*(3), 248–251.

Weaver, K., & Mitcham, C. (2008). Nursing concept analysis in North America: State of the art. *Nursing Philosophy, 9*(2), 180–194.

Weaver, K., Morse, J., & Mitcham, C. (2008). Ethical sensitivity in professional practice: Concept analysis. *Journal of Advanced Nursing, 62*(5), 607–618.

Whitehead, D. (2004). Health promotion and health education: Advancing the concepts. *Journal of Advanced Nursing, 47*(3), 311–320.

Wilson, J. (1963). *Thinking with concepts.* Cambridge, United Kingdom: Cambridge University Press.

CHAPTER 4

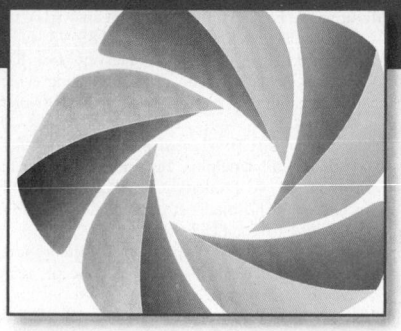

Theory Development

Structuring Conceptual Relationships in Nursing

Melanie McEwen

Jill Watson is enrolled in a master's nursing program and is beginning work on her thesis. As an occupational health nurse at a large telecommunication manufacturing company for the past 7 years, Jill has concentrated much of her practice on health promotion. She has organized numerous health fairs, led countless health help sessions, regularly posted health information on intranet bulletin boards, and provided screening programs for many illnesses. Despite her efforts to improve the health of the workers, many still smoke, are overweight, do not exercise, and have other deleterious lifestyle habits. Realizing that lack of information about health-related issues is not a problem, Jill has focused on trying to understand why people choose not to engage in positive health practices. As a result, she became interested in the concept of motivation.

In one of her early courses in her master's program, Jill completed an analysis of the concept of health motivation. During this exercise, she defined the concept; identified antecedents, consequences, and empirical referents; and developed a number of case studies, including a model case, a related case, and a contrary case.

As her studies progressed, Jill reviewed the literature from nursing, psychology, and sociology on health beliefs and health motivation and discovered several related theories. The Health Belief Model appeared to best explain her impressions of the issues at hand, but the model had not been developed for nursing and did not completely fit her concept of the variables and issues in health motivation. For her thesis, she decided to modify the Health Belief Model to focus on the concept of health motivation and to develop an instrument to measure the variables she had generated in her earlier work.

In nursing, theories are systematic explanations of events in which constructs and concepts are identified; relationships are proposed; and predictions are made to describe, explain, predict, or prescribe practice and research (Dickoff, James, & Wiedenbach, 1968; Streubert & Carpenter, 2011). Without nursing theory, nursing activities and interventions are guided by rote, tradition, some outside authority, or hunches, or they may simply be random.

Theories are not discovered; rather, they are constructed or developed to describe, explain, or understand phenomena or solve nagging problems (e.g., Why don't people apply knowledge of positive health practices?). In the past, nursing leaders saw theory development as a means of clearly establishing nursing as a profession, and throughout the last 50 years, many nursing scholars developed models and theories to guide nursing practice, nursing research, nursing administration and management, and nursing education. As discussed in Chapter 2, these models and theories have been created at different levels (grand, middle range, practice) and for different purposes (description, explanation, prediction, etc.).

Theory development seeks to help the nurse understand practice in a more complete and insightful way and provides a method of identifying and expressing key ideas about the essence of practice. Theories help organize existing knowledge and aid in making new and important discoveries to advance practice (Walker & Avant, 2011). As illustrated earlier in the case study, development and application of nursing theory are essential to revise, update, and refine the practice of nursing and to further advance the profession.

Overview of Theory Development

Several terms related to the creation of theory are found in the nursing literature. Theory construction, theory development, theory building, and theory generation are sometimes used synonymously or interchangeably. In other cases (Cesario, 1997; Walker & Avant, 2011), authors have differentiated the constructs or subsumed one term as a component or process within another. In this chapter, the term *theory development* is used as the global term to refer to the processes and methods used to create, modify, or refine a theory. *Theory construction* is used to describe one of the final steps of theory development in which the components of the theory are organized and linkages specified.

Theory development is a complex, time-consuming process that covers a number of stages or phases from inception of concepts to testing of theoretical propositions through research (Powers & Knapp, 2011). In general, the process of theory development begins with one or more concepts that are derived from within a discipline's metatheory or philosophy. These concepts are further refined and related to one another in propositions or statements that can be submitted to empirical testing (Chinn & Kramer, 2011; Peterson, 2013; Reynolds, 1971).

Categorizations of Theory

As described in Chapter 2, theories are often categorized using different criteria. Theories may be grouped based on scope or level of abstraction (grand theory, middle range theory, practice theory), the purpose of the theory, or the source or discipline in which the theory was developed.

Categorization Based on Scope or Level of Abstraction

An overview of "levels of theory" was presented in Chapter 2. In nursing, theories are often viewed based on scope or level of abstraction, where the most global or abstract level is the philosophical, or metatheory, level, followed by grand theory, middle range theory, and practice theory. In the early years of nursing theory (1950 to 1980), theory development was largely at the metatheory and grand theory levels. Recently, however, there has been a significant shift with recognition of the need to focus more on middle range and practice (situation-specific) theories that are more relevant to nursing practice and more amenable to testing through research. The following sections will review and expand on each level of theory.

Philosophy, Worldview, or Metatheory

Metatheory refers to the philosophical and methodologic questions related to developing a theoretical base for nursing. It has also been termed "worldview" by some (Hickman, 2011). According to Walker and Avant (2011), metatheory deals with the processes of generating knowledge and debating broad issues related to the nature of theory, types of theory needed, and suitable criteria for theory evaluation. Chapter 1 discussed a number of philosophical issues related to a worldview or metatheory in nursing, including epistemology, research methods, and related questions.

Grand Theories

In nursing, grand theories are composed of relatively abstract concepts that are not operationally defined and attempt to explain or describe very comprehensive aspects of human experience and response. Grand theories consist of conceptual frameworks defining broad perspectives for practice and ways of looking at nursing phenomena based on these perspectives. They provide global viewpoints for nursing practice, education, and research, but they are limited because of their generality and abstractness. Indeed, because of their level of abstraction, these theories are often considered to be difficult to apply to the daily practice of nurses and are difficult to test (Hickman, 2011; Higgins & Moore, 2000; Peterson, 2013; Walker & Avant, 2011).

Early grand nursing theories focused on the nurse–client relationship and the role of the nurse. Later grand theories expanded to more encompassing concepts (holistic perspective, interpersonal relations, social systems, and health). Recent grand theories have attempted to address phenomenologic aspects of nursing (caring, transcultural issues) (Moody, 1990). Chapters 6 to 9 provide an examination of grand nursing theories.

Middle Range Theories

The need for practice disciplines to develop middle range theories was first proposed in the field of sociology in the 1960s. In nursing, development of middle range theory is growing to fill the gaps between grand nursing theories and nursing practice.

Compared to grand theories, middle range theories contain fewer concepts and are limited in scope. Within the scope of middle range theories, however, some degree of generalization is possible across specialty areas and settings. Propositions are clear, and testable hypotheses can be derived. Middle range theories cover such concepts as pain, symptom management, cultural issues, and health promotion (Higgins & Moore, 2000; Peterson, 2013; Walker & Avant, 2011). Chapters 10 and 11 provide a detailed discussion of middle range theories and their application in nursing.

Practice Theories

Practice theories (microtheories, situation-specific, or prescriptive theories) explain prescriptions or modalities for practice. The essence of practice theory is a defined or identified goal and descriptions of interventions or activities to achieve this goal (Walker & Avant, 2011). Practice theories can cover particular elements of a specialty, such as oncology nursing, obstetric nursing, or operating room nursing, or they may relate to another aspect of nursing, such as nursing administration or nursing education. Such theories typically describe specific elements of nursing care, such as cancer pain relief, or a specific experience, such as dying and end-of-life care.

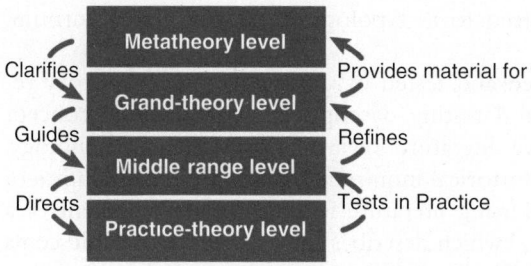

Figure 4-1 Relationship among levels of theory. (From Walker, L. O., & Avant, K. C. (2011). *Strategies for theory construction in nursing* (5th ed.). Upper Saddle River, NJ: Prentice-Hall. Reprinted by permission of Pearson Education, Inc., Upper Saddle River, NJ.)

Practice theories contain few concepts, are narrow in scope, and explain a relatively small aspect of reality. They are derived from middle range theories, practice experiences, comprehensive literature reviews, and empirical testing (Peterson, 2013). Furthermore, when the concepts and statements are operationally defined, they may be tested by appropriate research strategies (Higgins & Moore, 2000). Chapters 12 and 18 cover practice—or situation-specific—theories in more detail.

Relationship Among Levels of Theory in Nursing

Walker and Avant (2011) state that the four levels of theory may be linked in order to direct and focus the discipline of nursing. As they describe, metatheory (worldview or philosophy) clarifies the methodologies and roles for each subsequent level of theory development (grand, middle range, and practice). Each level of theory provides material for further analysis and clarification at the level of metatheory. Grand nursing theories guide the phenomena of concern at the middle range level. Middle range theories assist in refinement of grand theories and direct prescriptions of practice theories. Practice theories are constructed from scientifically based propositions about reality and test the empirical validity of those propositions as they are incorporated into client care (Higgins & Moore, 2000). Figure 4-1 illustrates the relationships among the levels of theory in nursing.

Categorization Based on Purpose

As discussed in Chapter 2, Dickoff and James (1968) described four kinds of theory: factor-isolating theories (descriptive theories), factor-relating theories (explanatory theories), situation-relating theories (predictive theories), and situation-producing theories (prescriptive theories). Each higher level of theory builds on the lower levels (Dickoff et al., 1968), and each is reviewed and expanded upon in the following sections.

Descriptive Theories

Descriptive theories describe, observe, and name concepts, properties, and dimensions, but they typically do not explain the interrelationships among the concepts or propositions, and they do not indicate how changes in one concept affect other concepts. According to Barnum (1998), descriptive theory is the first and most important level of theory development because it determines what will be perceived as the essence of the phenomenon under study. Subsequent theory development expands or refines those elements and specifies relationships that are determined to be important in the descriptive phase. Thus, it is critical that the most significant constituents of the phenomenon be recognized and named in this earliest phase of theory development.

The two types of descriptive theory are naming and classification. *Naming theories* describe the dimension or characteristics of a phenomenon. *Classification theories* describe dimensions or characteristics of a phenomenon that are structurally interrelated and are sometimes referred to as typologies or taxonomies (Barnum, 1998; Fawcett, 1999).

Descriptive theories are generated and tested by descriptive or explanatory research. Techniques for generating and testing descriptive theory include concept analysis, case studies, comprehensive literature review, surveys, phenomenology, ethnography, grounded theory, and historical inquiry (Fawcett, 1999). Examples of descriptive theory found in recent nursing literature include the development of a conceptual model of "almost normal," which describes the experience of adolescents living with implantable cardioverter defibrillators (phenomenology) (Zeigler & Tilley, 2011); development of a model for understanding caregiving changes among poor, chronically ill Mexicans (ethnography) (Robles-Silva, 2008); and the proposed middle range theory of nursing presence (comprehensive literature review) (McMahon & Christopher, 2011). In other examples, a case study approach was used by Zauderer (2008) to examine the phenomenon of "altered maternal–newborn attachment" and by Davidson (2010) to develop a middle range theory to support families of intensive care unit (ICU) patients.

Explanatory Theories

Explanatory theory is the second level in theory development. Once phenomena have been identified and named, they can be viewed in relation to other phenomena. Explanatory theories relate concepts to one another and describe and specify some of the associations or interrelations between and among the concepts. Further, explanatory theories attempt to tell how or why the concepts are related and may deal with causality, correlations, and rules that regulate interactions (Barnum, 1998; Dickoff et al., 1968).

Explanatory theories can be developed only after the parts of the phenomena have been identified and tested, and they are generated and tested by correlational research. Correlational research requires collection or measurement of data gathered by observation or self-report instruments that will yield either qualitative or quantitative data (Fawcett, 1999). Explanatory theories may also be generated by processes involving in-depth integrative/systematic and rigorous review of extant research literature. Examples of explanatory theories from recent nursing literature include development of a theory describing women's attitudes towards physical activity (Im, Stuifbergen, & Walker, 2010) and an examination of resilience among operating room nurses (Gillespie, Chaboyer, Wallis, & Grimbeek, 2007). In a qualitative study, Greco, Nail, Kendall, Cartwright, and Messecar (2010) developed a theoretical model of "guarding against cancer" describing and explaining the interaction of factors and beliefs that lead to how older women make decisions to be screened for breast cancer. Similarly, using grounded theory methodology, Doering and Durfor (2011) developed a model of "persevering toward normalcy after childbirth" that explained the processes of managing fatigue, accessing social support, and maximizing sleep as families with infants adjust the routines of the infant and the family while they progress toward "normalcy."

Predictive Theories

Predictive theories describe precise relationships between concepts and are the third level of theory development. Predictive theories presuppose the prior existence of the more elementary types of theory. They result after concepts are defined and relational statements are generated and are able to describe future outcomes consistently. Predictive theories include statements of causal or consequential relatedness (Dickoff et al., 1968).

Predictive theories are generated and tested by experimental research involving manipulation of a phenomenon to determine how it affects or changes some dimension or characteristic of another phenomenon (Fawcett, 1999). Different research designs may be used in this process. These include pretest–posttest designs, quasi-experiments, and true experiments. These research studies produce quantifiable data that are statistically analyzed. Examples of predictive theories include a model examining patient satisfaction with nurse practitioner care (Green & Davis, 2005), a theory of family interdependence that predicted the relationships between spirituality and psychological well-being among elders and their family caregivers (Kim, Reed, Hayward, Kang, & Koenig, 2011), and a model predicting physical activity in older adults with hypertension (Lee & Laffrey, 2006). In an interesting work, Tourangeau (2005) synthesized research literature from multiple sources to propose a theoretical model predicting patient mortality. She identified the following contributing or determining factors to mortality: nurses' staffing, burnout, satisfaction, skill mix, experience, and role support, as well as such factors as physician expertise, hospital location, and patient characteristics (e.g., age, gender, comorbidity, socioeconomic status, and chronicity).

Prescriptive Theories

Prescriptive theories are perceived to be the highest level of theory development (Dickoff et al., 1968). Prescriptive theories prescribe activities necessary to reach defined goals. In nursing, prescriptive theories address nursing therapeutics and predict the consequence of interventions (Meleis, 2012). Prescriptive theories have three basic components: (1) specified goals or outcomes, (2) explicit activities to be taken to meet the goal, and (3) a survey list that articulates the conceptual basis of the theory (Dickoff et al., 1968).

According to Dickoff and colleagues (1968), the outcome or goal of a prescriptive theory serves as the norm or standard by which to evaluate activities. The goal must articulate the context of the situation, and this provides the basis for testing to determine whether the goal has been achieved. The specified actions or activities are those nursing interventions that should be taken to realize the goal. The goal will not be realized without the activity, and prescriptions for activities directly affect the goals.

The survey list augments and supplements the prescribed activities. In addition, it serves to prepare for future prescriptive activities. The survey list asks six questions about the prescribed activity that relate to the delineated goal (Box 4-1). In current vernacular, as practice guidelines based on research, evidence-based practice (EBP) consists of many attributes of prescriptive theory. This will be discussed in more detail in Chapter 12.

Examples of prescriptive theory are becoming more common in the literature, enhanced by the expanding volume of nursing research and increasing calls for EBP. In one work, Ade-Oshifogun (2012) presented a research tested and supported model to assist

Box 4-1 Survey List of Questions for Prescriptive Theories

1. Who performs the activity? (agency)
2. Who or what is the recipient of the activity? (patiency)
3. In what context is the activity performed? (framework)
4. What is the end point of the activity? (terminus)
5. What is the guiding procedure, technique, or protocol of the activity? (procedure)
6. What is the energy source for the activity? (dynamics)

Source: Dickoff, James, & Weidenbach (1968).

and support clinicians to develop interventions to reduce or minimize truncal obesity in people with chronic obstructive pulmonary disease (COPD). The descriptions of feeding, pelvic floor exercise, therapeutic touch, and latex precautions are only a few of many excellent examples of nursing interventions presented by Bulechek, Butcher, Dochterman, and Wagner (2012). Lastly, Finnegan, Shaver, Zenk, Wikie, and Ferrans (2010) developed the "symptom cluster experience profile" framework to anticipate symptom clusters and derive interventions and clinical practice guidelines among survivors of childhood cancers.

Categorization Based on Source or Discipline

Theories may be classified based on the discipline or source of origin. As briefly discussed in Chapter 1, many of the theories used in nursing are borrowed, shared, or derived from theories developed in other disciplines. Because nursing is a human science and a practice discipline, incorporation of shared theories into practice and modification of them for use and testing are common.

Nurses use theories and concepts from the behavioral sciences, biologic sciences, and sociologic sciences, as well as learning theories and organizational and management theories, among others. In many cases, these concepts and theories will overlap. For example, adaptation and stress are concepts found in both the behavioral and biologic sciences, and multiple theories have been developed using these concepts. Additionally, some theories defy placement in one discipline but relate to many. These include such basic concepts as systems theory, change theory, and chaos.

This book discusses a number of theories and concepts organized in terms of sociologic sciences, behavioral sciences, biomedical sciences, administration and management sciences, and learning theories. Table 4-1 presents examples of theories from

Table 4-1 Shared Theory Used in Nursing Practice and Research

Disciplines	Examples of Theories Used by Nurses
Theories from sociologic sciences	Family systems theory Feminist theory Role theory Critical social theory
Theories from behavioral sciences	Attachment theory Theories of self-determination Lazarus and Folkman's theory of stress, coping, and adaptation Theory of planned behavior
Theories from biomedical sciences	Pain Self-regulation theory Immune function Symptomology Germ theory
Theories from administration and management sciences	Donabedian's quality framework Theories of organizational behavior Models of conflict and conflict resolution Job satisfaction
Learning theories	Bandura's social cognitive learning theory Developmental learning theory Prospect theory

each of these areas. Although by no means exhaustive, Chapters 13 through 17 provide information on many of the shared theories commonly used in nursing practice, research, education, and administration.

Components of a Theory

A theory has several components, including purpose, concepts and definitions, theoretical statements, structure/linkages and ordering, and assumptions (Chinn & Kramer, 2011; Hardin & Bishop, 2010; Powers & Knapp, 2011). Creation of conceptual models is also a component of theory development that is promoted to further explain and define relationships, structure, and linkages.

Purpose

The purpose of a theory explains why the theory was formulated and specifies the context and situations in which it should be applied. The purpose might also provide information about the sociopolitical context in which the theory was developed, circumstances that influenced its creation, the theorist's past experiences, settings in which the theory was formulated, and societal trends. The purpose of the theory is usually explicitly described and should be found within the discussion of the theory (Chinn & Kramer, 2011).

Concepts and Conceptual Definitions

Concepts and concept development are described in detail in Chapter 3. Concepts are linguistic labels that are assigned to objects or events and are considered to be the building blocks of theories. The theoretical definition defines the concept in relation to other concepts and permits the description and classification of phenomena. Operationally defined concepts link the concept to the real world and identify empirical referents (indicators) of the concept that will permit observation and measurement (Chinn & Kramer, 2011; Hardin & Bishop, 2010; Walker & Avant, 2011). Theories should include explicit conceptual definitions to describe and clarify the phenomenon and explain how the concept is expressed in empirical reality.

Theoretical Statements

Once a concept is fully developed and presented, it can be combined with other concepts to create statements to describe the real world. Theoretical statements, or propositions, are statements about the relationship between two or more concepts and are used to connect concepts to devise the theory. Statements must be formulated before explanations or predictions can be made, and development of statements asserting a connection between two or more concepts introduces the possibility of analysis (Hardin & Bishop, 2010). The several types of theoretical statements include propositions, laws, axioms, empirical generalizations, and hypotheses (Table 4-2).

Theoretical statements can be classified into two groups. The first group consists of statements that claim the *existence* of phenomena referred to by concepts (existence statements). The second group describes *relationships* between concepts (relational statements) (Reynolds, 1971).

Table 4-2 Types of Relationship Statements

Type of Statement	Characteristics
Axioms	Consist of a basic set of statements or propositions that state the general relationship between concepts. Axioms are relatively abstract; therefore, they are not directly observed or measured.
Empirical generalizations	Summarize empirical evidence. Empirical generalizations provide some confidence that the same pattern will be repeated in concrete situations in the future under the same conditions.
Hypotheses	Statements that lack support from empirical research but are selected for study. The source of hypotheses may be a variation of a law or a derivation from an axiomatic theory, or they may be generated by a scientist's intuition (a hunch). All concepts in a hypothesis must be measurable, with operational definitions in concrete situations.
Laws	Well-grounded, with strong empirical support and evidence of empirical regulatory. Laws contain concepts that can be measured or identified in concrete settings.
Propositions	Statements of a constant relationship between two or more concepts or facts.

Sources: Hardy (1973); Jacox (1974); Reynolds (1971).

Existence Statements

Existence statements and definitions relate to specific concepts and make existence claims about that concept (e.g., that chair is brown or that man is a nurse). Each statement has a concept and is identified by a term that is applied to another object or phenomena. Existence statements serve as adjuncts to relational statements and clarify meanings in the theory. Existence statements are also termed *nonrelational statements* and may be right or wrong depending on the circumstances (Reynolds, 1971).

Relational Statements

Existence statements can only name and classify objects. Knowing the existence of one concept may be used to convey information about the existence of other concepts. Relational statements assert that a relationship exists between the properties of two or more concepts. This relationship is basic to development of theory and is expressed in terms of relational statements that explain, predict, understand, or control.

Like concepts, statements may have different levels of abstraction (theoretical and operational). The more general statements contain theoretically defined concepts. If the theoretical concepts are replaced with operational definitions, then the statement is "operationalized." The two broad groups of relational statements are those that describe an *association* between two concepts and those that describe a *causal relationship* between two concepts (Reynolds, 1971).

Associational or Correlational Relationships. Associational statements describe concepts that occur or exist together (Reynolds, 1971; Walker & Avant, 2011). The nature of the association/correlation may be positive (when one concept occurs or is high, the other concept occurs or is high). For example, as the external temperature rises during the summer, consumption of ice cream increases. An example in human beings is a positive correlation between height and weight—as people get taller, in general their weight will increase.

The association may be neutral when the occurrence of one concept provides no information about the occurrence of another concept. For example, there is no correlation between gender and scores on a pharmacology examination. Finally, the association may be negative. In this case, when one concept occurs or is high, the other concept is low and vice versa. For example, failure to use condoms regularly is associated with an increase in the occurrence of sexually transmitted infections.

Causal Relationships. In causal relationships, one concept is considered to cause the occurrence of a second concept. For example, as caloric intake increases, weight increases. In scientific research, the concept or variable that is the cause is typically referred to as the independent variable and the variable that is affected is referred to as the dependent variable.

In science, there is often disagreement about whether a relationship is causal or simply highly correlated. A classic example is the relationship between cigarette smoking and lung cancer. As early as the 1940s, an association between smoking and lung cancer was recognized, but not until the 1980s was it determined that smoking actually *caused* lung cancer. Likewise, genetic predisposition is *associated* with development of heart disease; it has not been shown to *cause* heart disease.

Structure and Linkages

Structuring the theory by logical arrangement and specifying linkages of the theoretical concepts and statements is critical to the development of theory. The structure of a theory provides overall form to the theory. Theory structuring includes determination of the order of appearance of relationships, identification of central relationships, and delineation of direction, strength, and quality of relationships (Chinn & Kramer, 2011).

Although theoretical statements assert connections between concepts, the rationale for the stated connections needs to be developed. Theoretical linkages offer a reasoned explanation of why the variables in the theory may be connected in some manner, which brings plausibility to the theory. When developed operationally, linkages contribute to the testability of the theory by specifying how variables are connected. Thus, conceptual arrangement of statements and linkages can lead to hypotheses (Hardin & Bishop, 2010).

Assumptions

Assumptions are notations that are taken to be true without proof. They are beliefs about a phenomenon that one must accept as true to accept a theory, and although they may not be empirically testable, they can be argued philosophically. The assumptions of a theory are based on what the theorist considers to be adequate empirical evidence to support propositions, on accepted knowledge, or on personal beliefs or values (Jacox, 1974; McKenna & Slevin, 2008; Powers & Knapp, 2011). Assumptions may be in the form of factual assertions or they may reflect value positions. Factual assumptions are those that are known through experience. Value assumptions assert or imply what is right, or good, or ought to be (Chinn & Kramer, 2011).

In a given theory, assumptions may be implicit or explicit. In many nursing theories, they must be "teased out." Furthermore, it is often difficult to separate assumptions that are implicit or integrated into the narrative of the theory from relationship statements (Powers & Knapp, 2011).

Models

Models are schematic representations of some aspect of reality. Various media are used in construction of models; they may be three-dimensional objects, diagrams, geometric formulas, or words. Empirical models are replicas of observable reality (e.g., a plastic model of a uterus or an eye). Theoretical models represent the real world through language or symbols and directional arrows.

In a classic work, Artinian (1982) described the rationale for creating a theoretical or conceptual model. She determined that models help illustrate the processes through which outcomes occur by specifying the relationships among the variables in graphic form where they can be examined for inconsistency, incompleteness, or errors. By creating a model of the concepts and relationships, it is possible to trace the effect of certain variables on the outcome variable rather than making assertions that each variable under study is related to every other variable. Furthermore, the model depicts a process that starts somewhere and ends at a logical point. Using the model, a person should be able to explain what happened, predict what will happen, and interpret what is happening. Finally, Artinian stated that once a model has been conceptually illustrated, the phenomenon represented can be examined in different settings testing the usefulness and generalizability of the underlying theory. The figure in the exemplar at the end of the chapter shows a model illustrating the relationships between the variables of the Perceived Access to Breast Health Care in African American Women Theory.

Theory Development

Several factors are vital for nurses to examine the process of theory development. First, an understanding of the relationship among theory, research, and practice should be recognized. Second, the nurse should be aware that there are various approaches to theory development, based on the source of initiation (i.e., practice, theory, or research). Finally, the process of theory development should be understood. Each of these factors is discussed in the following sections.

Relationship Among Theory, Research, and Practice

Many nurses lack a true understanding of the interrelationship among theory, research, and practice and its importance to the continuing development of nursing as a profession (Pryjmachuk, 1996). As early as the 1970s, nursing scholars commented on the relationships among theory, research, and practice. Indeed, at that time nursing leaders urged that nursing research be combined with theory development to provide a rational basis for practice (Flaskerud, 1984; Moody, 1990).

In applied disciplines such as nursing, practice is based on the theories that are validated through research. Thus, theory, research, and practice affect each other in a reciprocal, cyclical, and interactive way (Hickman, 2011; Marrs & Lowry, 2006) (Figure 4-2).

Relationship Between Theory and Research

Research validates and modifies theory. In nursing, theories stimulate nurse scientists to explore significant problems in the field of nursing. In doing so, the potential for the development of nursing knowledge increases (Meleis, 2012). Theories can be used to formulate a set of generalizations to explain relationships among variables.

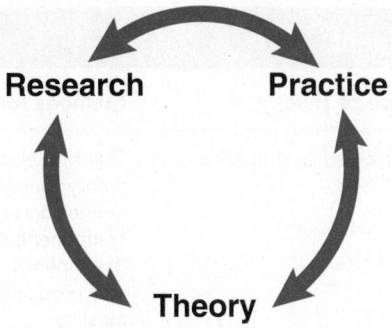

Figure 4-2 Research–theory–practice cycle.

When empirically tested, the results of research can be used to verify, modify, disprove, or support a theoretical proposition.

Relationship Between Theory and Practice

Theory guides practice. One of the primary uses of theory is to contribute insights about nursing practice situations through provision of goals for assessment, diagnosis, and intervention. Likewise, through practice, nursing theory is shaped, and guidelines for practice evolve. Theory renders practice more efficient and more effective, and the ultimate benefit of theory application in nursing is the improvement in client care (Meleis, 2012).

Relationship Between Research and Practice

Research is the key to the development of a discipline. Middle range and practice theories may be tested in practice through clinical research (Hickman, 2011). If individual practitioners are to develop expertise, they must participate in research. In summary, there is a need to encourage nurses to test and refine theories and models to develop their own personal models of practice (Marrs & Lowry, 2006; Pryjmachuk, 1996).

Approaches to Theory Development

Several different approaches may be used to initiate the process of theory development. Meleis (2012) cites four major strategies differentiated by their origin (theory, practice, or research) and by whether sources from outside of nursing were used to develop the theory. These approaches are theory to practice to theory, practice to theory, research to theory, and theory to research to theory. She then proposes employment of an integrated approach to theory development. Table 4-3 summarizes these different approaches.

Theory to Practice to Theory

The theory to practice to theory approach to theory development begins with a theory (typically non-nursing) that describes a phenomenon of interest (Meleis, 2012). This approach assumes that the theory can help describe or explain the phenomenon, but it is not completely congruent with nursing and/or is not directly defined for nursing practice. Thus, the focus of the theory is different from the focus needed for nursing.

Using the theory to practice to theory strategy, the nurse would select a theory that may be used to explain or describe a clinical situation (e.g., adaptation, stress, health beliefs). The nurse could modify concepts and consider relationships between concepts that were not proposed in the original theory. To accomplish this, the nurse would need to (a) have a basic knowledge of the theory; (b) analyze the theory by

Table 4-3 Strategies for Theory Development

Origin of Theory	Basis for Development	Type of Theory	Methods for Development
Theory–practice–theory	An existing theory non-nursing that can help describe and explain a phenomenon, but the theory is not complete or not completely developed for nursing	Borrowed or shared theory	Theorist selects a non-nursing theory; analyzes the theory; defines and evaluates each component; and redefines assumptions, concepts, and propositions to reflect nursing
Practice–theory	Existing theories are not useful in describing the phenomenon of interest; theory is derived from clinical situations	Grounded theory	Researcher observes phenomenon of interest, analyzes similarities and differences, compares and contrasts responses, and develops concepts and linkages
Research–theory	Development of theory is based on research; theories evolve from replicated and confirmed research findings	Scientific theory	Researcher selects a common phenomenon, lists and measures characteristics of the phenomenon in a variety of situations, analyzes the data to determine if there are patterns that need further study, and formalizes patterns as theoretical statements
Theory–research–theory	Theory drives the research questions; the result of the research informs and modifies the theory	Theory testing	Theorist defines a theory and determines propositions for testing; the theory is modified, refined, or further developed based on research findings; in some cases, a new theory will be formed

Source: Meleis (2012).

reducing it into components where each component is defined and evaluated; (c) use assumptions, concepts, and propositions to describe the clinical area; (d) redefine assumptions, concepts, and propositions to reflect nursing; and (e) reconstruct a theory using exemplars representing the redefined assumptions, concepts, and propositions (Meleis, 2012). Examples of a theory to practice to theory strategy include Benner's use of Dreyfus's Model of Skill Acquisition to describe novice to expert practice (Benner, 2001) and Roy's use of Helson's Adaptation Theory to describe human responses (Roy & Roberts, 1981). Other examples of theory to practice to theory in recent nursing literature include a work that applied the Theory of Planned Behavior to develop a situation-specific theory of breastfeeding (Nelson, 2006) and Davidson's (2010) middle range theory, facilitated sensemaking, which supports families of ICU patients. The latter was derived from the work of Karl Weick (2001), an expert in organizational psychology.

Practice to Theory

If no appropriate theory appears to exist to describe or explain a phenomenon, theories may be inductively developed from clinical practice situations. The practice to theory approach is based on the premise that in a given situation, existing theories are not useful in describing the phenomenon of interest. It assumes that the phenomenon is important enough to pursue and that there is a clinical understanding about it that has not been articulated. Furthermore, insight gained from describing the phenomenon has potential for enhancing the understanding of other similar situations through development of a set of propositions (Meleis, 2012).

This strategy is a grounded theory approach, which begins with a question evolving from a practice situation. It relies on observation of new phenomena in a practice situation, development of concepts, and then labeling, describing, and articulating properties of these concepts. To accomplish this, the researcher observes the phenomenon, analyzes similarities and differences, and then compares and contrasts responses. Following this, the researcher may develop concepts and propositional statements and propose linkages (Meleis, 2012). Examples of the practice to theory strategy of theory development include a situation-specific theory of Caucasian cancer patients' pain experience (Im, 2006), a theory of "bridging worlds" to assist caregivers to meet emotional needs of dying patients (Law, 2009), and a proposed model of "becoming normal," which describes the emotional process of recovery from stroke (Gallagher, 2011). Finally, Falk-Rafael and Betker (2012) developed the "critical caring theory" following detailed interviews of practice accounts of 25 public health nurses, and Drake, Luna, Georges, and Steege (2012) created the "hospital nurse force theory" from detailed reflection and literature review to guide hospital nursing practice and support research to address the association between nursing fatigue and patient harm.

Research to Theory

The research to theory strategy is the most accepted strategy for theory development in nursing, largely due to the early emphasis on empiricism described in Chapter 1. For empiricists, theory development is considered a product of research because theories evolve from replicated and confirmed research findings. The research to theory strategy assumes that there is truth in real life, that the truth can be captured through the senses, and that the truth can be verified (Meleis, 2012). Furthermore, the purpose of scientific theories is to describe, explain, predict, or control a part of the empirical world.

In the research to theory strategy for theory development, the researcher selects a phenomenon that occurs in the discipline and lists characteristics of the phenomenon. A method to measure the characteristics of the phenomenon is developed and implemented in a controlled study. The results of the measurement are analyzed to determine if there are any systematic patterns, and once patterns have been discovered, they are formalized into theoretical statements (Meleis, 2012). Examples of the research to theory strategy from nursing include the development of the "guarding against cancer" model, which was developed from a grounded theory study of women to identify how women with a family history of breast cancer decide to be screened through mammography (Greco et al., 2010), and the Adolescent Support Model (Sauls & Grassley, 2011), which was developed following three research studies comparing the nurse's perspective with the pregnant adolescent's perspective to promote interventions to enhance adolescents' breastfeeding experiences.

Theory to Research to Theory

In the theory to research to theory approach, theory drives the research questions and the results of the research are used to modify the theory. In this approach, the theorist will begin by defining a theory and determining propositions for testing. If carried through, the research findings may be used to further modify and develop the original theory (Meleis, 2012).

In this process, a theory is selected to explain the phenomenon of interest. The theory is a framework for operational definitions, variables, and statements. Concepts are redefined and operationalized for research. Findings are synthesized and used to modify, refine, or develop the original theory or, in some cases, to create a new theory. The goal is to test, refine, and develop theory and to use theory as a framework for research and theory modification. The researcher/theorist concludes the investigation with a refined, modified, or further developed explanation of the theory (Meleis, 2012). Examples of the theory to research to theory approach from recent nursing literature include a theory of genetic vulnerability developed from Roy's Adaptation Model using grounded theory methodology (Hamilton & Bowers, 2007), and Dunn's (2005) middle range theory of adaptation to chronic pain, which was also derived from Roy's Adaptation Model. Another example is the theory of diversity of human field pattern, which was developed from Martha Rogers' Science of Unitary Human Beings using a quantitative research design (Hastings-Tolsma, 2006).

Integrated Approach

An integrated approach to theory development describes an evolutionary process that is particularly useful in addressing complex clinical situations. It requires gathering data from the clinical setting, identifying exemplars, discovering solutions, and recognizing supportive information from other sources (Meleis, 2012).

Integrated theory development is rooted in clinical practice. Practice drives the basic questions and provides opportunities for clinical involvement in research that is designed to answer the questions. In this process for theory development, hunches and conceptual ideas are communicated with other clinicians or participants to allow for critique and further development. Among other strategies, the integrated approach uses skills and tools from clinical practice, various research methods, clinical diaries, descriptive journals, and collegial dialogues in developing a framework or conceptualization (Meleis, 2012).

Process of Theory Development

The process of theory development has been described in some detail by several nursing scholars (Jacox, 1974; Walker & Avant, 2011). Despite slight variations related to terminology and sequencing, the sources are similar in explaining the processes used to develop theory. The three basic steps are concept development, statement/proposition development, and theory construction. Chinn and Kramer (2011) add two additional steps that involve validating, confirming, or testing the theory and applying theory in practice. Each of the steps is described in the following sections, and Table 4-4 summarizes the theory development process.

Concept Development: Creation of Conceptual Meaning

This first step or process of theory development involves creating conceptual meaning. This provides the foundation for theory development and includes specifying, defining, and clarifying the concepts used to describe the phenomenon of interest (Jacox, 1974).

Table 4-4 Process of Theory Development

Step	Description
Concept development	Specifying, defining, and clarifying the concepts used to describe a phenomenon of interest
Statement development	Formulating and analyzing statements explaining relationships between concepts; also involves determining empirical referents that can validate them
Theory construction	Structuring and contextualizing the components of the theory; includes identifying assumptions and organizing linkages between and among the concepts and statements to form a theoretical structure
Testing theoretical relationships	Validating theoretical relationships through empirical testing
Application of theory in practice	Using research methods to assess how the theory can be applied in practice; research should provide evidence to evaluate the theory's usefulness

Creating conceptual meaning uses mental processes to create mental structures or ideas to be used to represent experience. This produces a tentative definition of the concept(s) and a set of criteria for determining if the concept(s) exists in a particular situation (Chinn & Kramer, 2011). Methods of concept development are described in detail in Chapter 3.

Statement Development: Formulation and Validation of Relational Statements

Relational statements are the skeletons of theory; they are the means by which the theory comes together. The process of formulation and validation of relational statements involves developing the relational statements and determining empirical referents that can validate them.

After a statement has been delineated initially, it should be scrutinized or analyzed. Statement analysis is a process described by Walker and Avant (2011) to thoroughly examine relational statements. Statement analysis classifies statements and examines the relationships between the concepts and helps direct theoretical construction. There are seven steps in the process of statement analysis (Box 4-2). Following the process of statement analysis, the statements are refined and may be operationalized.

Box 4-2 Steps in Statement Analysis

1. Select the statement to be analyzed.
2. Simplify the statement.
3. Classify the statement.
4. Examine concepts within the statement for definition and validity.
5. Specify relationship between concepts.
6. Examine the logic.
7. Determine stability.

Source: Walker & Avant (2011).

Theory Construction: Systematic Organization of the Linkages

The third stage in theory development involves structuring and contextualizing the components of the theory. This includes formulating systematic linkages between and among concepts, which results in a formal, coherent theoretical structure. The format used depends on what is known or assumed to be true about the phenomena in question (Chinn & Kramer, 2011). Aspects of theory construction include identifying and defining the concepts; identifying assumptions; clarifying the context within which the theory is placed; designing relationship statements; and delineating the organization, structure, or relationship among the components.

Theory synthesis is a theory construction strategy developed by Walker and Avant (2011). In theory synthesis, concepts and statements are organized into a network or whole. The purposes of theory synthesis are to represent a phenomenon through an interrelated set of concepts and statements, to describe the factors that precede or influence a particular phenomenon or event, to predict effects that occur after some event, or to put discrete scientific information into a more theoretically organized form.

Theory synthesis can be used to produce a compact, informative graphic representation of research findings on a topic of interest, and synthesized theories may be expressed in several ways such as graphic or model form. The three steps in theory synthesis are summarized in Box 4-3.

Validating and Confirming Theoretical Relationships in Research

Chinn and Kramer (2011) include the process of validating and confirming theoretical relationships as a component of theory development. Validating theoretical relationships involves empirically refining concepts and theoretical relationships, identifying empirical indicators, and testing relationships through empirical methods. In this step, the focus is on correlating the theory with demonstrable experiences and designing research to validate the relationships. Additionally, alternative explanations are considered based on the empirical evidence.

Validation and Application of Theory in Practice

An important final step in theory development identified by Chinn and Kramer (2011) is applying the theory in practice. In this step, research methods are used to assess how the theory can be applied in practice. The theoretical relationships are examined in the practice setting and results are recorded to determine how well the

Box 4-3 Steps in Theory Synthesis

1. Select a topic of interest and specify focal concepts (may be one concept/variable or a framework of several concepts).
2. Conduct a review of the literature to identify related factors and note their relationships. Identify and record relationships indicating whether they are bidirectional, unidirectional, positive, neutral or negative, weak or ambiguous, or strong in support evidence.
3. Organize concepts and relational statements into an integrated representation of the phenomena of interest. Diagrams may be used to express the relationships among the concepts.

Source: Walker & Avant (2011).

Link to Practice 4-1

Where Do I Begin?

An experienced emergency department (ED) RN wants to conduct a research study on "frequent flyers in the ED" (i.e., patients who return multiple times for the same or similar health problem) and is not sure how to proceed.

Following the guidelines in the chapter, the nurse should begin with developing the concept. For this step, he or she can search the health literature. Has a concept study of "frequent flyer" been published? If not, he or she can perform a formal or informal concept analysis, following one of the strategies presented in Chapter 3. If an analysis of "frequent flyers" has been published, the nurse might use it to set up the next steps—statement development and theory construction.

In the second and third steps, the nurse should continue to search the literature to learn all he or she can about the various aspects of "frequent flyers" and related phenomena. What studies have been published on patients who return to the ED repeatedly during a short period of time? What characteristics or diagnoses are typically reported? What other factors are usually found? How do they present? How do ED personnel care for them? From this review, the nurse can propose linkages between and among the various concepts/characteristics and draft a conceptual model. This might send him or her back to the literature to search for other, potentially related terms and phenomena. The literature and published studies can also lead him or her to instruments or tools that have been developed to measure some of the concepts and phenomena. Following these steps, the nurse can develop a research study to try to validate and refine the conceptual linkages. Completion and publication of research will contribute to the evidence that can then be used to improve nursing practice.

theory achieves the desired outcomes. The research design should provide evidence of the effect of the interventions on the well-being of recipients of care. Questions to be considered in this step include: Are the theory's goals congruent with practice goals? Is the intended context of the theory congruent with the practice situation? Are explanations of the theory sufficient for use in the nursing situation? Is there research evidence supporting use of the theory? See Link to Practice 4-1 for more information on the process of theory development.

Summary

Jill Watson, the nurse/graduate student introduced in the case study at the beginning of this chapter, was unable to identify a theory or conceptual model that completely met the needs for her study on health motivation. Because of this, she determined that it would be appropriate and feasible to use theory development techniques to revise an existing theory to use in her research project.

Theory development is an important but complex and time-consuming process. This chapter has presented a number of issues related to the process of theory development. These issues included the purpose of developing theory and the components of a theory. Discussion focused on concepts, theoretical statements, assumptions, and model development and explained the relationships among theory, research, and practice. Finally, the process of theory development was presented.

Key Points

- In nursing, theories are constructed or developed to describe, explain, or understand phenomena to help solve clinical problems or improve practice outcomes.
- Nursing theory can be categorized based on level (grand theory, middle range theory, or practice theory), based on purpose (descriptive theories, explanatory theories, predictive theories, or prescriptive theories), or based on source or background.
- Components of theories include purpose, concepts, definitions, theoretical statements, structure/linkages, assumptions, and often a diagram or model.
- There is a reciprocal relationship among theory, research, and practice that is critical for professional nurses to recognize and understand.
- Several approaches to theory development (e.g., theory to practice to theory, theory to research to theory, practice to theory, and research to theory) are found in the nursing literature.
- The process of theory development often follows these steps: concept development, statement development, theory construction, validation/confirmation of relationships in research, and validation/application of theory in practice.

To further illustrate the process of theory development, a summary report of a theory recently published in the nursing literature is presented. In the following exemplar, each of the components of the theory is clearly identified. In addition, Chapter 5 expands on the process of theory development by examining the processes of theory analysis and evaluation.

THEORY DEVELOPMENT EXEMPLAR

Garmon, S. C. (2012). Theory of perceived access to breast health care in African American women. *Advances in Nursing Science, 35*(2), E13–E23.

Garmon developed the Perceived Access to Breast Health Care in African American Women Theory to help direct future research studies exploring the relationship between access to care and utilization of preventive services related to breast health care.

Scope of theory: Middle range

Purpose:

The Perceived Access to Breast Health Care in African American Women Theory was developed to "propose an alternative view of access to breast health care and to demonstrate the importance of testing the relationships between culture, definitions of health, health behaviors, and practices and their influence on the perception of access to breath health care in AAW [African American women]" (p. E16).

Concepts and definitions are listed in the following table.

Concept	Definition
Culture	Combination of age, ethnicity, race, gender, socioeconomic status, religious beliefs, family history, and geographical origin that shapes and guides the values, beliefs, practices, thinking, decisions, and actions of individuals.
Health	A state of well-being that is culturally defined, valued, and practiced and that reflects the ability of individuals or groups to perform their daily role activities in a culturally satisfactory way.
Health promotion	Behavior(s) aimed at increasing the level of well-being and actualization of health.
Health protection	Behavior(s) aimed at decreasing the likelihood of experiencing health problems by active protection or early detection of health problems in the asymptomatic stage.
Health behaviors and practices	Culturally guided activities that are performed by an individual to help maintain his or her definition of health and well-being. These include health promotion and disease prevention breast care practices.
Access	The perceived necessity, availability, and appropriateness of breast health care provided by the health care delivery system, which purposes to assist an individual in maintaining his or her cultural definition of health and well-being
Perception of availably of care	Influenced by economic factors such as location of care; fit with time schedules; fit with family; and fit with cultural beliefs, values, and expectations.
Perception of necessity of care	Influenced by incorporation of health promotion and disease prevention into definitions of health, symptomatology, and cultural definitions of severity and personal and family priorities.
Perception of appropriateness of care	Influenced by fit of the breast health care with cultural values, beliefs, and practices; interactions and relationships with providers of care; and previous experience associated with breast cancer and breast health care.

Theoretical Statement and Linkages

1. Culture shapes the definition of health.
2. Perceived access to breast health care is postulated to be a product of three subconcepts: necessity, availability, and appropriateness of care.
3. Health behaviors and practices are a function of the perception of necessity of care, the availably of care, and the appropriateness of care.
4. When (a) the definition of health includes perspectives of health promotion and disease prevention; (b) health behaviors and practices include breast health practices; and (c) access to breast health care is perceived as necessary, available, and appropriate, then breast cancer diagnosis is likely to occur in its early stages.
5. Delayed diagnosis of breast cancer influences cultural beliefs, values, and practices and also reshapes individual definitions of health, health practices, and behaviors.

Model: Garmon's schematic diagram illustrates the main concepts and their interrelationships. It also depicts how perceptions may lead to either early or delayed diagnosis of breast cancer.

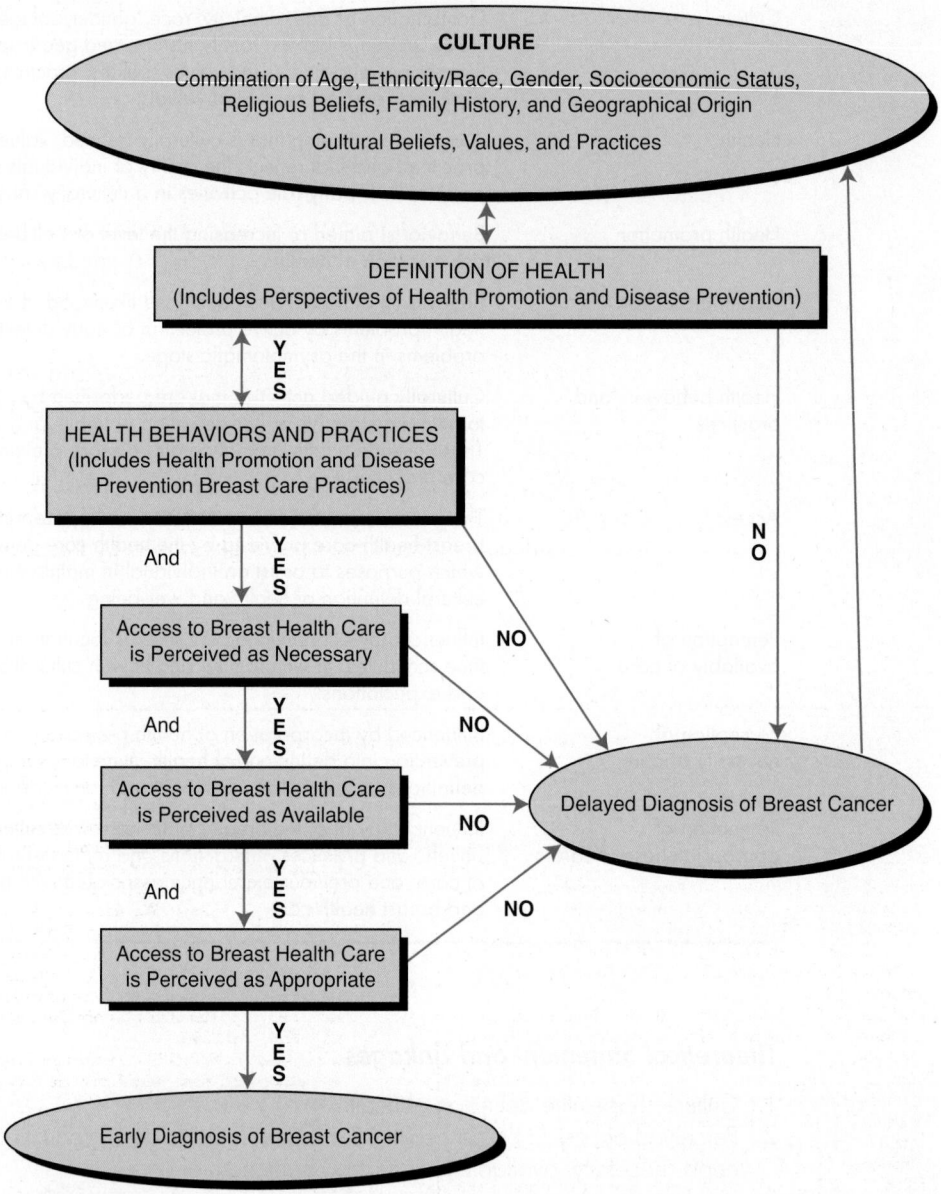

A theory of perceived access to breast health care in African American women (Garmon, 2012, p. E19).

Assumptions

1. Definitions of health care are shaped by culture and determine an individual's participation in health promotion and disease prevention strategies.
2. Perceived access to necessary care will result in seeking breast health care for health promotion and disease prevention.
3. Seeking breast health care in a health care delivery system with perceived appropriate and available care will result in diagnosis of breast cancer in its early stages.

Implications for Nursing

The theory of perceived access provides nurses with an opportunity for testing the relationships among culture; health definitions; health practices; and perceived necessity, availability, and appropriateness of breast cancer screening. The theory may aid in the discovery of the culturally appropriate approaches for promoting breast health care.

Learning Activities

1. Find an example of a nursing theory in a current book or periodical. Review the theory and classify it based on scope or level of abstraction (grand theory, middle range theory, or practice theory), the purpose of the theory (describe, explain, predict, or control), and the source or discipline in which the theory was developed.
2. Find an example of a middle range nursing theory (see Chapter 10 or 11 for ideas). Following the preceding exemplar, identify the components of the theory (e.g., scope of the theory, purpose, concepts and definitions, etc.).
3. Find an example of a middle range theory that does not contain a model. With classmates, try to create a model that depicts the relationships between and among the concepts. Discuss the challenges posed by this exercise.

REFERENCES

Ade-Oshifogun, J. B. (2012). Model of functional performance in obese elderly people with chronic obstructive pulmonary disease. *Journal of Nursing Scholarship, 44*(3), 232–241.

Artinian, B. (1982). Conceptual mapping: Development of the strategy. *Western Journal of Nursing Research, 4*(4), 379–393.

Barnum, B. S. (1998). *Nursing theory: Analysis, application, evaluation* (5th ed.). Philadelphia: Lippincott Williams & Wilkins.

Benner, P. (2001). *From novice to expert: Excellence and power in clinical nursing practice* (Commemorative edition). Upper Saddle River, NJ: Prentice-Hall.

Bulechek, G. M., Butcher, H. K., Dochterman, G. M., & Wagner, C. (2012). *Nursing interventions classification* (6th ed.). St. Louis: Mosby.

Cesario, S. (1997). The impact of the electronic domain on theory construction. *Journal of Theory Construction and Testing, 1*(2), 60–63.

Chinn, P. L., & Kramer, M. K. (2011). *Integrated knowledge developing in nursing* (7th ed.). St. Louis: Mosby.

Davidson, J. E. (2010). Facilitated sensemaking: A strategy and new middle-range theory to support families of intensive care unit patients. *Critical Care Nurse, 30*(6), 28–34.

Dickoff, J., & James, P. (1968). A theory of theories: A position paper. *Nursing Research, 17*(3), 197–203.

Dickoff, J., James, P., & Wiedenbach, E. (1968). Theory in a practice discipline part II: Practice oriented research. *Nursing Research, 17*(6), 545–554.

Doering, J., & Durfor, S. L. (2011). The process of "persevering toward normalcy" after childbirth. *MCN, 36*(4), 258–266.

Drake, D. A., Luna, M., Georges, J. M., & Steege, L. M. B. (2012). Hospital nurse force theory: A perspective of nurse fatigue and patient harm. *Advances in Nursing Science, 35*(4), 305–314.

Falk-Rafael, A., & Betker, C. (2012). The primacy of relationships: A study of public health nursing practice from a critical caring perspective. *Advances in Nursing Science, 35*(4), 315–332.

Fawcett, J. (1999). *The relationship of theory and research* (3rd ed.). Philadelphia: F. A. Davis.

Finnegan, L., Shaver, J. L., Zenk, S. N., Wikie, D. J., & Ferrans, C. E. (2010). The symptom cluster experience profile framework. *Oncology Nursing Forum, 37*(6), E377–E385.

Flaskerud, J. H. (1984). Nursing models as conceptual frameworks for research. *Western Journal of Nursing Research, 6*(2), 153–155.

Gallagher, P. (2011). Becoming normal: A grounded theory study on the emotional process of stroke recovery. *Canadian Journal of Neuroscience Nursing, 33*(3), 24–31.

Gillespie, B. M., Chaboyer, W., Wallis, M., & Grimbeek, P. (2007). Resilience in the operating room: Developing and testing of a resilience model. *Journal of Advanced Nursing, 59*(4), 427–438.

Greco, K. E., Nail, L. M., Kendall, J., Cartwright, J., & Messecar, D. C. (2010). Mammography decision making in older women with a breast cancer family history. *Journal of Nursing Scholarship, 42*(3), 348–356.

Green, A., & Davis, S. (2005). Toward a predictive model of patient satisfaction with nurse practitioner care. *Journal of the American Academy of Nurse Practitioners, 17*(4), 139–148.

Hamilton, R. J., & Bowers, B. J. (2007). The theory of genetic vulnerability: A Roy model exemplar. *Nursing Science Quarterly, 20*(3), 254–264.

Hardin, S. R., & Bishop, S. M. (2010). Theory development process. In M. R. Alligood & A. M. Tomey (Eds.), *Nursing theorists and their work* (7th ed., pp. 36–49). St. Louis: Mosby.

Hardy, M. E. (1973). The nature of theories. *Theoretical foundations for nursing*. New York: MSS Information Systems.

Hastings-Tolsma, M. (2006). Toward a theory of diversity of human field pattern. *Visions, 14*(2), 34–46.

Hickman, J. S. (2011). An introduction to nursing theory. In J. B. George (Ed.), *Nursing theories: The base for professional nursing practice* (6th ed., pp. 1–22). Upper Saddle River, NJ: Pearson Education.

Higgins, P. A., & Moore, S. M. (2000). Levels of theoretical thinking in nursing. *Nursing Outlook, 48*(4), 179–183.

Im, E. O. (2006). A situation-specific theory of Caucasian cancer patients' pain experience. *Advances in Nursing Science, 29*(3), 232–244.

Im, E. O., Stuifbergen, A. K., & Walker, L. (2010). A situation-specific theory of midlife women's attitudes toward physical activity (MAPA). *Nursing Outlook, 58*(1), 52–58.

Jacox, A. K. (1974). Theory construction in nursing: An overview. *Nursing Research, 23*(1), 4–13.

Kim, S., Reed, P. G., Hayward, R. D., Kang, Y., & Koenig, H. G. (2011). Spirituality and psychological well-being: Testing a theory of family interdependence among family caregivers and their elders. *Research in Nursing & Health, 34*(1), 103–115.

Law, R. (2009). 'Bridging worlds': Meeting the emotional needs of dying patients. *Journal of Advanced Nursing, 65*(12), 2630–2641.

Lee, Y. S., & Laffrey, S. C. (2006). Predictors of physical activity in older adults with borderline hypertension. *Nursing Research, 55*(2), 110–120.

McMahon, M. A., & Christopher, K. A. (2011). Toward a mid-range theory of nursing presence. *Nursing Forum, 46*(2), 71–81.

Marrs, J., & Lowry, L. W. (2006). Nursing theory and practice: Connecting the dots. *Nursing Science Quarterly, 19*(1), 44–50.

McKenna, H. P., & Slevin, O. D. (2008). *Vital notes for nurses: Nursing models, theories and practice*. Oxford, United Kingdom: Blackwell Publishing.

Meleis, A. I. (2012). *Theoretical nursing: Development and progress* (5th ed.). Philadelphia: Lippincott Williams & Wilkins.

Moody, L. E. (1990). *Advancing nursing science through research*. Newbury Park, CA: Sage Publications.

Nelson, A. M. (2006). Toward a situation-specific theory of breastfeeding. *Research and Theory for Nursing Practice: An International Journal, 20*(1), 9–19.

Peterson, S. J. (2013). Introduction to the nature of nursing knowledge. In S. J. Peterson and T. S. Bredow (Eds.), *Middle range theories: Application to nursing research* (3rd ed., pp. 3–41). Philadelphia: Lippincott Williams & Wilkins.

Powers, B. A., & Knapp, T. R. (2011). *Dictionary of nursing theory and research* (4th ed.). New York: Springer.

Pryjmachuk, S. (1996). A nursing perspective on the interrelationships between theory, research and practice. *Journal of Advanced Nursing, 23*, 679–684.

Reynolds, P. D. (1971). *A primer in theory construction*. New York: Macmillan.

Robles-Silva, L. (2008). The caregiving trajectory among poor and chronically ill people. *Qualitative Health Research, 18*(3), 358–368.

Roy, C., & Roberts, S. (1981). *Theory construction in nursing: An adaptation model*. Englewood Cliffs, NJ: Prentice-Hall.

Sauls, D. J., & Grassley, J. (2011). Development of the adolescent support model. *Journal of Theory Construction & Testing, 15*(1), 24–28.

Streubert, H. J., & Carpenter, D. R. (2011). *Qualitative research in nursing: Advancing the humanistic imperative* (5th ed.). Philadelphia: Lippincott Williams & Wilkins.

Tourangeau, A. E. (2005). A theoretical model of the determinants of mortality. *Advances in Nursing Science, 28*(1), 58–69.

Walker, L. O., & Avant, K. C. (2011). *Strategies for theory construction in nursing* (5th ed.). Upper Saddle River, NJ: Prentice-Hall.

Weick, K. E. (2001). *Making sense of the organization*. London, United Kingdom: Blackwell Publishers.

Zauderer, C. R. (2008). A case study of postpartum depression & altered maternal–newborn attachment. *The American Journal of Maternal Child Nursing, 33*(3), 172–177.

Zeigler, V. I., & Tilley, D. S. (2011). Almost normal: A practice-oriented conceptual model of adolescent living with implantable cardioverter defibrillators. *Journal of Theory Construction & Testing, 14*(1), 23–27.

CHAPTER 5

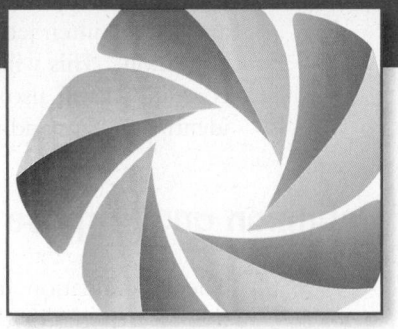

Theory Analysis and Evaluation

Melanie McEwen

Jerry Thompson is nearing completion of his master's degree in nursing. He is currently a case manager for a home health agency, and his goal is to become an agency director after he completes his degree. For his research application project, Jerry wants to compare the effectiveness of health teaching in the hospital setting with the effectiveness of health teaching in the home setting. He has identified several areas to examine. These include the quality and type of health information provided, professional competencies of the nurses providing the information, the client's support system, and environmental resources. Outcome variables he will measure focus on utilization of health care (e.g., length of time on home health service, hospital readmissions, development of complications).

As his research project began to take shape, Jerry realized he needed a conceptual framework to help him set it up and organize it. His advisor suggested Pender's Health Promotion Model. To determine if the model would be appropriate for his study, Jerry obtained the latest edition of Pender's book (Pender, Murdaugh, & Parsons, 2010), which described the model in depth. He then read commentaries in nursing theory books that analyzed her work and completed a literature search to find examples of research studies using the Health Promotion Model as a conceptual framework. After he had compiled the information, Jerry summarized his findings by using Whall's (2005) criteria for analysis and evaluation of middle range theories.

This exercise helped Jerry gain insight into the major concepts of the model and let him examine its important assumptions and linkages. From the evaluation, he determined that the model would be appropriate for use as the conceptual framework for his research study.

As nurses began to participate in the processes of theory development in the 1960s, they realized that there was a corresponding need to identify criteria or develop mechanisms to determine if those theories served their intended purpose. As a result, the first method to describe, analyze, and critique theory was published in 1968. Over the following decades, a number of methods or techniques for theory evaluation were proposed. A general understanding of these methods will help nurses select an evaluation method for theory, which is appropriate to the stage of theory development and for the intended application of the theory (research, practice, administration, or education). This will, in turn, help ensure that the theory is valid and is being used correctly. It will also provide information for developing and testing new theories by identifying gaps and inconsistencies.

Definition and Purpose of Theory Evaluation

Theory evaluation has been defined as the process of systematically examining a theory. Criteria for this process are variable, but they generally include examination of the theory's origins, meaning, logical adequacy, usefulness, generalizability, and testability. Theory evaluation does not generate new information outside the confines of the theory, but it often leads to new insights about the theory being examined.

In short, theory evaluation identifies a theory's degree of usefulness to guide practice, research, education, and administration. Such evaluation gives insight into relationships among concepts and their linkages to each other and allows the reviewer to determine the strengths and weaknesses of a theory. It also assists in identifying the need for additional theory development or refinement. Finally, theory evaluation provides a systematic, objective way of examining a theory that may lead to new insights and new formulations that will add to the body of knowledge and thereby affects practice or research (Walker & Avant, 2011). The ultimate goal of theory evaluation is to determine the potential contribution of the theory to scientific knowledge.

In nursing practice, theory evaluation may provide a clinician with additional knowledge about the soundness of the theory. It also helps identify which theoretical relationships are supported by research, provides guidelines for the choice of appropriate interventions, and gives some indication of their efficacy. In research, theory evaluation helps clarify the form and structure of a theory being tested or will allow the researcher to determine the relevance of the content of a theory for use as a conceptual framework, as described in the case study. Evaluation will also identify inconsistencies and gaps in the theory when used in practice or research (Walker & Avant, 2011). See Link to Practice 5-1 for another example.

Link to Practice 5-1

The Synergy Model for Patient Care

The Synergy Model for Patient Care was developed by the American Association of Critical Care Nurses (AACN) to be used as the basis for the AACN's certification examination (Curley, 1998). Although the model was explicitly designed to be used to direct nursing care for critically ill patients in the acute care settings (practice), it has also been used in numerous research studies, as well as in many different types of settings and for varying types of patients.

When considering its original intended purpose, what processes or methods might a nurse use to determine the Synergy Model's suitability for:

- Directing nursing practice in a high school or occupational health setting?
- Working with elders in a long-term care facility?
- Planning care for a home-based hospice patient?
- Guiding a research study in a pediatric hospital?

Various methods have been outlined to assist with this process. The methods are described by several overlapping terms or terms that are used in different ways by different authors. For example, theory analysis, theory description, theory evaluation, and theory critique all describe the process of critically reviewing a theory to assess its relevance and applicability to nursing practice, research, education, and administration. In this chapter, "theory evaluation" is used as a global term to discuss the process of reviewing theory.

Theory evaluation has been described as a single-phase process (theory analysis) by Alligood (2010) as well as Hardy (1974) (theory evaluation), a two-phase process (theory analysis and theory critique/evaluation) by Fawcett and DeSanto-Madeya (2013) and Duffey and Muhlenkamp (1974), or a three-phase process (theory description, theory analysis, and theory critique/evaluation) by scholars including Meleis (2012) and Moody (1990). It should be noted that the methods are similar whether they describe one, two, or three phases. A three-phase process is outlined briefly in the following section. Later sections provide more detailed discussions of each phase.

Theory Description

Theory description is the initial step in the evaluation process. In theory description, the works of a theorist are reviewed with a focus on the historical context of the theory (Hickman, 2011). In addition, related works by others are examined to gain a clear understanding of the structural and functional components of the theory. The structural components include assumptions, concepts, and propositions. The functional components consist of the concepts of the theory and how they are used to describe, explain, predict, or control (Meleis, 2012; Moody, 1990).

Theory Analysis

Theory analysis is the second phase of the evaluation process. It refers to a systematic process of objectively examining the content, structure, and function of a theory. Theory analysis is conducted if the theory or framework has potential for being useful in practice, research, administration, or education. Theory analysis is a nonjudgmental, detailed examination of a theory, the main aim of which is to understand the theory (Fawcett & DeSanto-Madeya, 2013; Meleis, 2012).

Theory Evaluation

Theory evaluation, or theory critique, is the final step of the process. Evaluation follows analysis and assesses the theory's potential contribution to the discipline's knowledge base (Fawcett & DeSanto-Madeya, 2013; Walker & Avant, 2011). In theory evaluation, critical reflection involves ascertaining how well a theory serves its purpose, with the process of evaluation resulting in a decision or action about use of the theory (Chinn & Kramer, 2011). This includes consideration of how the theory is used to direct nursing practice and interventions and whether or not it contributes to favorable outcomes (Hickman, 2011).

Historical Overview of Theory Analysis and Evaluation

Since the late 1960s, a number of nursing scholars have published systems or methods for theory analysis/evaluation. Table 5-1 provides a list of these works. Basic components of the processes described by each are presented in the following sections.

Table 5-1 Publications of Methods for Nursing Theory Analysis and Evaluation

Nursing Scholar	Dates of Publications	Techniques Described (Most Recent Publication)
Rosemary Ellis	1968	Characteristics of significant theories
Margaret Hardy	1974, 1978	Theory evaluation
Mary Duffey and Ann Muhlenkamp	1974	Theory analysis and theory evaluation
Barbara Barnum (Stevens)	1979, 1984, 1990, 1994, 1998	Theory evaluation—internal criticism, external criticism
Lorraine Walker and Kay Avant	1983, 1988, 1995, 2005, 2011	Theory analysis
Jacqueline Fawcett	1980, 1993, 1995, 2000, 2005, 2013	Theory (conceptual framework) analysis and theory (conceptual framework) evaluation
Peggy Chinn and Maeona Kramer (Jacobs)	1983, 1987, 1991, 1995, 1999, 2004, 2008, 2011	Theory description and critical reflection
Afaf Meleis	1985, 1991, 1997, 2007, 2012	Theory description, theory analysis, theory critique
Joyce Fitzpatrick and Ann Whall	1989, 1996, 2005	Analysis and evaluation of practice theory, middle range theory, and nursing models
Sharon Dudley-Brown	1997	Theory evaluation

It should be noted that most of the processes/methods for theory analysis and theory evaluation were implicitly or explicitly developed to review grand nursing theories and conceptual frameworks. Only in recent years have the processes and methods been applied to middle range theories and, rarely, practice theories. This observation, however, does not negate the need for analysis and evaluation (whether formal or informal) of middle range and practice theories. Furthermore, the processes should be applicable to all levels of theory.

Characteristics of Significant Theories: Ellis

Probably the first nursing scholar to document criteria for analyzing theories for use by nurses was Rosemary Ellis. Although not specifically describing a process or method of theory analysis or evaluation, Ellis (1968) identified characteristics of significant theories. The characteristics she specified were scope, complexity, testability, usefulness, implicit values of the theorist, information generation, and meaningful terminology. Her discussion of these characteristics produced the foundation on which later writers developed their criteria.

Theory Evaluation: Hardy

A few years after Ellis, Margaret Hardy (1974) wrote that theory should be evaluated according to certain universal standards. In her writings, Hardy provided a more detailed description of criteria for theory evaluation and presented personal insight on the processes needed. Criteria or standards she suggested for theory evaluation were as follows:

- Meaning and logical adequacy
- Operational and empirical adequacy
- Testability
- Generality
- Contribution to understanding
- Predictability
- Pragmatic adequacy

In a later work (1978), Hardy discussed logical adequacy (diagramming) and stated that because a theory is a set of interrelated concepts and statements, its structure can be analyzed for internal consistency by examining the syntax of the theory as well as its content. Diagramming involves identifying all major theoretical terms (concepts, constructs, operational definitions, and referents). Once identified, each component can be represented by a symbol, and a model may be drawn illustrating relationships or linkages between or among the terms. These linkages should specify the direction, the type of relationship (whether positive or negative), and the form of the relationship.

According to Hardy (1974), empirical adequacy is the single most important criterion for evaluating a theory applied in practice. Assessing empirical adequacy requires reviewing literature and critically reading relevant research; it is necessary to determine if hypotheses testing the theory are clearly deduced from the theory. The entire body of relevant studies should be evaluated in terms of the extent to which it supports the theory or a part of the theory. Finally, the criteria of usefulness and significance refer to the theory's use in controlling, altering, or manipulating major variables and conditions specified by the theory to realize a desired outcome.

Theory Analysis and Theory Evaluation: Duffey and Muhlenkamp

Writing at approximately the same time as Hardy, Duffey, and Muhlenkamp (1974) published a two-phase approach to critically examining nursing theory. Theory analysis was the first phase, for which they posited four questions for examination. For theory evaluation, they suggested six additional questions (Box 5-1).

Box 5-1 Questions for Theory Analysis and Theory Evaluation: Duffey and Muhlenkamp

Theory Analysis

1. What is the origin of the problem(s) with which the theory is concerned?
2. What methods were used in theory development (induction, deduction, synthesis)?
3. What is the character of the subject matter dealt with by the theory?
4. What kind of outcomes of testing propositions are generated by the theory?

Theory Evaluation

1. Does the theory generate testable hypotheses?
2. Does the theory guide practice or can it be used as a body of knowledge?
3. Is the theory complete in terms of subject matter and perspective?
4. Are the biases or values underlying the theory made explicit?
5. Are the relationships among the propositions made explicit?
6. Is the theory parsimonious?

Box 5-2 Theory Evaluation Criteria: Barnum

Internal Criticism
Clarity
Consistency
Adequacy
Logical development
Level of theory development

External Criticism
Reality convergence (how the theory relates to the real world)
Utility
Significance
Discrimination (differentiation between nursing and other health professions)
Scope
Complexity

Theory Evaluation: Barnum

Barbara Barnum (Stevens) first published her ideas for theory evaluation in 1979. Subsequent editions were published in 1984, 1990, 1994, and 1998. Barnum suggested a method of theory evaluation that differentiates internal and external criticisms. Internal criticism examines how the components of the theory fit with each other; external criticism examines how a theory relates to the extant world. Box 5-2 lists points to be examined for both.

Theory Analysis: Walker and Avant

Lorraine Walker and Kay Avant first presented their detailed methods for theory analysis in 1983. Their work was subsequently revised in 1988, 1995, 2005, and 2011. Building on a multiphase background of concept and statement development, which involves concept and statement analysis, synthesis, and derivation, they expanded the processes to include theory analysis. Table 5-2 gives a brief synopsis of the process of theory analysis they propose.

Theory Analysis and Evaluation: Fawcett

Jacqueline Fawcett (1980, 1993, 1995, 2000, 2005; Fawcett & DeSanto-Madeya, 2013) used a two-phase process for analysis and evaluation of theories and conceptual frameworks. In her writings, she noted that analysis is a nonjudgmental, detailed examination of a theory. In Fawcett's most recent work (Fawcett & DeSanto-Madeya, 2013), components of the analysis process include the theory's origins, unique focus, and content. The theory's "origins" refers to the historical evolution of the model/theory, the author's motivation, philosophical assumptions about nursing, the author's inclusion of works of nursing and non-nursing scholars, and the worldview reflected by the model.

The unique focus refers to distinctive views of the metaparadigm concepts, different problems in nurse–patient situations or interactions, and differences in modes of nursing interventions. She notes that theories can be categorized as developmental,

Table 5-2 Theory Analysis: Walker and Avant

Step	Questions or Tasks
Determine the origins of the theory.	Identify the basis of the original development of the theory. Why was it developed? Was the process of development inductive or deductive? Is there evidence to support or refute the theory?
Examine the meaning of the theory.	Identify concepts. Examine definitions and their use (theoretical and operational definitions). Identify statements. Examine relationships.
Analyze the logical adequacy of the theory.	Determine if scientists agree on predictive ability of the theory. Determine if the content makes sense. Identify any logical fallacies.
Determine the usefulness of the theory.	Is the theory practical and helpful to nursing? Does it contribute to understanding and predicting outcomes?
Define the degree of generalizability.	Is the theory highly generalizable or specific?
Determine if the theory is parsimonious.	Can the theory be stated briefly and simply or is it complex?
Determine the testability of the theory.	Can the theory be supported with empirical data? Can testable hypotheses be generated from the theory?

Source: Walker & Avant (2011).

systems, interaction, needs, client-focused, person–environment interaction–focused, or nursing therapeutics–focused. The content of the model is examined to analyze the abstract and general concepts and propositions. Fawcett's method of theory analysis specifically identifies whether and how the concepts and propositions of the metaparadigm (nursing, environment, health, and person) are included in the theory. Representative questions to be addressed relative to the content include: "How are human beings defined and described? How is environment defined and described? How is health defined? . . . What is the goal of nursing? . . . and What statements are made about the relations among the four metaparadigm concepts?" (Fawcett & DeSanto-Madeya, 2013, p. 49).

Theory evaluation requires judgments to be made about a theory's significance based on how it satisfies certain criteria (Fawcett & DeSanto-Madeya, 2013). The process of theory evaluation includes review of previously published critiques, research reports, and reports of practical application of the theory. During the process of theory evaluation, the criteria to be examined are the explication of the origins of the theory, the comprehensiveness of the content, its logical congruence, how well it can lead to generation of new theory, and its legitimacy. The legitimacy is determined by reviewing the theory's social utility, social congruence, and social significance. The final step in theory evaluation is to examine the theory's contribution to the discipline of nursing.

Theory Description and Critique: Chinn and Kramer

Peggy Chinn and Maeona Kramer (Jacobs) initially wrote on the processes used to analyze theory in 1983. They used the terms theory description and critical reflection to describe a two-phase process. Theory description has six elements: purpose, concepts, definitions, relationships, structure, and assumptions. Table 5-3 presents these elements and their defining characteristics.

Critical reflection of a theory involves determining how well a theory serves its purpose. Critical reflection analyzes clarity and consistency of the theory as well

Table 5-3 Components of Theory Description: Chinn and Kramer

Component	Characteristics
Purpose	The purpose of the theory should be stated explicitly or at least be identifiable in the text of the theory.
Concepts	The concepts of the theory should be linguistically expressed.
Definitions	Meanings of concepts are conveyed in theoretical definitions; these definitions give character to the theory.
Relationships	Concepts are structured into a systematic form that links each concept with others.
Structure	The relationships are linked to form a whole when the ideas of the theory interconnect; structure makes it possible to follow the reasoning of the theory.
Assumptions	Assumptions refer to underlying truths that determine the nature of concepts, definitions, purpose, relationship, and structure; may not be explicitly stated.

Source: Chinn & Kramer (2011).

as its complexity, generality, accessibility, and importance. In assessing clarity and consistency, Chinn and Kramer's (2011) critical reflection would examine:

- Semantic clarity—Are the concepts defined? Do the concepts establish empirical meaning?
- Semantic consistency—Are the concepts used consistently? Are the concepts congruent with their definitions?
- Structural clarity—Are the connections and reasoning within the theory understandable?
- Structural consistency—Is the structure of the theory consistent in its form?
- Simplicity or complexity—Is the theory simple? Is the theory complex?
- Generality—Does the theory cover a wide scope of experiences and phenomena?
- Accessibility—How accessible is the theory? How well are concepts grounded in empirically identifiable phenomena?
- Importance—How can the theory contribute to nursing practice, research, and education?

Theory Description, Analysis, and Critique: Meleis

According to Meleis (1985, 2007, 2012), there are three stages involved in theory evaluation: theory description, theory analysis, and theory critique. During the process of theory description, the reviewer closely examines the structural and functional components of the theory. The structural components include assumptions (implicit and explicit), concepts, and propositions. The functional assessment considers the anticipated consequence of the theory and its purpose. Components that should be examined are the focus of the theory and how it addresses the client, nursing, health, the nurse–client interactions, environment, nursing problems, and nursing therapeutics.

Theory analysis involves considering important variables that may have influenced the development of the theory. These include the theorist, paradigmatic origins of the theory, and internal dimensions of the theory. During the analysis procedure, Meleis (2012) recommends reviewing external and internal factors that influenced the theorist, as well as the theorist's experiential background, educational background, and employment history. Likewise, a reconstruction of the professional and academic networks that surrounded the theorist while the theory was evolving should be examined.

Second, Meleis argues that careful consideration of use of theories from other fields or paradigms is to be encouraged. To identify the paradigm(s) from which the theory may have evolved, or to recognize other theorists who may have influenced the development of the theory, the reviewer would consider references, educational and experiential background of the theorist, and the sociocultural context of the theory as it was developed.

Finally, internal dimensions of the theory should be analyzed. This will provide information about the rationale on which the theory is built, systems of relationships, content of the theory, goal of the theory, scope of the theory, context of the theory, abstractness of the theory, and method of development.

Critique of a theory may follow analysis, and Meleis (2012) identified five elements to consider in this phase: the relationship between structure and function, diagram of the theory, circle of contagiousness, usefulness, and external components. The relationship between structure and function involves evaluating the theory's clarity and consistency, level of simplicity or complexity, and tautology/teleology. In assessing the tautology of the theory, the reviewer would observe for needless repetition of an idea in different parts of the theory, which Meleis claims will decrease the clarity of the theory. Teleology occurs when definitions of concepts, conditions, and events are described by consequences rather than properties and dimensions; this should be avoided.

Although not all theories contain models graphically or pictorially depicting the structure of the theory, Meleis (2012) states that theories and models are enhanced by visual representation. The reviewer should determine if the model does indeed help clarify linkages among the concepts and propositions and, thereby, enhance clarity of the theory.

The circle of contagiousness refers to whether, and to what extent, the model or theory has been adopted by other experts in the field. In evaluating usefulness, Meleis suggests analysis of the theory's usefulness in practice, research, education, and administration.

The final component of this method is the review of external components of the theory. These include implicit and explicit personal values of both the theorist and the critic. It also refers to congruence with other professional values as well as with social values. Finally, the critic would determine whether the theory has social significance.

Analysis and Evaluation of Practice Theory, Middle Range Theory, and Nursing Models: Whall

Whall (2005) is the only nurse scholar to explicitly outline three separate criteria for analysis and evaluation for the three levels of nursing theory. In her most recent edition, she noted that middle range and practice theories have achieved status equal to that of nursing conceptual models, but it has only been nursing models that have been systematically examined. Following this observation, she outlined distinct, although similar, criteria for evaluation of all three levels of nursing theory using a three-phase approach that reviews basic considerations, internal analysis and evaluation, and external analysis and evaluation.

According to Whall (2005), practice theory is produced from practice and deduced from middle range theory as well as from research. Because practice theory is designed for immediate application to practice, questions regarding the fit with empirical data are important in the evaluation process. Operational definitions and descriptions of how to apply practice theory are also important. Internal analysis of practice theory may be accomplished by diagramming the interrelationships of all concepts to detect lapses and inconsistencies in the theory's structure. The assumptions of the theory should be considered in light of historical and current perspectives of nursing. This should include ethical and cultural implications of the theory. External analysis should compare standards of care with the theory and examine nursing research to determine if it supports the theory, is neutral, or is in opposition.

Analysis and evaluation of middle range theory modifies the guidelines used for nursing conceptual models. It examines whether the theory fits with the existing nursing perspective and domains. Propositional statements should be examined to determine if they are causal or associative in nature, to assess their relative importance, and to find missing linkages between concepts. It is suggested that diagramming of the relationships may help identify missing relationships. Concepts should be operationally defined to support empirical adequacy. External analysis refers to congruence with more global theories and other related middle range theories. Examination of ethical, cultural, and social policy implications is crucial.

Whall (2005) believes nursing conceptual models should be assessed from a postmodern view. In addition, conceptual models should consider the major paradigm concepts (person, environment, health, and nursing) as well as additional concepts specific to the model. Analysis should examine whether the definitions of the concepts and statements are consistently used throughout the model and whether the interrelationships among the concepts are consistent. Internal analysis considers the assumptions and philosophical basis of the model and looks at the uniformity of discussion throughout the model. External consistency examines the model in relation to views external to the model (i.e., whether the model is being evaluated consistent with other nursing conceptual models and with nursing intervention classification systems). Table 5-4 lists some of the questions for consideration by Whall in analysis and evaluation of all three levels of nursing theory.

Theory Evaluation: Dudley-Brown

One of the most contemporary methods for theory evaluation was presented by Dudley-Brown (1997), who strongly relied on Kuhn's (1977) criteria for theory evaluation. In this method, evaluation should consider accuracy, consistency, fruitfulness, simplicity/complexity, scope, acceptability, and sociocultural utility.

To Dudley-Brown (1997), *accuracy* is essential because the theory should describe nursing as it exists today—not the nursing of the future or of the past. The theory should contain a worldview of nursing consistent with the present reality. *Consistency* relates to the importance of the nursing theory being internally consistent. There should be logical order: Terms, concepts, and statements should be used consistently and defined operationally.

Another criterion Dudley-Brown (1997) identifies for evaluation is *fruitfulness.* For this criterion, the theory should be useful in generating information and significant in contributing to the development of nursing knowledge.

Simplicity/complexity is a fourth criterion for evaluation. Both simple and complex theories are needed. In general, a theory should be balanced and logical. The theory should describe the phenomenon consistently in terms of simplicity or complexity.

Scope is a fifth criterion because theories of both broad and limited scope are needed. Scope should be dependent on the phenomenon and its context. Acceptance

Table 5-4 Criteria for Analysis and Evaluation of Theory: Whall

Level of Theory	Basic Considerations	Internal Analysis and Evaluation	External Analysis and Evaluation
Practice theory	Can the concepts be operationalized? Are operationalized concepts congruent with empirical data? Do statements lead to directives for nursing care? Are statements sufficient to practice and not contradictory?	Are there gaps or inconsistencies within the theory that may lead to conflicts and difficulties? Are assumptions congruent with nursing's historical perspective? Are assumptions congruent with ethical standards and social policy? Are assumptions in conflict with given cultural groups?	Is the theory produced with existing nursing standards? Is the theory consistent with existing standards of education within nursing? Is the theory related to nursing diagnoses and nursing intervention practices? Is the theory supported by existing research internal and external to nursing?
Middle range theory	What are the definitions and relative importance of major concepts? What is the type and relative importance of major theoretical statements?	What are the assumptions of the theory? What is the relationship of the theory to philosophy of science positions? Are concepts related/not related via statements? Is there internal consistency and congruency of all component parts of the theory? What is the empirical adequacy of the theory? Has the theory been examined in practice and research, and has it held up to this scrutiny?	What is the congruency with related theory and research internal and external to nursing? What is the congruence with the perspective of nursing, the domains, and the persistent questions? What ethical, cultural, and social policy issues are related to the theory?
Nursing models	What are the definitions of person, nursing, health, and environment? What are additional understandings of the metaparadigm concepts? What are the interrelationships among the metaparadigm concepts? What are the descriptions of other concepts found in the model?	What are the underlying assumptions of the model? What are the definitions of other components of the model? What is the relative importance of basic concepts or other components of the model? What are the analyses of internal and external consistency? What are the analyses of adequacy?	Is nursing research based on the model or related to the model? Is nursing education based on the model or related to the model? Is nursing practice based on the model? What is the relationship to existing nursing diagnoses and interventions systems?

refers to the adoption of the theory by others. Theories should be useful in practice, education, research, or administration.

Sociocultural utility is the final criterion for evaluation. Social congruence encompasses the beliefs, values, and expectations of different cultures. The theory should be measured against the criterion of social utility according to the culture for which it was proposed. Theories proposed for Western societies need to be evaluated for their philosophical and theoretical relevance in other societies and cultures.

Comparisons of Methods

Several authors (Dudley-Brown, 1997; Moody, 1990; Meleis, 2012) have compared many of the theory analysis and evaluation methods described here. A number of similarities can be found between and among all the methods. Table 5-5 provides a list of the methods reviewed and criteria specified by each author. It is important to note that different authors use different terms for similar concepts; thus, some interpretation of meaning of terms was necessary for the comparison.

As Table 5-5 shows, the most common criteria identified among the theory evaluation methods were an examination of complexity/simplicity (7 of 9) and scope/generality (7 of 9 methods). Other common criteria were inclusion of meaningful terminology, definitions of concepts (6 of 9), consistency (6 of 9), contribution to understanding (5 of 9), usefulness (6 of 9), testability (4 of 9), logical adequacy (4 of 9), and validity/accuracy/empirical adequacy (4 of 9). Criteria mentioned in only one or two methods were implicit values of the theorist, information generation, reality convergence, discrimination between nursing and other health professions, consequences, method of development, correspondence to existing standards, origins of the theory, context, pragmatic adequacy, and application of or to nursing therapeutics.

There appears to be an evolution of the processes over the past three decades. Similarities of criteria were evident based on time of initial writing. Ellis, Duffey and Muhlenkamp, and Hardy were the first nurses to describe the processes of theory evaluation, and their criteria are similar. The methods proposed by Walker and Avant are also consistent with those of Hardy and Ellis. Fawcett's model is similar to Chinn and Kramer's approach and to Barnum's internal criticism criteria. Meleis and Whall present the most detailed methods. Meleis' system has three components (description, analysis, and critical reflection) and Whall's examines three levels of theory. Barnum and Whall are similar in that they describe separate internal and external dimensions. The later works of Whall, Meleis, and Dudley-Brown are similar because they include characteristics of circle of contagion and consideration of social and cultural significance as evaluation criteria.

Most methods for analysis and evaluation were developed and used to review grand nursing theories. Indeed, a literature review resulted in no published report of theory evaluation in nursing beyond those in nursing theory textbooks. Books that focus on analysis and evaluation of grand nursing theories include those by Alligood and Tomey (2010), Fawcett (1993, 1995, 2000, 2005, 2013), Fitzpatrick and Whall (2005), George (2002, 2011), Masters (2012), and Parker and Smith (2010). Alligood and Tomey (2010), Parker and Smith (2010), Peterson and Bredow (2013), and Smith and Liehr (2013) also analyze/evaluate selected middle range nursing theories in their works.

Synthesized Method of Theory Evaluation

Following the detailed review and comparison of the many methods for theory analysis and evaluation, a method specifically designed to evaluate middle range and practice theories was developed (Box 5-3). These criteria were synthesized from the works of noted nursing scholars described earlier and are intended to be contemporary and responsive to both recent and anticipated changes in use of theory in nursing practice, research, education, and administration.

Table 5-5 Comparison of Theory Evaluation Criteria

Evaluation Criteria	Ellis	Hardy	Barnum	Walker and Avant	Fawcett	Chinn and Kramer	Meleis	Whall	Dudley-Brown
Complexity/simplicity	X		X	X	X	X	X		X
Testability	X	X		X	X				
Generality/scope	X	X	X	X	X	X			X
Usefulness	X	X	X	X		X	X		
Contribution to understanding		X	X		X	X			X
Implicit values	X						X		
Information generation	X								
Meaningful terminology (definitions)	X			X	X	X	X	X	
Logical adequacy		X	X	X				X	
Validity/accuracy/empirical adequacy		X			X			X	X
Predictability/tested		X				X		X	
Origins				X	X		X		
Clarity		X			X	X			
Consistency		X		X	X	X	X	X	
Context				X		X			
Pragmatic adequacy				X			X		
Reality convergence		X							
Discrimination		X							
Metaparadigm concepts					X	X	X		
Assumptions					X	X	X		
Purpose					X	X			
Consequences						X			
Nursing therapeutics interventions					X	X	X		
Method of development						X			
Circle of contagion						X	X	X	
Social/cultural significance					X	X	X	X	
Correspondence to standards/professional values						X	X		

Box 5-3 Synthesized Method for Theory Evaluation

Theory Description

What is the purpose of the theory (describe, explain, predict, prescribe)?
What is the scope or level of the theory (grand, middle range, practice/situation specific)?
What are the origins of the theory?
What are the major concepts?
What are the major theoretical propositions?
What are the major assumptions?
Is the context for use described?

Theory Analysis

Are concepts theoretically and operationally defined?
Are statements theoretically and operationally defined?
Are linkages explicit?
Is the theory logically organized?
Is there a model/diagram? Does the model contribute to clarifying the theory?
Are the concepts, statements, and assumptions used consistently?
Are outcomes or consequences stated or predicted?

Theory Evaluation

Is the theory congruent with current nursing standards?
Is the theory congruent with current nursing interventions or therapeutics?
Has the theory been tested empirically? Is it supported by research? Does it appear to be accurate/valid?
Is there evidence that the theory has been used by nursing educators, nursing researchers, or nursing administrators?
Is the theory relevant socially?
Is the theory relevant cross-culturally?
Does the theory contribute to the discipline of nursing?
What are implications for nursing related to implementation of the theory?

Summary

Nurses in clinical practice, as well as graduate students like Jerry Thompson from the case study, should know how to analyze or evaluate a theory to determine if it is reliable and valid and to determine when and how to apply it in practice, research, administration, or education. This chapter has presented and analyzed a number of different methods for evaluation of theory. Like many issues in the study of use of theory in nursing, the process of theory evaluation, although important, is often confusing. In addition, with very few exceptions, the methods or techniques were developed and used almost exclusively to analyze and evaluate grand nursing theories. It is hoped that with the current emphasis on development and use of both practice and middle range theories, there will be a concurrent emphasis on the analysis and evaluation of those theories. In this chapter, the most commonly used methods were described in some detail and compared. Following this comparison, a synthesized and simplified method for examination of theory was presented.

Key Points

- Theory evaluation is the process of systematically examining a theory; the intent of evaluation is to determine how well the theory guides practice, research, education, or administration.
- The process of theory evaluation typically includes examination of the theory's origins, meaning, logical adequacy, usefulness, generalizability, and testability. Additional criteria are also considered, depending on which process or technique is being used.
- Several different methods for theory analysis/theory evaluation have been proposed in the nursing literature.
- The Synthesized Method for Theory Evaluation was derived from other published methods and is intended to be used to evaluate middle range and practice theories.

To further help the reader understand the theory evaluation process, this chapter presents an exemplar of the synthesized method for theory evaluation.

THEORY EVALUATION EXEMPLAR: THEORY OF CHRONIC SORROW

Primary References for the Theory of Chronic Sorrow

Burke, M. L., Eakes, G. G., & Hainsworth, M. A. (1999). Milestones of chronic sorrow: Perspectives of chronically ill and bereaved persons and family caregivers. *Journal of Family Nursing, 5*(4), 374–387.

Eakes, G. G. (1993). Chronic sorrow: A response to living with cancer. *Oncology Nursing Forum, 20*(9), 1327–1334.

Eakes, G. G. (1995). Chronic sorrow: The lived experience of parents of chronically mentally ill individuals. *Archives of Psychiatric Nursing, 9*(2), 77–84.

Eakes, G. G. (2013). Chronic sorrow. In S. J. Peterson and T. S. Bredow (Eds.), *Middle range theories: Application to nursing research* (3rd ed., pp 96-107). Philadelphia: Lippincott Williams & Wilkins.

Eakes, G. G, Burke, M. L., & Hainsworth, M. A. (1998). Middle-range theory of chronic sorrow. *Image: Journal of Nursing Scholarship, 30*(2), 179–185.

References for Examples of Application of the Theory of Chronic Sorrow in Practice and Research

Bowes, S., Lowes, L., Warner, J., & Gregory, J. W. (2009). Chronic sorrow in parents of children with type 1 diabetes. *Journal of Advanced Nursing, 65*(5), 992–1000.

Gordon, J. (2009). An evidence-based approach for supporting parents experiencing chronic sorrow. *Pediatric Nursing, 35*(2), 115–123.

Hobdell, E. (2004). Chronic sorrow and depression in parents of children with neural tube defects. *Journal of Neuroscience Nursing, 36*(2), 82–84.

Hobdell, E. F., Grant, M. L., Valencia, I., Mare, J., Kothare, S. V., Legido, A., & Khurana, D. S. (2007). Chronic sorrow and coping in families of children with epilepsy. *Journal of Neuroscience Nursing, 39*(2), 76–83.

Isaksson, A. K., & Ahlstrom, G. (2008). Managing chronic sorrow: Experiences of patients with multiple sclerosis. *Journal of Neuroscience Nursing, 40*(3), 180–192.

Kendall, L. C. (2005). The experience of living with ongoing loss: Testing the Kendall chronic sorrow instrument (Doctoral dissertation, Virginia Commonwealth University).

Melvin, C. S., & Heater, B. S. (2004). Suffering and chronic sorrow: Characteristics and a paradigm for nursing interventions. *International Journal for Human Caring, 8*(2), 41–47.

Schreier, A. M., & Droes, N. S. (2010). Georgene Gaskill Eakes, Mary Lermann Burke, and Margaret A. Hainsworth: Theory of Chronic Sorrow. In M. R. Alligood & A. M. Tomey (Eds.), *Nursing theorists and their work* (7th ed., pp. 656-672). St. Louis: Mosby.

Smith, C. S. (2009). Substance abuse, chronic sorrow, and mothering loss: Relapse triggers among female victims of child abuse. *Journal of Pediatric Nursing, 24*(5), 401–410.

Theory Description

Scope of theory: Middle range

Purpose of theory: Explanatory theory—"to explain the experiences of people across the lifespan who encounter ongoing disparity because of significant loss" (Eakes, Burke, & Hainsworth, 1998, p. 179).

Origins of theory: "Chronic sorrow" appeared in the literature in 1962 to describe recurrent grief experienced by parents of children with disabilities. A number of research projects were conducted in the 1980s and 1990s describing chronic sorrow among various groups with loss situations. The resulting Theory of Chronic Sorrow, therefore, was inductively developed using concept analysis, extensive review of the literature, critical review of research, and validation in 10 qualitative studies of various loss situations (Eakes et al., 1998; Eakes, 2013).

Major concepts: Chronic sorrow, loss experience, disparity, trigger events (milestones), external management methods, internal management methods. All are defined and explained.

Major theoretical propositions are as follows:

1. Disparity between a desired relationship and an actual relationship or a disparity between current reality and desired reality is created by loss experiences.
2. Trigger events bring the negative disparity into focus or exacerbate the experience of disparity.
3. For individuals with chronic or life-threatening illnesses, chronic sorrow is most often triggered when the individual experiences disparity with accepted norms (social, developmental, or personal).
4. For family caregivers, disparity between the idealized and actual is associated with developmental milestones.
5. For bereaved individuals, disparity from the ideal is created by the absence of a person who was central in the life of the bereaved.

Major assumptions: Not stated

Context for use: "Experienced by individuals across the lifespan"; implied that it may be used in multiple settings and nursing situations.

Theory Analysis

Theoretical definitions for major concepts:

Chronic sorrow—the periodic recurrence of permanent, pervasive sadness or other grief-related feelings associated with ongoing disparity resulting from a loss experience

Loss experience—a significant loss, either actual or symbolic, that may be ongoing, with no predictable end, or a more circumscribed single-loss event

Disparity—a gap between the current reality and the desired as a result of a loss experience

Trigger events or milestones—a situation, circumstance, or condition that brings the negative disparity resulting from the loss into focus or exacerbates the disparity

External management methods—interventions provided by professionals to assist individuals to cope with chronic sorrow

Internal management methods—positive personal coping strategies used to deal with the periodic episodes of chronic sorrow

Operational definitions for major concepts: No operational definitions are provided in the original works.

Statements theoretically defined: Theoretical propositions are implicitly stated in the body of the text.

Statements operationally defined: Theoretical propositions are not operationally defined.

Linkages explicit: Linkages are described in the text and explicated in the model.

Logical organization: Theory is logically organized and described in detail.

Model/diagram: A model is provided and assists in explaining linkages of the concepts.

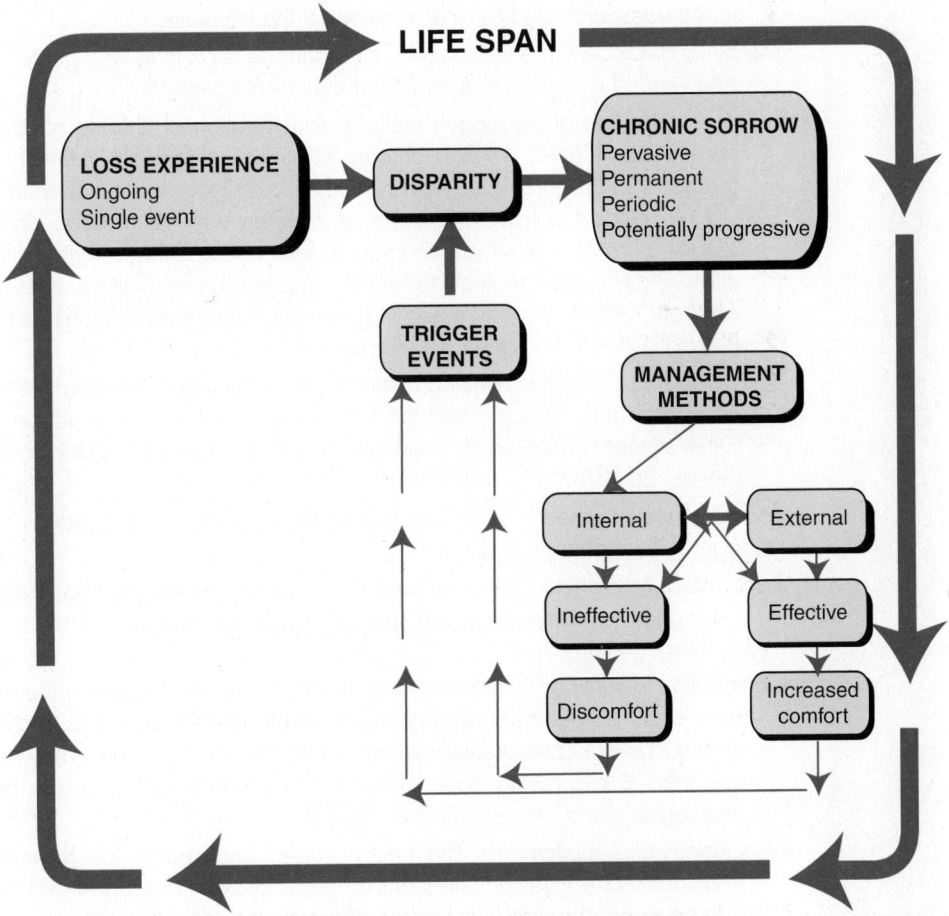

Theoretical model of chronic sorrow. (Source: Eakes, G. G., Burke, M. L., & Hainsworth, M. A. (1998). Middle range theory of chronic sorrow. Image: Journal of Nursing Scholarship, 30(2), 179–184. Used with permission of John Wiley & Sons LTD, Publisher.)

Consistent use of concepts, statements, and assumptions: Concepts and propositions are used consistently. Assumptions are not explicitly addressed.

Predicted or stated outcomes or consequences: Anticipated outcomes are stated in the model.

Theory Evaluation

Congruence with nursing standards: The theory appears congruent with nursing standards. A number of articles were identified in recent nursing literature describing how the construct of chronic sorrow has been identified among various aggregates (Eakes, 2013).

Congruence with current nursing interventions or therapeutics: Literature-based descriptions of application of components of the theory in nursing practice include caring for bereaved persons and family caregivers (Burke, Eakes, & Hainsworth, 1999), a discussion of caring for children with type 1 diabetes (Bowes, Lowes, Warner, & Gregory, 2009), interventions for community nurses to help assist families resolving chronic sorrow (Gordon, 2009), and interventions for suffering related to chronic sorrow (Melvin & Heater, 2004).

Evidence of empirical testing/research support/validity: The theory was derived from multiple research studies and a review of the literature.

The Burke/CCRCS Chronic Sorrow Questionnaire is an interview guide comprising 10 open-ended questions that explore the theory's concepts.

Research using the questionnaire includes investigation of chronic sorrow among cancer patients (Eakes, 1993), chronic sorrow in chronically mentally ill individuals (Eakes, 1995), chronic sorrow in women who were victims of child abuse (Smith, 2009), chronic sorrow in parents of children with neural tube defects (Hobdell, 2004), chronic sorrow and coping in families of children with epilepsy (Hobdell et al., 2007), and chronic sorrow among patients with multiple sclerosis (Isaksson & Ahlstrom, 2008). Further, a second instrument designed to measure chronic sorrow (Kendall, 2005) has been developed.

Use by nursing educators, nursing researchers, or nursing administrators: The references listed previously indicate that the theory has been used in practice and research. Other studies have cited the work of Eakes and colleagues related to chronic sorrow (Eakes, 2013).

Social relevance: Theory is relevant to individuals, families, and groups, irrespective of age or socioeconomic status.

Transcultural relevance: Theory is potentially relevant across cultures; theorist notes that "relevance for various cultural groups should be explored" (Eakes et al., 1998, p. 184).

Contribution to nursing: Authors note that the theory is applicable to different groups, but more study is needed to test the theory and to identify strategies to reduce disparity created by loss (prescriptive interventions). Despite the relative newness of the theory, there is a growing body of nursing literature reporting on use both related to interventions and research (Eakes, 2013).

Conclusions and implications: The theory is useful and appropriate for nurses practicing in a variety of settings. Implications for research were described and implications for education can be inferred. Further development of the theory is warranted to better explicate relationships and operationalize the concepts and propositions to allow testing.

Learning Activities

1. Obtain the original works of two of the nursing scholars whose theory analysis/evaluation strategies are discussed. Use the strategies to evaluate a recently published middle range nursing theory (see Chapter 11 for examples). How are the conclusions similar? How are they different?
2. For one of the nursing scholars who has published several versions or editions of her work (e.g., Fawcett, Chinn and Kramer, Meleis), obtain a copy of the oldest version and a copy of the most recent version and compare the strategies suggested. Have they changed?
3. Search the literature for examples of published accounts of nursing theory evaluation or theory analysis. Share your findings with classmates.

REFERENCES

Alligood, M. R. (2010). Introduction to nursing theory: Its history, significance and analysis. In M. R. Alligood & A. M. Tomey (Eds.), *Nursing theorists and their work* (7th ed., pp. 3–15). St. Louis: Mosby.

Alligood, M. R., & Tomey, A. M. (2010). *Nursing theorists and their work* (7th ed.). St. Louis: Mosby.

Barnum, B. S. (1984). *Nursing theory: Analysis, application, evaluation* (2nd ed.). Boston: Little Brown.

Barnum, B. S. (1990). *Nursing theory: Analysis, application, evaluation* (3rd ed.). Glenview, IL: Scott, Foresman/Little, Brown Higher Education.

Barnum, B. S. (1994). *Nursing theory: Analysis, application, evaluation* (4th ed.). Philadelphia: Lippincott Williams & Wilkins.

Barnum, B. S. (1998). *Nursing theory: Analysis, application, evaluation* (5th ed.). Philadelphia: Lippincott Williams & Wilkins.

Chinn, P. L., & Kramer, M. K. (1991). *Theory and nursing: A systematic approach* (3rd ed.). St. Louis: Mosby.

Chinn, P. L., & Kramer, M. K. (1995). *Theory and nursing: A systematic approach* (4th ed.). St. Louis: Mosby.

Chinn, P. L., & Kramer, M. K. (1999). *Theory and nursing: Integrated knowledge development* (5th ed.). St. Louis: Mosby.

Chinn, P. L., & Kramer, M. K. (2004). *Integrated theory and knowledge development in nursing* (6th ed.). St. Louis: Mosby.

Chinn, P. L., & Kramer, M. K. (2008). *Integrated theory and knowledge development in nursing* (7th ed.). St. Louis: Mosby.

Chinn, P. L., & Kramer, M. K. (2011). *Integrated theory and knowledge development in nursing* (8th ed.). St. Louis: Mosby.

Curley, M. A. Q. (1998). Patient-nurse synergy: Optimizing patients' outcomes. *American Journal of Critical Care, 7*(1), 64–72.

Dudley-Brown, S. L. (1997). The evaluation of nursing theory: A method for our madness. *International Journal of Nursing Studies, 34*(1), 76–83.

Duffey, M., & Muhlenkamp, A. F. (1974). A framework for theory analysis. *Nursing Outlook, 22*(9), 570–574.

Ellis, R. (1968). Characteristics of significant theories. *Nursing Research, 17*(3), 217–222.

Fawcett, J. (1980). A framework of analysis and evaluation of conceptual models of nursing. *Nurse Educator, 5*(6), 10–14.

Fawcett, J. (1993). *Analysis and evaluation of nursing theories.* Philadelphia: F. A. Davis.

Fawcett, J. (1995). *Analysis and evaluation of conceptual models of nursing* (3rd ed.). Philadelphia: F. A. Davis.

Fawcett, J. (2000). *Analysis and evaluation of contemporary nursing knowledge: Nursing models and theories.* Philadelphia: F. A. Davis.

Fawcett, J. (2005). *Contemporary nursing knowledge: Analysis and evaluation of nursing models and theories* (2nd ed.). Philadelphia: F. A. Davis.

Fawcett, J., & DeSanto-Madeya, S. (2013). *Contemporary nursing knowledge: Analysis and evaluation of nursing models and theories* (3rd ed.). Philadelphia: F. A. Davis.

Fitzpatrick, J. J., & Whall, A. (2005). *Conceptual models of nursing: Analysis and application* (4th ed.). Upper Saddle River, NJ: Prentice-Hall.

George, J. B. (2002). *Nursing theories: The base for professional nursing practice* (5th ed.). Upper Saddle River, NJ: Prentice-Hall.

George, J. B. (2011). *Nursing theories: The base for professional nursing practice* (6th ed.). Upper Saddle River, NJ: Pearson.

Hardy, M. E. (1974). Theories: Components, development, evaluation. *Nursing Research, 23,* 100–107.

Hardy, M. E. (1978). Perspectives on nursing theory. *Advances in Nursing Science, 1*(1), 27–48.

Hickman, J. S. (2011). An introduction to nursing theory. In J. B. George (Ed.), *Nursing theories: The base for professional nursing practice* (6th ed., 1–22). Upper Saddle River, NJ: Pearson.

Kuhn, T. S. (1977). Second thoughts on paradigms. In F. Suppe (Ed.), *The structure of scientific theory* (pp. 459–482). Urbana, IL: University of Illinois Press.

Masters, K. (2012). *Nursing theories: A framework for professional practice.* Sudbury, MA: Jones & Bartlett Learning.

Meleis, A. I. (1985). *Theoretical nursing: Development and progress.* Philadelphia: J. B. Lippincott.

Meleis, A. I. (2007). *Theoretical nursing: Development and progress* (4th ed.). Philadelphia: Lippincott Williams & Wilkins.

Meleis, A. I. (2012). *Theoretical nursing: Development and progress* (5th ed.). Philadelphia: Lippincott Williams & Wilkins.

Moody, L. E. (1990). *Advancing nursing science through research.* Newbury Park, CA: Sage.

Parker, M. E., & Smith, M. C. (2010). *Nursing theories & nursing practice* (3rd ed.). New York: F. A. Davis.

Pender, N. J., Murdaugh, C. L., & Parsons, M. H. (2010). *Health promotion in nursing practice* (6th ed.). Upper Saddle River, NJ: Prentice-Hall.

Peterson, S. J., & Bredow, T. S. (2013). *Middle range theories: Application to nursing research* (3rd ed.). Philadelphia: Lippincott Williams & Wilkins.

Smith, M. J., & Liehr, P. R. (2013). *Middle range theory for nursing* (3rd ed.). New York: Springer.

Stevens, B. J. (1979). *Nursing theory: Analysis, application, evaluation.* Boston: Little, Brown.

Walker, L. O., & Avant, K. (1983). *Strategies for theory construction in nursing.* Norwalk, CT: Appleton-Century-Crofts.

Walker, L. O., & Avant, K. (1988). *Strategies for theory construction in nursing* (2nd ed.). Norwalk, CT: Appleton & Lange.

Walker, L. O., & Avant, K. (1995). *Strategies for theory construction in nursing* (3rd ed.). Norwalk, CT: Appleton & Lange.

Walker, L. O., & Avant, K. (2005). *Strategies for theory construction in nursing* (4th ed.). Upper Saddle River, NJ: Prentice-Hall.

Walker, L. O., & Avant, K. (2011). *Strategies for theory construction in nursing* (5th ed.). Upper Saddle River, NJ: Prentice-Hall.

Whall, A. L. (2005). The structure of nursing knowledge: Analysis and evaluation of practice, middle range and grand theory. In J. J. Fitzpatrick & A. L. Whall (Eds.), *Conceptual models of nursing: Analysis and application* (3rd ed., pp. 13–51). Upper Saddle River, NJ: Prentice-Hall.

UNIT II

Nursing Theories

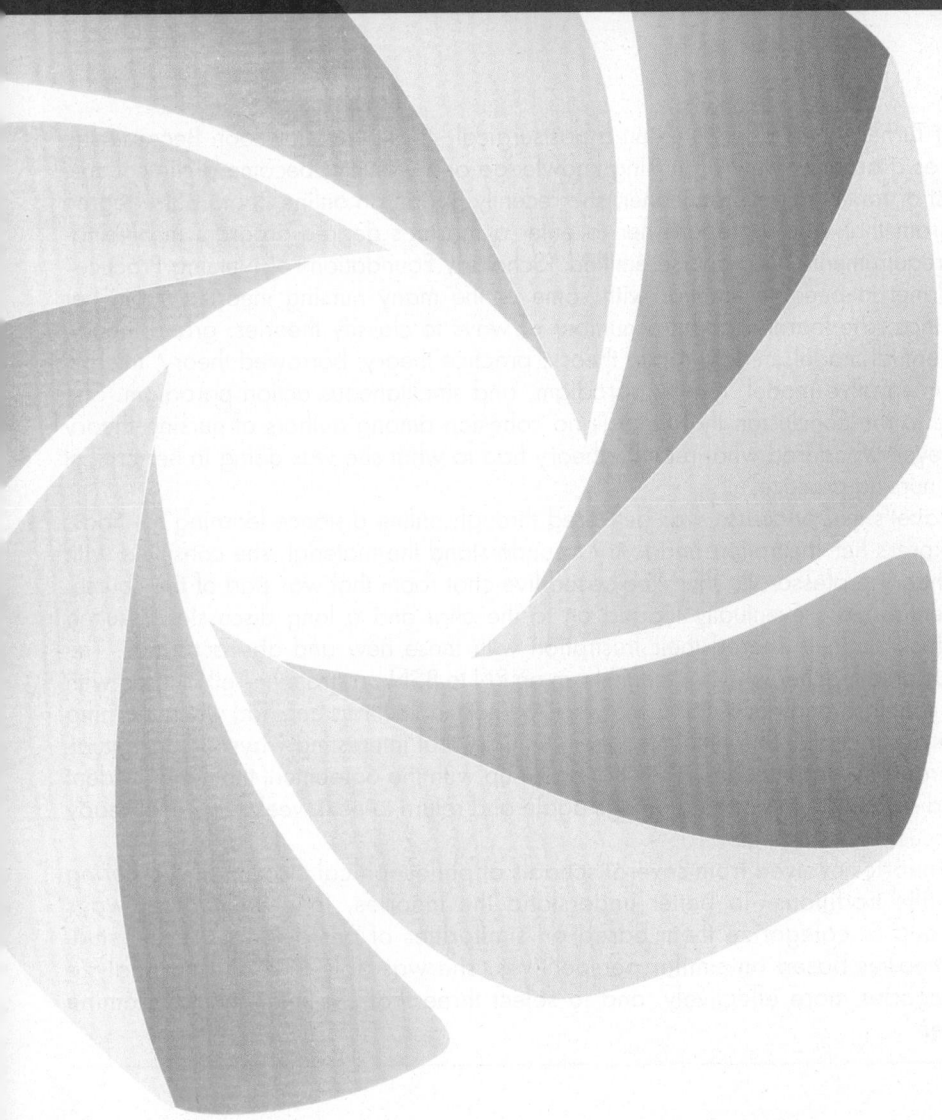

CHAPTER 6

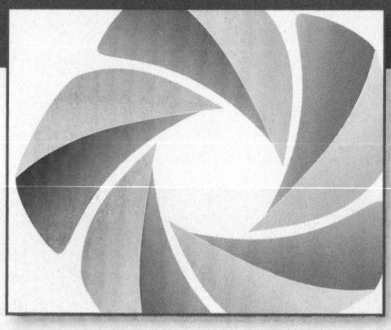

Overview of Grand Nursing Theories

Evelyn M. Wills

Janet Turner works as a nurse on a postsurgical, cardiovascular floor. Because she desires a broader view of nursing knowledge and wants to become a clinical specialist or family nurse practitioner, she recently began an online RN to BSN degree program that would prepare her to enter a master's degree program in nursing. The requirements for a course entitled "Scholarly Foundations of Nursing Practice" led Janet to become familiar with some of the many nursing theories. From her readings, she learned about a number of ways to classify theories: grand theory, conceptual model, middle range theory, practice theory, borrowed theory, interactive–integrative model, totality paradigm, and simultaneous action paradigm. She came to the conclusion that there is no cohesion among authors of nursing theory and even wondered what relation theory had to what she was doing in her critical care nursing practice.

Janet's theory course was delivered through online distance learning methods. To express her frustration and to try to understand the material, she consulted with her theory professor via the Web-based live chat room that was part of the course. The entire class eventually logged on to the chat and a long discussion resulted in which students shared their frustration with these new and abstract ideas. The instructor, a teacher who had come from an RN to BSN program herself, shared with them that frustration and confusion were the normal feelings one had when learning these abstractions. She presented them with several interesting ways to conceptualize grand nursing theories. The chat broke up with the agreement that each student would review the assigned readings again and return to next week's live chat ready to discuss their findings.

Theories evolved from several schools of philosophical thought and *differing* scientific traditions. To better understand the theories, Janet looked for ways to group or categorize them based on similarities of perspective. As she studied theories based on similar perspectives, she was able to read and analyze the theories more effectively, and to select three that she intended to examine further.

In Chapter 2, the reader was introduced to grand nursing theories and given a brief historical overview of their development. Fawcett and DeSanto-Madeya (2013) distinguish between conceptual models and grand theories, and this chapter discusses that differentiation in an effort to assist nursing students to understand the material. According to Fawcett and DeSanto-Madeya (2013), conceptual models are broad formulations of philosophy that are based on an attempt to include the whole of nursing reality as the scholar understands it. The concepts and propositions are abstract and not likely to be testable in fact. Grand nursing theories, by contrast, may be derived from conceptual models and are the most complex and widest in scope of the levels of theory; they attempt to explain broad issues within the discipline. Grand theories are composed of relatively abstract concepts and propositions that are less abstract than those of conceptual models (p. 15) and may not be directly amenable to testing (Butts, 2011; Fawcett & DeSanto-Madeya, 2013; Higgins & Moore, 2000). They were developed through thoughtful and insightful appraisal of existing ideas as opposed to empirical research and may provide the basis for scholars to produce innovative middle range or practice theories (Figure 6-1).

The grand nursing theories guide research and assist scholars to integrate the results of numerous diverse investigations so that the findings may be applied to education, practice, further research, and administration. Eun-Ok and Chang (2012), in their review of literature, found support for the idea that grand theories have an important place in nursing, for example, in research and clinical practice. They also found that theorists are further refining concepts and theories. They stated that theories are "essential for our discipline at multiple levels" (p. 162). Eun-Ok and Chang (2012) also noted that the grand theories provide a background of philosophical reasoning

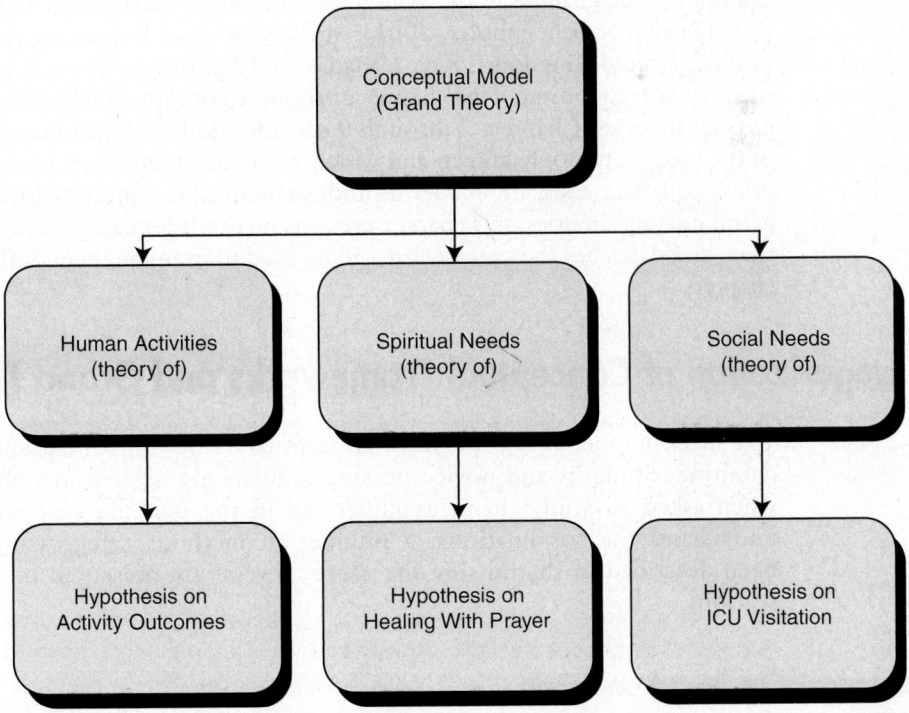

Figure 6-1 Relationship of conceptual model, theory, and hypotheses.

that allows nurse scientists to develop organizing principles for research or practice, sometimes referred to as middle range theory (middle range theories will be discussed in Chapters 10 and 11.) One of the most important benefits of invoking theories in education, administration, research, and practice has been the systematization of those domains of nursing activity.

Practitioners are more likely to succeed in analyzing research results using meta-analysis for evidence-based practice (EBP) when the research fits into a particular theoretical framework. Cody (2003) stated that "nursing theory guided practice can be shown to enhance health and quality of life when it is implemented with strong, well-qualified guidance" (p. 167). Mark, Hughes, and Jones (2004) echoed his beliefs and posited that theory-guided research results not only in greater patient safety but also in more predictable outcomes. These beliefs among nursing scientists provide clear direction that theory-guided research is necessary for evaluating nursing interventions in practice.

Over the last five decades of theory development, review of the health care literature demonstrates that changes in health care, society, and the environment, as well as changes in population demographics (e.g., aging, urbanization, and increase in minorities), led to a need to renew or update existing theories and to develop different theories. In fact, some theoretical writers would exclude the grand theory–middle range theory–microtheory relationship in favor of value-based and socially attuned constructions of nursing knowledge that fit contemporary understanding of human interactions (Risjord, 2010).

Health care delivery is a constantly changing process, and to be relevant to health care, theories require constant renewal and reevaluation. Indeed, many established nursing theorists continue to write, reevaluate, and improve their theories in light of these changes. Inspiration for many of the newer theories is linked not only to the changes in the health sciences but also to changes in society worldwide (Boykin & Schoenhofer, 2001). Such theorists as Roper, Logan, and Tierney (2000) (United Kingdom), Ray (Canada), and Martinson (Norway) have achieved worldwide recognition. This chapter introduces conceptual frameworks and grand nursing theories. Chapters 7 through 9 provide additional information about some of the more commonly known and widely recognized nursing frameworks and theories. To better assist the reader in understanding the conceptual frameworks and grand nursing theories, this chapter presents methods for categorizing or classifying them and describes the criteria that will be used to examine them in the subsequent chapters.

Categorization of Conceptual Frameworks and Grand Theories

The sheer number and scope of the conceptual frameworks and grand theories are daunting. Students and novice nursing scholars are understandably intimidated when asked to study them, as illustrated in the opening case study. To help understand the formulations, a number of methods categorizing them have been described in the nursing literature. Several are presented in the following sections.

Categorization Based on Scope

One of the most logical ways to categorize grand nursing theories is by scope. For example, Alligood and Tomey (2010) organized theories according to the scope of the theory. The categories they used were philosophies, nursing models, nursing theories, theories, and middle range nursing theories (pp. xv–xviii). Pokorny (2010) considered the writings of nursing theorists Peplau; Henderson; Abdellah; Wiedenbach; Hall; Travelbee; Barnard; Adam; Roper, Logan, and Tierney; and Ida Jean (Orlando) Pelletier (hereafter referred to as Orlando) as of historical significance (Alligood & Tomey, 2010, p. xv). Only Henderson, Abdellah, and Orlando will be presented in this unit. They considered the works of Nightingale, Watson, Ray, Martinson, Benner, and Katie Eriksson to be philosophies, explaining that those theorists had developed philosophies that were derived through "analysis, reasoning and logical presentation" (Alligood & Tomey, 2010, p. 6). These philosophies may form a basis for professional scholarship and help guide our understanding of nursing phenomena. (Eriksson, Martinson, and Ray are not included in the current volume because of space requirements.)

Alligood and Tomey (2010) considered the works of Levine, Rogers, Orem, King, Neuman, Roy, and Johnson as nursing conceptual models. Nursing conceptual models "specify a perspective from which to view phenomena specific to the discipline of nursing" (p. 223).

Boykin and Schoenhofer; Melies; Pender; Leininger; Newman; Parse; Helen Erickson, Tomlin, and Swain; and Husted and Husted are classified by Alligood and Tomey (2010) as nursing theories; works that apply to nursing practice and form "ways to describe, explain, or predict relationships among the concepts of nursing phenomena" (p. 391). Alligood and Tomey (2010) made the point that some of these theories evolved from the more global philosophical frameworks or grand theories.

Categorization Based on Nursing Domains

Meleis (2012) did not categorize according to levels of theory (e.g., grand theory, middle range theory, and practice theory). Rather, she categorized theories based on schools of thought or nursing domains: needs theorists; interaction theorists; outcomes theorists, as they developed in various eras; and finally caring/becoming theorists in the current era (see Table 6-1).

She further defined each school of thought according to the major influences of that genre. The needs theorists, according to Meleis (2012), are Abdellah, Henderson, and Orem. The interaction theorists are King, Orlando, Paterson and Zderad, Peplau, Travelbee, and Wiedenbach, and the outcome theorists are Johnson, Levine, Rogers, and Roy (Meleis, 2012). She lists the caring/becoming theorists as Watson and Parse. Each school of thought has certain concepts and defining properties to Meleis.

Meleis (2012) directs us to view areas of agreement among the schools of thought: the focus on the client/patient, who requires a nurse to assist in meeting the vicissitudes and wellness experiences of life, and the ideal that nurses have means to assist human beings. Further, the schools of thought share the ideal that nurses' focus is on human beings and on discovering ways to meet health and illness situations.

Categorization Based on Paradigms

A *paradigm* is a worldview or an overall way of looking at a discipline and its science. It is seen as a universal view of life, rather than just a model or principle of a theory. Kuhn (1962, 1996), a theoretical physicist turned science historian,

Table 6-1 Meleis' 2012 Method of Categorizing Theories

	Theorist's School			
Element	**Needs**	**Interaction**	**Outcome**	**Caring/Becoming**
Focus	Problems, nurse's function	Interaction, illness as experience	Energy, balance, stability, homeostasis, outcomes of care	Human–universe health process, meaning, mutual relations, unitary being
Human being	Set of needs, problems, developmental being	Interacting, set of needs, validated needs, human experience/ meaning	Adaptive, developmental being	Man-living-health, continuously becoming, continuous person/environment relationship
Patient	Needs deficit	Helpless being, human experience/ meaning	Lacks adaptation, systems deficiency	Unique human being, transformation, transcendence, disharmony between spirit–body–mind–soul, sense of incongruence
Orientation	Illness/disease	Illness/disease	Illness/disease	Health, humanbecoming: both client and nurse
Nurse's role	Depends on medical practice, begin independent function, fulfills needs requisites	Helping process, self: therapeutic agent, nursing process	External regulatory mechanism	Connect, be present, extract meaning
Decision maker	Health care provider	Health care provider	Health care provider	Mutual between health care provider and client

Source: Meleis (2012).

awakened the scientific community to revolutions in understanding what he called paradigm shifts. Paradigm shifts occur when empirical reality no longer fits the existing theories of science. As an example, he cited Einstein's theory of general relativity, which came about when the extant theories no longer fit the evidence that was being generated regarding matter and energy (Kuhn, 1962).

Recent scientific revolutions in health disciplines have changed the way scientists view human beings and their health. For example, immunotherapy and gene therapy are currently being studied extensively. Human genes have been mapped and this knowledge has impacted areas of life as varied as ethics, law, pharmacology, and medicine. The impact of these new ideas and research on health care delivery is, in effect, a paradigm shift.

Nursing scientists are finding that the theories that have guided practice in the past are no longer sufficient to explain, predict, or guide current practice. Further, older theories may not be helpful in developing nursing science

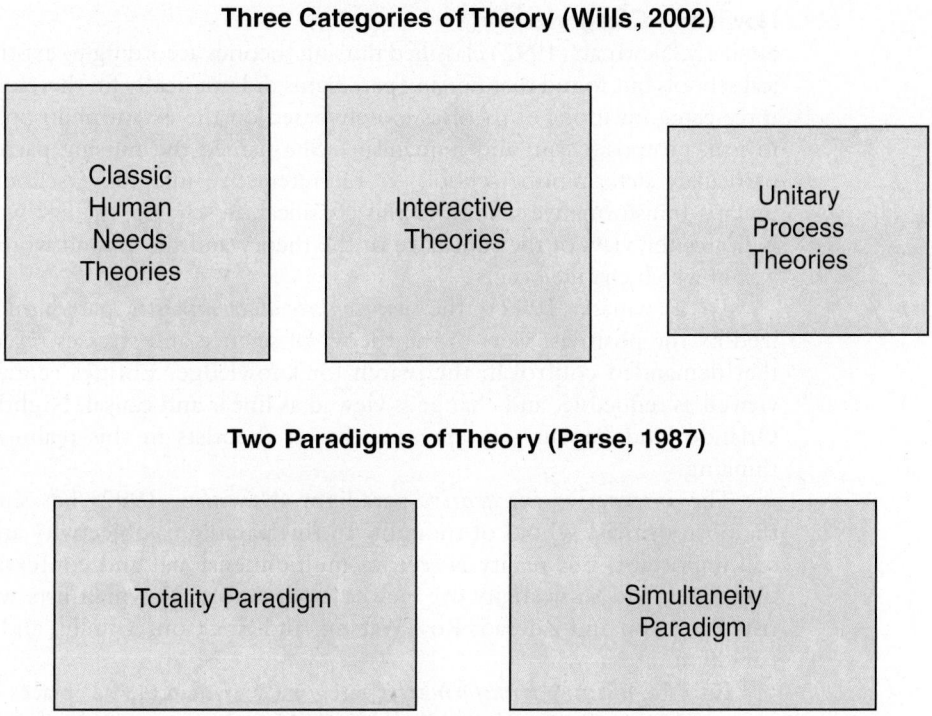

Figure 6-2 Comparison of categories (paradigms) of theories.

because scholars working in nursing's new paradigm are finding evidence that distinguishes nursing science from the sciences that nurses have traditionally consulted to explain the discipline, that is, anthropology, biology, chemistry, physics, psychology, sociology, and medicine (Cody, 2000; Newman, 2008). The following sections outline how three modern nursing scholars (Parse, Newman, and Fawcett) have categorized nursing theories based on paradigms or worldviews (Figure 6-2).

Parse's Categorization

Parse (1995) categorized the various nursing theories into two basic paradigms. These she termed the *totality paradigm* and the *simultaneity paradigm*, and she later added the *humanbecoming paradigm* (humanbecoming is all one word) (Parse, 2013). The totality paradigm includes all theoretical perspectives in which humans are biopsychosocial-spiritual beings, adapting to their environment, in whatever way the theory defines environment. The simultaneity paradigm, on the other hand, includes the theoretical perspectives in which humans are identified as unitary beings, which are energy systems in simultaneous, continuous, mutual process with, and embedded in, the universal energy system. Using this classification scheme, the works of Orem, Roy, Johnson, and others would fit within the totality paradigm, and the works of theorists such as Parse, Rogers, and Newman are within the simultaneity paradigm. Recently, Parse noted that Rogers' and Newman's theories differed from her current thinking sufficiently that she named a third paradigm. She calls the new paradigm the *humanbecoming* paradigm (Parse, 2013). This new paradigm will be discussed in Chapter 9.

Newman's Categorization

Similarly, Newman (1992) classified nursing theories according to existing philosophical schools but found that nursing paradigms did not neatly fit; therefore, she created three categorizations of theories loosely based on the extant philosophies (i.e., positivism, postpositivism, and humanism). She named the nursing paradigms (1) the particulate–deterministic school, (2) the interactive–integrative school, and (3) the unitary–transformative school. In this classification scheme, the first word in the pair indicates the view of the substance of the theory and the second word indicates the way in which change occurs.

To Newman (1992), the *particulate–deterministic* paradigm is characterized by the positivist view of the theory of science and stresses research methods that demanded control in the search for knowledge. Entities (e.g., humans) are viewed as reducible, and change is viewed as linear and causal. Nightingale, Orem, Orlando, and Peplau are representative of theorists in this realm of theoretical thinking.

The *interactive–integrative* paradigm (Newman, 1992) has similarities with the postpositivist school of thought. In this paradigm, objectivity and control are still important, but reality is seen as multidimensional and contextual, and both objectivity and subjectivity are viewed as desirable. Newman lists works of theorists Patterson and Zderad; Roy, Watson, and Erickson; Tomlin; and Swain in this paradigm.

Into the *unitary–transformative* category, Newman (1992) places her works and those of Martha E. Rogers and Parse. Each of these theorists views humans as unitary beings, which are self-evolving and self-regulating. Humans are embedded in, and constantly and simultaneously interacting with, a universal, self-evolving energy system. These theorists agree that human beings cannot be known by the sum of their parts; rather, they are known by their patterns of energy and ways of being apart and distinct from others.

Fawcett's Categorization

Fawcett and DeSanto-Madeya (2013) simplified Newman's (1992) categorization of theories when they created three categories of worldview based on the treatment of change in each theory. The categories Fawcett and DeSanto-Madeya delineated were (1) reaction, (2) reciprocal interaction, and (3) simultaneous action (Fawcett & DeSanto-Madeya, 2013). Like Newman (1992), they showed that each category coincided with a philosophical tradition.

In describing the *reaction* worldview, Fawcett and DeSanto-Madeya (2013) indicated that these theories classify humans as biopsychosocial-spiritual beings who react to the environment in a causal way. The interaction changes predictably and controllably as humans survive and adapt. They argued that in these theories, phenomena must be objective and observable and may be isolated and measured.

In the *reciprocal interaction* worldview, humans are viewed as holistic, active, and interactive with their environments, with the environments returning interactions (Fawcett, 1993; Fawcett & DeSanto-Madeya, 2013). Fawcett noted that these theorists viewed reality as multidimensional, dependent on context (i.e., the surrounding conditions), and relative. This means that change is probabilistic (based on chance) and a result of multiple antecedent factors. The reciprocal interaction theories support the study of both objective and subjective phenomena, and both qualitative and quantitative research methods are encouraged, although controlled research methods and inferential statistical techniques are most frequently used to analyze empirical data (Fawcett & DeSanto-Madeya, 2013).

Table 6-2 Fawcett's Categorization of Nursing Theories

Paradigm	Characteristics
Reaction	Humans are biopsychosocial–spiritual beings. Humans react to their environment in a causal way. Change is predictable as humans survive and adapt.
Reciprocal interaction	Humans are holistic beings. Humans interact reciprocally with their environment. Reality is multidimensional, contextual, and relative.
Simultaneous action	Humans are unitary beings. Humans and their environment are constantly interacting, changing, and evolving. Change is unidirectional and unpredictable.

In the third category of grand theories, the *simultaneous action* worldview, Fawcett and DeSanto-Madeya (2013) report that human beings are viewed as unitary, are identified by patterns in mutual rhythmical interchange with their environments, are changing continuously, and are evolving as self-organized fields. She states that in the simultaneous action paradigm, change is in a single direction (unidirectional) and is unpredictable in that beings progress through organization to disorganization on the way to more complex organization. In this paradigm, knowledge and pattern recognition are the phenomena of interest.

This categorization explained the major differences among the many current and past nursing theories and conceptual models (Fawcett, 2005; Fawcett & DeSanto-Madeya, 2013). Table 6-2 summarizes the grand theory categorization scheme. Table 6-3 compares the classification methods of Fawcett and DeSanto-Madeya (2013), Meleis (2007, 2012), Newman (1995), and Parse (1995).

Table 6-3 Classification of Grand Theories by Current Theory Analysts

Theory Analyst	Source	Basis for Typology	Categories
Fawcett	Philosophy	Worldviews	Reaction Reciprocal interaction Simultaneous action
Meleis	Patient care philosophy	Metaparadigm concepts Schools of thought	Nursing clients Human being–environment interactions Interactions Needs, interaction, outcomes, caring
Newman	Paradigm	Philosophical schools	Particulate–deterministic Interactive–integrative Unitary–transformative
Parse	Paradigm	Difference between worldviews	Totality Simultaneity–humanbecoming

Sources: Fawcett (2000, 2005); Fawcett and DeSanto-Madeya (2013); Meleis (2012); Newman (1995); Parse (1995, 2013).

Specific Categories of Models and Theories for This Unit

For this book, the conceptual models and grand nursing theories were categorized based on distinctions that are similar to those presented by Fawcett (2005), Fawcett and DeSanto-Madeya (2013), and Newman (1992). Chapters 7 through 9 thus present analyses of models and theories according to the following classifications: (1) the human needs theories (which relate to Fawcett's reaction category), (2) the interactive theories, and (3) the unitary process theories.

The theories discussed in Chapter 7 are based on a classical needs perspective and are among the earliest theories and models derived for nursing science. They include the works of Nightingale, Henderson, Johnson, and others. In Chapter 8, each of the perspectives has human interactions as the basis of their content, regardless of the era in which they were developed. The works of Roy, Watson, King, and others are also included in Chapter 8. Finally, the simultaneous process theories (i.e., simultaneity theories) are described in Chapter 9. The theorists presented include Rogers, Newman, and Parse. Table 6-4 summarizes the theories that are presented in Chapters 7 through 9.

Analysis Criteria for Grand Nursing Theories

Describing how models and theories can be employed in nursing practice, research, administration/management, and education necessitates a review of selected elements through theory analysis. Seven criteria were selected for description and analysis of grand theories in this unit. As described in Chapter 5, these seven chosen criteria were among the earliest enumerated by Ellis (1968) and Hardy (1978) and promoted by Walker and Avant (2005), Fawcett (1993, 1995), and Fawcett and DeSanto-Madeya (2013).

Complete analysis of each theory was not performed; instead, the presentation of the models and theories in Chapters 7 through 9 is largely descriptive rather than analytical or evaluative. Each theory's ease of interpretation and application is also briefly critiqued. The criteria used for reviewing the grand theories in these three chapters are listed in Box 6-1. Each criterion is also discussed briefly in the following sections.

Table 6-4 Categorization of Grand Nursing Theories for Chapters 7–9

Human Needs	Models and Theories Interactive Process	Unitary Process
Abdellah	Artinian	Newman
Henderson	Erickson, Tomlin, and Swain	Parse
Johnson	King	Rogers
Nightingale	Levine	
Neuman	Roy	
Orem	Roy, Watson	

Box 6-1 Review Criteria for Descriptive Analysis of Grand Nursing Theories

Background of the theorist
Philosophical underpinnings of the theory
Major assumptions, concepts, and relationships
Usefulness
Testability
Parsimony
Value in extending nursing science

Background of the Theorist

A review of the background of the theorist is likely to reveal the foundations of the theorist's ideas. The individual's educational experiences, in particular, may be relevant to the development of the theory. At one time, higher education, particularly university education, was open only to the children of financially secure families and often limited to nonminorities. Only in the years after the 1960s were scholarships for students with financial hardships and students of ethnic minorities readily available. In addition, nursing graduate programs were not widely available in most parts of the United States before the creation of federal programs in the late 1960s. Because of the limited availability of graduate nursing programs, the majority of the early nursing scholars who developed conceptual models and grand theories received graduate education in disciplines other than nursing. As a result, the earliest nursing models and theories reflected the paradigms that were accepted in the scholar's educative discipline at the time in which they studied or wrote.

The nurse scholar's experience and specialty also influenced the theoretical perspective. For example, Orlando and Peplau were psychiatric nurses who were educated in the first half of the 20th century. Their graduate education in psychology was tempered by the focus of psychology at that time—that of the logical–positivist era, which emphasized reductionistic principles and was mathematically based. Later scholars (e.g., Fawcett, Parse, Fitzpatrick, and Newman) received their doctoral credentials within the discipline of nursing. The writings of these scholars reflect the scientific thought processes, knowledge base, and current thinking of the discipline at the time of their writing as well as their personal perspectives and experiences.

The placement of the author of the model or theory in historical and conceptual perspective promotes understanding of the extant views of science during the time in which the theorist wrote. Only in the most exceptional of cases are scholars not likely to be influenced by the times in which they formulated their work. One exception to this was Martha Rogers. Interestingly, the discipline of nursing was deep in the positivist era in the 1960s when she began her work; the hard sciences (i.e., physics and chemistry), however, had entered the postpositivist era, which posited the idea that change is inherent in a growing discipline. Rogers' (1970) theory did not fit easily into the concurrent paradigm of nursing science of that time and was rejected by many in favor of more intermediate thinking that corresponded to that of the postpositivist thinkers.

Philosophical Underpinnings of the Theory

The background of the scholar most likely contributed heavily to the philosophical basis and paradigmatic origins of the model or theory. Historically, nursing theories of the 1950s and 1960s corresponded to the reaction (Fawcett & DeSanto-Madeya, 2013) worldview. In the late 1960s through the early 1980s, the reciprocal interaction worldviews began to take precedence, and by the 1990s, the unitary process perspectives began to achieve importance, although the earlier paradigms were still influential (Fawcett & DeSanto-Madeya, 2013). It is important to note that most of the scholars who adhered to the interaction worldviews were working and writing in the 1950s, before their ideas achieved general recognition in the profession. The simultaneous action scholars, beginning with Rogers and followed by Parse and Newman, developed their ideas in the 1970s and 1980s and continuously grew their theories as each was influenced by modern thinking and technology.

The fundamental philosophies and the disciplines in which the scholars were educated are reflected in their works. Those educated in the social sciences, for example, incorporated some of the characteristics, concepts, and assumptions of those disciplines in their works. Personal philosophies are also reflected in written views on humans, science, environment, and health. Whether written from the positivist philosophy of science or the postpositivist or modern worldviews, the philosophical viewpoints that form the basis of the works are indicated by the chosen concepts. A component of theory analysis is to point out the underlying philosophy and review the consistency with which the writer demonstrates attention to that background.

Major Assumptions, Concepts, and Relationships

Examination of the major assumptions, concepts, and relationships of the model or theory is vital because they are the substance of the formulation. These components will direct practice, assist with selection of concepts to be studied, and generate collateral theories for the discipline of nursing (Walker & Avant, 2011). Whether the assumptions are spelled out or merely inferred indicates the strength of the theory in elucidating its content. The concepts, carefully defined and explained, along with their derivation, assist the analyst in determining the essence of the model or theory. The relationships between and among the concepts, their strength, and whether they are positive, negative, or neutral indicate the structure of the theory (Walker & Avant, 2011).

Usefulness

Conceptual models and grand theories are reputed not to be particularly useful in directing nursing practice because of their scope and level of abstraction and because they were created through the analytical, logical, and philosophical understandings of a single theorist (Alligood & Tomey, 2010). The reality is that although many of the conceptual models and grand theories cannot be tested in a single research project, they have been useful in guiding nursing scholarship and practice and in providing the structure from which testable theories may be derived. Grand nursing theories, more often than conceptual models, are likely to provide the basis for concrete theories, with specifically defined concepts and highly derived relationships that may be more easily applied in clinical practice, nursing education, research, or nursing administration (Fawcett & DeSanto-Madeya, 2013).

Testability

To be useful, theories should be disprovable (Shuttleworth, 2008); that is, they can be questioned and tested in the real world through research. Because the major purposes of nursing theory are to guide research, practice, education, and administration, the theory must be subjected to examination. Theories that are capable of being tested make the most reliable guides for scholarly work (Walker & Avant, 2011). Many grand theories are not testable in totality, but they may generate theories that are testable from their conceptual matter, assumptions, or structure. The grand theories that are likely to generate middle range theories and practice theories, as well as theoretical models for research, are those most likely to fulfill the requirement of testability and have the ability to continue to generate new and useful models (Kim, 2006).

Parsimony

Parsimony is a criterion that is important because the more complex the theory, the less easily it is comprehended. Parsimony does not indicate that a theory is simplistic; in fact, often the more parsimonious the theory, the more depth the theory may have. For example, the standard of parsimony in a theory is Einstein's theory of relativity (Cody, 2012), which can be reduced to the formula $E = Mc^2$. Although the theory has only three concepts (E = energy, M = matter, and c^2 = the speed of light squared) (Einstein, 1961), the explanation of this theory is extremely complicated indeed.

Considering the complexity of nurses' primary subjects of interest, human beings in health and illness, it is unlikely that any of the grand nursing theories could ever approximate the mathematical elegance of Einstein's theory of relativity. Parsimonious theoretical constructions, however, provide nurses in research, administration, practice, and education with broad general categories into which to conceptualize problems and therefore may assist in the derivation of methods of problem solving. Indeed, the more elegant and universal a conceptual model or grand theory, the more global it is in contributing to the science of nursing.

Value in Extending Nursing Science

Ultimately, the value of any nursing theory, not just of grand theory, is its ability to extend the discipline and science of nursing. Understanding the nature of human beings and their interaction with the environment, and the impact of this interaction on their health, will help direct holistic and comprehensive nursing interventions that improve health and well-being. Improvement in nursing care is ultimately the reason for formulating theory. Further, the value of the theory in adding to and elaborating nursing science is an important function of grand theory (Fawcett & DeSanto-Madeya, 2013). Questions to be answered when analyzing any theory include: Does the theory generate new knowledge? Can the theory suggest or support new avenues of knowledge generation beyond those that already exist? Does the theory suggest a disciplinary future that is growing and changing? Can the theory assist nurses to respond to the rapid change and growth of health care? (Walker & Avant, 2011).

The Purpose of Critiquing Theories

Critiquing theory is a necessary part of the process when a scholar is selecting a theory for some disciplinary work. Determining whether a grand theory holds promise or value for the effort at hand and whether middle range theories, which are useful in research, practice, education, or administration, can be generated from it is a product of critique.

When a nursing student confronts the overarching ideals of the profession for the first time, it is not at all unlikely that the feeling is complete and overwhelming confusion and even disorientation. As in the case of Janet and her quest for advanced education, frustration was a new feeling to her. Her work in the critical care unit was focused and based on evidence and followed an ordered medical model, whereas the newness of this conceptually based study of theories left her disgruntled. The understanding displayed by her instructor, who had felt similar feelings during her education and who ascribed to the pattern that nurses learn together, was calming and set the stage for Janet to begin to learn the basics of the science of nursing, the theoretical underpinnings of the profession.

It is likely that a nursing student may find it difficult to critique the work of nursing's grand theorists considering the advanced educational attainment of the theorists. Yet, determining the usefulness of the theory to a project is important. The user of the theory must comprehend the paradigm of the theory, believe in the concepts and assumptions from which it is built, and be able to internalize the basic philosophy of the theorist. It is hardly beneficial to attempt to use a theory that one cannot accept or understand or one that seems inappropriate in the current time or place. The choice of a theoretical framework or model must fit with the student's or scholar's personal ideals, and this requires the student or scholar to critique the theory for its value in extending the selected professional work.

One problem that arises among both novice and experienced scholars is combining theories from competing paradigms. Often, the work generated from these efforts is confusing and obfuscating; it does not generate clear results that extend the thinking within either paradigm (Todaro-Franceschi, 2010). Therefore, the conscientious student or scholar selects theories that relate to the same paradigm in science, philosophy, and nursing when combining theories to guide research or practice. Wide reading in the discipline of nursing and the scientific literature of the disciplines from which the theorist has generated ideas will assist in preventing such errors. Theory review and extraction from the grand theories can result in work that satisfies the scholarly impulse in each of us, guides the research process, provides structure for safe and effective practice, and extends the science of nursing.

Summary

Grand theories are global in their application to the discipline of nursing and have been instrumental in helping to develop nursing science. Because of their diversity, their complexity, and their differing worldviews, learning about grand nursing theories can be confusing and frustrating, as illustrated by the experiences of Janet, the student nurse from the opening case study. To help make the study of grand theories more logical and rewarding, this chapter presented several methods for categorizing the grand theories on the basis of scope, basic philosophies, and needs of the discipline. It has also presented the criteria that will be used to describe grand nursing theories in subsequent chapters.

Chapters 7 through 9 discuss many of the grand nursing theories that have been placed into the three defined paradigms of nursing. These analyses are meant to be descriptive to allow the student to choose from different paradigms and the theories contained within them to further their work. The student or scholar must recognize that health care is constantly changing and that some theories may no longer seem applicable, whereas other theories are timeless in their abstraction. Before selecting a theory to guide practice, research, or other endeavors, it is the student's responsibility to obtain and read the theory in its latest iteration by the theorist, read analyses by other scholars in the discipline, and become thoroughly familiar with the theory.

Key Points

- Nursing scholars and nursing leaders have developed philosophies, conceptual frameworks, and grand theories to make the very complex study of nursing clear for both students and practitioners.
- The purpose of theory is to systematize nursing education and practice so that no important element of nursing care is forgotten.
- Reviewing and critiquing nursing theories is important, as nurse scholars, nurse educators, and nurse researchers use theories for the purposes of directing and coordinating practice, education, and research.
- Using nursing theories to guide their work allows practitioners, educators, and researchers to base their work on a system that allows critique of the outcomes of their work.
- Working within a paradigm, rather than combining disparate paradigms, prevents confusion because nursing paradigms relate to paradigms in other sciences.

Learning Activities

1. During an online classroom, debate similarities and differences in the several theoretical categorization schemes put forth by the different theory analysts discussed in this chapter. Which system appears to be the easiest to understand?
2. Does categorizing or classifying grand theories as the writers have done assist in studying and understanding them? Why or why not?
3. With classmates, critique theory-based research articles and decide whether they will yield believable evidence. Do the authors ascribe to the same or similar theoretical worldviews (paradigms)? Do you think that having differing paradigms will make a difference in your group's ability to identify the evidence needed for safe nursing practice?

REFERENCES

Alligood, M. R., & Tomey, A. M. (2010). *Nursing theorists and their work* (7th ed.). Maryland Heights, MO: Mosby Elsevier.

Boykin, A., & Schoenhofer, S. O. (2001). *Nursing as caring: A model for transforming practice.* Boston: Jones & Bartlett.

Butts, J. B. (2011). Components and levels of abstraction in nursing knowledge. In J. B. Butts & K. L. Rich (Eds.), *Philosophies and theories for advanced nursing practice* (Ch. 5, pp. 89–112). Sudbury, MA: Jones & Bartlett.

Cody, W. K. (2000). Paradigm shift or paradigm drift? *Nursing Science Quarterly, 13*(2), 93–102.

Cody, W. K. (2003). Nursing theory as a guide to practice. *Nursing Science Quarterly, 16*(3), 225–231.

Cody, W. K. (2012). A brave and startling truth: Parse's human-becoming school of thought in the context of the contemporary nursing discipline. *Nursing Science Quarterly, 25*(1), 7–10.

Einstein, A. (1961). *Relativity.* New York: Crown.

Ellis, R. (1968). Characteristics of significant theories. *Nursing Research, 17*(3), 217–222.

Eun-Ok, I., & Chang, S. J. (2012). Current trends in nursing theories. *Journal of Nursing Scholarship, 44*(2), 156–164.

Fawcett, J. (1993). *Analysis and evaluation of nursing theories.* Philadelphia: Davis.

Fawcett, J. (1995). *Analysis and evaluation of conceptual models of nursing* (3rd ed.). Philadelphia: Davis.

Fawcett, J. (2000). *Analysis and evaluation of contemporary nursing knowledge: Nursing models and theories.* Philadelphia: Davis.

Fawcett, J. (2005). *Contemporary nursing knowledge: Analysis and evaluation of nursing models and theories* (2nd ed). Philadelphia: Davis.

Fawcett, J., & DeSanto-Madeya, S. (2013). *Contemporary nursing knowledge: Analysis and evaluation of nursing models and theories* (3rd ed.). Philadelphia: Davis.

Hardy, M. E. (1978). Perspectives on nursing theory. *Advances in Nursing Science, 1*(1), 27–48.

Higgins, P. A., & Moore, S. M. (2000). Levels of theoretical thinking in nursing. *Nursing Outlook, 48*(4), 179–183.

Kim, H. S. (2000). *The nature of theoretical thinking in nursing* (2nd ed.). New York: Springer.

Kim, H. S. (2006). The concept of holism. In H. S. Kim & I. Kollak (Eds.), *Nursing theories: Conceptual & philosophical foundations.* New York: Springer.

Kuhn, T. S. (1962). *The structure of scientific revolutions.* Chicago: University of Chicago Press.

Kuhn, T. S. (1996). *The structure of scientific revolutions* (3rd ed.). Chicago: University of Chicago Press.

Mark, B., Hughes, I., & Jones, C. (2004). The role of theory in improving patient safety and quality health care. *Nursing Outlook, 52*(1), 11–16.

Meleis, A. I. (2007). *Theoretical nursing: Development and progress* (4th ed.). Philadelphia: Lippincott Williams & Wilkins.

Meleis, A. I. (2012). *Theoretical nursing: development and progress* (5th ed.). Philadelphia: Lippincott Williams & Wilkins.

Newman, M. A. (1992). Prevailing paradigms in nursing. *Nursing Outlook, 40*(1), 10–13, 32.

Newman, M. A. (1995). *A developing discipline: Selected works of Margaret Newman.* New York: National League for Nursing Press.

Newman, M. A. (2008). *Transforming presence: The difference that nursing makes.* Philadelphia: Davis.

Parse, R. R. (Ed.). (1995). *Illuminations: The human becoming theory in practice and research.* New York: National League for Nursing Press.

Parse, R. R. (2013). Living Quality: A humanbecoming phenomenon. *Nursing Science Quarterly, 26*(2), 111–115.

Pokorny, M. E. (2010). Nursing theorists of historical significance. In M. R. Alligood & A. M. Tomey (Eds.), *Nursing theorists and their work* (7th ed., pp. 54–68). Maryland Heights, MO: Mosby Elsevier.

Risjord, M. (2010). *Nursing knowledge: Science, practice, and philosophy.* Ames, IA: Wiley-Blackwell.

Rogers, M. E. (1970). *An introduction to the theoretical basis of nursing.* Philadelphia: Davis.

Roper, N., Logan, W., & Tierney, A. J. (2000). *The Roper-Logan-Tierney Model of Nursing: Based on activities of living.* London, United Kingdom: Churchill Livingston.

Shuttleworth, M. (2008). *Falsifiability.* Retrieved from http://www.explorable.com/falsifiability

Todaro-Franceschi, V. (2010). Two paradigms, different fruit: Mixing apples with oranges. *Visions: The Journal of Rogerian Nursing Science, 17*(1), 44–51.

Walker, L. O., & Avant, K. (2005). *Strategies for theory construction in nursing* (4th ed.). Upper Saddle River, NJ: Pearson.

Walker, L. O., & Avant, K. (2011). *Strategies for theory construction in nursing* (5th ed.). Upper Saddle River, NJ: Pearson.

CHAPTER 7

Grand Nursing Theories Based on Human Needs

Evelyn M. Wills

Donald Crawford is an intensive care unit (ICU) clinical nurse specialist (CNS) who has just completed his graduate degree. Donald strongly believes that evidence guiding nursing practice should be experiential and measurable, and during his master's program, he derived a system for evaluation of the needs of the seriously ill individuals for whom he cared. He also devised a way to diagram the disease pathophysiology for many of his patients based on the Neuman Systems Model (Neuman & Fawcett, 2009).

During his graduate studies, Donald began to apply concepts and principles from Neuman's model in his practice with encouraging results. He observed that the model helped predict what would happen next with some patients and helped him define patient's needs, predict outcomes, and prescribe nursing interventions more accurately. In particular, he appreciated how Neuman focused on identification and reduction of stressors through nursing interventions and liked the construct of prevention as intervention. Using his position as CNS, he is developing a proposal to implement his methods throughout the ICU to help other nurses apply Neuman's model in managing patient care.

The earliest theorists in nursing drew from the dominant worldviews of their time, which were largely related to the medical discoveries from the scientific era of the 1850s through 1940s (Artinian, 1991). During those years, nurses in the United States were seen as handmaidens to doctors, and their practice was guided by disease theories of medical science. Even today, much of nursing science remains based in the positivist era with its focus on disease causality and a desire to produce measurable outcome data. Evidence-based medicine is the current means of enacting the positivist focus on research outcomes for effective clinical therapeutics (Cody, 2013).

In an effort to define the uniqueness of nursing and to distinguish it from medicine, nursing scholars from the 1950s through the 1970s developed a number of nursing theories. In addition to medicine, the majority of these early works were strongly influenced by the needs theories of social scientists (e.g., Maslow). In needs-based theories, clients are typically considered biopsychosocial beings who are the sum of their parts, who are experiencing disease or trauma, and who need nursing care. Further, clients are thought of as mechanistic beings, and if the correct information can be gathered, the cause or source of their problems can be discerned and measured. At that point, interventions can be prescribed that will be effective in meeting their needs (Dickoff, James, & Wiedenbach, 1968). Evidence-based nursing fits with these theories completely and comfortably.

The grand theories and models of nursing described in this chapter focus on meeting clients' needs for nursing care. These theories and models, like all personal statements of scholars, have continued to grow and develop over the years; therefore, several sources were consulted for each model. The latest writings of and about the theories were consulted and are presented. As much as possible, the description of the model is either quoted or paraphrased from the original texts. Some needs theorists may have maintained their theories over the years with little change; others have updated and adapted theirs to later ideas and methods. Nevertheless, new research has often extended the original work. Students are advised to consult the literature for the newest research using the needs theory of interest.

It should be noted that a concerted attempt was made in this book to ensure that the presentation of the works of all theorists is balanced. Some theories (e.g., Orem and Neuman) are more complex than others, and the body of information is greater for some than for others. As a result, the sections dealing with some theorists are a little longer than others. This does not imply that shorter works are inferior or less important to the discipline.

Finally, all theory analysts, whether novice or expert, will comprehend theories and models from their own perspectives. If the reader is interested in using a model, the most recent edition of the work of the theorist should be obtained and used as the primary source for any projects. All further works using the theory or model should come from researchers using the theory in their work. Current research writings are one of the best ways to understand the development of the needs theories.

Florence Nightingale: Nursing: What It Is and What It Is Not

Nightingale's model of nursing was developed before the general acceptance of modern disease theories (i.e., the germ theory) and other theories of medical science. Nightingale knew the germ theory (Beck, 2005), and prior to its wide publication she had deduced that cleanliness, fresh air, sanitation, comfort, and socialization were necessary to healing. She used her experiences in the Scutari Army Hospital in Turkey and in other hospitals in which she worked to document her ideas on nursing (Beck, 2005; Dossey, 2000; Selanders, 1993; Small, 1998).

Nightingale was from a wealthy family, yet she chose to work in the field of nursing, although it was considered a "lowly" occupation. She believed nursing was her call from God, and she determined that the sick deserved civilized care, regardless of their station in life (Nightingale, 1860/1957/1969).

Through her extensive body of work, she changed nursing and health care dramatically. Nightingale's record of letters is voluminous, and several books have been written analyzing them (Attewell, 2012; Dossey, Selanders, Beck, & Attewell, 2005). She wrote many books and reports to federal and worldwide agencies. Books she wrote that are especially important to nurses and nursing include *Notes on Nursing: What It Is and What It Is Not* (original publication in 1860; reprinted in 1957 and 1969), *Notes on Hospitals* (published in 1863), and *Sick-Nursing and Health-Nursing*, originally published in Hampton's *Nursing of the Sick*, 1893) (Reed & Zurakowski, 1996) and reprinted *in toto* in Dossey et al. (2005a), to name but a small portion of her great body of works. Much of her work is now available, where once it was kept out of circulation; perhaps because of the sheer volume and perhaps because she originally asked that her papers all be destroyed at her death. She later recanted that request (Bostridge, 2011; Cromwell, 2013).

Background of the Theorist

Nightingale was born on May 12, 1820, in Florence, Italy; her birthday is still honored in many places. She was privately educated in the classical tradition of her time by her father, and from an early age, she was inclined to care for the sick and injured (Bostridge, 2011; Dossey, 2000, 2005a; Selanders, 1993). Although her mother wished her to lead a life of social grace, Nightingale preferred productivity, choosing to school herself in the care of the sick. She attended nursing programs in Kaiserswerth, Germany, in 1850 and 1851 (Bostridge, 2011; Dossey et al., 2010; Small, 1998), where she completed what was at that time the only formal nursing education available. She worked as the nursing superintendent at the Institution for Care of Sick Gentlewomen in Distressed Circumstances, where she instituted many changes to improve patient care (Cromwell, 2013; Dossey, 2000; Selanders, 1993; Small, 1998).

During the Crimean War, she was urged by Sidney Herbert, Secretary of War for Great Britain, to assist in providing care for wounded soldiers. The dire conditions of British servicemen had resulted in a public outcry that prompted the government to institute changes in the system of medical care (Small, 1998). At Herbert's request, Nightingale and a group of 38 skilled nurses were transported to Turkey to provide nursing care to the soldiers in the hospital at Scutari Army Barracks. There, despite daunting opposition by army physicians, Nightingale instituted a system of care that reportedly cut casualties from 48% to 2% within approximately 2 years (Bostridge, 2011; Dossey, 2000, 2005a; Selanders, 1993; Zurakowski, 2005).

Early in her work at the army hospital, Nightingale noted that the majority of soldiers' deaths was caused by transport to the hospital and conditions in the hospital itself. Nightingale found that open sewers and lack of cleanliness, pure water, fresh air, and wholesome food were more often the causes of soldiers' deaths than their wounds; she implemented changes to address these problems (Small, 1998). Although her recommendations were known to be those that would benefit the soldiers, physicians in charge of the hospitals in the Crimea blocked her efforts. Despite this, by her third trip to the Crimea, Nightingale had been appointed the supervisor of all the nurses (Bostridge, 2011; Dossey, 2000).

At Scutari, she became known as the "lady with the lamp" from her nightly excursions through the wards to review the care of the soldiers (Audain, 1998; Bostridge, 2011). To prove the value of the work she and the nurses were doing, Nightingale instituted a system of record keeping and adapted a statistical reporting method known as the *polar area diagram* (Audain, 2007; O'Connor & Robertson, 2003), or Cock's Comb model, to analyze the data she so rigorously collected (Small, 1998). Thus, Nightingale was the first nurse to collect and analyze evidence that her methods were working.

On her return to England from Turkey, Nightingale worked to reform the Army Medical School, instituted a program of record keeping for government health statistics and assisted with the public health system in India. The effort for which she is most remembered, however, is the Nightingale School for Nurses at St. Thomas'

Hospital. This school was supported by the Nightingale Fund, which had been instituted by grateful British citizens in honor of her work in the Crimea (Bostridge, 2011; Cromwell, 2013; O'Connor & Robertson, 2003; Selanders, 1993).

Philosophical Underpinnings of the Theory

Nightingale's work is considered a broad philosophy. Zurakowski (2005) indicates it is a "perspective" (p. 21). By contrast, Selanders (2005a) states that her work is a foundational philosophy (p. 66). Dossey (2005a) demonstrates that the three tenets of Nightingale's philosophy are "healing, leadership, and global action" (p. 1). Dossey states that "her basic tenet was healing and secondary to it are the tenets of leadership and global action which are necessary to support healing at its deepest level" (p. 1). Nightingale's work has influenced the nursing profession and nursing education for nearly 160 years. To Nightingale, nursing was the domain of women but was an independent practice in its own right. Nurses were, however, to practice in accord with physicians, whose prescriptions nurses were faithfully to carry out (Nightingale, 1893/1954). Nightingale did not believe that nurses were meant to be subservient to physicians. Rather, she believed that nursing was an independent profession or a calling in its own right (Selanders, 1993). Nightingale's educational model is based on anticipating and meeting the needs of patients and is oriented toward the works a nurse should carry out in meeting those needs. Nightingale's philosophy was inductively derived, abstract yet descriptive in nature, and is classified as a grand theory or philosophy by most nursing writers (Alligood & Tomey, 2010; Dossey, 2000; Selanders, 1993, 2005a).

Major Assumptions, Concepts, and Relationships

Nightingale was an educated gentlewoman of the Victorian era. The language she used to write her books—*Notes on Nursing: What It Is and What It Is Not* (1860/1957/1969) and *Sick-Nursing and Health-Nursing* (1893/1954)—was cultured, flowing, logical in format, and elegant in style. She wrote numerous letters, many of which are still available. These were topical, direct and yet abstract, and addressed a plethora of topics, such as personal care of patients and sanitation in army hospitals and communities, to name only a few (Bostridge, 2011; Cromwell, 2013; Dossey, 2005b; Selanders, 2005b).

Nightingale (1860/1957/1969) believed that five points were essential in achieving a healthful house: "pure air, pure water, efficient drainage, cleanliness, and light" (p. 24). She thought buildings should be constructed to admit light to every occupant and to allow the flow of fresh air. Further, she wrote that proper household management makes a difference in healing the ill and that nursing care pertained to the house in which the patient lived, and to those who came into contact with the patient, as well as to the care of the patient.

Although the metaparadigm concepts had not been so labeled until over 130 years later, Nightingale (1893/1954) addressed them—human, environment, health, and nursing—specifically in her writings. She believed that a healthy environment was essential for healing. For example, noise was harmful and impeded the need of the person for rest, and noises to avoid included caregivers talking within the hearing of the individual, the rustle of the wide skirts (common at the time), fidgeting, asking unnecessary questions, and a heavy tread while walking. Nutritious food, proper beds and bedding, and personal cleanliness were variables Nightingale deemed essential, and she was convinced that social contact was important to healing. Although the germ theory had been proposed, Nightingale's writings do not specifically refer to it. Her ideals of care, however, indicate that she recognized and agreed that cleanliness prevents morbidity (Nightingale, 1999).

Nightingale believed that nurses must make accurate observations of their patients and report the state of the patient to the physician in an orderly manner. She explained that nurses should think critically about the care of the patient and do what was appropriate and necessary to assist the patient to heal. Nursing was seen as a way "to put the constitution in such a state as that it will have no disease, or that it can recover from disease" (Nightingale, 1893/1954, p. 3), which will "put us in the best possible conditions for nature to restore or to preserve health—to prevent or to cure disease or injury" (p. 357). She believed that nursing was an art, whereas medicine was a science, and stated that nurses were to be loyal to the medical plan but not servile. Throughout her writings, Nightingale enumerated tasks that nurses should complete to care for ill individuals, and many of the tasks she outlined are still relevant today (Nightingale, 1860/1957/1969).

Health was defined in her treatise, *Sickness-Nursing and Health-Nursing* (1893/1954), as "to be well but to be able to use well every power we have" (p. 357). It is apparent throughout that volume that health meant more than the mere absence of disease, a view that placed Nightingale ahead of her time (Selanders, 1993).

Usefulness

Nightingale wrote on hospitals, nursing, and community health in the 19th and into the 20th century, and her works served as the basis of nursing education in Britain and in the United States for over a century. King's College Hospital and St. Thomas' Hospital in London, England, were the initial nursing programs developed by Nightingale, and she maintained a special interest in St. Thomas' Hospital during most of her life (Small, 1998). Nursing programs that used the Nightingale method in the United States included Bellevue Hospital in New York, New Haven Hospital in Connecticut, and Massachusetts Hospital in Boston. Indeed, the influence of Nightingale's methods is felt in nursing programs to the present (Pfettscher, 2006).

A resurgence in attention to Nightingale's philosophy is noteworthy. Jacobs (2001) discussed the attribute of human dignity as a central phenomenon uniting nursing theory and practice, two areas that were extensively treated by Nightingale in her own writings. Cromwell (2013) discussed Nightingale's early feminism and her willingness to fight local and federal authorities to procure humane treatment for British soldiers of the time. She showed how Nightingale continued her works for the British army long after returning from the Bosporus. Many other contemporary writers and researchers have displayed an intense interest in Nightingale's work and its applicability to modern nursing (Beck, 2010; Dossey, 2010; Hoyt, 2010; McElligott, 2010; Neils, 2010; Rew & Sands, 2010; Selanders, 2010; Wagner & Whaite, 2010); indeed, two full issues of a recent journal were published solely of articles inspired by Nightingale. Non-nurses have written about her work as well (Attewell, 2010; Karpf, 2010; Weyneth, 2010), and educators worldwide continue to use her ideals in teaching nurses (Haddad & Santos, 2011 [Portugal]).

Testability

Nightingale's theory can be the source of testable hypotheses because she treated concrete as well as abstract concepts. Research that is conversant with her ideas of care includes research on noise (Tailor-Ford, Catlin, LaPlant, & Weinke, 2008), environment (Pope, 1995), and spirituality (Tanyi & Werner, 2008). Current researchers have written about her statistical work (McDonald, 2010; Rew & Sands, 2010), showing that it stands up to modern thinking as it did in the 19th century. Indeed, research around the globe is still progressing using her work as a basis (Burkhart & Hogan, 2008).

Parsimony

In her work, Nightingale succinctly stated what she believed was important in caring for ill individuals. Furthermore, in one small volume, she includes information about nursing care, patient needs, proper buildings in which the sick are to be treated, and the administration of hospitals.

Value in Extending Nursing Science

Nightingale was a noted nurse of her time. She was a consultant who promoted the collection and analyses of health statistics. She was deeply involved in nursing education and promoting the science of public health (Bostridge, 2011; Cromwell, 2013; Small, 1998), hospital administration, community health, and global health (Dossey, 2005a). Nightingale's legacy continues to be important to nursing scholars, and her vast contributions continue to enlighten nursing science. Current Nightingale scholars include Attewell (2012), Bostridge (2011), Cromwell (2013), Dossey et al. (2005), Jacobs (2001), and many others who have contributed to the understanding of her multitudinous works. Nightingale's work was revolutionary for its impact on nursing and health care. Furthermore, her many works continue to present effective guidelines for nurses.

Virginia Henderson: The Principles and Practice of Nursing

Virginia Avenal Henderson was a well-known nursing educator and a prolific author. In 1937, Henderson and others created a basic nursing curriculum for the National League for Nursing in which education was "patient centered and organized around nursing problems rather than medical diagnoses" (Henderson, 1991, p. 19). In 1939, she revised Harmer's classic textbook of nursing for its fourth edition and later wrote the fifth edition, incorporating her personal definition of nursing (Henderson, 1991). Although she was retired, she was a frequent visitor to nursing schools well into her 90s. O'Malley (1996) states that Henderson is known as the modern-day mother of nursing. Her work influenced the nursing profession in America and throughout the world.

Background of the Theorist

Henderson was born in Missouri but spent her formative years in Virginia. She received a diploma in nursing from the Army School of Nursing at Walter Reed Hospital in 1921 and worked at the Henry Street Visiting Nurse Service for 2 years after graduation. In 1923, she accepted a position teaching nursing at the Norfolk Protestant Hospital in Virginia, where she remained for several years. In 1929, Henderson determined that she needed more education and entered Teachers College at Columbia University, where she earned her bachelor's degree in nursing in 1932 and a master's degree in 1934. Subsequently, she joined Columbia as a member of the faculty, where she remained until 1948 (Herrmann, 1998). "Ms. Virginia," as she was known to her friends, died in 1996 at the age of 98 (Allen, 1996). Because of her importance to modern nursing, the Sigma Theta Tau International Nursing Library is named in her honor.

Philosophical Underpinnings of the Theory

Henderson was educated during the empiricist era in medicine and nursing, which focused on patient needs, but she believed that her theoretical ideas grew and matured through her experiences (Henderson, 1991). Henderson was introduced to physiologic principles during her graduate education, and the understanding of these principles was the basis for her patient care (Henderson, 1965, 1991). The theory presents the patient as a sum of parts with biopsychosocial needs, and the patient is neither client nor consumer. Henderson stated that "Thorndike's fundamental needs of man" (Henderson, 1991, p. 16) had an influence on her beliefs.

Although her major clinical experiences were in medical-surgical hospitals, she worked as a visiting nurse in New York City. This experience enlarged Henderson's view to recognize the importance of increasing the patient's independence so that progress after hospitalization would not be delayed (Henderson, 1991). Henderson was a nurse educator, and the major thrust of her theory relates to the education of nurses.

Major Assumptions, Concepts, and Relationships

Henderson's concept of nursing was derived from her practice and education; therefore, her work is inductive. Henderson did not manufacture language to elucidate her theoretical stance; she used correct, scholarly English in all of her writings. She called her definition of nursing her "concept" (Henderson, 1991, pp. 20–21).

Assumptions

The major assumption of the theory is that nurses care for patients until patients can care for themselves once again (Henderson, 1991). She assumes that patients desire to return to health, but this assumption is not explicitly stated. She also assumes that nurses are willing to serve and that "nurses will devote themselves to the patient day and night" (p. 23). A final assumption is that nurses should be educated at the university level in both arts and sciences.

Concepts

The major concepts of the theory relate to the metaparadigm (i.e., nursing, health, patient, and environment). Henderson believed that "the unique function of the nurse is to assist the individual, sick or well, in the performance of those activities contributing to health or its recovery (or to a peaceful death) that he would perform unaided if he had the necessary strength, will or knowledge. And to do this in such a way as to help him gain independence as rapidly as possible" (Henderson, 1991, p. 21). She defined the patient as someone who needs nursing care but did not limit nursing to illness care. She did not define environment, but maintaining a supportive environment is one of the elements of her 14 activities. Health was not explicitly defined, but it is taken to mean balance in all realms of human life. The concept of nursing involved the nurse attending to 14 activities that assist the individual toward independence (Box 7-1).

Box 7-1 Henderson's 14 Activities for Client Assistance

1. Breathe normally.
2. Eat and drink adequately.
3. Eliminate body wastes.
4. Move and maintain desirable postures.
5. Sleep and rest.
6. Select suitable clothes—dress and undress.
7. Maintain body temperature within normal range by adjusting clothing and modifying environment.
8. Keep the body clean and well groomed and protect the integument.
9. Avoid dangers in the environment and avoid injuring others.
10. Communicate with others in expressing emotions, needs, fears, or opinions.
11. Worship according to one's faith.
12. Work in such a way that there is a sense of accomplishment.
13. Play or participate in various forms of recreation.
14. Learn, discover, or satisfy the curiosity that leads to normal development and health and use the available health facilities.

Source: Henderson (1991, pp. 22–23).

Usefulness

Nursing education has been deeply affected by Henderson's clear vision of the functions of nurses. The principles of Henderson's theory were published in the major nursing textbooks used from the 1930s through the 1960s, and the principles embodied by the 14 activities are still important in evaluating nursing care in the 21st century. Other concepts that Henderson proposed have been used in nursing education from the 1930s until the present (O'Malley, 1996).

Testability

Henderson supported nursing research but believed that it should be clinical research (O'Malley, 1996). Much of the research before her time had been on educational processes and on the profession of nursing itself, rather than on the practice and outcomes of nursing, and she worked to change that.

Each of the 14 activities can be the basis for research. Although the statements are not written in testable terms, they may be reformulated into researchable questions. Further, the theory can guide research in any aspect of the individual's care needs.

Parsimony

Henderson's work is parsimonious in its presentation, but complex in its scope. The 14 statements cover the whole of the practice of nursing, and her vision about the nurse's role in patient care (i.e., that the nurse perform for the patient those activities the patient usually performs independently until the patient can again adequately perform them) contributes to that complexity.

Value in Extending Nursing Science

From a historical standpoint, Henderson's concept of nursing enhanced nursing science; this has been particularly important in the area of nursing education.

Her contributions to nursing literature extended from the 1930s through the 1990s. Her work has had an international impact on nursing research by strengthening the focus on nursing practice and confirming the value of tested interventions in assisting individuals to regain health. Internationally, researchers continue to direct their work with Virginia Henderson's model as a framework. Researchers from Japan, the Netherlands, Poland, and Turkey teamed up to create the Care Dependency Scale using Henderson's components of nursing care (Dijkstra et al., 2012), and Medina, Ruiz–Lozano, Delgado, & Vila (2012) found the "need theory of Henderson valuable in creating a patient valuation model for a mobile device for nursing" (p. 10479).

Faye G. Abdellah: Patient-Centered Approaches to Nursing

Faye Abdellah was one of the first nursing theorists. In one of her earliest writings (Abdellah, Beland, Martin, & Matheney, 1960), she referred to the model created by her colleagues and herself as a framework. Her writings spanned the period from 1954 to 1992 and include books, monographs, book chapters, articles, reports, forewords to books, and conference proceedings.

Background of the Theorist

Abdellah earned her bachelor's degree in nursing, master's degree, and doctorate from Columbia University, and she completed additional graduate studies in science at Rutgers University. She served as the Chief Nurse Officer and Deputy U.S. Surgeon General, U.S. Public Health Service before retiring in 1993 with the rank of Rear Admiral. She has been awarded many academic honors from both civilian and military sources (Abdellah & Levine, 1994). She retired from her position as dean of the Graduate School of Nursing, Uniformed Services University of the Health Sciences in 2000.

Philosophical Underpinnings of the Theory

Abdellah's patient-centered approach to nursing was developed inductively from her practice and is considered a human needs theory (Abdellah et al., 1960). The theory was created to assist with nursing education and is most applicable to education and practice (Abdellah et al., 1960). Although it was intended to guide care of those in the hospital, it also has relevance for nursing care in community settings.

Major Assumptions, Concepts, and Relationships

The language of Abdellah's framework is readable and clear. Consistent with the decade in which she was writing, she uses the term "she" for nurses, "he" for doctors and patients, and refers to the object of nursing as "patient" rather than client or consumer (Abdellah et al., 1960). Interestingly, she was one of the early writers who referred to "nursing diagnosis" (Abdellah et al., 1960, p. 9) during a time when nurses were taught that diagnosis was not a nurse's prerogative.

Assumptions

There are no openly stated assumptions in Abdellah's early work (Abdellah et al., 1960), but in a later work, she added six assumptions. These relate to change and anticipated changes that affect nursing; the need to appreciate the interconnectedness of social enterprises and social problems; the impact of problems such as poverty, racism, pollution,

Box 7-2 Abdellah's 21 Nursing Problems

1. To maintain good hygiene and physical comfort
2. To promote optimal activity, exercise, rest, and sleep
3. To promote safety through prevention of accidents, injury, or other trauma and through the prevention of the spread of infection
4. To maintain good body mechanics and prevent and correct deformities
5. To facilitate the maintenance of a supply of oxygen to all body cells
6. To facilitate the maintenance of nutrition of all body cells
7. To facilitate the maintenance of elimination
8. To facilitate the maintenance of fluid and electrolyte balance
9. To recognize the physiologic responses of the body to disease conditions
10. To facilitate the maintenance of regulatory mechanisms and functions
11. To facilitate the maintenance of sensory function
12. To identify and accept positive and negative expressions, feelings, and reactions
13. To identify and accept the interrelatedness of emotions and organic illness
14. To facilitate the maintenance of effective verbal and nonverbal communication
15. To promote the development of productive interpersonal relationships
16. To facilitate progress toward achievement of personal spiritual goals
17. To create and maintain a therapeutic environment
18. To facilitate awareness of self as an individual with varying physical, emotional, and developmental needs
19. To accept the optimum possible goals in light of physical and emotional limitations
20. To use community resources as an aid in resolving problems arising from illness
21. To understand the role of social problems as influencing factors in the cause of illness

Source: Abdellah et al. (1960).

education, and so forth on health and health care delivery; changing nursing education; continuing education for professional nurses; and development of nursing leaders from underserved groups (Abdellah, Beland, Martin, & Matheney, 1973).

Abdellah and colleagues (1960) developed a list of 21 nursing problems (Box 7-2). They also identified 10 steps to identify the client's problems and 10 nursing skills to be used in developing a treatment typology.

According to Abdellah and colleagues (1960), nurses should do the following:

1. Learn to know the patient.
2. Sort out relevant and significant data.
3. Make generalizations about available data in relation to similar nursing problems presented by other patients.
4. Identify the therapeutic plan.
5. Test generalizations with the patient and make additional generalizations.
6. Validate the patient's conclusions about his nursing problems.
7. Continue to observe and evaluate the patient over a period of time to identify any attitudes and clues affecting his or her behavior.
8. Explore the patient's and family's reaction to the therapeutic plan and involve them in the plan.
9. Identify how the nurse feels about the patient's nursing problems.
10. Discuss and develop a comprehensive nursing care plan.

Abdellah and colleagues (1960) distinguished between nursing diagnoses and nursing functions. Nursing diagnoses were a determination of the nature and extent of nursing problems presented by individuals receiving nursing care, and functions were nursing activities that contributed to the solution for the same nu problem. Other concepts central to her work were (1) health care team (a gr of health professionals trained at various levels, and often at different institution working together to provide health care); (2) professionalization of nursing (requires that nurses identify those nursing problems that depend on the nurse's use of his or her capacities to conceptualize events and make judgments about them); (3) patient (individual who needs nursing care and who is dependent on the health care provider); and (4) nursing (a service to individuals and families and to society, which helps people cope with their health needs) (Abdellah et al., 1960).

Usefulness

The patient-centered approach was constructed to be useful to nursing practice, with the impetus for it being nursing education. Abdellah's publications on nursing education began with her dissertation; her interest in education of nurses continues into the present.

Abdellah also published work on nursing, nursing research, and public policy related to nursing in several international publications. She has been a strong advocate for improving nursing practice through nursing research and has a publication record on nursing research that dates from 1955 to the present. Box 7-3 lists only a few of Abdellah's many publications.

Testability

Abdellah's work is a conceptual model that is not directly testable because there are few stated directional relationships. The model is testable in principle, though, because testable hypotheses can be derived from its conceptual material. One work (Abdellah & Levine, 1957) was identified that described the development of a tool to measure client and personnel satisfaction with nursing care.

Parsimony

Abdellah and colleagues' model (1960, 1973) touches on many factors in nursing but focuses primarily on the perspective of nursing education. It defines 21 nursing problems, 10 steps to identifying client's problems, and 10 nursing skills. Because of its focus and complexity, it is not particularly parsimonious.

Box 7-3 Examples of Abdellah's Publications

Abdellah, F. G., Beland, I. L, Martin, A., & Matheney, R. V. (1968). *Patient-centered approaches to nursing* (2nd ed.). New York: MacMillan.

Abdellah, F. G. (1972). Evolution of nursing as a profession: Perspective on manpower development. *International Nursing Review, 19*, 3.

Abdellah, F. G. (1986). The nature of nursing science. In L. H. Nicholl (Ed.), *Perspectives on nursing theory.* Boston: Little, Brown.

Abdellah, F. G. (1987). The federal role in nursing education. *Nursing Outlook, 35*(5), 224–225.

Abdellah, F. G. (1991). Public policy impacting on nursing care of older adults. In E. M. Baines (Ed.), *Perspectives on gerontological nursing.* Newbury, CA: Sage Publications.

Abdellah, F. G., & Levine, E. (1994). *Preparing nursing research for the 21st century.* New York: Springer.

Nursing Science

model has contributed to nursing science as an early effort to change cation. In the early years of its application, it helped to bring structure and nization to what was often a disorganized collection of lectures and experiences. She categorized nursing problems based on the individual's needs and developed a typology of nursing treatment and nursing skills. Finally, she posited a list of characteristics that described what was distinctly nursing, thereby differentiating the profession from other health professions. Hers was a major contribution to the discipline of nursing, bringing it out of the era of being considered simply an occupation into Nightingale's ideal of becoming a profession.

Dorothea E. Orem: The Self-Care Deficit Nursing Theory

Dorothea Orem was born in Baltimore, Maryland. She received her diploma in nursing from Providence Hospital School of Nursing in Washington, DC, and her baccalaureate degree in nursing from Catholic University in 1939. In 1945, she also earned her master's degree from Catholic University (Taylor, 2006).

Background of the Theorist

Orem held a number of positions as private duty nurse, hospital staff nurse, and educator. She was the director of both the School of Nursing and Nursing Service at Detroit's Providence Hospital until 1949, moving from there to Indiana where she served on the Board of Health until 1957. She assumed a role as a faculty member of Catholic University in 1959, later becoming acting dean (Taylor, 2006).

Orem's interest in nursing theory was piqued when she and a group of colleagues were charged with producing a curriculum for practical nursing for the Department of Health, Education, and Welfare in Washington, DC. After publishing the first book on her theory in 1971, she continued working on her concept of nursing and self-care. She had numerous honorary doctorates and other awards as members of the nursing profession have recognized the value of the self-care deficit theory (Taylor, 2006). Dr. Orem died in 2007 after a period of failing health. Nurses will remember her as one of the pioneers of nursing theory (Bekel, 2007).

Philosophical Underpinnings of the Theory

Orem (1995) denied that any particular theorist provided the basis for the Self-Care Deficit Nursing Theory (SCDNT). She expressed interest in several theories, although she references only Parsons' structure of social action and von Bertalanfy's system theory (Orem, 1995). Taylor, Geden, Isaramalai, and Wongvatunyu (2000), however, stated that the ontology of Orem's SCDNT is the school of moderate realism, and its focus is on the person as agent; the SCDNT is a highly developed formalized theoretical system of nursing. Currently, the theory is referred to as self-care science and nursing theory (Taylor & Renpenning, 2011). Taylor and Renpenning make a case for the scientific basis of the life work that was Orem's magnum opus and quote from her works extensively.

Major Assumptions, Concepts, and Relationships

Orem's theory changed to fit the times most notably in the concept of the individual and of the nursing system. The original theory, however, remains largely intact.

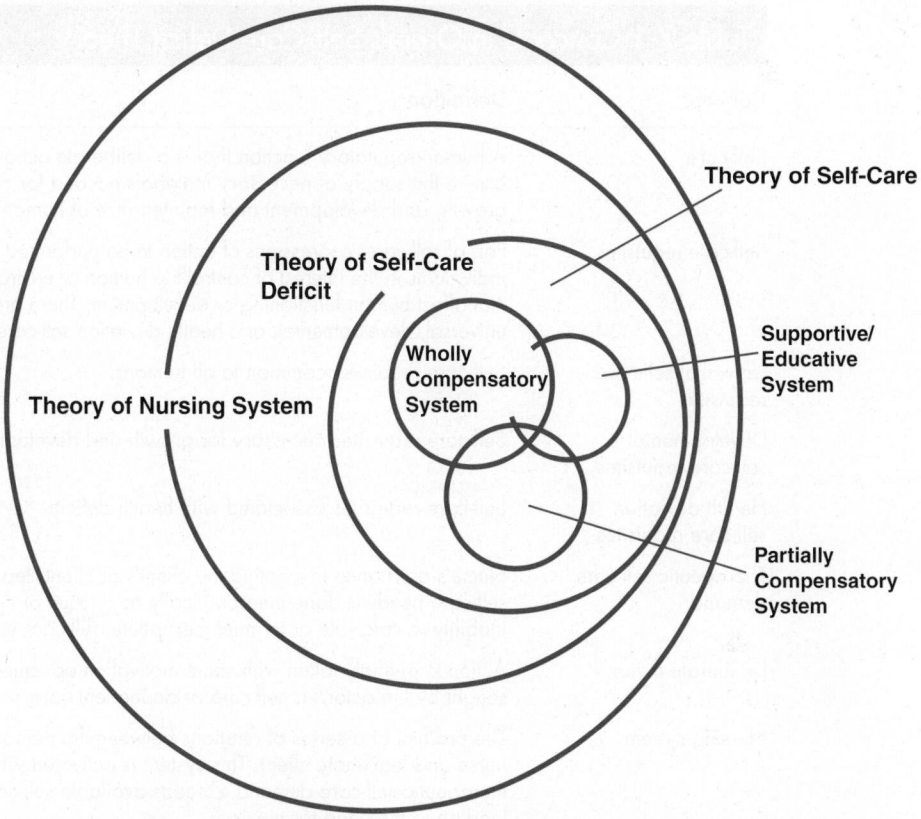

Figure 7-1 Self-care deficit nursing theory. (Source: Orem, D. [2001]. *Nursing: Concepts of practice* [6th ed.]. St. Louis: Mosby.)

Orem (2001) delineates three nested theories: theories of self-care, self-care deficit, and nursing systems (Figure 7-1). The theory of nursing systems is the outer or encompassing theory, which contains the theory of self-care deficit. The theory of self-care is a component of the theory of self-care deficit.

Concepts

Orem (1995, 2001) defined the metaparadigm concepts as follows:

> *Nursing is seen as an art through which the practitioner of nursing gives specialized assistance to persons with disabilities which makes more than ordinary assistance necessary to meet needs for self-care. The nurse also intelligently participates in the medical care the individual receives from the physician.*
>
> *Humans are defined as "men, women, and children cared for either singly or as social units," and are the "material object" (p. 8) of nurses and others who provide direct care.*
>
> *Environment has physical, chemical, and biological features. It includes the family culture and community.*
>
> *Health is "being structurally and functionally whole or sound" (p. 96). Also, health is a state that encompasses both the health of individuals and of groups, and human health is the ability to reflect on one's self, to symbolize experience, and to communicate with others.*

Table 7-1 Concepts in Orem's Self-Care Deficit Theory

Concept	Definition
Self-care	A human regulatory function that is a deliberate action to supply or ensure the supply of necessary materials needed for continued life, growth, and development and maintenance of human integrity.
Self-care requisites	Part of self-care; expressions of action to be performed by or for individuals in the interest of controlling human or environmental factors that affect human functioning or development. There are three types: universal, developmental, and health deviation self-care requisites.
Universal self-care requisites	Self-care requisites common to all humans.
Developmental self-care requisites	Self-care requisites necessary for growth and development.
Health deviation self-care requisites	Self-care requisites associated with health deficits.
Therapeutic self-care demand	Nurse's assistance in meeting the client's or client dependent's self-care needs is done therapeutically as a result of the client's inability to calculate or to meet therapeutic self-care needs.
Deliberate action	Action knowingly taken with some motivation or some outcome sought by the actor, as self-care or dependent care.
Nursing system	The product of a series of relations between the persons: legitimate nurse and legitimate client. This system is activated when the client's therapeutic self-care demand exceeds available self-care agency, leading to the need for nursing.
Product of nursing	Nursing has two products: An intellectual product (the design for helping the client) A system of care of long or short duration for persons requiring nursing

Source: Orem (1995).

Numerous additional concepts were formulated for Orem's theory; Table 7-1 lists some of the more significant ones.

Relationships

An underlying premise of Orem's theory is the belief that humans engage in continuous communication and interchange among themselves and their environments to remain alive and to function. In humans, the power to act deliberately is exercised to identify needs and to make needed judgments. Furthermore, mature human beings experience privations in the form of action in care of self and others involving making life-sustaining and function-regulating actions. Human agency is exercised in discovering, developing, and transmitting to others ways and means to identify needs for, and make inputs into, self and others. Finally, groups of human beings with structured relationships cluster tasks and allocate responsibilities for providing care to group members who experience privations for making required deliberate decisions about self and others (Orem, 1995).

Usefulness

Numerous colleges and schools of nursing base their curricula on the SCDNT. Georgetown University School of Nursing; Oakland University School of Nursing;

The University of Missouri, Columbia; and the University of Florida, Gainesville, for example, all have curricula based on Orem's SCDNT (Taylor, 2006, 2011). Hospitals in several areas of the country have based nursing care on Orem's theory, and it has been applied to an ambulatory care setting. Such medical conditions as arthritis or gastrointestinal and renal diseases, and such areas of practice as community nursing, critical care, cultural concepts, maternal–child nursing, medical-surgical nursing, pediatric nursing, perioperative nursing, and renal dialysis, among other specialties have used Orem's theory to structure care (Taylor, 2006, 2011). Orem's SCDNT has received international interest and has been used in many countries including Great Britain, Germany, Japan, the Netherlands, Norway, Sweden, and New Zealand. Moreover, numerous publications define methods for using Orem's SCDNT in practice, research, and education.

Orem was a prolific author and her writings spanned five decades. In addition to her detailed description of her theory (Orem, 1971, 1985a, 1991, 1995, 2001), she authored an analysis of hospital nursing service (Orem, 1956) and illustrations for self-care for the rehabilitation client (Orem, 1985b). Further evidence of the usefulness of Orem's work is the International Orem Society, which celebrates the work of Dr. Orem. Their journal, *Self-Care, Dependent-Care & Nursing*, indicates the value to nurses across the globe (Biggs, 2008).

Testability

Many nursing research studies have used Orem's theory as a conceptual framework or as a source of testable hypotheses. Further, over the years, many research studies have tested elements of the theory. The researchers have studied people with diminished self-care agency across age and social groups, in numerous situations, and in many countries. Most research into the SCDNT is descriptive, and the theory has not been subject to testing in its entirety (Taylor, 2006; Taylor & Renpenning, 2011). Box 7-4 lists some of the recent research studies using the SCDNT.

Box 7-4 Orem's Theory in Nursing Research, Practice, and Education

Burdette, L. (2012). Relationship between self-care agency, self-care practices and obesity among rural midlife women. *Self-Care, Dependent-Care & Nursing, 19*(1), 5–14.

Davidson, S. (2012). Challenging RN-BSN students to apply Orem's theory to practice. *Self-Care, Dependent-Care & Nursing, 19*(1), 15–19.

Fleck, L. M. (2012). The nutrition self-care inventory. *Self-Care, Dependent-Care & Nursing, 19*(1), 26–34.

Luxton, D. D., Armstrong, C. M., Fanelli, E., & Thomas, E. K., (2011). Attitudes and awareness of web-based self-care resources in the military: A preliminary survey study. *Telemedicine and E-health, 17*, 580–583.

Pickens, J. (2012). Development of self-care agency through enhancement of motivation in people with schizophrenia. *Self-Care, Dependent-Care & Nursing, 19*(1), 47–52.

Thi, T. L. (2012). An analysis of self-care knowledge of hepatitis B patients. *Self-Care, Dependent-Care & Nursing, 19*(1), 41–46.

Wanchai, A., Armer, J. M., & Stewart, B. R. (2010). Self-care agency using complementary and alternative medicine (CAM) among breast cancer survivors. *Self-Care, Dependent-Care & Nursing, 18*(1), 10–18.

Parsimony

Orem's (2001) SCDNT is complex. It consists of three nested theories, many presuppositions, and propositions in each of the individual theories. Revisions of the theory from the original (1971) have improved the organization; however, its complexity has increased in response to societal needs throughout the several editions.

Value in Extending Nursing Science

The SCDNT has been the basis for many college and university nursing curricula (Orem, 1995, 2001). It has been used in practice situations and extensively in research projects, theses, and dissertations (Taylor, 2011). The practical applicability of the theory is attractive to graduate students because it is perceived as a realistic reflection of nursing practice.

Dorothy Johnson: The Behavioral System Model

Dorothy Johnson began her work on the Behavioral System Model in the late 1950s and wrote into the 1990s. The focus of her model is on needs, the human as a behavioral system, and relief of stress as nursing care.

Johnson (1968, 1990) reported that her work began as a study of the knowledge that identified nursing while synthesizing content for nursing curricula at the graduate and undergraduate levels. She wanted the curricula to be focused on nursing rather than derived from the knowledge bases of other health care disciplines (Johnson, 1959a, 1959b, 1997). Indeed, she believed that nursing, although relying on the contributions of other sciences, is a discrete science and a unique discipline.

Johnson's model was deductively derived through long study of other theories and applying them to nursing (Johnson, 1997). Her goal was to conceptualize nursing for education of nurses at all levels (Johnson, 1990, 1997), and the model emanated from her practice, study, and teaching experiences.

Although Johnson did not write a book on her theory, she did write several chapters and articles that explained her theoretical framework. Box 7-5 lists a sampling of these writings.

Box 7-5 Examples of Johnson's Writings on Nursing Theory

Johnson, D. E. (1959a). A philosophy of nursing. *Nursing Outlook, 7*(4), 198–200.

Johnson, D. E. (1959b). The nature of nursing science. *Nursing Outlook, 7*(5), 291–294.

Johnson, D. E. (1968). Theory in nursing: Borrowed and unique. *Nursing Research, 17*(3), 206–209.

Johnson, D. E. (1974). Development of a theory: A requisite for nursing as a primary health profession. *Nursing Research, 23*(5), 372–377.

Johnson, D. E. (1980). The behavioral system model for nursing. In J. P. Riehl & C. Roy (Eds.), *Conceptual models for nursing practice* (pp. 207–216). New York: Appleton-Century-Crofts.

Johnson, D. E. (1990). The behavioral system model for nursing. In M. E. Parker (Ed.), *Nursing theories in practice* (pp. 23–32). New York: National League for Nursing Press.

Background of the Theorist

Dorothy Johnson was reared in Savannah, Georgia and received a bachelor's degree in nursing from Vanderbilt University. She earned a master's degree in public health from Harvard in 1948 and returned to Vanderbilt to begin her teaching career. In 1949, she joined the nursing faculty of the University of California at Los Angeles (UCLA). She retired from UCLA in 1977 and now lives in Florida.

Philosophical Underpinnings of the Theory

Johnson stated that Nightingale's work inspired her model. Nightingale's philosophical leanings prompted Johnson to consider the person experiencing a disease more important than the disease itself (Johnson, 1990). She reported that she derived portions of her theory from the works of Selye on stress, Grinker's theory of human behavior, and Buckley and Chin on systems theories (Johnson, 1980, 1990).

Major Assumptions, Concepts, and Relationships

Assumptions

Assumptions of Johnson's model are both stated and derived. There are four assumptions about human behavioral subsystems. First is the belief that drives serve as focal points around which behaviors are organized to achieve specific goals. Second, it is assumed that behavior is differentiated and organized within the prevailing dimensions of set and choice. Third, the specialized parts or subsystems of the behavioral system are structured by dimensions of goal, set, choice, and actions; each has observable behaviors. Finally, interactive and interdependent subsystems tend to achieve and maintain balance between and among subsystems through control and regulatory mechanisms (Grubbs, 1980).

Concepts

Although she adopted concepts from other disciplines, Johnson modified and defined them to apply specifically to nursing situations. This was an evolving process as shown in her writings (Johnson, 1959a, 1959b, 1968, 1974, 1980, 1990).

The metaparadigm concepts are apparent in Johnson's writings. Nursing is seen as "an external regulatory force which acts to preserve the organization and integration of the patient's behavior at an optimal level under those conditions in which the behavior constitutes a threat to physical or social health, or in which illness is found" (Johnson, 1980, p. 214). The concept of human was defined as a behavioral system that strives to make continual adjustments to achieve, maintain, or regain balance to the steady state that is adaptation (Johnson, 1980).

Health is seen as the opposite of illness, and Johnson (1980) defines it as "some degree of regularity and constancy in behavior, the behavioral system reflects adjustments and adaptations that are successful in some way and to some degree . . . adaptation is functionally efficient and effective" (pp. 208, 209). Environment is not directly defined, but it is implied to include all elements of the surroundings of the human system and includes interior stressors. Other concepts defined in Johnson's model are listed in Table 7-2.

Table 7-2 Concepts in Johnson's Behavioral System Theory

Concept	Definition
Behavioral system	Man is a system that indicates the state of the system through behaviors
Boundaries	The point that differentiates the interior of the system from the exterior
Function	Consequences or purposes of actions
Functional requirements	Input that the system must receive to survive and develop
Homeostasis	Process of maintaining stability
Instability	State in which the system output of energy depletes the energy needed to maintain stability
Stability	Balance or steady state in maintaining balance of behavior within an acceptable range
Stressor	A stimulus from the internal or external world that results in stress or instability
Structure	The parts of the system that make up the whole
System	That which functions as a whole by virtue of organized independent interaction of its parts
Subsystem	A minisystem maintained in relationship to the entire system when it or the environment is not disturbed
Tension	The system's adjustment to demands, change or growth, or to actual disruptions
Variables	Factors outside the system that influence the system's behavior, but which the system lacks power to change

Source: Grubbs (1980).

Relationships

Johnson (1980) delineated seven subsystems to which the model applied. These are as follows:

1. Attachment or affiliative subsystem—serves the need for security through social inclusion or intimacy
2. Dependency subsystem—behaviors designed to get attention, recognition, and physical assistance
3. Ingestive subsystem—fulfills the need to supply the biologic requirements for food and fluids
4. Eliminative subsystem—functions to excrete wastes
5. Sexual subsystem—serves the biologic requirements of procreation and reproduction
6. Aggressive subsystem—functions in self and social protection and preservation
7. Achievement system—functions to master and control the self or the environment

Finally, there are three functional requirements of humans in Johnson's (1980) model. These are:

1. To be protected from noxious influences with which the person cannot cope
2. To be nurtured through the input of supplies from the environment
3. To be stimulated to enhance growth and prevent stagnation

Usefulness

That Johnson's model is useful for nursing practic
in several articles and chapters. Damus (1980), D
described situations in which Johnson's model has
tice. Other authors have used the theory to apply
example, Benson (1997) used Johnson's model as
of fear of crime on an elder person's health, healt
life. Fruehwirth (1989) applied Johnson's model
caregivers for individuals with Alzheimer disease.

Testability

Parts of Johnson's model have been tested or used to direct nursing research. Indeed, more than 20 research studies have been identified using Johnson's model. Turner-Henson (1992), for example, used Johnson's model as a framework to examine how mothers of chronically ill children perceived the environment (i.e., whether it was supportive, safe, and accessible). Poster, Dee, and Randell (1997) used Johnson's theory as a conceptual framework in a study of client outcome evaluation; they found that the nursing theory made it possible to prescribe nursing care and to distinguish it from medical care. Derdiarian and Schobel (1990) used Johnson's model to develop an assessment tool for individuals with AIDS.

Aspects of Johnson's model have been tested in nursing research. In one study, Derdiarian (1990) examined the relationship between the aggressive/protective subsystem and the other six model subsystems.

Parsimony

Johnson (1980) was able to explicate her entire model in a single short chapter in an edited book. Relatively few concepts are used in the theory, and they are commonly used terms. Additionally, the relationships are clear; therefore, the model is considered to be parsimonious.

Value in Extending Nursing Science

Johnson's model has been used in nursing practice and research to a significant extent. In addition, her work has been used as a curriculum guide for a number of schools of nursing (Grubbs, 1980; Johnson, 1980, 1990), and it has been adapted for use in hospital situations (Dee, 1990). Finally, her work inspired the work of at least two other grand nursing theorists, Betty Neuman and Sister Calista Roy, who were her students.

Betty Neuman: The Neuman Systems Model

Since the 1960s, Betty Neuman has been recognized as a pioneer in the field of nursing, particularly in the area of community mental health. She developed her model while lecturing in community mental health at UCLA and first published it in 1972 under the title, "A Model for Teaching the Total Person Approach to Patient Problems" (Murray, 1999; Neuman & Fawcett, 2002). Since that time, she has been a prolific writer, and her model has been used extensively in colleges of nursing, beginning with Neumann College's baccalaureate nursing program in Aston, Pennsylvania. Numerous other nursing programs have organized their curricula around her model both in the United States and internationally (Neuman & Fawcett, 2009).

The major elements in this review of the Neuman Systems Model are taken from the third and fourth editions of her book (Neuman, 1995; Neuman & Fawcett, 2009), with references to earlier writings to show development of the model over time. The model was deductively derived and emanated from requests of graduate students who wanted assistance with a broad interpretation of nursing (Neuman, 1995).

Neuman's model uses a systems approach that is focused on the human needs of protection or relief from stress (Neuman & Fawcett, 2009). Neuman believed that the causes of stress can be identified and remedied through nursing interventions. She emphasized the need of humans for dynamic balance that the nurse can provide through identification of problems, mutually agreeing on goals, and using the concept of prevention as intervention. Neuman's model is one of only a few considered prescriptive in nature. The model is universal, abstract, and applicable for individuals from many cultures (Neuman, 1995; Neuman & Fawcett, 2009).

Background of the Theorist

Betty Neuman was born in 1924 on a farm near Lowell, Ohio. In 1947, she earned her nursing diploma from People's Hospital School of Nursing, Akron, Ohio, and moved to California shortly thereafter. She earned a bachelor's degree in nursing from UCLA and also studied psychology and public health. In 1966, she earned a master's degree in mental health and public health consultation, also from UCLA, then earned her doctorate in clinical psychology in 1985 from Pacific Western University. She worked as a hospital staff nurse, a head nurse, and an industrial nurse and consultant before becoming a nursing instructor. She has taught medical-surgical nursing, critical care, and communicable disease nursing at the University of Southern California Medical Center in Los Angeles and at other colleges in Ohio and West Virginia (Neuman & Fawcett, 2002).

Philosophical Underpinnings of the Theory

Neuman used concepts and theories from a number of disciplines in the development of her theory. In her works, she referred to Chardin and Cornu on wholeness in systems, von Bertalanfy and Lazlo on general systems theory, Selye on stress theory, and Lazarus on stress and coping (Neuman, 1995; Neuman & Fawcett, 2009).

Major Assumptions, Concepts, and Relationships

Concepts

Neuman (1995; Neuman & Fawcett, 2009) adhered to the metaparadigm concepts and has developed numerous additional concepts for her model. In her work, she defined human beings as a "client/client system, as a composite of variables . . . physiological, psychological, sociocultural, developmental, and spiritual (Neuman & Fawcett, 2009, p. 16). The ring structure is a "basic structure of protective concentric rings, for retention attainment or maintenance of system stability and integrity. . ." (Neuman & Fawcett, 2009, p. 16). Environment to Neuman is a structure of concentric rings representing the three environments, internal, external, and created environments, all of which influence the client's adaptation to stressors. Health is defined as "a continuum; wellness and illness are at opposite ends.... Health for the client is equated with optimal system stability that is the best possible wellness state at any given time" (p. 23). "Variances from wellness or varying degrees of system instability are caused by stressor invasion of the normal line of defense" (p. 24). Finally, in the nursing component, the major concern is to maintain client system stability through accurately assessing environmental and other stressors and assisting in client adjustments to maintain optimal wellness. Table 7-3 lists

Table 7-3 Concepts in Neuman's Systems Model

Concept	Definition
Basic structure	Common client survival factors and unique individual characteristics representing basic system energy resources.
Boundary lines	The flexible line of defense is the outer boundary of the client system.
Content	The variables of person in interaction with the internal and external environment comprise the whole client system.
Degree of reaction	The amount of system instability resulting from stressor invasion of the normal line of defense.
Entropy	A process of energy depletion and disorganization moving the system toward illness or possible death.
Flexible line of defense	A protective, accordion-like mechanism that surrounds and protects the normal line of defense from invasion by stressors.
Goal	Stability for the purpose of client survival and optimal wellness.
Input/output	The matter, energy, and information exchanged between client and environment that is entering or leaving the system at any point in time.
Lines of resistance	Protection factors activated when stressors have penetrated the normal line of defense, causing a reaction symptomatology.
Negentropy	A process of energy conservation that increases organization and complexity, moving the system towards stability or a higher degree of wellness.
Normal line of defense	An adaptational level of health developed over time and considered normal for a particular individual client or system; it becomes a standard for wellness–deviance determination.
Open system	A system in which there is a continuous flow of input and process, output, and feedback. It is a system of organized complexity where all elements are in interaction.
Prevention as intervention	Intervention modes for nursing action and determinants for entry of both client and nurse into the health care system.
Reconstitution	The return and maintenance of system stability, following treatment of stressor reaction, which may result in a higher or lower level of wellness.
Stability	A state of balance or harmony requiring energy exchanges as the client adequately copes with stressors to retain, attain, or maintain an optimal level of health, thus preserving system integrity.
Stressors	Environmental factors, intra-, inter-, and extrapersonal in nature, that have potential for disrupting system stability. A stressor is any phenomenon that might penetrate both the flexible and normal lines of defense, resulting in either a positive or negative outcome.
Wellness/illness	Wellness is the condition in which all system parts and subparts are in harmony with the whole system of the client. Illness indicates disharmony among the parts and subparts of the client system.

Source: Neuman (1995).

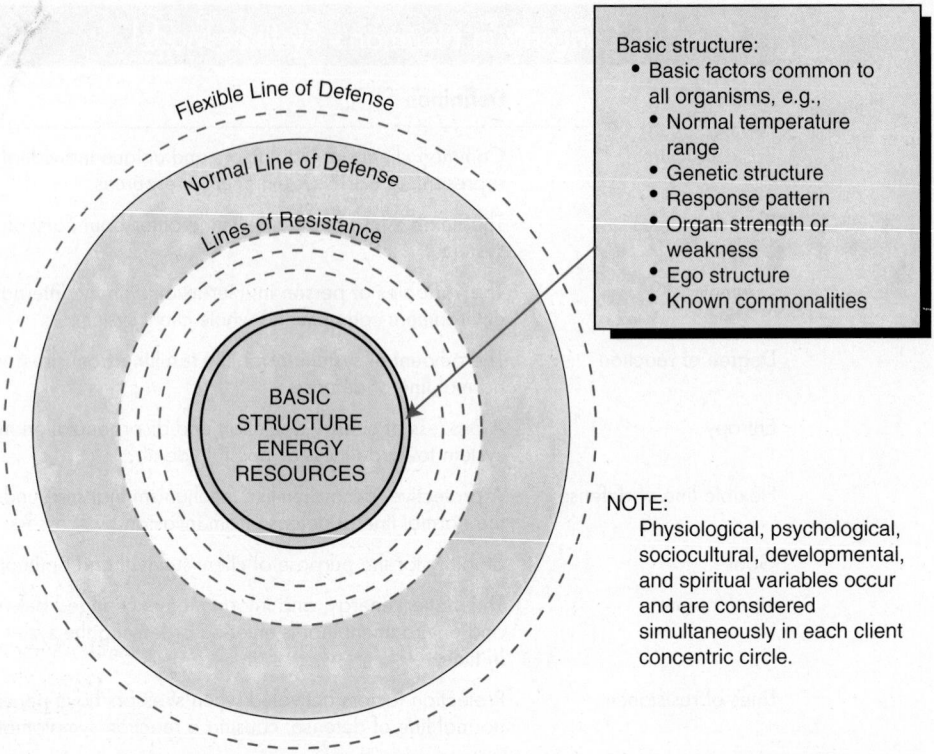

Figure 7-2 The Neuman systems model. (Source: Neuman, B., & Fawcett, J. [2002]. *The Neuman systems model* [4th ed.]. Upper Saddle River, NJ: Pearson Education, Inc. Used with permission of Betty Neuman, RN, PhD, FAAN.)

selected additional concepts from Neuman's model, and Figure 7-2 offers a visual representation.

Relationships

Neuman defined five interacting variables: physiologic, psychological, sociocultural, developmental, and spiritual. These five variables function in time to attain, maintain, or retain system stability. The model is based on the client's reaction to stress as it maintains boundaries to protect client stability (Neuman & Fawcett, 2009).

Neuman (1995; Neuman & Fawcett, 2009) delineated a three-step nursing process model in which nursing diagnosis (the first step) assumes that the nurse collects an adequate database from which to analyze variances from wellness to make the diagnoses. Nursing goals, which are determined by negotiation with the client, are set in the second step. Appropriate prevention as intervention strategies are decided in that step. The third step, nursing outcomes, is the step in which confirmation of prescriptive change or reformulation of nursing goals is evaluated. The nurse links the client, environment, health, and nursing. The findings feed back into the system as applicable. A table of prevention as intervention strategies clarifies what comprises the nursing actions to affect this type of intervention. Neuman outlined 10 propositions or assumptions of the model (Box 7-6).

Usefulness

Neuman's model has been used extensively in nursing education and nursing practice. In her latest work, she provides a number of specific examples of the systems

Box 7-6 Assumptions of Neum

1. Each client system is unique, a compos given range of responses.
2. Many known, unknown, and universal stres for disturbing a client's usual stability level or interrelationships of client variables at any poin which a client is protected by the flexible line of a to stressors.
3. Each client/client system has evolved a normal range ment that is referred to as a normal line of defense. The can be used as a standard from which to measure health a
4. When the flexible line of defense is no longer capable of pro client system against an environmental stressor, the stressor bre normal line of defense.
5. The client, whether in a state of wellness or illness, is a dynamic co interrelationships of the variables. Wellness is on a continuum of avai to support the system in an optimal state of system stability.
6. Implicit within each client system are internal resistance factors known as resistance, which function to stabilize and realign the client to the usual well state.
7. Primary prevention relates to general knowledge that is applied in client assessment and intervention, in identification, and in reduction or mitigation of possible or actual risk factors associated with environmental stressors to prevent possible reaction.
8. Secondary prevention relates to symptomatology following a reaction to stressors, appropriate ranking of intervention priorities, and treatment to reduce their noxious effects.
9. Tertiary prevention relates to the adjustive processes taking place as reconstitution begins and maintenance factors move the client back in a circular manner toward primary prevention.
10. The client as a system is in dynamic, constant energy exchange with the environment.

processes (Neuman & Fawcett, 2009). The Neuman Systems Model is in place in numerous states of the United States and internationally in countries as diverse as Taiwan and the Netherlands. It reportedly has been initiated to guide nursing practice for the management of patient care in the areas of medicine and surgery, mental health, women's health, pediatric nursing, community as client, and gerontology. Graduate students, in particular, find Neuman's model realistic to define their practice.

Because of its utility and popularity as a model, it has been monitored by a group called the Neuman Systems Model Trustees Group, Inc. This group meets periodically to discuss research and practice related to the model and to promote exchange of information and ideas. Neuman's model is in use as a guide in a plethora of nursing schools at all levels; a partial listing is included in Neuman and Fawcett (2009).

Testability

Although the Neuman model is not testable in its entirety, it gives rise to directional hypotheses that are testable in research. As a result, it has been used as a conceptual

Box 7-7 Examples of Nursing Research Studies Using Neuman's Systems Model

Cobb, R. K. (2012). How well does spirituality predict health status in adults living with HIV disease: A Neuman systems model study. *Nursing Science Quarterly, 25*(4), 347–355.

Elmore, D. H. (2010). Empirical testing of the Neuman systems nursing education model: Exploring the created environment of registered nursing students in Nevada's colleges and universities. Doctoral Dissertation, University of Nevada at Las Vegas: UMI Order AAI3412367.

Formanek-Hess, R., & Weinland, J. A. D. (2012). The life-changing impact of peripartum cardiomyopathy: An analysis of online postings. *MCN, 37*(4), 241–246.

Lowry, L. W. (2012). A qualitative descriptive study of spirituality guided by the Neuman systems model. *Nursing Science Quarterly, 25*(4), 356–361.

Lucki, M. M., Napier, D. E., & Wagner, C. (2012). Preoperative care management of patients with hip fractures during the wait time between emergency department discharge and operating room admission for surgical repair. *Orthopaedic Nursing, 31*(5), 281–286.

Gigliotti, E. (2012). New advances in the use of Neuman's lines of defense and resistance in quantitative research. *Nursing Science Quarterly, 25*(4), 336–340.

Pines, E. W., Rauschhuber, M. L., Norgan, G. H., Cook, J. D., Canchola, L., Richardson, C., & Jones, M. E. (2012). Stress resiliency, psychological empowerment and conflict management styles among baccalaureate nursing students. *Journal of Advanced Nursing, 68*(7), 1482–1493.

framework extensively in nursing research, and aspects of the model have been empirically tested. Intermediate theories using the Neuman Systems Model have been developed and are being tested. Box 7-7 lists a few of the many nursing research studies that have used Neuman's Systems Model.

Parsimony

Neuman's model is complex, and many parts of the model function in multiple ways. The description of the model's parts can be confusing; therefore, the model is not considered to be parsimonious. Neuman and Fawcett (2009), however, have developed intermediate diagrams to clarify the interactions among parts of the model and to facilitate its use. The definitions are well developed in the latest edition of the model, and the assumptions (propositions), although multileveled, are well organized.

Value in Extending Nursing Science

The Neuman Systems Model has extended nursing science as a needs and causality-focused framework. It appeals to nurses who consider the client to be a holistic individual who reacts to stressors because it predicts the outcomes of interventions to strengthen the lines of defense against stress, which may destabilize the system. Neuman's model is useful not only in the acute critical care area because of the focus on attaining, regaining, and maintaining system stability (Neuman, 1990) but also in community health situations because of its focus on prevention as intervention (Neuman, 1995; Neuman & Fawcett, 2009).

Summary

The human needs nursing theories were among the earliest of the nursing theories. In general, these theories followed the philosophical school of thought of the time by considering the person to be a biopsychosocial being and focusing on meeting the individual's needs.

Donald Crawford, the nurse from the opening case study, illustrated how a human needs–based model can be used to help direct client care through anticipating or predicting client needs and determining desirable outcomes. Many other nurses in a variety of settings use these models and theories to direct care for their clients.

It should be noted that succeeding generations of nursing theorists based their models and theories on the works discussed here. Indeed, these theories were building blocks on which the profession of nursing depended during the last half of the 20th century and into the 21st century.

Key Points

- Needs theorists generally come from the positivist school of thought philosophically, and therefore the theories fit well with medical theories of care.
- The needs theories of nursing work well with the current emphasis on evidence-based practice because of the bias toward experimental science.
- The first nursing theorists mainly focused on the human needs of their patients/clients.
- Florence Nightingale is respected as the mother of modern professional nursing. She brought nursing out of the servant position it held in the 19th century and into the respected professional status it holds currently.
- Virginia Henderson is often seen as the mother of American professional nursing. She was a prolific author and researcher. Her concept of nursing is still used in clinical and community health care.
- Faye Abdellah provided nurses with one of the first academic nursing theories. She was a prolific author and researcher. She categorized nursing problems based on the individual's needs and developed a typology of nursing treatment and nursing skills. Finally, she posited a list of characteristics that described what was distinctly nursing.
- Dorothea Orem provided one of the first theories that gave the patient/client the responsibility for self-care. Her ideas allowed patients to resume more normal lives with respect to their self-care agency.
- Dorothy Johnson was a teacher of nursing at all levels. Her theoretical work inspired many other nurses to become theoretical thinkers.
- Betty Neuman gave nurses the systems model with its lines of defense against stress. She believed that the causes of stress can be identified and remedied through nursing interventions. She developed the concept of prevention as intervention. Neuman's model is one of only a few considered prescriptive in nature.
- The needs theorists' works are still in daily use in education, in clinical nursing, and in clinical nursing research.

Learning Activities

1. Discuss how the needs-based theories fit into the current health care system and in the specialty in which you currently practice.
2. Discuss the usefulness of one of the models/theories in this chapter to evidence-based practice. How would you and colleagues present your evidence?
3. Choose one of the models discussed in this chapter and demonstrate its use in the care of a selected client. Write a nursing care plan using the model. Define all elements of the nursing care plan using the language and the assumptions/propositions of the model.
4. Obtain the work of one of the theorists described in this chapter. Outline a research study testing components of the model.
   a. Determine which major concepts or propositions of the model can be tested.
   b. Define the elements of the model to be tested in the research project.
   c. Develop a hypothesis statement that examines the model's propositions in a sample from an acute care or community setting.

REFERENCES

Abdellah, F. G., Beland, I. L., Martin, A., & Matheney, R. V. (1960). *Patient-centered approaches to nursing.* New York: MacMillan.

Abdellah, F. G., Beland, I. L., Martin, A., & Matheney, R. V. (1973). *New directions in patient-centered nursing.* New York: MacMillan.

Abdellah, F. G., & Levine, E. (1957). Developing a measure of patient and personnel satisfaction with nursing care. *Nursing Research, 5*(2), 100–108.

Abdellah, F. G., & Levine, E. (1994). *Preparing nursing research for the 21st century.* New York: Springer.

Allen, M. P. (1996). *Tribute to Virginia Avernal Henderson, 1897–1996 from the Interagency Council on Information Resources for Nursing (ICIRN).* Retrieved from http//www.sandiego.edu/nursing/theory/henderson.htm.

Alligood, M. R., & Tomey, A. M. (2010). *Nursing theorists and their work.* (7th ed.). Maryland Heights, MO: Mosby Elsevier.

Artinian, N. T. (1991). Philosophy of science and family nursing theory development. In A. L. Whall & J. Fawcett (Eds.), *Family theory development in nursing.* Philadelphia: F. A. Davis.

Attewell, A. (2010). Florence Nightingale's relevance to nurses. *Journal of Holistic Nursing, 28*(1), 101–106.

Attewell, A. (2012). *Illuminating Florence: Finding Nightingale's legacy in your practice.* Indianapolis, IN: Sigma Theta Tau International.

Audain, C. (1998). *Florence Nightingale.* Retrieved from www.scottla.edu/lriddle/women/nitegale.htm.

Audain, C. (2007). *Biographies of women mathematicians: Florence Nightingale.* Retrieved from www.agnesscott.edu/Lriddle/WOMEN/nitegale.htm.

Beck, D. M. (2005). Sick-nursing and health-nursing: Nightingale established our broad scope of practice in 1893. In B. M. Dossey, L. C. Selanders, D. M. Beck, & A. Attewell (Eds.), *Florence Nightingale today: Healing leadership global action.* Silver Spring, MD: American Nurses Association.

Beck, D. M. (2010). Expanding our Nightingale horizon: Seven recommendations for 21st century nursing practice. *Journal of Holistic Nursing, 28*(4), 317–326.

Bekel, G. (2007). Dorothea E. Orem—1914–2007. *Nursing Science Quarterly, 20*(4), 302.

Benson, S. (1997). The older adult and fear of crime. *Journal of Gerontological Nursing, 23*(10), 24–31.

Biggs, A. (2008). "Toast Crumbs"—memories of Dorothea Orem. *Self-Care, Dependant Care & Nursing, 16*(2), 5–6.

Bostridge, M. (2011). *Florence Nightingale: The making of an icon.* New York: Farrar, Straus and Giroux.

Burkhart, L., & Hogan, N. (2008). An experiential theory of spiritual care in nursing practice. *Qualitative Health Research, 18*(7), 928–938.

Cody, W. K. (2013). *Philosophical and theoretical perspectives for advanced nursing practice* (5th ed.). Burlington, MA: Jones & Bartlett Learning.

Cromwell, J. L. (2013). *Florence Nightingale, Feminist.* Jefferson, NC: McFarland & Company, Inc. Publishers.

Damus, K. (1980). An application of the Johnson behavioral system model for nursing practice. In J. P. Riehl & C. Roy (Eds.), *Conceptual models for nursing practice* (2nd ed., pp. 274–289). New York: Appleton-Century-Crofts.

Dee, V. (1990). Implementation of the Johnson model: One hospital's experience. In M. E. Parker (Ed.), *Nursing theories in practice* (pp. 33–44). New York: National League for Nursing.

Derdiarian, A. K. (1990). The relationships among the subsystems of Johnson's behavioral system model. *Image: Journal of Nursing Scholarship, 22*(4), 219–224.

Derdiarian, A. K., & Schobel, D. (1990). Comprehensive assessment of AIDS patients using the behavioral systems model for nursing practice instrument. *Journal of Advanced Nursing, 15*(4), 436–446.

Dickoff, J., James, P., & Wiedenbach, E. (1968). Theory in a practice discipline. Part 1: Practice-oriented theory. *Nursing Research, 17*(5), 415–435.

Dijkstra, A., Yönt, G. H., Korhan, E. A., Muszalik, M., Kedziora-Kornatowsa, K., & Suzuki, M. (2012). The care dependency scale for measuring basic human needs: An international comparison. *Journal of Advanced Nursing, 68*(10), 2341–2348.

Dossey, B. M. (2000). *Florence Nightingale, mystic, visionary, healer.* Springhouse, PA: Springhouse.

Dossey, B. M. (2005a). Florence Nightingale's three tenets: Healing, leadership, global action. In B. M. Dossey, L. C. Selanders, D. M. Beck, & A. Attewell (Eds.), *Florence Nightingale today: Healing leadership global action.* Silver Spring, MD: American Nurses Association.

Dossey, B. M. (2005b). Florence Nightingale's 13 formal letters to her nurses (1872–1900). In B. M. Dossey, L. C. Selanders, D. M. Beck, & A. Attewell (Eds.), *Florence Nightingale today: Healing leadership global action.* Silver Spring, MD: American Nurses Association.

Dossey, B. (2010). Florence Nightingale: Her Crimean fever and chronic illness. *Journal of Holistic Nursing, 28*(1), 38–53.

Dossey, B. M., Selanders, L. C., Beck, D. M., & Attewell, A. (2005). *Florence Nightingale today: Healing leadership global action.* Silver Spring, MD: American Nurses Association.

Fruehwirth, S. E. S. (1989). An application of Johnson's behavioral model: A case study. *Journal of Community Health Nursing, 6*(2), 61–71.

Grubbs, J. (1980). The Johnson behavioral system model. In J. P. Riehl & C. Roy (Eds.), *Conceptual models for nursing practice* (2nd ed., pp. 217–254). New York: Appleton-Century-Crofts.

Haddad, V. C. N., & Santos, T. C. F. (2011). The Environmental theory by Florence Nightingale in the reaching of the Nursing School Anna Nery [Portugese]. *Escola Anna Nery Revista de Enfermagen, 15*(4), 765–761.

Henderson, V. (1965). The nature of nursing. *International Nursing Review, 12*(1). Reprinted in E. J. Halloran (Ed.). (1995). *A Virginia Henderson reader: Excellence in nursing* (pp. 213–223). New York: Springer.

Henderson, V. (1991). *The nature of nursing: Reflections after 25 years.* New York: National League for Nursing Press.

Herrmann, E. K. (Ed.). (1998). *Virginia Avenel Henderson: Signature for nursing.* Indianapolis, IN: Sigma Theta Tau International Center Nursing Press.

Holaday, B. (1980). Implementing the Johnson model for nursing practice. In J. P. Riehl & C. Roy (Eds.), *Conceptual models for nursing practice* (2nd ed., pp. 255–263). New York: Appleton-Century-Crofts.

Hoyt, S. (2010). Florence Nightingale's contribution to contemporary nursing ethics. *Journal of Holistic Nursing, 28*(4), 331–332.

Jacobs, B. B. (2001). Respect for human dignity: A central phenomenon to philosophically unite nursing theory and practice through consilience of knowledge. *Advances in Nursing Science, 24*(1), 17–35.

Johnson, D. E. (1959a). A philosophy of nursing. *Nursing Outlook, 7*(4), 198–200.

Johnson, D. E. (1959b). The nature of nursing science. *Nursing Outlook, 7*(5), 291–294.

Johnson, D. E. (1968). Theory in nursing: Borrowed and unique. *Nursing Research, 17*(3), 206–209.

Johnson, D. E. (1974). Development of a theory: A requisite for nursing as a primary health profession. *Nursing Research, 23*(5), 372–377. Reprinted in L. H. Nichol (Ed.). (1997). *Perspectives on nursing theory* (3rd ed., pp. 219–225). Philadelphia: Lippincott-Raven.

Johnson, D. E. (1980). The behavioral system model for nursing. In J. P. Riehl & C. Roy (Eds.), *Conceptual models for nursing practice* (pp. 207–216). New York: Appleton-Century-Crofts.

Johnson, D. E. (1990). The behavioral system model for nursing. In M. E. Parker (Ed.), *Nursing theories in practice* (pp. 23–32). New York: National League for Nursing Press.

Johnson, D. E. (1997). Author's comments. In L. H. Nichol (Ed.), *Perspectives on nursing theory* (3rd ed., pp. 225, 405). Philadelphia: Lippincott-Raven.

Karpf, T. (2010). She must be a saint, it's clear she's not a sinner. *Journal of Holistic Nursing, 28*(1), 8–9.

McDonald, L. (2010). Florence Nightingale: Passionate statistician. *Journal of Holistic Nursing, 28*(1), 92–98.

McElligott, D. (2010). Healing: The journey from concept to nursing practice. *Journal of Holistic Nursing, 28*(4), 251–259.

Medina, J., Ruiz-Lozano, M. D., Delgado, M., & Vila, A. (2012). A fuzzy temporal rule-based system for handling the nursing process on mobile devices. *Expert Systems with Applications, 39*(12), 10479–10488.

Murray, P. J. (1999). *Betty Neuman: Biographical details.* Retrieved from http://www.lemmus.demon.co.uk/neu-man1.htm

Neils, P. E. (2010). The influence of Nightingale rounding by the liaison nurse on surgical patient families with attention to differing cultural needs. *Journal of Holistic Nursing, 28*(4), 235–243.

Neuman, B. M. (1990). The Neuman systems model: A theory for practice. In M. E. Parker (Ed.), *Nursing theories in practice* (pp. 241–261). New York: National League for Nursing Press.

Neuman, B. (1995). *The Neuman systems model* (3rd ed.). Stamford, CT: Appleton & Lange.

Neuman, B., & Fawcett, J. (2002). *The Neuman systems model* (4th ed.). Upper Saddle River, NJ: Prentice-Hall.

Neuman, B., & Fawcett, J. (2009). *The Neuman systens model* (5th ed.). Upper Saddle River, NJ: Pearson Education, Inc.

Nightingale, F. (1893/1954). Sick-nursing and health-nursing. First printed in A. Burdett-Clouts (Ed.), *Women's mission: A series of congress papers of the philanthropic work of women by eminent writers.* New York: Charles Scribner's Sons. Reprinted in L. R. Seymer (Ed.). (1954). *Selected writings of Florence Nightingale.* New York: MacMillan.

Nightingale, F. (1860/1957/1969). *Notes on nursing: What it is and what it is not.* New York: Dover Publications.

Nightingale, F. (1999). Retrieved from http://www.sociology.uoguelph.ca/fnightingale/Introduction/ index.htm

O'Connor, J. J., & Robertson, E. F. (2003). Florence Nightingale. School of Mathematics and Statistics. Retrieved from http://www-history.mcs.st-andrews.ac.uk/Biographies/Nightingale.html

O'Malley, J. (1996). A nursing legacy: Virginia Henderson. *Advanced Practice Nursing Quarterly, 2*(2), v–vii.

Orem, D. E. (1956). *Hospital nursing service: An analysis.* Indianapolis, IN: Division of Hospital and Institutional Services of the Indiana State Board of Health.

Orem, D. E. (1971). *Nursing: Concepts of practice.* New York: McGraw-Hill.

Orem, D. E. (1985a). *Nursing: Concepts of practice* (3rd ed.). New York: McGraw-Hill.

Orem, D. E. (1985b). A concept of self-care for the rehabilitation client. *Rehabilitation Nurse, 10,* 33–36.

Orem, D. E. (1991). *Nursing: Concepts of practice* (4th ed.). St. Louis: Mosby.

Orem, D. E. (1995). *Nursing: Concepts of practice* (5th ed.). St. Louis: Mosby.

Orem, D. E. (2001). *Nursing: Concepts of practice* (6th ed.). St. Louis: Mosby.

Pfettscher, S. A. (2006). Florence Nightingale: Modern nursing. In A. M. Tomey & M. R. Alligood (Eds.), *Nursing theorists and their work* (6th ed., pp. 71–90). St. Louis: Mosby.

Pope, D. S. (1995). Music, noise, and the human voice in the nurse–patient environment. *Image: Journal of Nursing Scholarship, 27*(4), 291–296.

Poster, E. C., Dee, V., & Randell, B. P. (1997). The Johnson behavioral systems model as a framework for patient outcome evaluation. *Journal of the American Psychiatric Nursing Association, 3*(3), 73–80.

Reed, P. G., & Zurakowski, T. L. (1996). Nightingale: Foundations of nursing. In J. J. Fitzpatrick & A. L. Whall (Eds.), *Conceptual models of nursing: Analysis and application* (3rd ed.). Norwalk, CT: Appleton & Lange.

Rew, L., & Sands, D. (2010). Reflections: The joy of the research process. *Journal of Holistic Nursing, 28*(1), 99–100.

Selanders, L. C. (1993). *Florence Nightingale: An environmental adaptation theory.* Newbury Park, CA: Sage.

Selanders, L. C. (2005a). Nightingale's foundational philosophy of nursing. In B. M. Dossey, L. C. Selanders, D. M. Beck, & A. Attewell (Eds.), *Florence Nightingale today: Healing leadership global action.* Silver Spring, MD: American Nurses Association.

Selanders, L. C. (2005b). Social change and leadership: Dynamic forces for nursing. In B. M. Dossey, L. C. Selanders, D. M. Beck, & A. Attewell (Eds.), *Florence Nightingale today: Healing leadership global action.* Silver Spring, MD: American Nurses Association.

Selanders, L. C. (2010). The power of environmental adaptation: Florence Nightingale's original theory for nursing practice. *Journal of Holistic Nursing, 28*(1), 81–88.

Small, H. (1998). *Florence Nightingale avenging angel.* New York: St. Martin's Press.

Tailor-Ford, R., Catlin, A., LaPlant, M., & Weinke, C. (2008). Effect of a noise reduction program on a medical-surgical unit. *Clinical Nursing Research, 17*(2), 74–86.

Tanyi, R. A., & Werner, J. S. (2008). Women's experience of spirituality within endstage renal disease and hemodialysis. *Clinical Nursing Research, 17*(1), 32–49.

Taylor, S. G. (2006). Self-care deficit theory of nursing. In A. M. Tomey & M. R. Alligood (Eds.), *Nursing theorists and their work* (6th ed., pp. 267–296). St Louis: Mosby.

Taylor, S. G. (2011). Moving forward: Ramblings of an antique nurse. *Self-Care, Dependent-Care and Nursing, 16*(1), 61–65.

Taylor, S. G., Geden, E., Isaramalai, S., & Wongvatunyu, S. (2000). Orem's self-care deficit nursing theory: Its philosophic foundation and the state of the science. *Nursing Science Quarterly, 13*(2), 104–110.

Taylor, S. G., & Renpenning, K. (2011). *Self-care science, nursing theory and evidence-based practice.* New York: Springer.

Turner-Henson, A. (1992). Chronically ill children's mothers' perceptions of environmental variables. Doctoral dissertation, University of Alabama at Birmingham.

Wagner, D. J., & Whaite, B. (2010). An exploration of the nature of caring relationships in the writings of Florence Nightingale. *Journal of Holistic Nursing, 28*(4), 225–234.

Weyneth, C. C. (2010). The gift of Nightingale's presence. *Journal of Holistic Nursing, 28*(4), 333–339.

Zurakowski, T. L. (2005). Florence Nightingale: Pioneer in nursing knowledge development. In J. J. Fitzpatrick & A. L. Whall (Eds.), *Conceptual models of nursing: Analysis and application* (4th ed.). Upper Saddle River, NJ: Pearson.

CHAPTER 8

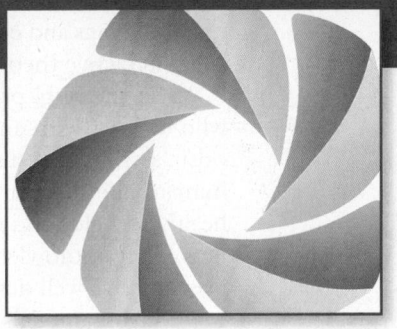

Grand Nursing Theories Based on Interactive Process

Evelyn M. Wills

Jean Willowby is a student in an RN to master of science in nursing program. She is working to become a pediatric nurse practitioner. For one of her practicum assignments, she must incorporate a nursing theory into her clinical work, using the theory as a guide. During an earlier course on theory, Jean read several nursing theories that focused on interactions between the client and the nurse and between the client and the health care system. She remembered that in the interaction models and theories, human beings are viewed as interacting wholes and client problems are seen as multifactorial.

The theories that stress human interactions best fit Jean's personal philosophy of nursing because they take into account the multitude of factors she believes to be part of clinical nursing practice. Like the perspective taken by interaction model theorists, Jean understands that, at times, the results of interventions are unpredictable and that many elements in the client's background and environment have an effect on the outcomes of interventions. She also acknowledges that there are many interactions between clients and their environments, both internal and external, some of which cannot be measured.

To better prepare for the assignment, Jean studied several of the human interaction models and theories, focusing most of her attention on the works of Roy and King. But after discussing her thoughts with her professor, she was referred to the Artinian Intersystem Model (AIM), a relatively new model by Barbara Artinian. After reviewing some of the precepts of the model, she thought that it appeared to best fit her pediatrics practice and determined that she would learn more about it.

As discussed in Chapter 6, interactive process nursing theories occupy a place between the needs-based theories of the 1950s and 1960s, most of which were philosophically grounded in the positivist school of thought, and the unitary process models, which are grounded in humanist philosophy, which expresses the belief that humans are unitary beings and energy fields in constant interaction with the universal energy field. The interactive theories are grounded in the postpositive schools of philosophy.

The theorists presented in this chapter believe that humans are holistic beings who interact with and adapt to situations in which they find themselves. These theorists ascribe to systems theory and agree that there is constant interaction between humans and their environments. In general, human interaction theorists believe that health is a value and that a continuum of health ranges from high-level wellness to illness. They acknowledge, however, that people with chronic illnesses may have healthy lives and live well despite their illnesses.

Nursing models that can be described as interactive process theories include Levine's Conservation Model; Artinian's Intersystem Model; Erickson, Tomlin, and Swain's Modeling and Role-Modeling; King's Systems Framework and Theory of Goal Attainment; Roy's Adaptation Model; and Watson's Philosophy and Science of Caring. Each is discussed in this chapter. The models treated in this chapter are not arranged historically; some date back to the 1960s, whereas some are relatively new. Levine's model is placed early in the chapter because it is one of the classic models.

An attempt was made to ensure that a balanced approach was used in presenting the works of these theorists. However, some of the theories are quite complex (e.g., those of Erickson, Tomlin, and Swain; King; and Roy), whereas others are quite parsimonious (e.g., those of Levine and Watson). Additionally, some of the models have been revised repeatedly (e.g., Artinian, King, Roy, and Watson). As a result, the sections dealing with some models are longer or more involved than others, but this does not imply that the works of any of the theorists discussed are more or less important to the discipline than others.

Myra Estrin Levine: The Conservation Model

The ideal of conservation pervades the background of some nurses' ideas (Mefford, 2004). Myra Levine (1973) stated that "nursing is a human interaction" (p. 237). Her model deals with the interactions of nurse and client. It considers multiple factorial interactions, which may produce predictable effects using probability as the reality.

Background of the Theorist

Myra Levine earned a diploma in nursing from Cook County School of Nursing in Chicago, Illinois, in 1944; a bachelor's degree in science at the University of Chicago in 1949; and a master of science in nursing from Wayne State University in Detroit, Michigan, in 1962. She held numerous clinical and education positions during her long career (Schaefer, 2010). She published *An Introduction to Clinical Nursing* in 1969; this work was revised in 1973 and again in 1989 (Levine, 1989). Levine enjoyed a long and productive career, which included a distinguished publication record. She died in 1996, at age 75, leaving a legacy to nursing of education, administration, and scholarship (Schaefer, 2002).

Philosophical Underpinnings of the Theory

Levine (1973) based the Conservation Model on Nightingale's idea that "the nurse created an environment in which healing could occur" (p. 239). She drew from the works of Tillich on the unity principle of life, Bernard on internal environment,

Cannon on the theory of homeostasis, and Waddington on the concept of homeorrhesis. The works of other scientists were also used. Four conservation principles form the basis of the model; these were synthesized from her scientific study and practice (Levine, 1990).

Major Assumptions, Concepts, and Relationships

The following four conservation principles are the major principles around which the model is constructed:

- The principle of the conservation of energy
- The principle of the conservation of structural integrity
- The principle of the conservation of personal integrity
- The principle of the conservation of social integrity
  (Levine, 1990, p. 331)

According to Levine's model, nursing interventions are based on conservation of the client's integrity in each of the conservation domains. The nurse is seen as a part of the environment and shares the repertoire of skill, knowledge, and compassion, assisting each client to confront environmental challenges in resolving the problems encountered in the client's own unique way. The effectiveness of the interventions is measured by the maintenance of client integrity (Levine, 1973, 1990).

Assumptions About Individuals

Each individual "is an active participant in interactions with the environment constantly seeking information from it" (Levine, 1969, p. 6).

The individual "is a sentient being and the ability to interact with the environment seems ineluctably tied to his sensory organs" (Levine, 1973, p. 450).

"Change is the essence of life and it is unceasing as long as life goes on. Change is characteristic of life" (Levine, 1973, p. 10).

Assumptions About Nursing

"Ultimately the decisions for nursing intervention must be based on the unique behavior of the individual patient" (Levine, 1973, p. 6).

"Patient-centered nursing care means individualized nursing care. It is predicated on the reality of common experience: every man is a unique individual, and as such he requires a unique constellation of skills, techniques and ideas designed specifically for him" (Levine, 1973, p. 23).

Concepts

Many concepts are discussed in the model. Major concepts are listed in Table 8-1.

Relationships

Relationships are not specifically stated but can be extracted from the descriptions given by Levine (1973). The relationships serve as the basis for nursing interventions and include:

1. Conservation of energy is based on nursing interventions to conserve energy through a deliberate decision as to the balance between activity and the person's available energy.
2. Conservation of structural integrity is the basis for nursing interventions to limit the amount of tissue involvement.

Table 8-1 Major Concepts of the Conservation Model

Concept	Definition
Environment	Includes both the internal and external environment.
Person	The unique individual in unity and integrity, feeling, believing, thinking, and whole.
Health	Patterns of adaptive change of the whole being.
Nursing	The human interaction relying on communication, rooted in the organic dependency of the individual human being in his [sic] relationships with other human beings.
Adaptation	The process of change and integration of the organism in which the individual retains integrity or wholeness. It is possible to have degrees of adaptation.
Conceptual environment	The part of the person's environment that includes ideas, symbolic exchange, belief, tradition, and judgment.
Conservation	Includes joining together and is the product of adaptation including nursing intervention and patient participation to maintain a safe balance.
Energy conservation	Nursing interventions based on the conservation of the patient's energy.
Holism	The singular, yet integrated response of the individual to forces in the environment.
Homeostasis	Stable state normal alterations in physiologic parameters in response to environmental changes; an energy-sparing state, a state of conservation.
Modes of communication	The many ways in which information, needs, and feelings are transmitted among the patient, family, nurses, and other health care workers.
Personal integrity	A person's sense of identity and self-definition. Nursing intervention is based on the conservation of the individual's personal integrity.
Social integrity	Life's meaning gained through interactions with others. Nurses intervene to maintain relationships.
Structural integrity	Healing is a process of restoring structural integrity through nursing interventions that promote healing and maintain structural integrity.
Therapeutic interventions	Interventions that influence adaptation in a favorable way, enhancing the adaptive responses available to the person.

Source: Adapted from Levine (1973).

3. Conservation of personal integrity is based on nursing interventions that permit the individual to make decisions for himself or herself or to participate in the decisions.
4. Conservation of social integrity is based on nursing interventions to preserve the client's interactions with family and the social system to which they belong.
5. All nursing interventions are based on careful and continued observation over time (abstracted from Levine, 1973).

Usefulness

Levine's (1973) model has been useful in nursing education. For example, it was used to develop a nursing undergraduate program at Allentown College of Saint Francis de Sales in Center Valley, Pennsylvania, where it was deemed to be compatible with the mission and philosophy of the college (Grindley & Paradowski, 1991). It was also used in the graduate program at the same school as the framework for development of the content of the graduate nursing courses (Schaefer, 1991a).

The emergency department at the Hospital of the University of Pennsylvania used the four conservation principles of Levine's model as an organizing framework for nursing practice (Pond & Taney, 1991). It was believed that use of the model strengthened communication and improved nursing care in the hospital through an atmosphere of collaboration among disciplines. The conservation principles were also found to be useful in directing nursing practice in the care of children (Dever, 1991). The concept of adaptation and the four conservation principles were particularly relevant, and conservation of personal and social integrity was especially important to the healing of the ill child. A concept analysis was published using Levine's conservation model to refine the concept of creativity for nursing practice (Fasnacht, 2003). Mefford (2004) based her theory of health promotion for preterm infants on Levine's conservation model.

Neswick suggested Levine's model as the theoretic basis for enterostomal therapy (ET) nursing. She integrated the four conservation principles into wound and ostomy care. The principles that she found useful are energy, structure, personal integrity, and social integrity. She found Levine's framework useful because of its holistic approach (Neswick, 1997).

Testability

Levine's (1990) Conservation Model has guided research studies internationally. Piccoli and Galvao (2005) investigated methods of assessing and preparing perioperative nursing patients, focusing on Levine's four conservation principles. Leach (2006) studied wound management in Australia using Levine's four principles and found that the model contributed to health and wholeness of the client and assisted in cost-effective care. Mock and colleagues (2007) stated that the model "provided a useful framework" (p. 509) for their investigation of nursing interventions to manage fatigue in cancer patients. The Canadian Association of Critical Care Nursing, which published the abstract of Vandall-Walker, Jensen, and Oberle (2006), cited Levine in their investigation of nursing support of family members of critically ill adults.

Conserving the cognitive integrity of hospitalized elderly was the focus of a research study by Foreman (1991). In that study, 71 participants were administered several cognitive measures by an interview process. The researchers stated that the four conservation principles were supported in their study. The model has been the guide for qualitative studies to understand clients in their whole state. Schaefer (1991b) reported a case study of a patient with congestive heart failure and found the model "pragmatic and parsimonious in studying the subject" (p. 130). Schaefer and Potylycki (1993) used Levine's model to study fatigue in patients with congestive heart failure with a focus on client adaptation.

Parsimony

The model is fairly parsimonious; however, there are a great many concepts with comparatively unspecified relationships and unstated assumptions. Four conservation principles comprise the model; these principles are succinctly stated. According to

Levine (1991), redundancy of the domains allows multiple means of configuring interventions. When domain redundancy is lost by the seriousness of disease, the options for intervention are limited. Practitioners and researchers using the model have considerable latitude to configure ways in which the model will be used or studied and to derive the theoretical structures that proceed from the model.

Value in Extending Nursing Science

Levine's (1973) Conservation Model has impacted the discipline of nursing in education, practice, and research, providing four defining principles that are sufficiently universal to allow research and practice in a large number of situations. The concept of holism, although not unique to this model, was proposed at an early stage in nursing's scientific history and has made an important difference in the care of clients.

Barbara M. Artinian: The Intersystem Model

The Intersystem Model was first published in 1983 as the Intersystem Patient-Care Model (Artinian, 1983) and was later expanded to the Intersystem Model (Artinian, 1991). It is currently in its third iteration and following refinement and revision, it became the basis for the curriculum at Azusa Pacific University in Azusa, California (Wood, 1997). The second edition of Artinian's work was published in 2011, expanded on the previous model, and was renamed the Artinian Intersystem Model (AIM). Its focus is the nursing process using the AIM (Artinian, 2011).

Background of the Theorist

Barbara Artinian received her bachelor's degree from Wheaton (IL) College; master's degrees from Case Western Reserve University in Cleveland, Ohio, and the University of California, Los Angeles (UCLA); and her doctorate from the University of Southern California. Influenced by her education as a sociologist, Artinian developed a nursing model that used an intersystems approach and focused on the interactions between client and nurse. She is currently professor emeritus of the School of Nursing at Azusa Pacific University, having taught graduate and undergraduate students in the areas of community health nursing, family theory, nursing theory, and qualitative research methods (Artinian, 2013).

Philosophic Underpinnings of the Theory

The Intersystem Model replaced Chrisman and Riehl's (1974, 1989) systems model at the School of Nursing at Azusa Pacific University. Several works were used in developing the components of the model. For example, *sense of coherence* (SOC), a social science construct proposed by Antonofsky, provided grounding for the concept *situational sense of coherence* (SSOC). The SSOC serves as a measure of the integrative potential of clients within the context of situations (Artinian, 1997a) (see Table 8-2 and Figure 8-1).

Additionally, the model of intrasystem analysis and intersystem interaction developed by Alfred Kuhn was refined by Artinian to explain client–nurse interaction processes in health care situations and for use in developing the nursing plan of care. Finally, the work of Maturana and Varela provided the conceptualization of the person as a perceiving, self-determining, self-regulating human system and explains the patient/client concept of the model (Artinian, 1997a).

Table 8-2 Relationship Between SOC and SSOC in Artinian's Model

Term	Definition
Sense of coherence (SOC)	The progenitor to the SSOC
Situational sense of coherence (SSOC)	The analytic structure for evaluating the effectiveness of interventions in the plan of care and the current level of health
Comprehensibility	The extent to which one perceives the stimuli present in the situational environment deriving from the internal and external environments as making cognitive sense, in that information is ordered, consistent, structured, and clear, versus disordered random or inexplicable
Meaningfulness	The extent to which one feels that the problem demands posed by the situation are worth investing energy in and are challenges for which meaning or purpose is sought rather than burdens.
Manageability	The extent to which one perceives that resources at one's disposal are adequate to meet the demands posed by stimuli present in the situation.

Source: Antonofski (1987) as cited in Artinian (1991, p. 199); Erdmann, C. M. (2003). The value of the Intersystem Model for cosmetic nursing practice. *Dermatology Nursing, 15*(4), 335–339.

Major Assumptions, Concepts, and Relationships

In the Intersystem Model, there is a differentiation between the human as a system (the intrasystem) and the interactive systems of individuals or groups, known as the intersystem (Artinian, 2011). The language of the Intersystem Model is scholarly English, and nonsexist language is used throughout.

Assumptions

A number of major assumptions of the model (Artinian, 1997a) are listed in Box 8-1.

Concepts

The Intersystem Model incorporates nursing's metaparadigm concepts of person, environment, and health and specifies the concept nursing action. Definitions for these concepts are presented in Table 8-3. Person is viewed as a "coherent being who continually strives to make sense of his or her world" (Artinian, 2011, p. 13). The person as an individual has biologic, psychosocial, and spiritual subsystems (Artinian, 2011). Person may also be an aggregate, meaning a group of people, such as a family, community, or other aggregates. Environment includes internal and external environments and specifies developmental environment and situational environment as important to the interaction (Artinian, 2011).

Health is viewed on a multidimensional continuum involving health/disease (Artinian, 2011, p. 15). The focus is on stability and adaptation, and Artinian developed the concept of SSOC to measure adaptation. Health is considered to be "a dynamic state of functioning within the limitations of the person" (Artinian, 1991, p. 10), and includes the element of effective adaptation that occurs through strengthening the SSOC. As a result, the model defines health as "a strong SSOC."

Nursing is specified as "nursing action," which is identified by the mutual communication, negotiation, organization, and priorities of both the client and nurse intrasystems. This is accomplished through intersystem interaction; feedback loops are necessary to produce a mutually determined plan of care (Artinian, 2011). One major

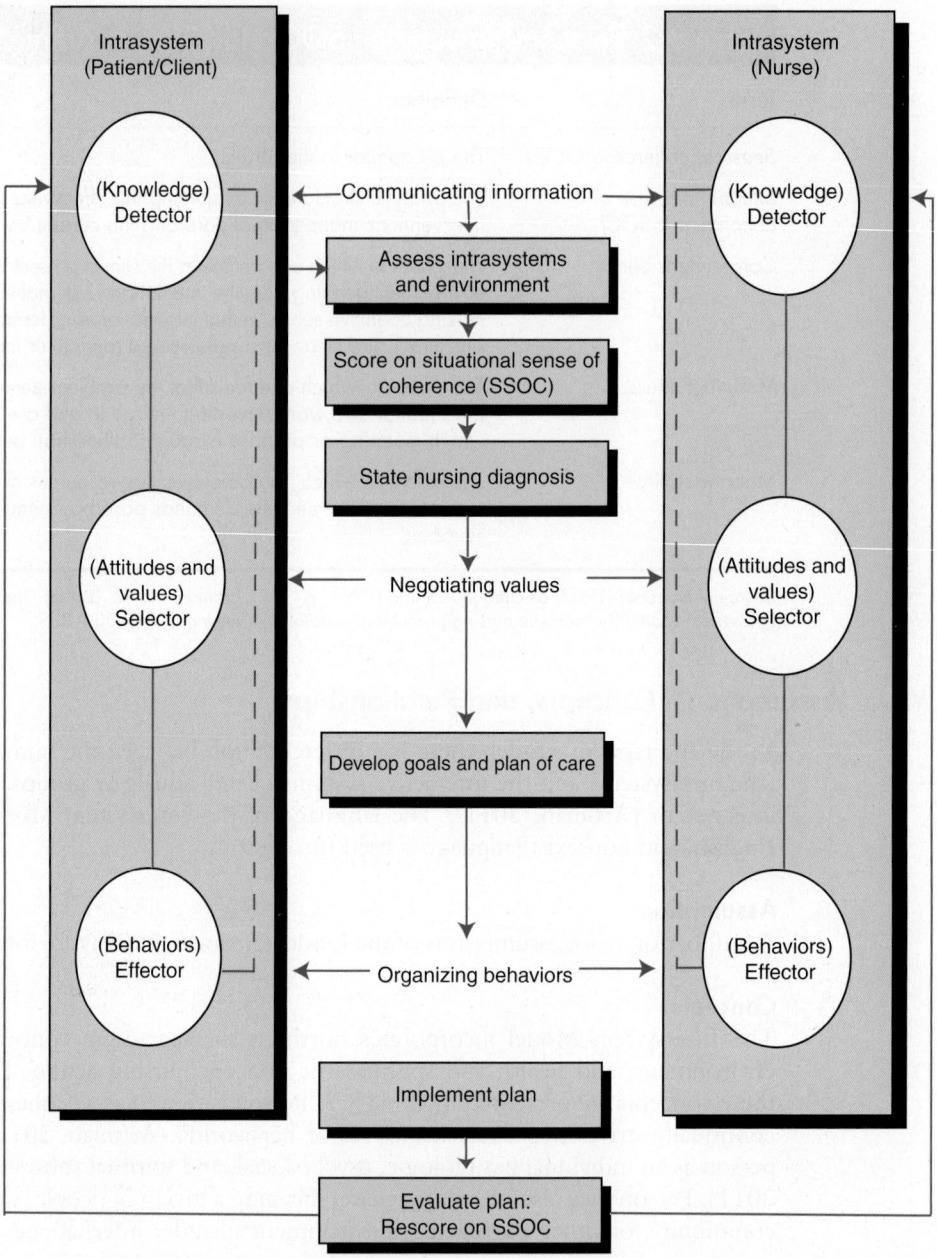

Figure 8-1 The Intersystem Model. (Source: Artinian, B. M. (1991). *Journal of Advanced Nursing*, p. 201 [Reprinted with permission by John Wiley & Sons, Inc.].)

innovation of this model is that client spirituality and values are important in the assessment of client needs and within the resulting nursing process.

Relationships

The Intersystem Model consists of two levels: the *intrasystem* and the *intersystem*. The intrasystem applies both to the client and to the nurse and focuses on the individual. The intersystem, by contrast, focuses on the interactions between the nurse and client (Artinian, 2011).

Box 8-1 Assumptions of Artinian's Intersystem Model

1. The human being exists within a framework of development and change, which is inherent to life.
2. The human's life is a unit of interrelated systems that is viewed as past and potential future.
3. Persons interact with the environment on the biologic level, and the senses are the mode of input from the environment; bodily functions are the mode for output.
4. The person's present can be seen in terms of his past and future.
5. The human spirit is at the center of the person's being, transcending time and affecting all aspects of life.
6. The nurse focuses on all aspects of the total person, systematically noting the interrelations of the systems and the relationships of the systems to time and environment.
7. The nursing process can take place only in the present.

Source: Artinian (1997a).

In the intrasystem model, three basic components comprise each intrasystem: the detector, selector, and effector. The detector processes information, the selector compares the situation with the attitudes and values of the individual, and the effector identifies behaviors relevant to the situation (Artinian, 1991, 1997a, 2011).

Table 8-3 Concepts of the Intersystem Model

Concept	Definition
Person	A coherent being who continually strives to make sense of his or her world. The person is a system, the subsystems of which are biologic, psychosocial, and spiritual. Subsystem configuration is such that "transactions among the subsystems result in emergent properties at the systemic level" (Artinian, 2011, p. 13).
Environment	The environment has two dimensions, developmental and situational. The developmental environment is "all the events, factors, and influences that affect the system . . . as it passes through its developmental stages" (p. 14). This developmental environment provides the context for other developmental arenas such as the healing environment. Situational environment occurs when the nurse and client interact, and this includes all the details of the encounter.
Health	Health is considered to be a multidimensional continuum. The client's situational sense of coherence (SSOC) is a reflection of the client's adaptation to crisis and is the factor that the nurse assesses and to which the nurse ministers in assisting the client to adapt. In the Intersystem Model, health is defined as having a strong SSOC, illness has a low SSOC, and adaptation moves the SSOC toward a higher level.
Nursing	Those actions (interventions) that are needed when the client enters the hospital environment. It is the goal of both the nurse and client to move the client to a higher SSOC. The nurse assesses the client's knowledge (comprehensibility of the problem), the available resources needed to manage the problem (manageability), and the client's motivation to meet the challenges posed by the problem (meaningfulness).

Source: Artinian (1997a).

The first step in an interaction in the intrasystem is to evaluate the detector domain, each person's knowledge of the problem. The detector incorporates knowledge about the internal environment (physical symptoms), social situations, the condition, treatment, and available resources. The selector allows the client and nurse to examine their attitudes and values in choosing a course of action that fits both patient/client and nurse. The effector is the behavioral level in which a response is selected from the repertoire of the behaviors available. This intrasystem level of the model provides the nurse with the capability of progressively clarifying with the client to bring about a mutual plan of care (Artinian, 2011).

The intersystem (Artinian, 1991, 1997a, 2011) is seen when client and nurse interact, which occurs when nursing assistance is required. Communication and negotiation between nurse and client lead to developing a plan of care. If the planned intervention is not effective, the determination is made that further assessment is necessary.

SOC and SSOC are the concepts that relate to health. In the intervention phase of the process, "input is the nurse–client interaction to change the SSOC if it is judged to be low" (Artinian, 1997a, p. 13). Outcomes are scored on the SSOC by changes in knowledge, values and beliefs, and behaviors.

Usefulness

The Intersystem Model is relatively new; nonetheless, examples in nursing literature describing its use in practice and education are available. Online searches indicate that Artinian's qualitative research method is being used in Central Africa (McCowan & Artinian, 2011), Europe, and the United States. A recent investigation by Giske and Artinian (2008) used classical grounded theory and studied adults aged 80 and older in a Norwegian hospital who were undergoing gastroenterologic studies. Findings indicate that participants were concerned with preparing themselves for life after their diagnosis, a difficult period for the participants.

Research on educational issues includes work by Cone, Artinian, and West (2011) on students at undergraduate and graduate levels. Cason and colleagues (2008) studied perceived barriers and supports for nursing students as seen by successful Hispanic health care professionals. They found that multiple barriers deter Hispanic students from success. Bond and colleagues (2008) followed up with a study of Hispanic students in baccalaureate nursing programs and found multiple barriers and supports. Critchley and Ball (2007) studied rheumatology patients using Artinian's (1998) descriptive qualitative method. Dover and Pfieffer (2006) studied spiritual care of Christian clients of parish nurses. They developed a theory of spirituality for work in parish nursing. Vukovitch and Artinian (2005) investigated mental health nurses who administered medications to psychiatric patients and their methods of avoiding coercion. The Glaserian grounded theory method of research was codified by Artinian for use specifically in nursing research and has been used by her students for more than 20 years (McCallin, 2012).

Testability

The Intersystem Model has not been fully tested. Research studies applying the model primarily involve using grounded theory methodology to examine the meanings of events and the person's reactions to those events in the effort to formulate theories and hypotheses (B. M. Artinian, personal communication, May 30, 2003).

The SSOC instrument has been used in research as a self-report instrument (Artinian, 1997b). Major themes that emerged from a study of patients with chronic obstructive pulmonary disease (COPD) by Milligan-Hecox (Artinian, 1997c) were "pacing, depending on others, clarifying values, maintaining independence, maintaining the struggle and accepting ambiguity" (p. 259). Other research efforts using the model included caring for cancer patients, COPD patients, and patients experiencing difficulties in managing illness situations (Artinian, 1997d).

Parsimony

The model developed by Artinian (1997a) is parsimonious and is explained in a logical and coherent way using two simple diagrams. It is not simplistic, however, and has multiple interacting elements. The more current model has expanded the diagrams to more thoroughly explain the aspects of the model as needed by both graduate and undergraduate students (Artinian, 2011).

Value in Extending Nursing Science

The Intersystem Model has value in guiding education and in implementing practice. Its innovation is attention to the spirituality, goals, and values of both the client and nurse. Nurses use it in diverse clinical settings, such as psychiatric care, acute care, and community nursing. Several chapters, three books by the author and associates, and numerous journal articles have been generated by this model (Artinian, 1997a; Artinian, 1998; Artinian, 2011; Artinian, Giske, & Cone, 2009; Giske & Artinian, 2008; Treolar & Artinian, 2001; Vukovitch & Artinian, 2005).

Helen C. Erickson, Evelyn M. Tomlin, and Mary Ann P. Swain: Modeling and Role-Modeling

Modeling and role-modeling (MRM) is considered by its authors to be a theory and a paradigm. They constructed the theory from a multiplicity of resources that explain nurses' interactions with clients.

Background of the Theorists

Helen Erickson earned a diploma in nursing from Saginaw General Hospital in Saginaw, Michigan. She earned a bachelor's degree in nursing, a master's degree in psychiatric nursing, and a doctorate in educational psychology from the University of Michigan. Her career spans positions in nursing practice and education, both in the United States and abroad. She chaired the adult health nursing curriculum in the graduate program at the University of Texas at Austin and was a Special Assistant to the Dean for Graduate Studies. She is professor emeritus of the University of Texas at Austin, chairs the board of directors of the American Holistic Nurses' Certification Corporation, and is active in the Society for the Advancement of Modeling and Role-Modeling (SAMRM) (Erickson, 2008). *Modeling and Role-Modeling: A Theory and Paradigm for Nursing* has been the lifework of Dr. Erickson and is now in its third printing (Erickson, 2008).

Evelyn M. Tomlin was educated at Pasadena City College in southern California and Los Angeles General Hospital School of Nursing. She received her bachelor's degree in nursing from the University of Southern California and her master's degree from the University of Michigan. She has had varied experiences in practice and education, including medical-surgical nursing, maternity, and pediatric nursing. Tomlin was a member of the faculty at the University of Michigan. In semiretirement from active nursing, she counsels homeless mothers in a religious-based environment (Erickson, 2010).

Mary Ann P. Swain was educated in psychology at DePauw University in Greencastle, Indiana, and earned master's and doctoral degrees from the University of Michigan. She taught research methods in psychology at DePauw University and at the University of Michigan. She also served as the director of the doctoral program in nursing at the University of Michigan for a year and assumed the role of chairperson of nursing research from 1977 to 1982. Later, she was professor of nursing research at the University of Michigan and, in 1983, was appointed the Associate Vice President for Academic Affairs at the same university. Swain currently resides in New York State and is a provost for the New York State University system (Erickson, 2006).

Philosophical Underpinnings of the Theory

A number of theoretical works served as the foundation for MRM. Indeed, MRM is a synthesis of the foundational works of Maslow, Milton Erickson, Piaget, Bowlby, Winnicott, Engel, Lindemann, Selye, Lazarus, and Seligman (Erickson, 2006).

Philosophically, Erickson, Tomlin, and Swain (1983) believe "that nursing is a process between the nurse and client and requires an interpersonal and interactive nurse–client relationship" (p. 43). For this reason, their work is considered to be human interaction theory.

Major Assumptions, Concepts, and Relationships

Assumptions

Assumptions about adaptation and nursing are proposed in the MRM theory; the authors state that adaptation "is an innate drive toward holistic health, growth, and development. Self-healing, recovery and renewal, and adaptation are all instinctual despite the aging process or inherent malformations" (Erickson et al., 1983, p. 47).

When describing nursing, it is assumed that (1) "nursing is the nurturance of holistic self-care"; (2) "nursing is assisting persons holistically to use their adaptive strengths to attain and maintain optimum biopsychosocial-spiritual functioning"; (3) "nursing is helping with self-care to gain optimum health"; and (4) "nursing is an integrated and integrative helping of persons to better care for themselves" (Erickson et al., 1983, p. 50).

Concepts

The MRM theory contains a detailed set of concepts, and a glossary is provided in their work that assists in its comprehension. Table 8-4 provides definitions for some of the major concepts.

Relationships

The active potential assessment model (APAM) directs nursing assessment in the MRM theory. The APAM is a synthesis of Selye's general adaptation syndrome and Engles' response to stressors (Erickson et al., 1983). The APAM assists the nurse in predicting a client's potential to cope and is used to assess three states: equilibrium, arousal, and impoverishment. Equilibrium has two facets: adaptive and maladaptive.

Table 8-4 Major Concepts of the Modeling and Role-Modeling Theory

Concept	Definition
Holism	The idea that "human beings have multiple interacting subsystems including genetic make up and spiritual drive, body, mind, emotion, and spirit are a total unit and act together, affecting and controlling one another interactively" (Erickson et al., 1983, p. 44).
Health	"The state of physical, mental, and social well-being, not merely the absence of disease or infirmity" (p. 46).
Lifetime growth and development	Lifetime growth and development are continuous processes. When needs are met, growth and development promote health.
Affiliated-individuation	The dependence on support systems while maintaining the independence of the individual.
Adaptation	The individual's response to external and internal stressors in a health- and growth-directed manner. The opposite is maladaptation, which is the taxing of the system when the individual is "unable to engage constructive coping methods or mobilize appropriate resources to contend with the stressor(s)" (p. 47).
Self-care	Knowledge, resources, and action of the client; knowledge considers what has made the client sick, what will make him or her well, and "the mobilization of internal resources, and acquisition of additional resources to gain, maintain, or promote an optimal level of holistic health" (p. 48).
Nursing	"The holistic helping of persons with their self-care activities in relation to their health—an interactive, interpersonal process that nurtures strengths to achieve a state of perceived holistic health" (p. 49).
Modeling	The process by which the nurse seeks to understand the client's unique model of the world.
Role-modeling	The process by which the nurse understands the client's unique model within the context of scientific theories and uses the model to plan interventions that promote health for the client.

Source: Erickson et al. (1983).

People in equilibrium have potential for mobilizing resources; those in maladaptive equilibrium have fewer resources.

Both arousal and impoverishment are considered to be states of stress in which mobilizing resources are expected. Persons in impoverishment have diminished or depleted abilities for mobilizing resources. People move between the states as their capacities to meet stress change. The APAM is considered dynamic rather than unidirectional and depends on the person's abilities to mobilize resources. Nursing interventions influence the person's ability to mobilize resources and move from impoverishment to equilibrium within the APAM (Erickson et al., 1983).

From the data collected, a client model is developed with a description of the functional relationship among the factors. Etiologic factors are analyzed, and possible therapeutic interventions are devised recognizing possible conflicts with treatment plans of other health professionals. Diagnoses and goals are established to complete the planning process (Erickson et al., 1983).

The success of the process is predicated on nurse's coming to know the client. The five aims of nursing interventions are building trust, promoting the client's positive orientation, promoting the client's control, affirming and promoting the client's strength, and setting health-directed mutual goals while meeting the client's needs (e.g., biophysical, safety and security, love and belonging, esteem, and self-esteem) (Erickson, 2010; Erickson et al., 1983).

Usefulness

Currently, the model is the basis for a series of conferences incorporating MRM into research, practice settings, and curricula. Adherents of the theory state that it is used in courses or in the curricula of several universities. These include Humboldt State University School of Nursing in Arcata, California; Metropolitan State University in St. Paul, Minnesota; and the University of Texas at Austin, Alternate Entry Program, where graduate nursing students use MRM as a unifying model (Modeling and Role-Modeling, 2008); St. Catherine's University, Associate Degree Program Minneapolis, MN; Washetnaw Community College AD-N Program, Ypsilanti MI; Portland Health Science Center, Portland, OR; Harding University, Pediatric Nursing Course, Searcy, AR; and East Carolina University, Greensboro, NC, RN to MSN program (retrieved from http://www.mrmnursingtheory.org).

Several institutions use the model for practice. The University of Texas Medical Branch at Galveston used the model to structure the academic/service model. The University of Michigan Medical Center, Brigham and Women's Hospital in Boston, and the University of Pittsburgh (PA) hospitals all used the MRM as a theoretical basis for practice (Erickson et al., 1998). Several examples demonstrate how MRM has been applied in nursing practice. One in particular, Baldwin (2004), used the model to describe effective nursing interventions to promote independence for clients with interstitial cystitis.

Testability

MRM provides assumptions and relationships that are amenable to testing and have been and continue to be tested in research. The model has been used by nurses who have studied with Erickson, Tomlin, and Swain, and many theses and dissertations have incorporated elements of the model. Box 8-2 lists some of the current works using MRM in research.

Box 8-2 Examples of Research Studies Using Modeling and Role-Modeling Theory

Koren, M. E., & Papamiditriou, C. (2013). Spirituality of staff nurses: Application of modeling and role modeling theory. *Holistic Nursing Practice, 27*(1), 37–44.

Haylock, P. J. (2010). Advanced cancer: A mind-body-spirit approach to life and living. *Seminars in Oncology Nursing, 26*(3), 183–194.

Beery, T., Baas, L. S., & Henthorn, C. (2007). Self-reported adjustment to implanted cardiac devices. *Journal of Cardiovascular Nursing, 22*(6), 516–524.

Nash, K. (2007). Evaluation of the empower peer support and education program for middle school-aged adolescents. *Journal of Holistic Nursing, 25*(1), 26–36.

Mitchel, J. B. (2007). Enhancing patient connectedness: Understanding the nurse-patient relationship. *International Journal for Human Caring, 11*(4), 79–82.

Parsimony

The MRM theory is not parsimonious. Its complexity, however, reflects human beings, to whom it applies. MRM incorporates several borrowed theories that are synthesized for use in nursing science. The many linkages among the concepts and multiple levels need to be addressed, and considerable explanation is needed to enhance understanding of the tenets of the theory for nursing practice and for client care activities. However, nurses who use the theory are grateful for the fit it has with their practice.

Value in Extending Nursing Science

In addition to the uses of MRM in nursing education, practice, and research, three middle range nursing theories have been based on MRM. Acton (1997) developed a model describing affiliated-individuation, Irvin and Acton (1996) described caregiver stress, and Rogers (1996) discussed the concept of facilitative affiliation.

MRM theory is used in education, practice, and research. The Society for Promoting MRM Theory was formed in 1988 to promote understanding and use of the theory. This group meets annually and maintains a website at http://www.mrmnursingtheory.org. Research has been completed with people of all ages and with those who are suffering from many different health problems. According to those who espouse the theory, its major attraction is that it is practical, reflects the domain of nursing, and is a realistic model for guiding research, practice, and education.

Imogene M. King: King's Conceptual System and Theory of Goal Attainment and Transactional Process

King's theory evolved from early writings about theory development. In her first book in 1971, she synthesized scholarship from nursing and related disciplines into a theory for nursing (King, 1971). She wrote the Theory of Goal Attainment in 1980. The most recent edition (King, 1995a) contains further refinements and more detailed explanation of the general nursing framework and the theory.

Background of the Theorist

Imogene King graduated from St. John's Hospital School of Nursing in St. Louis, Missouri, with a diploma in nursing in 1945. She received a bachelor of science in nursing education from St. Louis University in 1948 and a master of science in nursing from the same school in 1957. In 1961, she received the doctor of education degree from Teacher's College, Columbia University, in New York (Sieloff, 2006). She held a variety of staff nursing, educational, research, and administrative roles throughout her professional life. She worked as a research consultant for the Division of Nursing in the Department of Health, Education, and Welfare from 1964 to 1966 (I. M. King, personal communication, October 2005). King moved to Tampa, Florida in 1980, assuming the position of professor at the University of South Florida College of Nursing (Sieloff, 2006). She remained active in professional organizations for many years. She died in 2008 and has been celebrated by a plethora of her colleagues (Mensik, 2008; Mitchell, 2008; Smith, Wright, & Fawcet, 2008; Stevens & Messmer, 2008).

Philosophical Underpinnings of the Theory

The von Bertalanffy General Systems Model is acknowledged to be the basis for King's work. She stated that the science of wholeness elucidated in that model gave her hope that the complexity of nursing could be studied "as an organized whole" (King, 1995b, p. 23).

Major Assumptions, Concepts, and Relationships

King's conceptual system and theory contain many concepts and multiple assumptions and relationships. A few of the assumptions, concepts, and relationships are presented in the following sections. The scholar wishing to use King's model or theory is referred to the original writings as both the model and theory are complex (Figure 8-2).

Assumptions

The Theory of Goal Attainment lists several assumptions relating to individuals, nurse–client interactions, and nursing. When describing individuals, the model shows that individuals (1) are social, sentient, rational, reacting beings and (2) are controlling, purposeful, action oriented, and time oriented in their behavior (King, 1995b).

Regarding nurse–client interactions, King (1981) believed that (1) perceptions of the nurse and client influence the interaction process; (2) goals, needs, and values of the nurse and client influence the interaction process; (3) individuals have a right to knowledge about themselves; (4) individuals have a right to participate in decisions that influence their lives, health, and community services; (5) individuals have a right to accept or reject care; and (6) goals of health professionals and goals of recipients of health care may not be congruent.

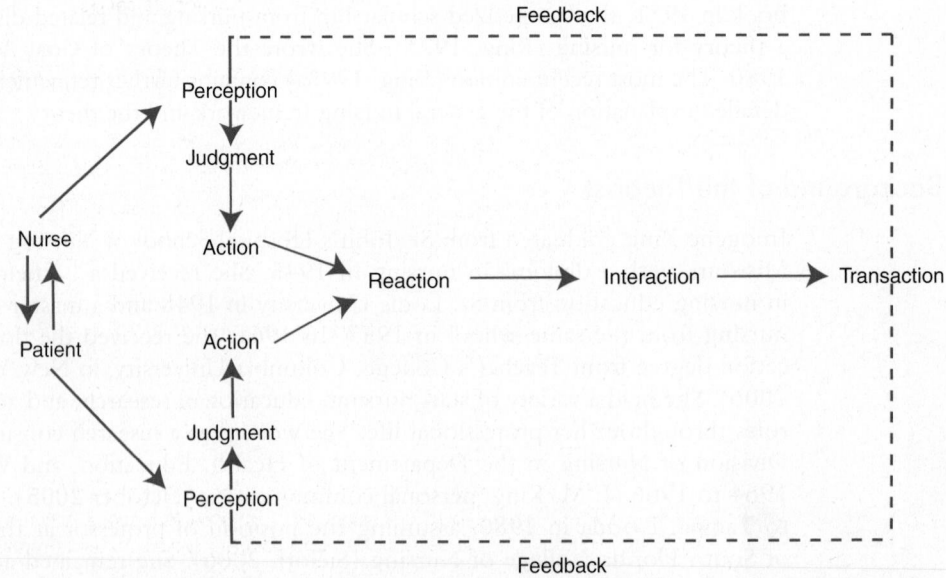

Figure 8-2 A model of nurse–patient interactions. (Source: King, I. M. (1981). *A theory for nursing: Systems, concepts, process*, p. 61 [Reprinted with permission of Sage Publications, Inc.].)

With regard to nursing, King (1981, 1995b) wrote that (1) nursing is the care of human beings; (2) nursing is perceiving, thinking, relating, judging, and acting *vis-a-vis* the behavior of individuals who come to a health care system; (3) a nursing situation is the immediate environment in which two individuals establish a relationship to cope with situational events; and (4) the goal of nursing is to help individuals and groups attain, maintain, and restore health. If this is not possible, nurses help individuals die with dignity.

Concepts

King's Theory of Goal Attainment defines the metaparadigm concepts of nursing as well as a number of additional concepts. Table 8-5 lists some of the major concepts.

Table 8-5 Major Concepts of the Theory of Goal Attainment

Concept	Definition
Nursing	A process of action, reaction, and interaction whereby nurse and client share information about their perceptions in the nursing situation. The nurse and client share specific goals, problems, and concerns and explore means to achieve a goal.
Health	A dynamic life experience of a human being, which implies continuous adjustment to stressors in the internal and external environment through optimum use of one's resources to achieve maximum potential for daily living.
Individuals	Social beings who are rational and sentient. Humans communicate their thoughts, actions, customs, and beliefs through language. Persons exhibit common characteristics such as the ability to perceive, to think, to feel, to choose between alternative courses of action, to set goals, to select the means to achieve goals, and to make decisions.
Environment	The background for human interactions. It is both external to and internal to the individual.
Perception	The process of human transactions with environment. It involves organizing, interpreting, and transforming information from sensory data and memory.
Communication	A process by which information is given from one person to another, either directly in face-to-face meetings or indirectly. It involves intrapersonal and interpersonal exchanges.
Interaction	A process of perception and communication between person and environment and between person and person represented by verbal and nonverbal behaviors that are goal-directed.
Transaction	A process of interactions in which human beings communicate with the environment to achieve goals that are valued; transactions are goal-directed human behaviors.
Stress	A dynamic state in which a human interacts with the environment to maintain balance for growth, development, and performance; it is the exchange of information between human and environment for regulation and control of stressors.

Source: King (1981).

Relationships

The Theory of Goal Attainment encompasses a great many relationships, many of them complex. King organized them into useful propositions that enhance the understanding of the relationships of the theory. A review of some relationships among the theory's concepts follows:

- Nurse and client are purposeful interacting systems.
- Nurse and client perceptions, judgments, and actions, if congruent, lead to goal-directed transactions.
- If perceptual accuracy is present in nurse–client interactions, transactions will occur.
- If nurse and client make transactions, goals will be attained.
- If goals are attained, satisfaction will occur.
- If goals are attained, effective nursing care will occur.
- If transactions are made in nurse–client interactions, growth and development will be enhanced.
- If role expectations and role performance as perceived by nurse and client are congruent, transactions will occur.
- If role conflict is experienced by nurse or client or both, stress in nurse–client interactions will occur.
- If nurses with special knowledge and skills communicate appropriate information to clients, mutual goal setting and goal attainment will occur (King, 1981, pp. 61, 149).

Usefulness

King's Theory of Goal Attainment has enhanced nursing education. For example, it served as a framework for the baccalaureate program at the Ohio State University School of Nursing, where it determined the content and processes taught at each level of the program (Daubenmire, 1989). Similarly, in Sweden, King's model was used to organize nursing education (Frey, Rooke, Sieloff, Messmer, & Kameoka, 1995). In more recent years, King's model has been useful in nursing education programs in Sweden, Portugal, Canada, and Japan (Sieloff, 2002, 2006).

King's conceptual system is an organizing guide for nursing practice. Joseph, Laughton, and Bogue (2011) examined the "sustainable adoption of whole-person care" (p. 989) in a Florida hospital guided by King's theory of goal attainment. Using a phenomenologic approach, they found that whole patient care was "lived" in their hospital as "relationship oriented patient care model" (p. 997). Gemmill and colleagues (2011) assessed nurses' knowledge about and attitudes toward ostomy care using King's theory of goal attainment to guide the research. Their findings included the finding that it is difficult for staff nurses to maintain their clinical abilities when there are few opportunities. Maintaining currency may require creative teaching interventions, such as simulations (Gemmill et al., 2011).

Hughes, Lloyd, and Clarke (2008) found King's model "a radical approach to process of nursing . . . in the United Kingdom" (p. 48). They found King's transaction process especially suited to nursing information systems.

Testability

Parts of the Theory of Goal Attainment have been tested, and a number of research studies reported in the literature used the model as a conceptual framework. For example, recent research includes that of Lockhart and Goodfellow (2009), who studied the effect of a 5-week head and neck surgical oncology practicum on nursing students' perceptions of facial disfigurement. With King's theory of goal attainment to guide their research, they presented the students with photographs of the surgical results, which they were to rank order as to amount of disfigurement. The researchers found that the students rated the female patients more disfigured than the males who had had the identical procedures. They also noted that central disfigurement was rated as greater than peripheral disfigurement.

An investigation in Brazil by Bezerra, da Silva, Guedes, and de Freitas (2010) analyzed perceptions of people about hypertension using King's model to structure their research. Their descriptive exploratory study found that the subjects feared complications yet were resigned to the changes in their lives necessitated by their disease. They also found that patients viewed nurses as helpful. The authors, however, noted that nurses need to take time to reflect on how they provide patient care.

Parsimony

The conceptual system and theory were presented together in several versions of King's writings and remain largely as written in 1981. The theory is not parsimonious, having numerous concepts, multiple assumptions, many statements, and many relationships on a number of levels. This complexity, however, mirrors the complexity of human transactions for goal attainment. The model is general and universal and can be the umbrella for many midrange and practice theories.

Value in Extending Nursing Science

In addition to application in practice and research described previously, King's work has been the basis for development of several middle range nursing theories. For example, the Theory of Goal Attainment was used by Rooda (1992) to develop a model for multicultural nursing practice. King's Systems Framework was reportedly used by Alligood and May (2000) to develop a theory of personal system empathy, and by Doornbos (2000) to derive a middle range theory of family health. Several Magnet status hospitals in the United States are using King's conceptual system in practice (I. M. King, personal communication, October 2005).

King's conceptual system and theory have been used internationally in Australia, Brazil, Canada, Pakistan, and Sweden, as well as in numerous university nursing programs in the United States, and have provided a foundation for many research studies. Her work has extended nursing science by its usefulness in education, practice, and research across international boundaries (King, 2001; Sieloff, 2006).

Sister Callista Roy: The Roy Adaptation Model

The Roy Adaptation Model (RAM) focuses on the interrelatedness of four adaptive systems. Like many of the models/theories in this unit, it is a deductive theory based on nursing practice. The RAM guides the nurse who is interested in physiologic adaptation as well as the nurse who is interested in psychosocial adaptation.

Background of the Theorist

Sister Callista Roy is a member of the Sisters of Saint Joseph of Carondelet. She received a BS in nursing from Mount Saint Mary's College in Los Angeles, California, an MS in nursing from UCLA, and a master's degree and doctorate in sociology from UCLA (Phillips, 2010). Roy first proposed the RAM while studying for her master's degree at UCLA, where Dorothy Johnson challenged students to develop conceptual models of nursing (Phillips, 2010; Roy, 2009). Her work is known internationally; she has presented at conferences in at least 30 countries and throughout the United States. She has received numerous honors and awards for her scholarly and professional work and is currently a professor and nurse theorist at Boston College's Connell School of Nursing (Roy, 2013).

Philosophical Underpinnings of the Theory

Johnson's nursing model was the impetus for the development of the RAM. Roy also incorporated concepts from Helson's adaptation theory, von Bertalanffy's system model, Rapoport's system definition, the stress and adaptation theories of Dohrenrend and Selye, and the coping model of Lazarus (Phillips, 2010).

Major Assumptions, Concepts, and Relationships

Assumptions

In the RAM, assumptions are specified as philosophical, scientific, and cultural (Roy, 2009, p. 31). Philosophical assumptions include:

- Persons have mutual relationships with the world and God.
- Human meaning is rooted in the omega point convergence of the universe.
- God is intimately revealed in the diversity of creation.
- Persons use human creative abilities of awareness, enlightenment, and faith.
- Persons are accountable for sustaining and transforming the universe (Roy, 2009, p. 31).

Scientific assumptions of the RAM for the 21st century include:

- Systems of matter and energy progress to higher levels of complex self-organization.
- Consciousness and meaning constitute person and environment integration.
- Self and environmental awareness is rooted in thinking and feeling.
- Human decisions account for integration of creative processes.
- Thinking and feeling mediate human action.
- System relationships include acceptance, protection, and fostering interdependence.
- Persons and the earth have common patterns and integral relationships.
- Person and environment transformations are created in human consciousness.
- Integration of human and environment results in adaptation (Roy, 2009, p. 1).

Cultural assumptions include:

- Cultural experiences influence how RAM is expressed.
- A concept central to the culture may influence the RAM to some extent.
- Cultural expressions of the RAM may lead to changes in practice activities such as nursing assessment (Roy, 2009, p. 31).
- As RAM evolves within a culture, implications for nursing may differ from experience in the original culture (Roy, 2009, p. 31).

All elements of the model are part of the care of clients and groups. The nurse undertakes a bi-level assessment to accurately define the problem and come to decisions on the plan of care. The process in formulating the nursing plan is intricate and is prescriptive in its objectives.

Table 8-6 Major Concepts of the Roy Adaptation Model

Concept	Definition
Environment	Conditions, circumstances, and influences that affect the development and behavior of humans as adaptive systems.
Health	A state and process of being and becoming integrated and whole.
Person	"The human adaptive system" and defined as "a whole with parts that function as a unity for some purpose. Human systems include people groups organizations, communities, and society as a whole" (Roy & Andrews, 1999, p. 31).
Goal of nursing	The "promotion of adaptation in each of the four modes" (p. 31).
Adaptation	The "process and outcome whereby thinking and feeling persons as individuals or in groups use conscious awareness and choice to create human and environmental integration" (p. 30).
Focal stimuli	Those stimuli that are the proximate causes of the situation.
Contextual stimuli	All other stimuli in the internal or external environment, which may or may not affect the situation.
Residual stimuli	Those immeasurable and unknowable stimuli that also exist and may affect the situation.
Cognator subsystem	"A major coping process involving four cognitive-emotive channels: perceptual and information processing, learning, judgment, and emotion" (p. 31).
Regulator subsystem	"A basic type of adaptive process that responds automatically through neural, chemical, and endocrine coping channels" (p. 46).
Stabilizer control processes	The structures and processes aimed at system maintenance and involving values and daily activities whereby participants accomplish the primary purpose of the group and contribute to the common purposes of the society.
Innovator control processes	The internal subsystem that involves structures and processes for growth.

Concepts

The RAM contains many defined concepts, including the metaparadigm concepts. Table 8-6 lists some of these.

Relationships

Roy's model is composed of four adaptive modes that constitute the specific categories that serve as framework for assessment (Figure 8-3). Through the four modes, "responses to and interaction with the client's environment are carried out and adaptation can be observed" (Roy, 2009, pp. 69–72).

They are the:

1. *Physiologic–physical mode:* Physical and chemical processes involved in the function and activities of living organisms; the underlying need is physiologic integrity: the degree of wholeness achieved through adaptation to changes in needs. In groups, this is the manner in which human systems manifest adaptation to basic operating resources (Roy, 2009, pp. 69–70).

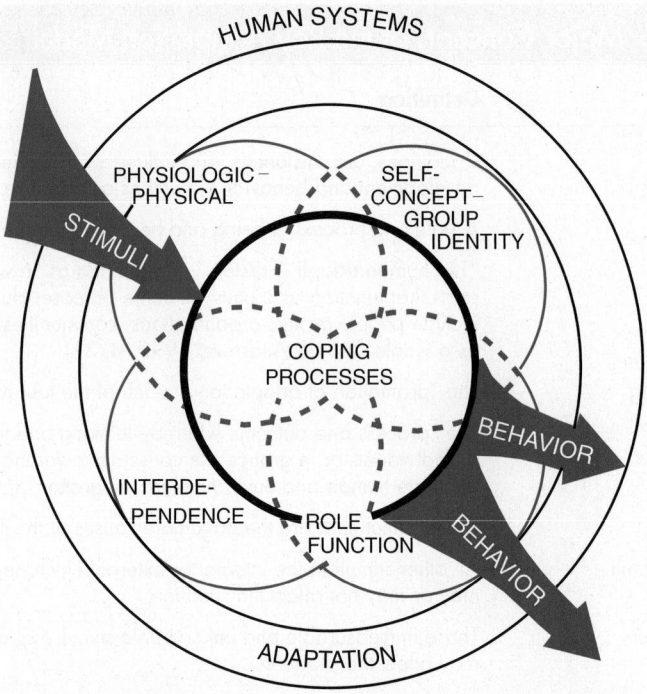

Figure 8-3 Diagrammatic representation of human adaptive systems. (Source: Roy, C., & Andrews, H. A. (1998). *The Roy adaptation model* (2nd ed., p. 114). Stamford, CT: Appleton & Lange [Reprinted with permission of Pearson Education, Inc, Upper Saddle River, NJ].)

2. *Self-concept–group identity mode:* Focuses on psychological and spiritual integrity and a sense of unity, meaning, and purposefulness in the universe (p. 70).
3. *Role function mode:* Refers to the roles that individuals occupy in society fulfilling the need for social integrity; it is knowing who one is, in relation to others (p. 70).
4. *Interdependence mode:* The close relationships of people and their purpose, structure, and development, individually and in groups and the adaptation potential of these relationships (Roy, 2009, p. 71).

Two subsystems require assessment in the RAM: the regulator and the cognator. These are coping subsystems that allow the client to adapt and make changes when stressed. The regulator is the physiologic coping subsystem, and the cognator is the cognitive–emotive coping subsystem (Roy, 2009). In her writing, *Extending the Roy Adaptation Model . . .* , Roy shows how the four modes work in communities and globally. She states that "this theoretical work . . . portends well . . . for nurse scholars to meet the challenges . . . for the nursing role in the global community" (Roy, 2011a, p. 350).

Usefulness

The RAM has been used extensively to guide practice and to organize nursing education. International conferences on the RAM have been conducted across the United States and abroad (Roy, 2009). The RAM was adopted as a component of the curricular framework of such widely diverse colleges and departments of nursing as Mount

Saint Mary's College, Department of Nursing; the University of Texas at Austin School of Nursing; Boston College School of Nursing; and the nurse practitioner program at the University of Miami in Florida. The RAM has also been implemented internationally at the University of Ottawa School of Nursing and in university schools of nursing in Japan and France (Phillips, 2010).

Among middle range nursing theories derived from the RAM are a longitudinal model of psychosocial determinants of adaptation (Ducharme, Richard, Duquette, Levesque, & Lachance, 1998); a middle range theory of psychological adaptation (Levesque, Ricard, Ducharme, Duquette, & Bonin, 1998); and another middle range nursing theory, the Urine Control Theory, by Jirovec, Jenkins, Isenberg, and Baiardi (1999). The RAM has also been tested and applied to practice in Latin America (Moreno-Fergusen, 2007).

Testability

The RAM is testable. Indeed, the Boston Based Adaptation Research in Nursing Society (BBARNS, 1999) reported that since the 1970s, 163 studies had been conducted using the model. *Note:* An international nursing society specifically focused on researching adaptation nursing, Roy Adaptation Association (RAA), replaced the BBARNS organization, which was based in Boston College School of Nursing (Roy, 2009). Roy (2011b) shows that not only the RAM but many middle range theories originating in the RAM also have grounded research in the past 25 years. She gives numerous instances of the use of the RAM in research in that period. Box 8-3 lists a few recent examples of nursing research using aspects of the RAM.

Parsimony

The RAM is not parsimonious because of its many elements, systems, structures, and concepts. However, Clarke, Barone, Hanna, and Senesac (2011) state that the RAM is "accessible, elegant and practical" (p. 338) in its presentation. It is complete and comprehensive, and it attempts to explain the reality of the clients so that nursing interventions can be specifically targeted. The nursing assessment is conducted on two levels and is extensive and complex. It requires assessment of the stimuli to which the client is responding and of the coping subsystems. It targets the client in the four adaptive modes, and an assessment must be made to determine how effectively the subsystems (i.e., cognator and regulator) are working.

Value in Extending Nursing Science

The RAM has been a valuable asset in extending nursing science. Dunn and Dunn (1997) summarized the impact of the RAM on nursing practice, education, and administration, stating that it has contributed significantly to the science and practice of nursing. Indeed, the RAM has generated hundreds of research studies and has contributed to nursing education for more than 35 years (Roy, 2009). Fredrickson (2011) states that chapters of the RAM society are present in such disparate areas such as several countries of South America as well as Japan, thus extending the reach of Roy's principles globally. Indeed, the RAM is used in almost every country in Europe, Asia, South America, and others as well (Clarke et al., 2011). Roy (2011a) states that ". . . the criteria for good . . . is to promote adaptation of individuals and groups; to transform a society to one that promotes dignity, and to sustain and transform th universe" (p. 346).

Box 8-3 Examples of Studies Using the Roy Adaptation Model

Ashktorab, T., Zabihi, R. E., Banaderakhshan, H., Zayeri, F., & Anbuhi, S. Z. (2011). Correlation between self-concept according to Roy Adaptation Model with adherence to therapeutic regimen in hypertensive out patients who attended one of the hospitals affiliated to Urmia University of Medical Sciences and health services. *Journal of Nursing and Midwifery, 21*(73), 59.

Cummins, J. (2011). Sharing a traumatic event: The experience of the listener and the storyteller within the dyad. *Nursing Research, 60*(6), 386–392.

Debiasi, L. B., Reynolds, A., & Buckner E. B. (2012). Assessing emotional well-being of children in a Honduran orphanage: Feasibility of two screening tools. *Pediatric Nursing, 38*(3), 169–176.

DeSanto-Madeya, S., & Fawcett, J. (2009). Toward understanding and measuring adaptation level in the context of the Roy adaptation model. *Nursing Science Quarterly, 22*(4), 355–359.

Heydari, A., Ahrari, S., & Vaghee, S. (2011). The relationship between self-concept and adherence to therapeutic regimens in patients with heart failure. *Journal of Cardiovascular Nursing, 26*(6), 475–480.

Kaur, H., & Mahal, R. (2012). A study of nurses acceptability for utilization of theory based nursing assessment tool. *International Journal of Nursing Education, 4*(2), 132–136.

Omrah, S., Saeed, A. M. A., & Simpson, J. (2012). Symptom distress of Jordanian patients with cancer receiving chemotherapy. *International Journal of Nursing Practice, 18*(2), 125–132.

Ordin, Y. S., Karayurt, O., & Wellard, S. (2013). Investigation of adaptation after liver transplantation using Roy's Adaptation Model. *Nursing and Health Sciences, 15*(1), 31–38.

Poirier, P., (2011). The impact of fatigue on role functioning during radiation therapy. *Oncology Nursing Forum, 38*(4), 457–465.

Rogers, C. E., Keller, C., Larkey, L. K., & Ainsworth, B. E. (2012). A randomized controlled trial to determine the efficacy of Sign Chi Do exercise on adaptation to aging. *Research in Gerontological Nursing, 5*(2), 101–113.

Jean Watson: Caring Science as Sacred Science

Jean Watson's (2008) *Philosophy and Science of Caring,* a recent publication, builds on her previous work, *Nursing: Human Science and Human Care: A Theory of Nursing.* This theory is one of the newest of nursing's grand theories, having only been completely codified in 1979, revised in 1985 (Watson, 1988), and broadened and advanced more recently (Watson, 2005, 2008). Watson called her earlier work a descriptive theory of caring and stated that it was the only theory of nursing to incorporate the spiritual dimension of nursing at the time it was first conceptualized. The theory was both deductive and inductive in its origins and was written at an abstract level of discourse.

It is somewhat difficult to categorize Watson's work with the works of other nursing theorists. It has many characteristics of a human interaction model, although it also incorporates many ideals of the unitary process theories, which are discussed in Chapter 9. Watson (2005) has always described the human as a holistic, interactive being and is now explicit in describing the human as an energy field and in explaining health and illness as manifestations of the human pattern (Watson, 2008), two tenets of the unitary process theories. Parse (2004) points out, however, that although theorists profess belief in unitary human beings, other definitions and relationships still separate theories from the interactive process paradigms and the unitary process nursing paradigms. Based on overall considerations, the philosophy and science of caring reflects the interactive process nursing theories.

Background of the Theorist

Jean Watson was born in West Virginia and attended Lewis Gale School of Nursing in Roanoke, Virginia. She earned a bachelor's degree in nursing, a master of science degree in psychiatric–mental health nursing, and a doctorate in educational psychology and counseling, all from the University of Colorado (Neill, 2002). Watson is an internationally published author, having written many books, book chapters, and articles about the science of human caring (Watson, 1994, 1996, 1999, 2005, 2008).

Watson is the former Dean of the School of Nursing at the University of Colorado, and she founded and directed the Center for Human Caring at the Health Sciences Center in Denver. She has received numerous awards and honors (Neill, 2002) and is currently Distinguished Professor of Nursing and Dean Emerita at the University of Colorado Denver College of Nursing and Anschutz Medical Center, "where she held an endowed chair in Caring Science for 16 years. She is a fellow of the American Academy of Nursing and past president of the National League for Nursing" (Watson Caring Science Institute and International Caring Consortium [WCSIICC], 2013). Some of her honors include Fetzer Institute Norman Cousins Award; an International Kellogg Fellowship in Australia; a Fulbright research award in Sweden; and 10 honorary doctoral degrees, including those from Sweden, United Kingdom, Spain, British Columbia and Quebec in Canada, and from Japan (WCSIICC, 2013).

Philosophical Underpinnings of the Theory

Watson (1988) noted that she drew parts of her theory from nursing writers, including Nightingale and Rogers. She also used concepts from the works of psychologists Giorgi, Johnson, and Koch, as well as concepts from philosophy. She reported being widely read in these disciplines and synthesized a number of diverse concepts from them into nursing as a science of human caring. In a recent work, Watson (2005) continues to "bridge paradigms and point toward transformative models for the 21st century" (p. 2).

Major Assumptions, Concepts, and Relationships

The value system that permeates Watson's (1988, 2008) theory of human caring includes a "deep respect for the wonders and mysteries of life" (1988, p. 34) and recognition that spiritual and ethical dimensions are major elements of the human care process. A number of assumptions are both stated and implicit in her theory. Additionally, several concepts were defined, refined, and adapted for it. From this, 10 carative factors were developed (Box 8-4; Watson, 1985, 2008).

Assumptions

Watson (2008) describes the tenets of caring science and sacred science. She proposed that caring and love are universal and mysterious "cosmic forces" that comprise the primal and universal psychic energy. Further, she believes that health professionals make social, moral, and scientific contributions to humankind and that nurses' caring ideal can affect human development. Further, she believes that it is critical in today's society to sustain human caring ideals and a caring ideology in practice, as there

Box 8-4 Watson's 10 Carative Factors

1. Humanistic–altruistic system of values
2. Faith–hope
3. Sensitivity to self and others
4. Developing helping–trusting, caring relationship
5. Expressing positive and negative feelings and emotions
6. Creative, individualized, problem-solving caring process
7. Transpersonal teaching–learning
8. Supportive, protective, and/or corrective, mental, physical, societal, and spiritual environment
9. Human needs assistance
10. Existential-phenomenologic and spiritual forces

Source: Watson (1999, 2005).

been a proliferation of radical treatment and "cure techniques," often without regard to costs or human considerations.

Explicit assumptions that were derived for Watson's (2005) work include:

- An ontologic assumption of oneness, wholeness, unity, relatedness, and connectedness.
- An epistemologic assumption that there are multiple ways of knowing.
- Diversity of knowing assumes all, and various forms of evidence can be included.
- A caring science model makes these diverse perspectives explicitly and directly.
- Moral-metaphysical integration with science evokes spirit; this orientation is not only possible but also necessary for our science, humanity, society-civilization, and world-planet.
- A caring science emergence, founded on new assumptions, makes explicit an expanding unitary, energetic worldview with a relational human caring ethic and ontology as its starting point (Watson, 2005, p. 28).

Concepts

Watson (1988) defined three of the four metaparadigm concepts (human being, health, and nursing). She coined several other concepts and terms that are integral to understanding the science of human caring (Table 8-7). Her 10 carative factors are caring needs specific to human experiences that should be addressed by nurses with their clients in the caring role. She continues to value those carative factors (Watson, 2008). The carative factors are listed in Box 8-4.

Relationships

Watson has refined and updated the relationships of the theory, bringing them closer to her current way of understanding human caring and spirituality. Her continued study has involved lengthy examination of her beliefs about caring, spirituality, and human and energy fields (Watson, 2005, 2008). The following are some of the relationships of the theory:

- A transpersonal caring field resides within a unitary field of consciousness and energy that transcends time, space, and physicality.
- A transpersonal caring relationship connotes a spirit-to-spirit unitary connection within a caring moment, honoring the embodied spirit of both practitioner and patient within a unitary field of consciousness.

Table 8-7 Major Concepts of the Science of Human Caring

Concept	Definition
Human being	A valued person to be cared for, respected, nurtured, understood, and assisted.
Health	Unity and harmony within the mind, body, and soul; health is associated with the degree of congruence between the self as perceived and the self as experienced.
Nursing	A human science of persons and human health–illness experiences that are mediated by professional, personal, scientific, esthetic, and ethical human care transactions.
Actual caring occasion	Involves actions and choices by the nurse and the individual. The moment of coming together in a caring occasion presents the two persons with the opportunity to decide how to be in the relationship—what to do with the moment.
Transpersonal	An intersubjective human-to-human relationship in which the nurse affects and is affected by the person of the other. Both are fully present in the moment and feel a union with the other; they share a phenomenal field that becomes part of the life history of both.
Phenomenal field	The totality of human experience of one's being in the world. This refers to the individual's frame of reference that can only be known to that person.
Self	The organized conceptual gestalt composed of perceptions of the characteristics of the "I" or "ME" and the perceptions of the relationship of the "I" or "ME" to others and to various aspects of life.
Time	The present is more subjectively real and the past is more objectively real. The past is prior to, or in a different mode of being, than the present, but it is not clearly distinguishable. Past, present, and future incidents merge and fuse.

Sources: Watson (1999); online site: http://www.uchsc.edu/ctrsinst/chc/index.html

- A transpersonal caring relationship transcends the ego level of both practitioner and patient, creating a caring field with new possibilities for how to be in the moment.
- The practitioner's authentic intentionality and consciousness of caring has a higher frequency of energy than noncaring consciousness, opening up connections to the universal field of consciousness and greater access to one's inner healer.
- Transpersonal caring is communicated via the practitioner's energetic patterns of consciousness, intentionality, and authentic presence in a caring relationship.
- Caring-healing modalities are often noninvasive, nonintrusive, natural-human, energetic environmental field modalities.
- Transpersonal caring promotes self-knowledge, self-control, and self-healing patterns and possibilities.
- Advanced transpersonal caring modalities draw upon multiple ways of knowing and being; they encompass ethical and relational caring, along with those intentional consciousness modalities that are energetic in nature (e.g., form, color, light, sound, touch, vision, scent) that honor wholeness, healing, comfort, balance, harmony, and well-being (Watson, 2005, p. 6).

Usefulness

Watson's works on the Theory of Human Caring and the Art and Science of Human Caring are used by nurses in diverse settings; for example, Brockopp and colleagues (2011) details an evidence-based, practice-based practice model rounded in Watson's theory of caring. The 10 carative factors are explicated throughout the hospital to provide a framework for nursing activities in this magnate hospital. The outcomes include 34 research projects, 9 published articles, and 9 funded research studies. Furthermore, the nurses "maintain high levels of work satisfaction, strong retention rates and a large percentage of associate-degree nurses return to school for baccalaureate degrees" (p. 511).

Hills and colleagues (2011) developed a text to promote caring science curriculum in nursing, which they called an emancipatory pedagogy for nursing. It is based on Watson's science of caring and explores an alternative method of student evaluation. Lukose (2011) developed a practice model for Watson's theory of caring that "can be used by nurse educators to teach staff nurses and students" (p. 27). Noel (2010) reviewed Watson's theory of human caring for occupational health and nursing and found it relevant in that context. The author also found that other disciplines are using the theory of human caring as their guiding principle in contact with people.

The University of Colorado School of Nursing implemented the model not only in its education programs (BSN, MSN, and PhD), but also in clinical practice at the Center for Human Caring (Watson, 1988). In addition, the School of Nursing at Georgia Southern University in Statesboro taught both undergraduate courses and the nurse practitioner program from the human caring philosophy (Watson, 1988). Writings that detail how Watson's work is used in nursing education include Bevis and Watson (1989), Leininger and Watson (1990), and Watson (1994). Furthermore, schools around the world are using Watson's science of caring in nursing education. They include Scandinavia (Wicklund-Gustin & Wagner, 2013), Japan (Ishikawa & Kawano, 2012), and throughout the United States in nursing curricula (Hills et al., 2011). Numerous nationwide community caring projects have made a difference in such areas as immediate care for victims of natural disasters, veterans returning from Iraq and Afghanistan, and homeless people (J. Laroussini, personal communication, March 2013).

Testability

Testing of Watson's theory and dissemination of findings are progressing. The science allows both quantitative and qualitative research methods. For example, Watson's work was used as the framework for a study by Perry (2009), who discussed findings from an investigation of nurses whom their colleagues identified as exemplary using a phenomenologic approach. Perry found that those nurses were also excellent clinical role models. The paper describes elements such as attending to the little things, making connections, and remaining lighthearted that made these nurses exemplary practitioners. Watson's Science of Caring has recently been researched by an extremely large number of nurses. Additional research articles are listed in Box 8-5.

Parsimony

Watson's theory is comparatively parsimonious. Although a number of new concepts and terms are defined, there are only 10 carative factors or areas to be addressed by nurses. In addition, there are six "working assumptions" (Watson, 2005, p. 28) and three considerations as to how to frame caring science.

Box 8-5 Examples of Research Using Watson's Model

Arslan-Ozkan, I., & Okumus, H. (2012). A model where caring and healing meets: Watson's theory of Human Caring. *Turkish Journal of Research & Development in Nursing, 14*(2), 61–72. (in Turkish with abstract translated).

Hermanns, M., Mastel-Smith, B., Lilly, M. L., Deardorff, K., & Price, C. (2009). Teaching theoretically based interventions: Use of life review. *International Journal of Human Caring, 13*(4), 44–49.

Hill, K. S. (2011). Work satisfaction, intent to stay, desires of nurses, and financial knowledge among bedside and advanced practice nurses. *Journal of Nursing Administration, 41*(5), 211–217.

Ishikawa, J., & Kawano, M. (2012). Caring practice of a psychiatric nursing in Japan—Analyzing from caring theory focusing on the inner process of the individual. *International Journal for Human Caring, 16*(3), 80–81.

Schmock, B. N., Breckenridge, D. M., & Benedict, K. (2009). Effect of sacred space environment on surgical patient outcomes: A pilot study. *International Journal for Human Caring, 13*(1), 49–59.

Suliman, W. A., Welmann, E., Omer, T., & Thomas, L. (2009). Applying Watson's nursing theory to assess patient perceptions of being cared for in a multicultural environment. *Journal of Nursing Research (Taiwan), 17*(4), 293–300.

Vandenhouten, C., Kubsch, S., Peterson, M., Murdock, J., & Lehrer, L. (2012). Watson's theory of transpersonal caring: Factors impacting nurses professional caring. *Holistic Nursing Practice, 26*(6), 326–334.

Wicklund-Gustin, L., & Wagner, L. (2013). The butterfly effect of caring—Clinical nursing teachers' understanding of self-compassion as a source to compassionate care. *Scandinavian Journal of Caring Sciences, 27*(1), 175–183.

Value in Extending Nursing Science

The Philosophy and Science of Caring (Watson, 2008) explicitly describes the connection between nursing and caring. It is used in education and in practice internationally and in numerous research studies. Collectively, findings present impressive indicators of the value of Watson's theory of caring to the discipline of nursing.

Summary

The models presented in this chapter all focus on human interactive processes as the basis for nursing care, research, and education. Some of the theories described (e.g., King and Levine) are among the oldest of the grand nursing theories, whereas others (e.g., Watson and Artinian) are among the most recently developed. There is a wide variety of complexity among the models, but each has demonstrated applicability to the discipline, and all are currently used in schools of nursing, hospital clinical and community settings, and nursing research.

Like Jean, the nurse in the opening case study, nurses in all settings will be able to relate to the perspective described by these theorists. Indeed, the premise that humans are adaptive, holistic beings, in constant interaction with their environment, is easily applied in nursing practice. Some philosophical bases, concepts, assumptions, and relationships (e.g., systems focus, adaptation, goal of nursing, and interaction) are relatively consistently held within the works of this group of theorists, whereas others (e.g., situational sense of coherence [Artinian], conservation principles [Levine], cognator and regulator subsystems [Roy], and carative factors [Watson]) are unique to just one theory. Evidence-based practice (EBP) fits well with these theories and models because they ascribe to outcomes-based quantitative and to reality-based qualitative research principles.

Nurses studying this group of theories will become aware of how they present and prescribe nursing practice. Many will undoubtedly consider adopting one as a basis for their own professional practice.

Key Points

1. The theories in this chapter depend on the ideal that nurses, other health care professionals, and patients are constantly interacting. The environment defined by most of these theorists is also foremost in individuals' interactions.
2. The theorists who have developed these theories and models generally include and provide definitions of the four metaparadigm concepts of person, health, environment, and nursing. Several also include spirituality among their concepts.
3. Most interactive process theories are practice-based and correspond closely to the work of nurses in clinical practice.
4. Several interactive process theories are well suited to and are chosen to guide EBP and research to gather that evidence.
5. Several of the theories and models in this group have been used or are being used to guide and structure educational programs in university nursing schools worldwide.

Learning Activities

1. Compare and contrast two of the models or theories presented in this chapter, considering their usefulness in practice, research, education, and administration. Share findings with classmates.
2. Select one of the models from this chapter and obtain the original work(s) of the theorist. From the work(s), outline a plan for a research study either using the work as the conceptual framework or testing components of the work.
   a. What concepts, assumptions, or relationships can be studied?
   b. To what population(s) can the work be applied?
   c. What concepts can be used as study variables?
3. Explain how a model of your choice can be used to guide evidence gathering through research for EBP.

REFERENCES

Acton, G. J. (1997). Affiliated-individuation as a mediator of stress and burden in caregivers of adults with dementia. *Journal of Holistic Nursing, 15*(4), 336–357.

Alligood, M. R., & May, B. A. (2000). A nursing theory of personal system empathy: Interpreting a conceptualization of empathy in King's interacting systems. *Nursing Science Quarterly, 13(3)*, 243–247.

Antonofski, A. (1987). *Unraveling the mystery of health: How people manage stress and stay well.* San Francisco: Jossey-Bass (as cited in Artinian, 1991).

Artinian, B. M. (1983). Implementation of the intersystem patient-care model in clinical practice. *Journal of Advanced Nursing, 8*(2), 117–124.

Artinian, B. M. (1991). The development of the intersystem model. *Journal of Advanced Nursing, 16*, 164–205.

Artinian, B. M. (1997a). Overview of the intersystem model. In B. M. Artinian & M. M. Conger (Eds.), *The intersystem model: Integrating theory and practice* (pp. 1–17). Thousand Oaks, CA: Sage.

Artinian, B. M. (1997b). Situational sense of coherence. In B. M. Artinian & M. M. Conger (Eds.), *The intersystem model: Integrating theory and practice* (pp. 18–30). Thousand Oaks, CA: Sage.

Artinian, B. M. (1997c). Research: Refining and testing the theoretical constructs of the intersystem model. In B. M. Artinian & M. M. Conger (Eds.), *The intersystem model: Integrating theory and practice* (pp. 225–269). Thousand Oaks, CA: Sage.

Artinian, B. M. (1997d). The nursing assessment decision grid. In B. M. Artinian & M. M. Conger (Eds.), *The intersystem model: Integrating theory and practice* (pp. 269–280). Thousand Oaks, CA: Sage.

Artinian, B. M. (1998). Grounded theory research: Its value for nursing. *Nursing Science Quarterly, 11*(1), 5–6.

Artinian, B. M. Personal communication. May 30, 2003.

Artinian, B. M. (2011). Theoretical background of the Artinian intersystem model. In B. M. Artinian, K. S. West, & M. M. Conger (Eds.). *The Artinian intersystem model* (2nd ed.). New York: Springer.

Artinian, B. M. (2013). *Curriculum vitae.* Retrieved from http://www.apu.edu/faculty/cvs/bartinian.pdf

Artinian, B. M., Giske, T., & Cone, P. H. (2009). *Glaserian grounded theory in nursing research: Trusting emergence.* New York: Springer.

Baldwin, C. M. (2004). Interstitial cystitis and self-care: Bearing the burden. *Urologic Nursing, 24*(2), 111–112.

Bevis, E. O., & Watson, J. (1989). *Toward a caring curriculum: A new pedagogy for nursing.* New York: National League for Nursing.

Bezerra, S. T. F., da Silva, L. de F., Guedes, M. V. C., & de Freitas, M. C. (2010). Perceptions of people about hypertension and concepts of Imogene King [Portugese]. *Revista Gaucha de Enfermagem, 31*(3), 499–507.

Bond, M. L., Gray, J. R., Baxley, S., Cason, C. L., Denke, L., & Moon, M. (2008). Voices of Hispanic students in baccalaureate nursing programs: Are we listening? *Nursing Education Perspectives, 29*(3), 136–142.

Brockopp, D., Schreiber, J., Hill, K., Altpeter, T., Moe, K., & Merritt, S. (2011). A successful evidence-based practice model in an acute care setting. *Oncology Nursing Forum, 38*(5), 509–511.

Boston Based Adaptation Research in Nursing Society. (1999). *Roy adaptation model-based research: 25 years of contributions to nursing science.* Indianapolis, IN: Center Nursing Press, Sigma Theta Tau International.

Cason, C., Bond, M. L., Gleason-Wynn, P., Coggin, C., Trevino, E., & Lopez, M. (2008). Perceived barriers and needed supports for today's Hispanic students in the health professions: Voices of seasoned Hispanic health care professionals. *Hispanic Care International, 6*(1), 41–50.

Chrisman, M., & Riehl, J. (1974). The systems-developmental stress model. In J. Riehl & C. Roy (Eds.), *Conceptual models for nursing practice* (pp. 247–266). New York: Appleton-Century-Crofts.

Chrisman, M., & Riehl, J. (1989). The systems-developmental stress model. In J. Riehl & C. Roy (Eds.), *Conceptual models for nursing practice* (3rd ed., pp. 247–268). New York: Appleton-Century-Crofts.

Clarke, P. N., Barone, S. H., Hanna, D., & Senesac, P. M. (2011). Roy's adaptation model. *Nursing Science Quarterly, 24*(4) 337–344.

Cone, P. H., Artinian, B. M., & West, K. S. (2011). The Artinian intersystem model in nursing school education. In B. M. Artinian, K. S. West, & M. M. Conger. (Eds.), *The Artinian intersystem model* (2nd ed.). New York: Springer.

Critchley, S., & Ball, E. (2007). Evaluation of the primary/secondary care interface in relation to primary care rheumatology service. *Quality in Primary Care, 15*(1), 33–36.

Daubenmire, M. J. (1989). A baccalaureate curriculum based on King's conceptual framework. In J. Riehl-Siska (Ed.), *Conceptual models for nursing practice* (3rd ed., pp. 167–178). Norwalk, CT: Appleton & Lange.

Dever, M. (1991). Care of children. In K. M. Schaefer & J. B. Pond (Eds.), *Levine's conservation model: A framework for nursing practice* (pp. 71–82). Philadelphia: Davis.

Doornbos, M. M. (2000). King's systems framework and family health: The derivation and testing of a theory. *Journal of Theory Construction and Testing, 4*(1), 20–26.

Dover, L., & Pfieffer, J. B. (2006). Spiritual care in Christian parish nursing. *Journal of Advanced Nursing, 57*(2), 213–221.

Ducharme, F., Richard, N., Duquette, A., Levesque, L., & Lachance, L. (1998). Empirical testing of a longitudinal model derived from the Roy adaptation model. *Nursing Science Quarterly, 119*(4), 149–159.

Dunn, H. C., & Dunn, D. G. (1997). The Roy adaptation model and its application to clinical nursing practice. *Journal of Ophthalmic Nursing and Technology, 16*(2), 74–78.

Erickson, H. L. (2008). *Biosketch.* Retrieved from http://www.unicornsunlimited.com

Erickson, M. E. (2010). Modeling and role-modeling. In M. R. Alligood & A. M. Tomey (Eds), *Nursing theorists and their work* (7th ed., pp. 536–559). St. Louis: Mosby.

Erickson, M. E., Caldwell-Gwin, J. A., Carr, L. A., Harmon, B. K., Hartman, K., Jarlsberg, C. R., et al. (1998). Helen C. Erickson, Evelyn M. Tomlin, Mary Ann P. Swain: Modeling and role-modeling. In A. M. Tomey & M. R. Alligood (Eds.), *Nursing theorists and their work* (pp. 387–406). St. Louis: Mosby.

Erickson, H. C., Tomlin, E. M., & Swain, M. A. P. (1983). *Modeling and role-modeling: A theory and paradigm for nursing.* Englewood Cliffs, NJ: Prentice-Hall.

Fasnacht, P. H. (2003). Creativity: A refinement of the concept for nursing practice. *Journal of Advanced Nursing, 41*(2), 195–202.

Foreman, M. D. (1991). Conserving cognitive integrity of hospitalized elderly. In K. M. Schaefer & J. B. Pond (Eds.), *Levine's conservation model: A framework for nursing practice* (pp. 134–149). Philadelphia: Davis.

Fredrickson, K. (2011). Callista Roy's adaptation model. *Nursing Science Quarterly, 24*(4), 301–303.

Frey, M. A., Rooke, L., Sieloff, C., Messmer, P. R., & Kameoka, T. (1995). King's framework and theory in Japan, Sweden, and the United States. *Image: Journal of Nursing Scholarship, 27*(2), 127–130.

Gemmill, R., Kravits, K., Oritz, M., Anderson, C., Lai, L., & Grant, M. (2011). What do surgical oncology staff nurses know about colorectal cancer ostomy care? *Journal of Continuing Education in Nursing, 42*(2), 81–88.

Giske, T., & Artinian, B. (2008). Patterns of "balancing between hope and despair" in the diagnostic phase: A grounded theory study of patients on a gastroenterology ward. *Journal of Advanced Nursing, 62*(1), 22–31.

Grindley, J., & Paradowski, M. B. (1991). Developing an undergraduate program using Levine's model. In K. M. Schaefer & J. B. Pond (Eds.), *Levine's conservation model: A framework for nursing practice* (pp. 199–208). Philadelphia: Davis.

Hills, M., Watson, J., Boykin, A., Touhy, T. A., Smith, M. C., Lewis, S., et al. (2011). *Creating a caring science curriculum: An emancipatory pedagogy for nursing.* New York: Springer.

Hughes, R., Lloyd, D., & Clarke, J. (2008). A conceptual model for nursing information. *International Journal of Nursing Technologies and Classifications, 29*(2), 48–56.

Irvin, B. L., & Acton, G. J. (1996). Stress mediation in caregivers of cognitively impaired adults: Theoretical model testing. *Nursing Research, 45*(3), 160–166.

Ishikawa, J., & Kawano, M. (2012). Caring practice of a psychiatric nurse in Japan—Analyzing from caring theory focusing on the inner process of the individual. *International Journal of Human Caring, 16*(3), 80–81.

Jirovec, M. M., Jenkins, J., Isenberg, M., & Baiardi, J. (1999). Urine control theory derived from Roy's conceptual framework. *Nursing Science Quarterly, 12*(3), 251–255.

Joseph, L. M., Laughton, D., & Bogue, R. (2011). An examination of the sustainable adoption of whole person care (WPC). *Journal of Nursing Management, 19*(8), 989–997.

King, I. (1971). *Toward a theory for nursing.* New York: Wiley.

King, I. (1981). *A theory for nursing, systems, concepts, process.* New York: Wiley.

King, I. M. (1995a). A systems framework for nursing. In M. A. Frey & C. L. Sieloff (Eds.), *Advancing King's systems framework and theory of nursing* (pp. 13–22). Thousand Oaks, CA: Sage.

King, I. M. (1995b). The theory of goal attainment. In M. A. Frey & C. L. Sieloff (Eds.), *Advancing King's systems framework and theory of nursing* (pp. 23–33). Thousand Oaks, CA: Sage.

King, I. M. (2001). Theory of goal attainment. In M. Parker (Ed.), *Nursing theories and nursing practice* (pp. 275–286). Philadelphia: Davis.

King, I. M. Personal communication. October 2005.

Laroussini, J. Personal communication. Ready for the return volunteer. March 2013.

Leach, M. J. (2006). Wound management: Using Levine's conservation model to guide practice. *Ostomy Wound Management, 52*(8), 74–76, 78–80.

Leininger, M., & Watson, J. (Eds.). (1990). *The caring imperative in education*. New York: National League for Nursing Press.

Levesque, L., Ricard, N., Ducharme, F., Duquette, A., & Bonin, J. (1998). Empirical verification of a theoretical model derived from the Roy adaptation model: Findings from five studies. *Nursing Science Quarterly, 11*(1), 31–39.

Levine, M. E. (1969). *Introduction to clinical nursing*. Philadelphia: Davis.

Levine, M. E. (1973). Introduction to patient-centered nursing care. (Reprinted from *Levine's conservation model*, pp. 237–259, by K. M. Schafer & J. B. Pond, 1991, Philadelphia: F. A. Davis).

Levine, M. E. (1989). The conservation principles of nursing: Twenty years later. In J. P. Riehl-Siska (Ed.), *Conceptual models for nursing practice* (3rd ed., pp. 325–337). Norwalk, CT: Appleton & Lange.

Levine, M. E. (1990). Conservation and integrity. In M. E. Parker (Ed.), *Nursing theories in practice* (pp. 189–201). New York: National League for Nursing Press.

Levine, M. E. (1991). The conservation principles: A model for health. In K. M. Schaefer & J. B. Pond (Eds.), *Levine's conservation model: A framework for nursing practice* (pp. 1–11). Philadelphia: Davis.

Lockhart, J. S., & Goodfellow, L. M. (2009). The effect of a 5-week head & neck surgical oncology practicum on nursing students' perceptions of facial disfigurement (part 1). *ORL-Head & Neck Nursing, 27*(3), 7–12.

Lukose, A. (2011). Developing a practice model for Watson's theory of caring. *Nursing Science Quarterly, 24*(1), 27–30.

McCallin, A. M. (2012). [Review of the book *Glaserian grounded theory in nursing research: Trusting emergence* by B. M. Artinian, T. Giske, & P. H. Cone]. *The Grounded Theory Review, 9*(2). Retrieved from http://www.groundedtheoryreview.com/2012/06/25/book-reviewartinian-b-m-giske-t-cone-p-h

McCowan, D. E., & Artinian, B. M. (2011). An emerging nursing program in a developing country. In B. M. Artinian, K. S. West, & M. M. Conger (Eds.), *The Artinian intersystem model: Integrating theory and practice for the professional nurse* (2nd ed., pp. 173–180). New York: Springer.

Mefford, L. C. (2004). A theory of health promotion for preterm infants based on Levine's conservation model of nursing. *Nursing Science Quarterly, 17*(3), 260–266.

Mensik, J. (2008). Nurses make a difference every day. *Arizona Nurse*, p. 2.

Mitchell, P. H. (2008). President's message: Legends and legacies. *Nursing Outlook, 56*(3), 97–98.

Mock, V., Ours, C., Hall, S., Bositis, A., Tillery, M., Belcher, A., et al. (2007). Using a conceptual model in nursing research—Mitigating fatigue in cancer patients. *Journal of Advanced Nursing, 58*(3), 503–512.

Moreno-Fergusen, M. E. (2007). Application of the Roy adaptation model in Latin America: Literature review. *Roy Adaptation Association Conference*, Los Angeles, CA.

Modeling and Role-Modeling. (2008). Retrieved from http://unicornsunlimited.com/modeling_and_rolemodeling.htm

Neill, R. M. (2002). Jean Watson: Philosophy and science of caring. In A. M. Tomey & M. R. Alligood (Eds.), *Nursing theorists and their work* (5th ed., pp. 144–164). St. Louis: Mosby.

Neswick, R. S. (1997). Myra E. Levine: A theoretic basis for ET nursing. *Journal of Wound Ostomy Continence Nursing, 24*(1), 6–9.

Noel, D. L. (2010). Occupational health nursing practice through the human caring lens. *AAOHN Journal, 58*(1), 17–26.

Parse, R. R. (2004). Editorial: The many meanings of unitary: A plea for clarity. *Nursing Science Quarterly, 17*(4), 293.

Perry, R. N. B. (2009). Role modeling excellence in clinical nursing practice. *Nurse Education in Practice, 9*(1), 36–44.

Phillips, K. D. (2010). Sister Callista Roy: Adaptation model. In M. R. Alligood & A. M. Tomey (Eds), *Nursing theorists and their work* (7th ed., pp. 335–365). St. Louis: Mosby.

Piccoli, M., & Galvao, C. M. (2005). Pre-operative nursing visit: Methodological proposal based on Levine's conceptual model [Portugese]. *Revista Electronica de Enfermagem, 7*(3), 365–371.

Pond, J. B., & Taney, G. (1991). Emergency care in a large university emergency department. In K. M. Schaefer & J. B. Pond (Eds.), *Levine's conservation model: A framework for nursing practice* (pp. 151–166). Philadelphia: Davis.

Rogers, S. (1996). Facilitative affiliation: Nurse–client interactions that enhance healing. *Issues in Mental Health Nursing, 17*(3), 171–184.

Rooda, L. A. (1992). The development of a conceptual model for multicultural nursing. *Journal of Holistic Nursing, 10*(4), 337–347.

Roy, C. (2009). *The Roy adaptation model* (3rd ed.). Upper Saddle River, NJ: Pearson.

Roy, C. (2011a). Extending the Roy adaptation model to meet changing global needs. *Nursing Science Quarterly, 24*(4), 345–351.

Roy, C. (2011b). Research based on the Roy adaptation model: Last 25 years. *Nursing Science Quarterly, 24*(4), 312–320.

Roy, C. (2013). Boston College, William F. Connell School of Nursing. (2013). *Featured faculty*. Retrieved from http://www.bc.edu/schools/son/faculty/featured/theorist.html

Roy, C., & Andrews, H. A. (1999). *The Roy Adaptation Model* (2nd ed.). Stamford, CT: Appleton & Lange.

Schaefer, K. M. (1991a). Developing a graduate program in nursing. In K. M. Schaefer & J. B. Pond (Eds.), *Levine's conservation model: A framework for nursing practice* (pp. 209–217). Philadelphia: Davis.

Schaefer, K. M. (1991b). Care of the patient with congestive heart failure. In K. M. Schaefer & J. B. Pond (Eds.), *Levine's conservation model: A framework for nursing practice* (pp. 119–130). Philadelphia: Davis.

Schaefer, K. M. (2010). Myra Estrin Levine: The conservation model. In M. R. Alligood & A. M. Tomey (Eds.), *Nursing theorists and their work* (7th ed., pp. 225–241). St. Louis: Mosby.

Schaefer, K. M., & Potylycki, M. J. S. (1993). Fatigue associated with congestive heart failure: Use of Levine's conservation model. *Journal of Advanced Nursing, 18*(2), 260–268.

Sieloff, C. L. (2002). Imogene King: Interacting systems framework and theory of goal attainment. In A. M. Tomey & M. R. Alligood (Eds.), *Nursing theorists and their work* (pp. 336–355). St. Louis: Mosby.

Sieloff, C. L. (2006). Imogene King: Interacting systems framework and middle range theory of goal attainment. In A. M. Tomey & M. R. Alligood (Eds.), *Nursing theorists and their work* (pp. 297–317). St. Louis: Mosby.

Smith, M., Wright, B. W., & Fawcet, J. (2008). In memory: A tribute to two giants of nursing conceptual models and theories. *Visions: Journal of Rogerian Nursing Science, 15*(1), 65–66.

Stevens, K. R., & Messmer, P. R. (2008). In remembrance of Imogene King, January 30, 1923–December 24, 2007: Imogene, a pioneer and dear colleague. *Nursing Outlook, 56*(3), 100–101.

Treolar, L., & Artinian, B. M. (2001). Populations affected by disability. In M. Neis & M. McEwen (Eds.), *Community health nursing*. Philadelphia: Saunders.

Vandall-Walker, V., Jensen, L., & Oberle, K. (2006). Lightening the load: Nursing support with family members of critically ill adults. *Dynamics of Critical Care: Canadian Association of Critical Care Nurses, 17*(2), 43–44.

Vukovitch, P. K., & Artinian, B. M. (2005). Justifying coercion. *Nursing Ethics, 12*(4), 370–380.

Watson, J. (1985). The *philosophy and science of caring* (Rev. ed.). Boulder, CO: Colorado Associated University Press.

Watson, J. (1988). *Nursing: Human science and human care: A theory of nursing*. New York: National League for Nursing Press.

Watson, J. (Ed.). (1994). *Applying the art and science of human caring*. New York: National League for Nursing Press.

Watson, J. (1996). Nursing, caring-healing paradigm. In D. Pesat (Ed.), *Capsules of comments in psychiatric nursing*. Chicago: Mosby-Year Book.

Watson, J. (1999). *Postmodern nursing and beyond*. London, United Kingdom: Churchill Livingstone.

Watson, J. (2005). *Caring science as sacred science*. Philadelphia: Davis.

Watson, J. (2008). *The philosophy and science of caring*. Boulder, CO: University Press of Colorado.

Watson Caring Science Institute and International Caring Consortium. (2013). *Faculty profile: Jean Watson*. Retrieved from http://www.watsoncaringscience.org/files/PDF/CV2012JeanWatsonJan_3_2013.pdf

Wicklund-Gustin, L., & Wagner, L. (2013). The butterfly effect of caring—Clinical nursing teachers' understanding of self-compassion as a source to compassionate care. *Scandinavian Journal of Caring Sciences, 27*(1), 175–183.

Wood, M. J. (1997). Foreword. In B. M. Artinian & M. M. Conger (Eds.), *The intersystem model* (pp. vii–viii). Thousand Oaks: Sage.

CHAPTER 9

Grand Nursing Theories Based on Unitary Process

Evelyn M. Wills

Kristin Kowalski is a hospice nurse who wishes to expand the scope of her therapeutic practice. She desires to delve more deeply into holistic health care, having recently completed courses of study in herbal medicine, touch therapy, and holistic nursing. Kristin is aware that to practice independently, she needs professional credentials that will be widely accepted; therefore, she applied to the graduate program of a nationally ranked nursing school at a large state university.

Because Kristin believes strongly in holistic nursing practice, for her master's degree she decided to focus her study of nursing theories on those that look at the whole person and have a broad, nontraditional view of health. She is particularly interested in Rosemarie Parse's Humanbecoming Paradigm because this viewpoint stresses the individual's way of being and becoming healthy and the nurse as an intersubjective presence.

Kristin is attracted to Parse's idea of true presence and wishes to further explore this concept as well as the rest of the perspective. She hopes to eventually apply it to her practice and use it as the research framework for her thesis. For her thesis, Kristin wants to examine the experiences of nurses who practice therapeutic touch. She desires to learn their perceptions of how therapeutic touch interventions help their clients. She also wants to learn more about Parse's research method and hopes to use it for her study.

The term *simultaneity paradigm* was first coined by nursing theorist Rosemarie Parse (1987) to describe a group of theories that adhered to a unitary process perception of human beings. This group of theorists believed that humans are unitary beings: energy systems embedded in the universal energy system. Within this group of theories, human beings are seen as unitary, "whole, open and free to choose ways of becoming" (Parse, 1998, p. 6), and health is described as continuous human environmental interchanges (Newman, 1994).

The unitary process nursing model and two corollary theories are described in this chapter: Science of Unitary Human Beings (Rogers, 1994), Health as Expanding Consciousness (Newman, 1999), and Humanbecoming School of Thought (Parse, 1998, 2010). The three are grouped together because they are significantly different in their concepts, assumptions, and propositions when compared to the theories described in Chapters 7 and 8. They are universal in scope and relatively abstract.

Martha Rogers: The Science of Unitary and Irreducible Human Beings

Martha E. Rogers first described her Theory of Unitary Man in 1961, and almost from the first, there has been widespread controversy and debate among nursing theorists and scholars regarding her work (Phillips, 1994). Prior to Rogers, it was rare that anyone in nursing viewed human beings as anything other than the receivers of care by nurses and physicians. Furthermore, the health care system was organized by specialization, in which nurses and other health providers focused on discrete areas or functions (e.g., a dressing change, medication administration, or health teaching) rather than on the whole person. As a result, it took many professionals working in isolation, none of whom knew the whole person, to care for patients. Rogers' (1970) insistence that the person was a "unitary energy system" in "continuous mutual interaction with the universal energy system" (p. 90) dramatically influenced nursing by encouraging nurses to consider each person as a whole (a unity) when planning and delivering care.

Background of the Theorist

Martha Rogers was born on May 12, 1914 (the anniversary of Florence Nightingale's birth) (Dossey, 2000) in Dallas, Texas. She earned a diploma in nursing from Knoxville General Hospital in 1936 and a bachelor's degree from George Peabody College in Nashville, Tennessee in 1937. She later received a master's degree in public health nursing from Teachers College, Columbia University in New York, and a master's degree in public health and a doctor of science from The Johns Hopkins University in Baltimore, Maryland (Gunther, 2010).

Rogers became the head of the Division of Nursing of New York University (NYU) in 1954, where she focused on teaching and formulating and elaborating her theory (Hektor, 1989). She was teacher and mentor to an impressive list of nursing scholars and theorists, including Newman and Parse, whose works are described later in the chapter. Rogers continued her work and writing until her death in March, 1994.

Philosophical Underpinnings of the Theory

The Science of Unitary and Irreducible Human Beings started as an abstract theory that was synthesized from theories of numerous sciences; therefore, it was deductively derived. Of particular importance was von Bertalanffy's theory on general systems, which contributed the concepts of entropy and negentropy and posited that open systems are characterized by constant interaction with the environment. The work of Rapoport provided a background on open systems, and the work of Herrick contributed to the premise of evolution of human nature (Rogers, 1994).

Rogers' synthesis of the works of these scientists formed the basis of her proposition that human systems are open systems, embedded in larger, open environmental systems. She also brought in other concepts, including the idea that time is unidirectional, that living systems have pattern and organization, and that man is a sentient, thinking being capable of awareness, feeling, and choosing. From all these theories, and from her personal study of nature, Rogers (1970) developed her original Theory of Unitary Man. She continuously refined and elaborated her theory, which she retitled Science of Unitary Humans (Rogers, 1986) and finally, shortly before her death, the Science of Unitary and Irreducible Human Beings (Rogers, 1994).

Major Assumptions, Concepts, and Relationships

Assumptions

Rogers presented several assumptions about man. These are as follows:

- Man is a unified whole possessing integrity and manifesting characteristics that are more than and different from the sum of his parts (Rogers, 1970, p. 47).
- Man and environment are continuously exchanging matter and energy with one another (Rogers, 1970, p. 54).
- The life process evolves irreversibly and unidirectionally along the space–time continuum (Rogers, 1970, p. 59).
- Pattern and organization identify man and reflect his innovative wholeness (Rogers, 1970, p. 65).
- Man is characterized by the capacity for abstraction and imagery, language and thought, sensation, and emotion (Rogers, 1970, p. 73).

Rogers (1990) later revised the term *man* to *human being* to coincide with the request for gender-neutral language in the social sciences and nursing science.

Concepts

In Rogers' work, the unitary human being and the environment are the focus of nursing practice. Other central components are energy fields, openness, pandimensionality, and pattern; these she identified as the "building blocks" (Rogers, 1970, p. 226) of her system. Rogers also derived three other components for the model, which served as a basis of her work. These were based on principles of homeodynamics and were termed *resonancy*, *helicy*, and *integrality* (Rogers, 1990) (Box 9-1). Definitions of the nursing metaparadigm concepts and other important concepts in Rogers' work are listed in Table 9-1.

Relationships

The Science of Unitary and Irreducible Human Beings is fundamentally abstract; therefore, specifically defined relationships differ from those in more linear theories. The major components of Rogers' model revolve around the building blocks (energy

Box 9-1 Principles of Homeodynamics Applied in Rogers' Theory

1. Resonancy is continuous change from lower to higher frequency wave patterns in human and environmental fields.
2. Helicy is continuous innovative, unpredictable, increasing diversity of human and environmental field patterns.
3. Integrality is continuous mutual human and environmental field processes.

Source: Rogers (1990, p. 8).

Table 9-1 Central Concepts of Rogers' Science of Unitary Human Beings

Concept	Definition
Human–unitary human beings	"Irreducible, indivisible, multidimensional energy fields identified by pattern and manifesting characteristics that are specific to the whole and which cannot be predicted from the knowledge of the parts" (p. 7).
Health	"Unitary human health signifies an irreducible human field manifestation. It cannot be measured by the parameters of biology or physics or of the social sciences" (p. 10).
Nursing	"The study of unitary, irreducible, indivisible human and environmental fields: people and their world" (p. 6). Nursing is a learned profession that is both a science and an art.
Environmental field	"An irreducible, indivisible, pandimensional energy field identified by pattern and integral with the human field" (p. 7).
Energy field	"The fundamental unit of the living and the non-living. Field is a unifying concept. Energy signifies the dynamic nature of the field; a field is in continuous motion and is infinite" (p. 7).
Openness	Refers to qualities exhibited by open systems; human beings and their environment are open systems.
Pandimensional	"A nonlinear domain without spatial or temporal attributes" (p. 28).
Pattern	"The distinguishing characteristic of an energy field perceived as a single wave" (p. 7).

Source: Rogers (1990).

fields, openness, pattern, and pandimensionality) and the principles of homeodynamics (resonancy, helicy, and integrality). These explain the nature of, and direction of, the interactions between unitary human beings and the environment.

Among the relationships that Rogers posited are that all things are integral in that their energy fields are in continuous mutual process and that pattern is the manifestation of the integrality of each entity and of the environmental energy field (Rogers, 1986). Other major relationships within Rogers' work are contained in the following statements:

> Humans and environment are interrelated in that neither "has an energy field," both are integral energy fields (Rogers, 1990, pp. 6–7).
> Manifestations of pattern emerge out of the human/environmental field mutual process and are continuously innovative (Rogers, 1990, p. 8).
> The group field is irreducible and indivisible to itself and integral with its own environmental field (Rogers, 1990, p. 8).

Nursing is concerned with maintaining and promoting health, preventing illness, and caring for the sick and the disabled. The purpose of nursing for Rogers (1986) is to help human beings achieve well-being within the potential of each individual, family, or group. Because human energy fields are complex, individualizing nursing services supports simultaneous human and environmental exchange, encouraging health (Rogers, 1990).

Usefulness

Rogers' theory is a synthesis of phenomena that are important to nursing. It is an abstract, unified, and highly derived framework and does not define particular hypotheses or theories. Rather, it provides a worldview from which nurses may derive theories and hypotheses and propose relationships specific to different situations. In essence, the theory allows many options for studying humans as individuals and groups and for studying various situations in health as manifestations of pattern and innovation. Rogers' model stresses the unitary experience and provides an abstract philosophical framework that can guide nursing practice.

Rogers' theory has been evident in nursing education, scholarship, and practice for more than four decades. In education, among other programs, it has guided the nursing curriculum at NYU, where Rogers was head of the Division of Nursing in the 1970s. This resulted in the education of numerous nurses who use her theory in practice internationally (Hektor, 1989). In the area of nursing scholarship, several noted nursing theorists (e.g., Fitzpatrick, 1989; Newman, 1994; Parse, 1998) derived theories from Rogers' work.

In other scholarly works, Barrett (1989) derived a theory of power for nursing practice from Rogers' theory. She used several of Rogers' concepts (e.g., energy fields, openness, pattern, and four-dimensionality [now *pandimensionality*]) and the principles of resonancy, helicy, and integrality to form the theory of power. The theory of power as knowing participation in change consisted of awareness, choices, freedom to act intentionally, and involvement in creating changes and was tested in research using Barrett's Power as Knowing Participation in Change Test. Barrett's (1986) theory has recently been used in research on patterning of pain and power with guided imagery by Lewandowski (2004), who found that guided imagery was effective in reducing pain for chronic pain sufferers. Farren (2010) found in a secondary analysis of data collected using Barrett's Power as Knowing Participation in Changes (PKPIC) tool with breast cancer survivors that the dimensions of power (awareness, choices, freedom to act with intention, and involvement in creating change) were responsible for all the variance. Moreover, the breast cancer survivors showed differing intensities of these dimensions. Farren reiterated the importance or awareness of PKPIC among nurses and other health care workers in assisting breast cancer survivors.

In practice settings, Rogerian practitioners employ the visible manifestations of Rogers' science. Madrid, Barrett, and Winstead-Fry (2010) studied the feasibility of using therapeutic touch with patients who were undergoing cerebral angiography. The design was a randomized, single blind clinical pilot study with outcome assessments of blood pressure, pulse, and respirations. The findings of this study were inconclusive, but the researchers followed up with exploration of the reasons and studied the implications for further research. Reed (2008) wrote about nursing time as a dimension of practice, research, and theory. In a nursing educational setting, Malinski and Todaro-Franceschi (2011) studied comeditation to reduce anxiety and facilitate relaxation. Their data from the qualitative study suggested that the participants reported feeling calmer, more relaxed, and balanced and centered after 1 month of practice. Their findings suggest that comeditation may help transform education in nursing programs, most of which have reputations as being stressful to students.

Testability

Because of the model's abstractness, Rogers' (1990) work is not directly testable, but it is testable in principle (Bramlett, 2010). Theories are being derived from the Science of Unitary Man and hypotheses to test those theories (Barrett, 1989; Cody, 1991; Kwekkeboom, Huseby-Moore, & Ward, 1998; Phillips, 1990).

Box 9-2 Examples of Research Studies Using Rogers' Theory

Farren, A. T. (2010). Power in breast cancer survivors: A secondary analysis. *Visions: The Journal of Rogerian Nursing Science, 17*(1), 29–43.

Gajowski, L. (2009). Sustaining Mom's expression of her identity using the Well-Being Picture scale. *Visions: The Journal of Rogerian Nursing Science, 16*(1), 48–53.

Kim, T. S. (2009). The theory of power as knowing participation in change: A literature review update. *Visions: The Journal of Rogerian Nursing Science, 16*(1), 19–25.

Phillips, B. B., & Bramlett, M. H. (2008). Integrated awareness: A key to the pattern of mutual process. *Visions: The Journal of Rogerian Nursing Science, 15*(2), 37–55.

Smith, M. C., Zahourek, R., Hines, M. E., Engebretson, J., & Wardell, D. W. (2013). Holistic nurses' stories of personal healing. *Journal of Holistic Nursing, 31*(3), 173–187. doi: 10.1177/0898010113477254.

Terwilliger, S. H., Gueldner, S. H., & Bronstein, L. (2012). A preliminary evaluation of the Well-Being Picture Scale–Children's Version (WPS-CV) in a sample of fourth and fifth graders. *Nursing Science Quarterly, 25*(2), 160–166.

Numerous research studies using Rogers' model have been completed and reported in the nursing literature. A plethora of these studies can be found in *Visions: The Journal of Rogerian Nursing Science*. In addition, a book, *Patterns of Rogerian Knowing* (Madrid, 1997) was published detailing a number of research studies. Madrid and Winstead-Fry (2001) found in a focused review of literature that from 1990 through 2000, 28 research studies on therapeutic touch were published in peer-reviewed journals, and 9 of them were based on the Science of Unitary Human Beings. Nine additional research studies included Rogers' model as explanation for the underlying processes of therapeutic touch and its relation to energy fields and energy transfer. Examples of some recent nursing studies using Rogers' theory are listed in Box 9-2.

Parsimony

This theory is relatively parsimonious. The model has five key definitions. These, combined with the three principles of homeodynamics and the six assumptions about human beings, are the major elements of the work. Despite its simplicity, however, it is difficult for many nurses to comprehend because the concepts are extremely abstract. Nurses who wish their research and practice to be guided by Rogers' model will benefit from studying with a Rogerian scholar who uses the model regularly.

Value in Extending Nursing Science

Rogers' contributions to nursing have been noted in the nursing literature, and she has had a significant influence on scientific inquiry in professional nursing practice. The major value of Rogers' work has been extending nursing science by challenging traditional ways of thinking about the world and nursing. She moved beyond a focus on such concepts and principles as adaptation, biopsychosocial beings, causal/probabilistic views, and the human-as-sum-of-parts thinking that had been common in nursing science (Parse, 2010; Phillips, 2010; Rogers, 1990). The contribution to nursing science of the Science of Unitary and Irreducible Human Beings is that it carries nursing into areas that are impossible to study using linear, three-dimensional, and reductionistic methods.

Margaret Newman: Health as Expanding Consciousness

Margaret Newman reported that she became interested in theory when asked to speak at a nursing conference in 1978 (George, 2010). She published a theory of health a year later (Newman, 1979) and *Health as Expanding Consciousness* in 1986. She revised this work in 1994 and 1999. Newman has published extensively on her theory and theoretical issues in books, book chapters, and articles (Newman, 1990a, 1990b, 1994, 1995, 1999, 2005, 2008a, 2008b).

Newman's *Health as Expanding Consciousness* is one of the most recent nursing theories; her work builds on the work of Rogers and others. Because of its similarity to Rogers' theory, particularly with regard to its conceptualizations of person, nursing, and the environment, it is included here among the unitary process theories. In 2008, Newman published a new, related work, which she entitled *Transforming Presence: The Difference Nursing Makes* (Newman, 2008a).

Background of the Theorist

As a young woman, Margaret Newman was involved in caring for her mother, who suffered from amyotrophic lateral sclerosis. She explained that it was during this period that she came to know her mother in ways that would have been impossible otherwise (Newman, 1986). This experience led Newman to study nursing, and she enrolled at the University of Tennessee, where she completed her bachelor's degree in 1962. She received a master's degree from the University of California, San Francisco in 1964, and a doctorate from NYU in 1971 (Brown, 2010).

Newman has served on the faculty at the University of Tennessee (which named her an outstanding alumna), NYU, Pennsylvania State University, and the University of Minnesota. She is currently professor emeritus at the University of Minnesota, Minneapolis. Her work has been recognized internationally, and she has received numerous awards and honors both in the United States and abroad (Jones, 2007b).

Philosophical Underpinnings of the Theory

While at NYU, Newman attended seminars taught by Martha Rogers, and she stated that Rogers' Science of Unitary Human Beings was the basis of her theory of Health as Expanding Consciousness. She also noted that, among others, Itzhak Bentov's explanation of the concept of evolution of consciousness, Arthur Young's work on pattern recognition, and David Bohm's theory of implicate order brought perspective to her thoughts and ideas (Newman, 1986).

Major Assumptions, Concepts, and Relationships

Assumptions

As a student of Rogers, Newman believed that "the human is unitary, that is, cannot be divided into parts, and is inseparable from the larger unitary field" (Newman, 1994, p. xviii). She saw humans as open energy systems in continual contact with a universe of open systems (i.e., the environment). Additionally, humans are continuously active in evolving their own pattern of the whole (i.e., health) and are intuitive as well as cognitive and affective beings (Marchione, 1995). She further posited that "persons as individuals, and human beings as a species, are identified by their patterns of consciousness" and that "the person does not possess consciousness—the person is consciousness" (Newman, 1999, p. 33).

In describing health, Newman (1994) explained that health encompasses illness or pathology and that pathologic conditions can be considered manifestations of the pattern of the individual. In addition, the pattern of the individual that eventually manifests itself as pathology is primary and exists prior to structural or functional changes; removal of the pathology in itself will not change the pattern of the individual. Finally, she noted an assumption that changes occur simultaneously and not in linear fashion (Newman, 1994).

Concepts

Newman built on Rogers' definitions for human and environment, but she redefined nursing and health. Health is an essential component of the theory of Health as Expanding Consciousness and is seen as a process of developing awareness of self and the environment together with increasing the ability to perceive alternatives and respond in a variety of ways (Newman, 1986). Nursing is described as "caring in the human health experience" (Newman, 1994, p. 139). Other central concepts in Newman's theory are pattern, pattern recognition, movement, and time and space. Definitions for these and other concepts specific to the theory are presented in Table 9-2.

Relationships

A fundamental proposition in Newman's model is the idea that health and illness are synthesized as "health." Indeed, the fusion of one state of being (disease) with its opposite (nondisease) results in what can be regarded as health (Newman, 1979, 2008a).

To Newman, health is pattern. *Pattern* is information that depicts the whole, and pattern recognition is essential. Pattern recognition involves moving from looking at parts to looking at patterns. Expanding consciousness occurs as a process of pattern recognition (insight) following a synthesis of contradictory events or disturbances in the flow of daily living. Pattern recognition comes from within the observer, and patterns unfold over time and cannot be predicted with certainty. Understanding the meaning of relationships through pattern recognition is important in providing care because patterns are the essence of a unitary view of health.

Newman (1979) also wrote of the interrelatedness of time, space, and movement. She explained that time and space have a complementary relationship, and movement is the means by which space and time become reality. Movement is seen as a reflection of consciousness; time is a function of movement; and time is a measure of consciousness (Newman, 2008b). Humans are in a constant state of motion and are constantly changing; movement through time and space gives modern people our unique perception of reality. Constant change is visible currently as technology; for example, smartphones and tablet computers can access e-books and e-libraries, giving people immediate access to high volumes of information. New technology, such as handheld laboratory testing and physical examination technology, is currently being used in clinics and physician and nurse practitioner offices. Such technology gives health professionals and other individuals immediate, conscious, and unrestricted access to information.

Access to information places people in constant contact with the whole world; indeed, instant communications, such as social media, have made it possible for people to respond immediately to a question, concern, or idea. Having information available at their fingertips lessens the need to try to remember telephone numbers and other facts that can be found easily online (Stein, 2013). In these

Table 9-2 Central Concepts of Newman's Health as Expanding Consciousness

Concept	Definition
Nursing	The act of assisting people to use the power within them to evolve toward higher levels of consciousness. Nursing is directed toward recognizing the patterns of the person in interaction with the environment and accepting the interaction as a process of evolving consciousness. Nursing facilitates the process of pattern recognition by a rhythmic connecting of the nurse with the client for the purpose of illuminating the pattern and discovering the rules of a higher level of organization.
Health	The expanding of consciousness; an evolving pattern of the whole of life. A unitary process, a fluctuating pattern of rhythmic phenomena that includes illness within the pattern of energy. Sickness can "be the shock that reorganizes the relationships of the person's pattern in a more harmonious way" (Newman, 1999, p. 11).
Person	A dynamic pattern of energy and an open system in interaction with the environment. Persons can be defined by their patterns of consciousness.
Consciousness	The information of the system; consciousness refers to the capacity of the system to interact with the environment and includes thinking, feeling, and processing the information embedded in physiologic systems.
Expanding consciousness	The evolving pattern of the whole. Expanding consciousness is the increasing complexity of the living system and is characterized by illumination and pattern recognition resulting in transformation and discovery. Expanding consciousness is health.
Integration via movement	The natural condition of living creatures. Consciousness is expressed in movement, which is the way that the organism interacts with the environment and exerts control over it. Movement patterns reflect and communicate the person's inner pattern and organization. Changes in the person's health patterns may be reflected in changes in their movement rhythms.
Pattern	Relatedness, which is characterized by movement, diversity, and rhythm. Pattern is a scheme, design, or framework and is seen in person–environment interactions. Pattern is recognized on the basis of variation and may not be seen all at once. It is manifest in the way one moves, speaks, talks, and relates with others.
Pattern recognition	The insight or recognition of a principle, realization of a truth, or reconciliation of a duality. Pattern recognition illuminates the possibilities for action and is the key to the process of evolving to a higher level of consciousness.
Time and space	Temporal patterns that are specific to individuals and define their ways of being within their world. Patterns of health may be detected in temporal patterns.

Sources: Marchione (1995); Newman (1999).

cases, currently expanding consciousness may be more important to them than memory.

Global positioning systems (GPS) allow people to be conscious of exactly where they are while traveling and allow the use of satellite information to determine their destination within mere feet of the actual place. GPS has almost obliterated the problem of being lost while en route to a destination.

Time, space, and movement have all changed in the past few years; indeed, "the person is the center of consciousness with information flow... [throughout] the universe" (Newman, 2008a, p. 36). Humans can only expect more and faster change as consciousness expands and our world of knowledge progresses.

Usefulness

Newman (1994) believed that theory must be derived from practice and theory must inform practice. To illustrate this relationship, she proposed a model for practice that she derived from her theory (Newman, 1990b).

Her work has been used by nurses in a number of settings, providing care for different types of clients and for a variety of interventions. For example, Newman (1995) reported that her theory guided her nursing practice with families. In another instance, her work was selected to direct practice among case managers at Tucson, Arizona's Carondelet, St. Mary's Hospital (Ethridge, 1991; Ethridge & Lamb, 1989). In describing the application of the theory in case management, Newman, Lamb, and Michaels (1991) explained that the theory–practice link helped facilitate the complementary link between nursing and medicine.

Pharris and Endo (2007) described the nature of Health as Expanding Consciousness with ill elders, groups and communities, and systems. In another example, Brown, Chen, Mitchell, and Province (2007) studied help-seeking by older husbands who were caring for wives with dementia using a grounded theory approach. They found that help-seeking for the sample was complex and gender-specific. They came to understand that interventions to assist the male caregivers must be gender-specific and complement their help-seeking patterns.

In other works, Neill (2005) completed an investigation into patterns of lives of women with multiple sclerosis. Jones (2007a) discussed Newman's theory in knowledge development for nursing practice, and Musker (2008) published her work on life transitions in menopausal women. These studies indicate that the ideal of health as expanding consciousness is useful for generating caring interventions in numerous populations.

Testability

Newman's theory has been the basis for an impressive number of doctoral dissertations. Other research projects have tested parts of the theory (i.e., time and movement) or used it as a framework. Most of the nursing studies using Newman's theory found in recent literature were qualitative in nature. Pickard (2000), for example, expanded Newman's praxis method, a hermeneutic dialectic process, "to include creative movement as a mode of expression" (p. 150). Findings indicated that movement supported women's self-awareness and expanding consciousness at midlife. The author also described activities of consciousness as choosing, balancing, accepting, and letting go. Pickard (2002) studied family reflections of living through sudden death of a child; Endo, Miyahara, Suzuki, and Ohmasa (2005) studied the process of partnering a researcher with a practicing nurse at a Japanese cancer center. They found that the nurses encountered a transformative experience with patients when the nursing interventions in everyday practice were enacted in the unitary perspective.

In other studies, Karian, Jankowski, and Beal (1998) examined the lived experience of survivors of childhood cancer by studying their patterns of interaction with family members and the environment. The researchers concluded that pattern recognition

Box 9-3 Examples of Research Studies Using Newman's Health as Expanding Consciousness

Endo, E., Takaki, M., Nitta, N., Abe, K., & Terashima, K. (2009). Identifying patterns in partnership with students who want to quit smoking. *Journal of Holistic Nursing, 27*(4), 256–265.

MacLeod, C. E. (2011). Understanding experiences of spousal caregivers with health as expanding consciousness. *Nursing Science Quarterly, 24*(3), 245–255.

MacNeil, J. M. (2012). The complexity of living with hepatitis: A Newman perspective. *Nursing Science Quarterly, 25*(3), 261–266.

Ness, S. M. (2009). Pain expression in the perioperative period: Insights from a focus group of Somali women. *Pain Management Nursing, 10*(2), 65–75.

Pierre-Louis, B., Akoh, V., White, P., & Pharris, M. D. (2011). Patterns in the lives of African American women with diabetes. *Nursing Science Quarterly, 24*(3), 227–236.

Smith, M. C. (2011). Integrative review of research related to Margaret Newman's theory of health as expanding consciousness. *Nursing Science Quarterly, 24*(3), 256–272.

Yang, A., Xiong, D., Vang, E., & Pharris, M. D. (2009). Hmong American women living with diabetes. *Journal of Nursing Scholarship, 41*(2), 139–148.

and insight into the meaning of the family pattern assisted in a process of transformation; most families found meaning in their patterns. Berry (2004) found a link between theory, research, and practice in her research with women maintaining weight loss. She found that a model of change supported the understanding of lifestyle change. Box 9-3 lists recent research studies that were conducted using Newman's model.

Parsimony

Newman's model consists of two major concepts: health and consciousness, and thus it seems parsimonious. Despite this seeming simplicity, however, the theory is one of great complexity (George, 2010). Those who do not comprehend the simultaneity paradigm may wander in its enfolded relationships. The real complexity relates to the nature of the relationships between and among the concepts and to its abstractness.

Value in Extending Nursing Science

The focus of Newman's work is on the person, client, individual, and family. It places the client and nurse as integrated actors in understanding the client's health as consciousness. It also requires the understanding that health and disease are the same and not separate in the life of the individual (Newman, 1994).

As illustrated by the examples from the literature presented, Newman's model has been successfully used in nursing practice and research. Newman's view can be applied in any setting, and research and practice application are underway to further verify its importance to the discipline (Jones, 2007b).

Rosemarie Parse: The Humanbecoming Paradigm

Rosemarie Parse is a noted nursing scholar and prolific author. She first published her theory of nursing, *Man-Living-Health,* in 1981, and has continually revised the work. In 1992, Parse changed the name to the Theory of Humanbecoming. She is the author of at least eight books and numerous articles. Her works have been translated into Danish, Finnish, French, German, Japanese, Korean, and other languages. She holds that humanbecoming has become a new paradigm, and the adherents to the scholarship of humanbecoming agree (Bournes, 2013; Parse, 2008, 2010, 2013; Smith, 2010).

Background of the Theorist

Parse was educated at Duquesne University in Pittsburgh, Pennsylvania, and earned her master's and doctoral degrees from the University of Pittsburgh. Some years later, she became dean of the College of Nursing at Duquesne, and she is currently professor emeritus at Loyola University in Chicago, Illinois. She is the founder and editor of *Nursing Science Quarterly* and president of Discovery International, which sponsors international nursing theory conferences. She is also the founder of the Institute of Humanbecoming, where she teaches the ontologic, epistemologic, and methodologic aspects of the humanbecoming school of thought. The humanbecoming perspective is honored and acknowledged in colleges of nursing worldwide. She has currently realized that although a student of Martha Rogers, her work has developed into a wholly new paradigm, and she has titled this the humanbecoming paradigm (Parse, 2010).

Philosophical Underpinnings of the Theory

Parse synthesized the Theory of Humanbecoming from principles and concepts from Rogers' work. She also incorporated concepts and principles from existential phenomenologic thought as expressed by Heidegger, Sartre, and Merleau-Ponty (Parse, 1981). The theory comes from her experience in nursing and from a synthesis of theoretical principles of human sciences.

Major Assumptions, Concepts, and Relationships

Assumptions

As with many of the major concepts, the major assumptions of Parse's theory originated with Rogers' Science of Unitary Human Beings and from existential phenomenology. Parse's thinking has brought her to a new ontology. Kuhn (1996) warned the scientific community that when the facts no longer support the current paradigm, the paradigm must change. For the humanbecoming perspective, a new paradigm has ascended. The language comes from the humanbecoming school of thought but has developed beyond that to a newer realm. Assumptions about humanbecoming paradigm are shown in Box 9-4.

Parse synthesized the nine assumptions of humanbecoming in four broad statements:

- Humanbecoming is structuring meaning, freely choosing the situation.
- Humanbecoming is configuring rhythmic humanuniverse patterns.
- Humanbecoming is cotranscending illimitably with emerging possibilities.
- Humanbecoming is humanuniverse co-creating a seamless symphony (Parse, 2013, p. 113).

Concepts

Parse builds on previous concepts and provides concepts and paradoxes that are found in this paradigm:

- Imaging: explicit–tacit; reflective–prereflective
- Valuing: confirming–not confirming

Box 9-4 Assumptions About Humans and Becoming From Parse's Humanbecoming Perspective

- The human with universe is coexisting while co-constituting rhythmic patterns.
- The human is open, freely choosing meaning with situation, bearing responsibility for decisions.
- The human is continuously co-constituting patterns of relating.
- The human is transcending illimitably with the possible.
- Becoming is human-living-health.
- Becoming is rhythmically co-constituting with humanuniverse.
- Becoming is the human's patterns of relating value priorities.
- Becoming is transcending with the possible.
- Becoming is the human's emerging.

Source: Parse (2008, p. 370).

- Languaging: speaking–being silent; moving–being still
  - Revealing–concealing: disclosing–not disclosing
  - Enabling–limiting: potentiating–restricting
  - Connecting–separating: attending–distracting
- Powering: pushing–resisting; affirming–not affirming; being–nonbeing
- Originating: certainty–uncertainty; conforming–not conforming
- Transforming: familiar–not familiar (Parse, 2013, p. 113)

Relationships

From the major concepts, Parse (1987) outlined three principles in the theory. These are updated and meaningful as enduring principles.

1. Structuring meaning is the imaging and valuing of languaging.
2. Configuring rhythmic patterns of relating the revealing–concealing and enabling–limiting of connecting–separating.
3. Cotranscending with the possible is powering and originating of transforming (Parse, 2010, p. 258).

Nurses guide individuals and families in choosing possibilities in changing the health process; this is accomplished by intersubjective participation with the clients. Practice focuses on illuminating meaning, and the nurse acts as a guide to choose possibilities in the changing health experiences (Parse, 1981, 2001, 2002, 2008).

Practitioners using Parse's method do not focus on changing an individual's behavior to fit a defined nursing process and do not attempt to label them with possibly erroneous nursing diagnoses. Rather, they practice from the understanding that the human–universe process involves the nurse's true presence with the person and the family. The nurse "dwells with the rhythms of the person and family" (Parse, 1995, p. 83) as they move through the experience. Nurses taking the time "to be fully present with the patient provides patient and nurse [who are] grounded in the humanbecoming theory"[sic] with meaningful and enlightening experiences (Smith, 2010, p. 216).

Usefulness

Parse's theory has been a guide for practice in health care settings in Canada, Finland, South Korea, Sweden, the United States, and other countries. Additionally, Parse's method for research, a descriptive phenomenologic method of inquiry, entitled "the human becoming hermeneutic method" (Barrett, 2002, p. 53), has been selected by nurse scholars in Australia, Canada, Denmark, Finland, Greece, Italy, Japan, South Korea, Sweden, the United Kingdom, and the United States. Legault and Ferguson-Pare (1999) discussed application of Parse's theory to guide practice in an acute care surgical setting. The authors concluded that there were positive patterns of change in nursing practice after implementing the guidelines; nursing care was more client-centered and more considerate of the individual and family experiences. Similarly, Kelley (1999) used Parse's theory to evaluate the practice of advanced practice nurses and found it to be beneficial. Practice regulation in one state, South Dakota, has adopted a decision-making model based on humanbecoming (Benedict, Bunkers, Damgaard, Hohman, & Vander Woude, 2000). This is the first theory-based model of this sort in the nation (Bournes, Bunkers, & Welch, 2004).

In education, Bunkers (2004) found that use of the Socratic method was effective in discussions with nursing students on concepts such as goodness, courage, and piety and in discussing topics that included "risk-taking in nursing, social justice issues in our classrooms ..., and teaching about the courage and fear that people experience in living their health" (p. 216).

Several examples were found that described the use of Parse's theory with regard to the concept of presence. Cody (1999) illustrated the importance of the concept of presence for nurses working with families living with HIV, and Cody, Hudepol, and Brinkman (1999) discussed presence in working with a pediatric client and his family. Finally, Jonas (1999) presented an intervention to enhance presence by using music to cope with dying.

Testability

The humanbecoming perspective is testable in principle, and many concepts that arise from it are being studied as the researchers develop perspectives on the human science of nursing (see Table 9-5). Parse believed that the science is as yet minimally developed and that the descriptive qualitative research method that she and other nursing scholars and researchers have developed is important to the discipline. Welch (2004) explored his experience using the method developed by Parse. His comments (Table 9-3) are important to students who wish to develop themselves as researchers within the method.

Research within Parse's method describes the lives, lived experiences, and ways of being of humans differently from research in the more reductionistic models. To study humanbecoming, Parse developed a research method similar to those of existential phenomenologists and derived specific steps that are rigorous and reproducible. The method involves dwelling with the information from the participant's perspective (dialogical engagement) and deriving themes from that data (extraction–synthesis), then synthesizing the meanings into a relevant whole through heuristic interpretation (Parse, 1987). The inductive research method Parse and others have created is a research strategy that values the lived experiences of humans as they go about their daily lives, cocreating their health in humanuniverse concert.

Researchers studying within the Parse method viewed hope from the perspective of persons worldwide, and a significant amount of their research has been published. Bunkers and Daly (1999) examined the lived experience of hope for families living with coronary disease in Australia. Hope was also described in persons from Wales (Pilkington & Millar, 1999) and persons in Finland (Toikkanen & Muurinen, 1999). In more recent works, Milton (2004) brings out the importance of patient's stories as referents of their lived experiences as they heal. Noh (2004) studied quality of life for

Table 9-3 Lessons From a Doctoral Dissertation

Lessons	Writings as He Worked Through the Process	Welch's Actions
Finding a focus for the study	Considered depression incurable and had other preconceived ideas.	Reviewed literature, thought through process. Came to view depression as a time for people to work through difficult times (p. 202).
Locating a philosophical approach to inquiry	Considered several different approaches to phenomenologic inquiry.	Realized the superficiality of his understanding but was unaware of the significance of the differences in the approaches.
Deciding on a phenomenologic position	Found himself at an impasse, different terms, philosophical stances. Read the works of Parse.	Developed a lexicon of terms to understand the world of phenomenology (p. 203).
	Walked in the desert of theoretical confusion and increasing disillusionment with lack of progress in 2 years.	Found humanbecoming method, but his advisors were not familiar with process and terminology of Parse's method.
	Discussion with Parse was a "watershed" in realizing that he needed to review the focus on the study and also his philosophical disposition toward adopting the humanbecoming perspective.	Attended Humanbecoming Institute in Pittsburgh. Dialogued with Parse and other scholars. Parse agreed to assist with dissertation as a second advisor.
Selecting participants for the study	Wanted to include only the best and most appropriate potential participants to tell their stories of taking life day by day.	Realized that his inclination to take only the best candidates would compromise the integrity of the study. Therefore, he decided he had to adhere to the established criteria and remain cognizant of his personal bias.
Engaging the participants	As each participant talked of taking life day by day, I sensed myself moving with the rhythms of their stories (p. 205).	Being with the participants in true presence as they shared their stories was a profound experience (p. 205).
Inadvertently straying from the humanbecoming path	Embracing the art of living humanbecoming was an affirming enterprise; however, learning the art of humanbecoming was difficult (p. 205).	Dr. Parse provided important feedback about the conduct of the first tape and it was subsequently excluded. Came to the understanding of the importance of maintaining rigor (p. 205).
Allowing the voice of the text to be heard	My initial attempts to move the essences of the participants' stories to the language of the researcher and engage in the process of heuristic interpretation could be described only as throwing seed on barren ground (p. 206).	"I realized that the process of abstraction is concept driven; in other words, language is a vehicle for expressing what has already been formulated in the mind's eye. The extraction–synthesis and heuristic interpretation processes of Parse's method were perceived as pathways to new levels of knowing in explicating the participants' lived experiences" (p. 206).

Table 9-3 Lessons From a Doctoral Dissertation *(continued)*

Lessons	Writings as He Worked Through the Process	Welch's Actions
Gleaning insights from the journey	**Being comfortable with the uncomfortable:** A willingness to learn from the experienced scholars and a preparedness to move with the rhythms of the humanbecoming school of thought. **Mapping the journey:** The telling of the researchers' experience is an opportunity for other researchers contemplating such endeavors (p. 206). **Rethinking authentic rigor:** Authentic rigor involves more than adhering strictly to an established set of protocols; it also requires the researcher to be the embodiment of humanbecoming. Living the spirit of humanbecoming has to engage in a seamless movement of researcher with participant, researcher with text, and researcher with reader in the process of cocreating new horizons of understanding of the phenomenon under study (p. 206).	"I feel comfortable about testing the boundaries of conventional scientific inquiry. I no longer feel the need to engage in academic debate concerning the primacy of particular research paradigms within the community of scholars. Of importance to me is keeping alive the creative process or inquiry even though at times doing so means being lost in the labyrinthine paths of creative discovery" (p. 207).

Source: Welch (2004). Reprinted by permission of SAGE Publications.

persons living with serious mental illness. Their research involved the lived experience of the person with mental illness and was conducted within the Parse method (based on existential phenomenology). Noh (2004) found that the meanings uncovered in the analysis were the paradoxes of living. A small sample of the numerous current studies of other aspects of human experience within Parse's humanbecoming perspective are listed in Box 9-5.

Parsimony

Parse's model is parsimonious and artistic, having nine assumptions, which have been synthesized to four working assumptions; four postulates; three principles; and numerous concept and paradoxes organized together in artful, logical, balanced ways to explain humanbecoming. With careful study, the perspective lends itself to scholarly research and debate. The theory may seem complicated because much of the terminology is unfamiliar to most nurses. Indeed, this is a new and working way of seeing nursing in the real world (Smith, 2010). Students who want this model to guide their research and practice might consider contacting Parse and or one of her students for assistance to fully understand this new paradigm. The rewards of expending the effort to think in this beautiful new worldview will provide great rewards to the diligent nurse (Bournes, 2013; Smith, 2010).

Box 9-5 Examples of Current Research Studies Using Parse's Humanbecoming Perspective

Bauman, S. (2013). Feeling bored: A Parse research method study with older adults. *Nursing Science Quarterly, 26*(1), 42–52.

Bournes, D. A. (2013). Cultivating a spirit of inquiry using a nursing leading-following model. *Nursing Science Quarterly, 26*(2), 182–188.

Bunkers, S. S. (2010). The lived experience of feeling sad. *Nursing Science Quarterly, 23*(3), 231–239.

Condon, B. B. (2013). Trying something new. *Nursing Science Quarterly, 26*(1), 68–77.

Doucet, T. J. (2012). Feeling strong: A Parse research method study. *Nursing Science Quarterly, 25*(1), 62–71.

Evans, J., Bell, J., Sweeney, A. E., Morgan, J. I., & Kelly, H. (2010). Confidence in critical care nursing. *Nursing Science Quarterly, 23*(4), 334–340.

Hart, J. D. (2013). Feeling grateful: A Parse research method study. *Nursing Science Quarterly, 26*(2), 156–166.

Ferrell, B. (2010). Palliative care research: Response to emergent society needs. *Nursing Science Quarterly, 23*(3), 221–223.

Thomas, K., Riggs, R., & Stothart, K. (2013). The meaning of changing expectations: A qualitative descriptive study. *Nursing Science Quarterly, 26*(1), 59–67.

Yu-O, Y., Chung-Hey, C., & Hui-Lai, C. (2010). Lao Lai Zi—Becoming a mother: Cultural implications with Parse's theory. *Nursing Science Quarterly, 23*(3), 240–244.

Value in Extending Nursing Science

The principal value of the humanbecoming perspective is the worldview that sees humans as intentional beings, freely choosing to live within paradoxical ways of being. It is a unique way to view health and gives insight into how individuals create their own destiny.

Practice and research in the humanbecoming perspective are quite different from those espoused in the other nursing perspectives. By living true presence with their clients, nurses guide and cocreate ways of being that enable choosing health. The amount of literature depicting use of Parse's work is multiplying rapidly, and support for the humanbecoming perspective is growing. It has become evident that time and continued research is having a significant effect on the adoption of the perspective to the discipline of nursing.

Summary

The models presented in this chapter are considerably different from those described in the previous chapters. Additionally, significant similarities and differences are evident among these three models. Table 9-4 summarizes some of these by comparing definitions of the metaparadigm concepts. As Table 9-4 shows, the conceptualization of human beings is similar because Rogers heavily influenced both Newman and Parse. On the other hand, Parse was more specific when describing the environment and Newman was much more explicit in her discussions of health. Perhaps the greatest difference, however, relates to how they view nurses and nursing. Those wishing to use these theories should study these concepts closely and seek to apply them in their practice and research. When employing the research methods, which are unique, close work with the researchers or their former students will assist the novice researcher to develop the depth of effort that is required (Welch, 2004).

Table 9-4 Comparison of Concepts Common to the Unitary Process Nursing Theories

Author and Model	Human	Health	Environment	Nursing
Rogers: Unitary Human Beings (Rogers, 1990)	A sentient, unitary being; a multidimensional irreducible energy field known by pattern manifestation, and who cannot be known by the sum of parts.	Signifies an irreducible human field manifestation.	"An irreducible, indivisible, multidimensional energy field identified by pattern ... integral with the human field" (p. 7).	A learned profession, a science and an art, whose uniqueness lies in concern for human beings.
Newman: Health as Expanding Consciousness (Newman, 1999)	Accepts the definition of human as stated by Rogers.	Health is a unitary process, a fluctuating pattern of rhythmic phenomena. Health includes illness within the pattern of energy.	Universal energy system as in Rogers' Science of Unitary Human Beings.	Assist persons to use innate power to evolve toward a higher level of consciousness. Nurses facilitate pattern recognition in this process.
Parse: Humanbecoming Paradigm (Parse, 2010)	Intentional beings involved with their world, having a fundamental nature of knowing, being present, and open to their world. The unitary human is one who "coparticipates in the universe in creating becoming and who is whole, open, free to choose ways of becoming" (p. 6).	A way of being in the world; it is not a continuum of healthy to ill, nor is it a dichotomy of health or illness, rather it is the living of day-to-day ways of being.	The world, the universe, and those who occupy spaces along with others who freely choose to be in the situation.	Guides humans toward ways of being, finding meaning in situations, and choosing ways of cocreating their own health. Nurses live true presence in the day-to-day of the person's life.

Nurses, such as Kristin from the opening case study, who prefer to view the person as a unitary being and who have a comprehensive view of health often find the theories from the simultaneity paradigm fascinating and helpful. These works have been extremely enlightening and helpful for the discipline of nursing, and all three have many adherents worldwide. A large and growing body of research explores patterns of lived experiences and health perspectives based on them, and the expanding topics of study currently enhance nursing science and will continue to do so into the future.

Key Points

- The simultaneity paradigm is an entirely different and nursing-centered way of studying nursing and humans.
- Martha E. Rogers and two of her students, Margaret Newman and Rosemarie Parse, have been active in providing education, collaborative communities, and the groundwork for students and nursing scientists who are currently working within the paradigm.

- Newman's Health as Expanding Consciousness is conversant with the current lives of the millennial age. Young people live an age of motion, information, and continuous communication. Expanding consciousness is the hallmark of this generation.
- Parse has recently determined that the humanbecoming school of thought is a paradigm of its own. This paradigm generates considerable nursing-focused research and scholarship.

Learning Activities

1. Select one of the theories described and apply it in developing comprehensive patterns of nursing care for young teenagers who are becoming first-time mothers. Consider all of the issues they encounter as they prepare for the birth of their babies. Share findings with classmates.
2. Select a different theory and apply it in developing comprehensive patterns of nursing care for the family of an elderly client with Alzheimer disease. Compare the two models for ease of application.
3. Reflect on a case or situation from your personal practice or experience. Apply one of the theories to the situation. How does the perspective from the theory alter how you view the situation? Are nursing interventions the same? Why or why not?
4. Construct a research question that fits one of the theories in this chapter. How will you name the research and construct the question? What would be a likely method of study in the theoretical perspective you have chosen?

REFERENCES

Barrett, E. A. M. (1986). Investigation of the principle of helicy: The relationship of human field motion and power. In V. M. Malinski (Ed.), *Explorations in Martha Rogers' science of unitary human beings* (pp. 173–188). Norwalk, CT: Appleton-Century-Crofts.

Barrett, E. A. M. (1989). A nursing theory of power for nursing practice. In J. Riehl-Siska (Ed.), *Conceptual models for nursing practice* (3rd ed., pp. 207–217). Norwalk, CT: Appleton & Lange.

Barrett, E. A. M. (2002). What is nursing science? *Nursing Science Quarterly, 15*(1), 51–60.

Benedict, L., Bunkers, S. S., Damgaard, G., Hohman, M., & Vander Woude, D. (2000). The South Dakota theory-based regulatory decisioning model. *Nursing Science Quarterly, 13*(2), 167–171.

Berry, D. (2004). An emerging model of behavior change in women maintaining weight loss. *Nursing Science Quarterly, 17*(3), 242–252.

Bournes, D. A. (2013). Cultivating a spirit of inquiry using a nursing leading-following model. *Nursing Science Quarterly, 26*(2), 182–188.

Bournes, E. A., Bunkers, S. S., & Welch, A. J. (2004). Human becoming: Scope and challenge. *Nursing Science Quarterly, 17*(3), 227–232.

Bramlett, M. H. (2010). What is nursing? What constitutes the Science of Unitary Human Beings? *Visions: The Journal of Rogerian Nursing Science, 17*(1), 6–7.

Brown, J. W. (2010). Margaret A. Newman: Health as expanding consciousness. In M. R. Alligood & A. M. Tomey (Eds.), *Nursing theorists and their work* (7th ed., pp. 480–502). St. Louis: Mosby.

Brown, J. W., Chen, S., Mitchell, C., & Province, A. (2007). Help-seeking by older husbands caring for wives with dementia. *Journal of Advanced Nursing, 59*(4), 352–360.

Bunkers, S. S. (2004). Socrates' questions: A focus for nursing. *Nursing Science Quarterly, 17*(3), 212–218.

Bunkers, S. S., & Daly, J. (1999). The lived experience of hope for Australian families living with coronary disease. In R. R. Parse (Ed.), *Hope: An international perspective* (pp. 45–61). Sudbury, MA: Jones & Bartlett and National League for Nursing Press.

Cody, W. K. (1991). Multidimensionality, its meaning and significance. *Nursing Science Quarterly, 4*, 140–141.

Cody, W. K. (1999). True presence with families living with HIV disease. In R. R. Parse (Ed.), *Illuminations: The human becoming theory in practice and research* (pp. 115–133). New York: National League for Nursing Press.

Cody, W. K., Hudepol, J. H., & Brinkman, K. S. (1999). True presence with a child and his family. In R. R. Parse (Ed.), *Illuminations: The human becoming theory in practice and research* (pp. 135–146). New York: National League for Nursing Press.

Dossey, B. M. (2000). *Florence Nightingale: Mystic, visionary, healer.* Springhouse, PA: Springhouse.

Endo, E., Miyahara, T., Suzuki, S., & Ohmasa, T. (2005). Partnering of researcher and practicing nurses for transformative nursing. *Nursing Science Quarterly, 18*(2), 138–145.

Ethridge, P. (1991). A nursing HMO: Carondelet St. Mary's experience. *Nursing Management, 22*(7), 22–27.

Ethridge, P., & Lamb, G. S. (1989). Professional nursing case management improves quality, access and costs. *Nursing Management, 20*(3), 30–35.

Farren, A. T. (2010). Power in breast cancer survivors: A secondary analysis. *Visions: The Journal of Rogerian Nursing Science, 17*(1), 29–43.

Fitzpatrick, J. J. (1989). A life perspective rhythm model. In J. J. Fitzpatrick & A. L. Whall (Eds.), *Conceptual model of nursing: Analysis and application* (2nd ed., pp. 401–407). Princeton, NJ: Appleton-Century-Crofts.

George, J. B. (2010). Health as expanding consciousness: Margaret Newman. In J. B. George (Ed), *Nursing theories: The base for professional nursing practice* (6th ed., pp. 519–538). Upper Saddle River, NJ: Pearson.

Gunther, M. E. (2010). Martha E. Rogers: Unitary human beings. In M. R. Alligood & A. M. Tomey (Eds.), *Nursing theorists and their work* (7th ed., pp. 242–264). St. Louis: Mosby.

Hektor, L. M. (1989). Martha E. Rogers: A life history. *Nursing Science Quarterly, 2*(2), 63–73.

Jonas, C. (1999). True presence through music for persons living with their dying. In R. R. Parse (Ed.), *Illuminations: The human becoming theory in practice and research* (pp. 97–104). New York: National League for Nursing Press.

Jones, D. A. (2007a). Newman's health as expanding consciousness. *Nursing Science Quarterly, 19*(4), 330–332.

Jones, D. (2007b). Margaret A. Newman over the years. *Nursing Science Quarterly, 20*(4), 306.

Karian, V. E., Jankowski, S. M., & Beal, J. A. (1998). Exploring the lived-experience of childhood cancer survivors. *Journal of Pediatric Oncology Nursing, 15*(3), 153–162.

Kelley, L. S. (1999). Evaluating change in quality of life from the perspective of the person: Advanced practice nursing and Parse's goal of nursing. *Holistic Nursing Practice, 13*(4), 61–70.

Kuhn, T. S. (1996). *The structure of scientific revolutions* (3rd ed.). Chicago: University of Chicago Press.

Kwekkeboom, K., Huseby-Moore, K., & Ward, S. (1998). Imagining ability and effective use of guided imagery. *Research in Nursing and Health, 21*(3), 189–198.

Legault, F., & Ferguson-Pare, M. (1999). Advancing nursing practice: An evaluation study of Parse's theory of human becoming. *Canadian Journal of Nursing Leadership, 12*(1), 30–35.

Lewandowski, W. A. (2004). Patterning of pain and power with guided imagery. *Nursing Science Quarterly, 17*(3), 233–241.

Madrid, M. (1997). *Patterns of Rogerian knowing.* New York: National League for Nursing Press.

Madrid, M., & Winstead-Fry, P. (2001). Nursing research on the health patterning modalities of therapeutic touch and imagery. *Nursing Science Quarterly, 14*(3), 187–194.

Madrid, M. M., Barrett, E. A. M., & Winstead-Fry, P. (2010). A study of the feasibility of introducing therapeutic touch into the operative environment with patients undergoing cerebral angiography. *Journal of Holistic Nursing, 28*(3), 168–174.

Malinski, V. M., & Todaro-Franceschi, V. (2011). Exploring co-meditation as a means of reducing anxiety and facilitating relaxation in a nursing school setting. *Journal of Holistic Nursing, 29*(4), 242–248.

Marchione, J. (1995). Margaret Newman: Health as expanding consciousness. In C. M. McQuiston & A. A. Webb (Eds.), *Foundations of nursing theory: Contributions of 12 key theorists* (pp. 261–316). Thousand Oaks, CA: Sage.

Milton, C. L. (2004). Stories: Implications for nursing ethics and respect for another. *Nursing Science Quarterly, 21*(4), 330–342.

Musker, K. M. (2008). Life patterns of women transitioning through menopause. *Nursing Science Quarterly, 17*(3), 208–211.

Neill, J. (2005). Recognizing patterns in the lives of women with multiple sclerosis. In C. Picard and D. Jones (Eds.), *Giving voice to what we know: Margaret Newman's theory of health as expanding consciousness in nursing practice, research, and education* (pp. 153–165). Sudbury, MA: Jones & Bartlett.

Newman, M. A. (1979). *Theory development in nursing.* Philadelphia: F. A. Davis.

Newman, M. A. (1986). *Health as expanding consciousness.* St. Louis: Mosby.

Newman, M. A. (1990a). Newman's theory of health as praxis. *Nursing Science Quarterly, 3*(1), 37–41.

Newman, M. A. (1990b). Toward an integrative model of professional practice. *Journal of Professional Nursing, 6,* 167–173.

Newman, M. A. (1994). *Health as expanding consciousness.* New York: National League for Nursing Press.

Newman, M. A. (1995). *A developing discipline: Selected works of Margaret Newman.* New York: National League for Nursing Press.

Newman, M. A. (1999). *Health as expanding consciousness* (2nd ed.). New York: National League for Nursing Press.

Newman, M. A. (2005). Caring in the human health experience. In C. Picard & D. Jones (Eds.), *Giving voice to what we know: Margaret Newman's Theory of health as expanding consciousness in nursing practice, research, and education* (pp. 3–9). Sudbury, MA: Jones & Bartlett.

Newman, M. A. (2008a). *Transforming presence: The difference that nursing makes.* Philadelphia: F. A. Davis.

Newman, M. A. (2008b). It's about time. *Nursing Science Quarterly, 21*(3), 225–229.

Newman, M. A., Lamb, G. S., & Michaels, C. (1991). Nurse case management: The coming together of theory and practice. *Nursing and Health Care, 12*(8), 404–408. Reprinted in M. A. Newman (Ed.). (1995). *A developing discipline: Selected works of Margaret Newman* (pp. 249–263). New York: National League for Nursing Press.

Noh, C. H. (2004). Meaning of the quality of life for persons living with serious mental illness: Human becoming practice with groups. *Nursing Science Quarterly, 17*(3), 220–225.

Parse, R. R. (1981). *Man-living-health: A theory of nursing.* New York: Wiley.

Parse, R. R. (1987). *Nursing science: Major paradigms and theories and critiques.* Philadelphia: Saunders.

Parse, R. R. (1995). *Illuminations: The human becoming theory in practice and research.* New York: National League for Nursing Press.

Parse, R. R. (1998). *The human becoming school of thought: A perspective for nurses and other health professionals.* Thousand Oaks, CA: Sage.

Parse, R. R. (2001). The human becoming school of thought. In M. Parker (Ed.), *Nursing theories and nursing practice* (pp. 227–238). Philadelphia: Davis.

Parse, R. R. (2002). Transforming healthcare with a unitary view of the human. *Nursing Science Quarterly, 15*(1), 46–50.

Parse, R. R. (2008). The human becoming leading following model. *Nursing Science Quarterly, 21*(4), 369–375.

Parse, R. R. (2010). Human dignity: A humanbecoming ethical phenomenon. *Nursing Science Quarterly, 23*(3), 256–262.

Parse, R. R. (2013). Living quality: A humanbecoming phenomenon. *Nursing Science Quarterly, 26*(2), 111–115.

Pharris, M. D., & Endo, E. (2007). Flying free: The evolving nature of nursing practice guided by the theory of health as expanding consciousness. *Nursing Science Quarterly, 20*(2), 136–140.

Phillips, J. R. (1990). Changing human potentials and future visions of nursing: A human field image perspective. In E. A. M. Barrett (Ed.), *Visions of Rogers' science-based nursing* (pp. 13–25). New York: National League for Nursing Press.

Phillips, J. R. (1994). Foreword. In V. M. Malinski, E. A. M. Barrett, & J. R. Phillips (Eds.), *Martha E. Rogers: Her life and her work* (pp. v–ix). Philadelphia: F. A. Davis.

Phillips, J (2010). Perspectives of Rogers' relative present. *Visions: The Journal of Rogerian Nursing Science, 17*(1), 8–18.

Pickard, C. (2000). Pattern of expanding consciousness in midlife women: Creative movement and the narrative as modes of expression. *Nursing Science Quarterly, 13*(2), 150–157.

Pickard, C. (2002). Family reflections on living through sudden death of a child: Cooperative inquiry grounded in Newman's health as expanding consciousness. *Nursing Science Quarterly, 15*(3), 242–250.

Pilkington, F. B., & Millar, B. (1999). The lived experience of hope with persons from Wales, UK. In R. R. Parse (Ed.), *Hope: An international human becoming perspective* (pp. 163–189). Sudbury, MA: Jones & Bartlett and National League for Nursing Press.

Reed, P. (2008). Nursing time: Research, practice, and theory dimensions. *Nursing Science Quarterly, 21*(3), 222–223.

Rogers, M. E. (1970). *An introduction to the theoretical basis of nursing*. Philadelphia: F. A. Davis.

Rogers, M. E. (1986). Science of unitary human beings. In V. M. Malinski (Ed.), *Explorations on Martha Rogers' science of unitary human beings* (pp. 3–8). Norwalk, CT: Appleton-Century-Crofts. Reprinted in V. M. Malinski, E. A. M. Barrett, & J. R. Phillips (Eds.). (1994). *Martha E. Rogers: Her life and her work* (pp. 233–238). Philadelphia: F. A. Davis.

Rogers, M. E. (1990). Nursing: The science of unitary, irreducible, human beings: Update 1990. In E. A. M. Barrett (Ed.), *Visions of Rogers' science-based nursing* (pp. 5–11). New York: National League for Nursing Press.

Rogers, M. E. (1994). Nursing science evolves. In M. Madrid & E. A. M. Barrett (Eds.), *Rogers' scientific art of nursing practice* (pp. 3–10). New York: National League for Nursing Press.

Smith, S. M. (2010). Humanbecoming: Not just a theory—it is a way of being. *Nursing Science Quarterly, 23*(3), 216–219.

Stein, J. (2013). The new greatest generation: Why millennials will save us all. *Time, 181*(19), 26–32, 34.

Toikkanen, T., & Muurinen, E. (1999). Tiovo: Hope for persons in Finland. In R. R. Parse (Ed.), *Hope: An international human becoming perspective* (pp. 79–96). Sudbury, MA: Jones & Bartlett and National League for Nursing Press.

Welch, A. J. (2004). The researcher's reflections on the research process. *Nursing Science Quarterly, 17*(3), 201–207.

CHAPTER 10

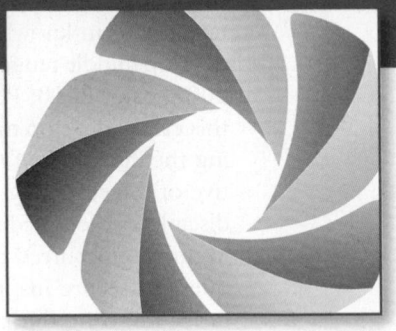

Introduction to Middle Range Nursing Theories

Melanie McEwen

Annette Cohen is a second-year graduate nursing student interested in starting her major research/scholarship project. For this project, she would like to develop some of her experiences in hospice nursing into a preliminary middle range theory of spiritual health. Annette has studied spiritual needs and spiritual care for many years but believes that the construct of spiritual health is not well understood. She views spiritual health as the result of the interaction of multiple intrinsic values and external variables within a client's experiences, and she believes that it is a significant contributing factor to overall health and well-being.

After reviewing theoretical writings dealing with spiritual nursing care, Annette found a starting point for her work in Jean Watson's Theory of Human Caring (Watson, 2005) because of its emphasis on spirituality and faith. From Watson's work, she was particularly interested in applying the concepts of "actual caring occasion" and "transpersonal" care. To develop the theory, Annette obtained a copy of Watson's most recent work and performed a comprehensive review of the literature covering theory development and the Theory of Human Caring. She then did an analysis of the concept of spiritual health. Combining the concept analysis and the literature review of Watson's work led to the development of assumptions and formal definitions of related concepts and empirical indicators. After conversing with her instructor, she concluded that her next steps were to construct relational statements and then draw a model depicting the relationships among the concepts that comprise spiritual health.

As discussed in Chapter 2, middle range nursing theories lie between the most abstract theories (grand nursing theories, models, or conceptual frameworks) and more circumscribed, concrete theories (practice theories, situation-specific theories, or microtheories). Compared to grand theories, middle range theories are more specific, have fewer concepts, and encompass a more limited aspect of the real world. Concepts are relatively concrete and can be operationally defined. Propositions are also relatively concrete and may be empirically tested.

The discipline of nursing recognizes middle range theory as one of the contemporary trends in knowledge development, and there is broad acceptance of the need to develop middle range theories to support nursing practice (Alligood, 2010; Fitzpatrick, 2003; Kim, 2010; Peterson, 2013). According to Morris (1996) and Suppe (1996), this call to develop middle range theory is consistent with the third stage of legitimizing the discipline of nursing. The first stage focuses on differentiation of the perspective of the emerging discipline, which is characterized by separation from antecedent disciplines (i.e., medicine) and the establishment of university-based education, which in nursing occurred during the 1950s and 1960s. The second stage is marked by the quest to secure institutional legitimacy and academic autonomy. This stage characterized nursing during the 1970s and through the 1980s, when pursuit of nursing's unique perspective on and clarification of the phenomena of interest to the discipline were stressed. The third stage began in the 1990s and is distinguished by increased attention to substantive knowledge development, which includes development and testing of middle range theories. This stage is expanding and evolving further to include evidence-based practice and situation-specific theories (see Chapter 12).

Middle range theories are increasingly being used in nursing research studies. Many researchers prefer to work with middle range theories rather than grand theories or conceptual frameworks because they provide a better basis for generating testable hypotheses and addressing particular client populations. A review of nursing research journals and dissertation abstracts indicates that nursing research is currently being used in the development and testing of a number of middle range theories, and middle range theories are frequently being used as frameworks for investigation. Furthermore, middle range theories are presently being refined on the basis of research results.

Despite the promotion of middle range theories in recent years, there is a lack of clarity regarding what constitutes middle range theory in nursing. According to Cody (1999), "It appears that almost any theoretical entity that is more concrete than the broadest of grand theories is considered middle range by someone" (p. 10). It has been noted that nursing theory textbooks (e.g., Alligood, 2010; Chinn & Kramer, 2011; Fawcett & DeSanto-Madeya, 2013; Parker & Smith, 2010) disagree to some degree on which theories should be labeled as middle range. Indeed, some authors list a few of the readily accepted grand theories (e.g., Parse, Newman, Peplau, and Orlando) as middle range. Others consider somewhat more circumscribed theories (e.g., Leininger, Pender, Benner and Erickson, Tomlin, and Swain) to be middle range, although the theory's authors may not agree. In essence, there has been a paucity of discussion on the subject and therefore there is little consensus. This issue is discussed in more detail later in the chapter.

Purposes of Middle Range Theory

Middle range theories were first suggested in the discipline of sociology in the 1960s and were introduced to nursing in 1974. At that time, it was observed that middle range theories were useful for emerging disciplines because they are more readily operationalized and addressed through research than are grand theories. More than 15 years elapsed, however, before there was a concerted call for middle range theory development in nursing (Blegen & Tripp-Reimer, 1997; Meleis, 2012).

Development of middle range theories is supported by the frequent critique of the abstract nature of grand theories and the difficulty of their application to practice and research. The function of middle range theories is to describe, explain, or predict phenomena, and, unlike grand theory, they must be explicit and testable. Thus, they are easier to apply in practice situations and to use as frameworks for research studies. In addition, middle range theories have the potential to guide nursing interventions and change conditions of a situation to enhance nursing care. Finally, a major role of middle range theory is to define or refine the substantive component of nursing science and practice (Higgins & Moore, 2000). Indeed, Lenz (1996) noted that practicing nurses are actually using middle range theories but are not consciously aware that they are doing so.

Each middle range theory addresses relatively concrete and specific phenomena by stating what the phenomena are, why they occur, and how they occur. In addition, middle range theories can provide structure for the interpretation of behavior, situations, and events. They support understanding of the connections between diagnosis and outcomes, and between interventions and outcomes (Fawcett & DeSanto-Madeya, 2013).

Enhancing the focus on middle range theories in nursing is supported by several factors. These include the observations that middle range theories

- are more useful in research than grand theories because of their low level of abstraction and ease of operationalization
- tend to support prediction better than grand theories due to circumscribed range and specificity of the concepts
- are more likely to be adopted in practice because their relative simplicity eases the process of developing interventions for identified health problems (Cody, 1999; Peterson, 2013)

Like theory in general, middle range theory has three functions in nursing knowledge development. First, middle range theories are used as theoretical frameworks for research studies. Second, middle range theories are open to use in practice and should be tested by research. Finally, middle range theories can be the scientific end product that expresses nursing knowledge (Suppe, 1996).

Characteristics of Middle Range Theory

Several characteristics identify nursing theories as middle range. First, the principal ideas of middle range theories are relatively simple, straightforward, and general. Second, middle range theories consider a limited number of variables or concepts; they have a particular substantive focus and consider a limited aspect of reality. In addition, they are receptive to empirical testing and can be consolidated into more wide-ranging theories. Third, middle range theories focus primarily on client problems and likely outcomes, as well as the effects of nursing interventions on client outcomes. Finally, middle range theories are specific to nursing and may specify an area of practice, age range of the client, nursing actions or interventions, and proposed outcomes (Meleis, 2012; Peterson, 2013).

The more frequently used middle range theories tend to be those that are clearly stated, easy to understand, internally consistent, and coherent. They deal with current nursing perspectives and address socially relevant topics that solve meaningful and persistent problems. In summary, middle range theories for nursing combine postulated relationships between specific, well-defined concepts with the ability to measure or objectively code concepts. Thus, middle range theories contain concepts and statements from which hypotheses may be logically derived and empirically tested, and they can be easily adopted to guide nursing practice. Table 10-1 compares characteristics of grand theory, middle range theory, and practice/situation-specific theory, and characteristics of middle range theory are shown in Box 10-1.

Table 10-1 Characteristics of Grand, Middle Range, and Practice/Situation-Specific Theories

Characteristic	Grand Theories	Middle Range Theories	Practice/Situation-Specific Theories
Complexity/abstractness, scope	Comprehensive, global viewpoint (all aspects of human experience)	Less comprehensive than grand theories, middle view of reality	Focused on a narrow view of reality, simple and straightforward
Generalizability/specificity	Nonspecific, general application to the discipline irrespective of setting or specialty area	Some generalizability across settings and specialties, but more specific than grand theories	Linked to special populations or an identified field of practice
Characteristics of concepts	Concepts abstract and not operationally defined	Limited number of concepts that are fairly concrete and may be operationally defined	Single, concrete concept that is operationalized
Characteristics of propositions	Propositions not always explicit	Propositions clearly stated	Propositions defined
Testability	Not generally testable	May generate testable hypotheses	Goals or outcomes defined and testable
Source of development	Developed through thoughtful appraisal and careful consideration over many years	Evolve from grand theories, clinical practice, literature review, and practice guidelines	Derived from practice or deduced from middle range or grand theory

Concepts and Relationships for Middle Range Theory

Middle range theories consist of two or more concepts and a specified relationship between the concepts. Middle range theories address phenomena (concepts) that are toward the middle of a continuum of scope with the metaparadigm concepts (nursing, person, health, environment) at one end and specific concrete actions or events (medication administration, preoperative teaching, electrolyte management, fall prevention) at the other. The concepts should be discrete, observable, and sufficiently abstract to be applied across multiple settings and used with clients with differing problems (Blegen & Tripp-Reimer, 1997). Examples from the nursing literature include theories describing health promotion, comfort, coping, resilience, uncertainty, pain, grief, fatigue, self-care, adaptation, self-transcendence, and transitions (Meleis, 2012; Peterson, 2013; Smith & Liehr, 2013).

Box 10-1 Characteristics of Middle Range Nursing Theory

Not comprehensive, but not narrowly focused
Some generalizations across settings and specialties
Limited number of concepts
Propositions that are clearly stated
May generate testable hypotheses

Middle range theories link discrete and observable phenomena
relationships statements. In middle range theory, relationships are ex
and, preferably, they are unidirectional. Relationships can be of severa
most common are causal relationships that state that a change in the value
able or concept is associated with a change in the value of another variable o concept (Peterson, 2013).

Categorizing Middle Range Theory

The question as to which nursing theories are middle range is not clear-cut. Middle range theory is more specific than grand theory but abstract enough to support both generalization and operationalization across a range of populations; this sets it apart from practice theory.

In a well-researched effort to describe the place of middle range theory in nursing, Liehr and Smith (1999) analyzed 22 middle range theories published during the previous decade. These theories were categorized as "high-middle," "middle," and "low-middle" based on their level of abstraction or degree of specificity. In the review, high-middle theories included concepts such as caring, growth and development, self-transcendence, resilience, and psychological adaptation. Middle theories included concepts such as uncertainty in illness, unpleasant symptoms, chronic sorrow, peaceful end of life, cultural brokering, and nurse-expressed empathy. Low-middle theories, those that are closer to practice or situation-specific theories, included hazardous secrets, women's anger, nurse midwifery care, acute pain management, helplessness, and intervention for postsurgical pain.

As mentioned, there is some debate on which theories should be considered middle range. Indeed, some theories *not* termed middle range more appropriately fit the criteria of middle range theory than a grand theory, and some theories that are labeled middle range better fit the criteria of situation-specific or practice theory. Chapter 11 presents a number of middle range nursing theories recently described in the literature, organized as high, middle, and low theories. It should be noted that the designations are arguably arbitrary and that one theory that is listed here as high-middle may be considered by others to be a grand theory. Likewise, another theory listed here as middle might be considered by others to be high-middle and so forth. Situation-specific theories and their relationship to evidence-based practice are discussed in more detail in Chapter 12.

Development of Middle Range Theory

Several methods for development of middle range theories have been identified in the nursing literature. Middle range theories emerge from combining research and practice and building on the work of others. Sources used to generate middle range theory include literature reviews, qualitative research, field studies, conceptual models, taxonomies of nursing diagnoses and interventions, clinical practice guidelines, theories from other disciplines, and statistical analysis of empirical data (Fawcett & DeSanto-Madeya, 2013; Peterson, 2013). Five approaches for middle range theory generation were identified by Liehr and Smith (1999) (Box 10-2). The following sections present examples describing the source and development process of middle range theories from each of the five approaches listed in Box 10-2.

Box 10-2 Approaches for Middle Range Theory Generation

1. Induction through research and practice
2. Deduction from research and practice or application of grand theories
3. Combination of existing nursing and non-nursing middle range theories
4. Derivation from theories of other disciplines that relate to nursing
5. Derivation from practice guidelines and standards rooted in research

Middle Range Theories Derived From Research and/or Practice

The most common sources for development of middle range nursing theories and models are nursing research and nursing practice. Grounded theory research and other qualitative methods in particular are frequently noted as sources for middle range theory development. Examples of middle range theories derived from qualitative research include the Theory of Normalizing Risky Sexual Behaviors (Weiss, Jampol, Lievano, Smith, & Wurster, 2008), a theory describing sustaining health in faith community nursing practice (Dyess & Chase, 2012), a theory for nursing care for patients at risk of suicide (Sun, Long, Boore, & Tsao, 2006), a theory describing humor use in nurse–patient interactions (McCreaddie & Wiggins, 2009), and a theory of career persistence in acute care (Hodges, Troyan, & Keeley, 2010).

Variations of the idea of development of middle range theory from research are fairly common. Theorists report combining qualitative research with literature review, concept analysis, concept synthesis, theory synthesis, and other techniques in the process of developing middle range theory. For example, Murrock and Higgins (2009) explained that they used statement and theory synthesis, along with literature review, to develop "the theory of music, mood and movement to improve health outcomes." In other works, Davidson (2010) developed "Facilitated Sensemaking" to support families of intensive care unit (ICU) patients following systematic literature review and synthesis, and Covell (2008) used concept analysis and theory derivation methods to develop a middle range theory of nursing intellectual capital. Eakes, Burke, and Hainsworth (1998) developed the middle range Theory of Chronic Sorrow from an extensive review of the literature and data gathered through 10 qualitative research studies.

Identification of middle range theories and models derived primarily from practice is more difficult. One example is the Theory of Unpleasant Symptoms (Lenz, Pugh, Milligan, Gift, & Suppe, 1997; Lenz, Suppe, Gift, Pugh, & Milligan, 1995), which was reportedly developed by integrating or melding existing practice and research information about a variety of symptoms. A second example is The Client Experience Model (Holland, Gray, & Pierce, 2011), which was reportedly developed through clinical observations in acute care settings using a practice-to-theory method.

Some models that describe areas of specialty nursing practice report being developed from combination of practice and another source, typically research or standards. One example of this technique is Benoit and Mion's (2012) model for pressure ulcer etiology in critically ill patients, which was constructed from combining a literature review and practice standards. The Omaha System, which is a model for community and home health nursing practice, is a second example. Martin (2005) explained that the conceptual framework for the Omaha System was a combination of practice, research, and literature review.

Another example of theory development combining practice with other elements is Rogers' (1994) model for occupational health nursing practice, which combined

NURSING EXEMPLAR 1: MIDDL THEORY DERIVED FROM RESEA PRACTICE

The process used to develop a middle range theory of caring was , Swanson (1991). Her purpose was to provide a definition of caring and describe its characteristics and to outline caring processes used by nurses.

Theory Development Process: The *theory of caring* was derived from three phenomenologic studies in perinatal nursing. The focus was on experiences of women who had miscarried, with an emphasis on patients and professionals in the newborn intensive care unit (NICU). In the first study, women who had recently miscarried were interviewed to learn about their perception of caring behaviors of others. Five caring processes (knowing, being with, doing for, enabling, and maintaining belief) were derived from this study and preliminary definitions were proposed.

A second study involved interviews and observation of care providers in a NICU. This study confirmed the five caring processes and allowed for refinement of the theoretical definitions. In the final study, interviews with 68 pregnant women who were considered to be at high risk from a social perspective were conducted. In that study, the five caring processes were reconfirmed, then slightly refined. Following that, subdimensions of each caring process were identified, the concept of caring was defined, and the theory was fully delineated.

practice experiences with standards. Lastly, Purnell (2000) explained that his Model for Cultural Competence was "developed from practice and working with staff and students in culturally diverse clinical settings" (p. 40). In addition to using practice experiences, he also detailed how concepts from many theories from other disciplines (e.g., organization/administration, anthropology, sociology, psychology, religion, and history) were incorporated into the model's development.

Middle Range Theory Derived From a Grand Theory

As explained previously, many nursing theorists and scholars agree that grand theories are difficult to apply in research and practice and suggest development of middle range theories derived from them. During the last two decades, several theories developed from grand theories have been published in the nursing literature. One example is a middle range theory of nurse-expressed empathy (Olson & Hanchett, 1997), which was derived from three relational statements taken from Orlando's model. These statements were developed into theoretical propositions focusing on nurse-expressed empathy. Two examples used Orem's theory. In one, Riegel, Jaarsma, and Stromberg (2012) developed the theory of self-care of chronic illness, patterning their notion of self-care from Orem's theory. Similarly, Rew (2003) developed a theory of self-care from experiences of homeless youth based on Orem's theory.

In other examples, Hastings-Tolsma (2006) developed the Theory of Diversity of Human Field Pattern from Martha Rogers' Science of Unitary Human Beings. Cazzell (2008) employed the Neuman Systems Model as a basis for the middle range theory of adolescent vulnerability to risk behaviors, and in another work, Polk (1997) cited the work of both Margaret Newman and Martha Rogers as sources contributing to her middle range theory of resilience.

Several middle range theories were found which were developed from the Roy Adaptation Model (RAM). In one example, Dobratz (2011) derived the theory of psychological adaptation in death and dying from a series of studies linked to the RAM, and in another example, Hamilton and Bowers (2007) developed the Theory of Genetic Vulnerability from Roy's work. Similarly, Smith and colleagues (2002) developed a theory describing caregiving effectiveness based on the structure and concepts from the RAM, and Whittemore and Roy (2002) used concept syntheses to integrate concepts and assumptions from the RAM to theoretically describe "adapting to diabetes mellitus." Finally, Roy's model was also used in the development of a middle range theory of caregiver stress (Tsai, 2003).

NURSING EXEMPLAR 2: MIDDLE RANGE THEORY DERIVED FROM A GRAND THEORY

Mefford (2004) used Levine's Conservation Model of Nursing to develop a Theory of Health Promotion for Preterm Infants. In this case, Levine's theory was used as a framework for nursing practice for the NICU to ensure that needs of both the infant and family are addressed.

Theory Development Process: To develop the Theory of Health Promotion for Preterm Infants, the theorist first described elements of Levine's Conservation Model internal and external environments, wholeness and conservation principles (conservation of energy, structural integrity, personal integrity, and social integrity) and applied these concepts in the NICU. She determined a "goal of restoring a state of wholeness, or health" (p. 260) (Figure 10-1).

Following initial development of the theory, its validity was tested in a retrospective study of 235 preterm infants. This study was designed to examine the influence of "consistency nursing care" on the health outcomes of the infants at discharge. Structural equation modeling demonstrated "strong support for the utility of this theory of health promotion . . . as a guide for nursing practice in the NICU" (p. 266). It was noted that the derived middle range theory validated Levine's work.

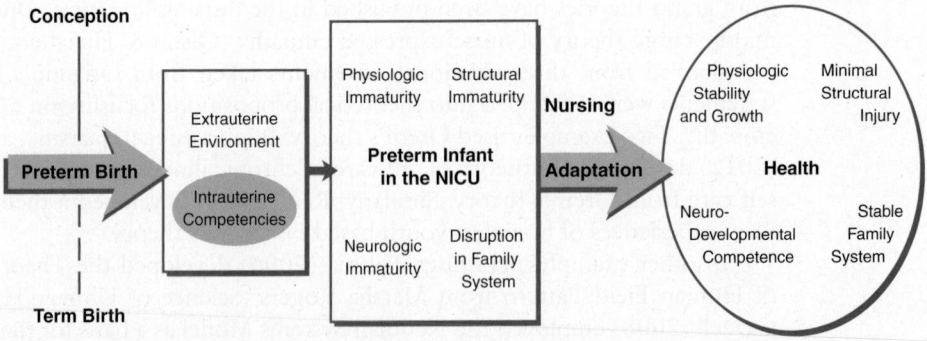

Figure 10-1 Conceptual diagram of Levine's conservation model of nursing. (From Mefford, L. C. (2004). A theory of health promotion for preterm infants based on Levine's Conservation Model of Nursing. *Nursing Science Quarterly, 17*(3), 261. Used with permission of SAGE Publications, Inc.)

Middle Range Theory Combining Existing Nursing and Non-Nursing Theories

Combining concepts or elements of multiple theories is common in middle range theory development. In many cases found in recent nursing literature, the author(s) of a middle range theory reported that they had derived their theory from both nursing and non-nursing theories. For example, Sousa and Zauszniewski (2005) used Orem's Self-Care Theory and Bandura's Self-Efficacy Theory to develop a theory of diabetes self-care management. Similarly, Ulbrich (1999) developed the Theory of Exercise as Self-Care through "triangulation of Orem's self-care deficit theory of nursing, the transtheoretical model of exercise behavior, and characteristics of a population at risk for cardiovascular disease" (p. 65). In another example, Reed (1991) used elements of Rogers' Science of Unitary Human Beings as the "nursing perspective of human development for . . . self-transcendence" (p. 65). For this theory, Rogers' work was used as a framework, and it was reportedly combined with concepts and elements from developmental psychologists, including Piaget and Fagin.

NURSING EXEMPLAR 3: MIDDLE RANGE THEORY COMBINING EXISTING NURSING AND NON-NURSING THEORIES

Dunn (2004) provided an excellent example of combining existing nursing and non-nursing theories in development of a middle range Theory of Adaptation to Chronic Pain. Her intention was to describe coping and pain control in elders with the purpose of maintaining their quality of life and functional ability.

Theory Development Process: Dunn wrote that the first step in developing her theory was to review and synthesize the theoretical knowledge related to pain in elders, coping with pain, religious coping, and spirituality. She reported identification of three theoretical models that addressed concepts related to pain control and coping in elders. These were Melzak and Wall's (1992) gate control theory of pain, Lazarus and Folkman's (1984) stress and coping theory, and Wallace, Benson, and Wilson's (1971) relaxation response. To ensure that the final model was applicable to nursing, she selected the RAM to guide the theory development process.

The second step reported by Dunn was to define assumptions for the theory; these were reportedly based on the assumptions from the four models from which the theory was drawn. Using the process of theoretical substraction, she then took concepts, relational statements, and propositions from the existing theories and arranged them into a diagram to represent the theoretical and operational systems. Finally, the concepts from the Adaptation to Chronic Pain model were linked to empirical indicators to provide a logical and consistent connection.

Middle Range Theory Derived From Non-Nursing Disciplines

A significant number of middle range nursing theories are developed from one or more non-nursing theories. Indeed, non-nursing theories, including those from the behavioral sciences, sociology, physiology, and anthropology, appear to be the most

Table 10-2 Middle Range Nursing Theories Derived From Behavioral Theories

Theory	Non-nursing Theory Source(s)
Commitment to Health Theory (Kelly, 2008)	Transtheoretical Model of Behavior Change
Recovery Alliance Theory of Mental Health Nursing (Shanley & Jubb-Shanley, 2007)	Humanistic Philosophy
Health Promotion Model (Pender, Murdaugh & Parsons, 2011)	Social Learning Theory and Expectancy-Value Theory
Theory of Care-Seeking Behavior (Lauver, 1992)	Health Belief Model and the Theory of Reasoned Action
Medication Adherence Model (Johnson, 2002)	Health Belief Model, Social Learning Theory, the Theory of Reasoned Action, and the Self-Regulation Model
Self-Efficacy in Nursing Theory (Lenz & Shortridge-Baggett, 2002)	Social Learning Theory
Health Behavior Self-Determinism (Cox, 1985)	Health Belief Model, Schuman Model
Cues to Participation in Prostate Screening (Nivens, Herman, Weinrich, & Weinrich, 2001)	Health Belief Model, Social Learning Theory
Model for Cross-Cultural Research (Poss, 2001)	Health Belief Model, Theory of Reasoned Action

common source for theory development, and many examples are evident. Kolcaba's (1994) Theory of Comfort, for example, was reportedly derived from a review of literature from medicine, psychiatry, ergonomics, and psychology, as well as from nursing literature and history. Benner (2001) explained that the Dreyfus model of skill acquisition, developed by a mathematician and a philosopher, was the primary source for her work. Mishel's Uncertainty in Illness Theory incorporated elements of chaos theory (Mishel & Clayton, 2003), and Mercer (1985) used role theory as the framework for her theory describing maternal role attainment.

Several middle range nursing theories have been derived from theories or models of behavioral change. Frequently cited are the Health Belief Model (Becker & Maiman, 1975; Rosenstock, 1990), the Theory of Reasoned Action (Ajzen & Fishbein, 1980), and the Social Learning/Social Cognitive Theory (Bandura, 1977, 1986), along with others. Table 10-2 lists some of these middle range theories and gives sources from which the theorist claims derivation of portions of their work.

NURSING EXEMPLAR 4: MIDDLE RANGE THEORY DERIVED FROM A NON-NURSING DISCIPLINE

McGahee, Kemp, and Tingen (2000) developed a theoretical model to study smoking behaviors and prevention interventions among preteens. They stated that the "theoretical framework was derived from the literature linking different concepts to smoking behaviors and from literature that supports recommended intervention methods" (p. 135). The theorists reportedly used Social Cognitive Theory and the Theory of Reasoned Action in designing their model.

Theory Development Process: In developing the model to study smoking behaviors, the theorists described a detailed study of the concepts and components of the two theories mentioned. They determined that Social Cognitive Theory helped explain the psychosocial dynamics underlying individual behaviors. It also described how behavior is determined by expectancies and incentives as perceived by the individual and the importance of self-efficacy beliefs in influencing behavior. From the Theory of Reasoned Action, the theorists learned the importance of intention, which is described as a function of attitudes and subjective norms. From this, they recognized the significance of measuring an individual's intention to perform a behavior rather than the behavior itself.

Four major concepts affecting smoking prevention intervention were identified and defined in the theory. The first concept is sociodemographics, which includes gender, ethnicity, and household composition. The second concept is internal factors, which includes subjective personal variables (e.g., attitude toward smoking), subjective norms (e.g., beliefs about whether others think the individual should smoke and motivation to comply with the opinions of others), and perception of refusal skills (self-reported judgment of how well the individual can successfully refuse offers to smoke). The third concept is external factors, which involves parental attitudes toward smoking and preteens' perceptions of how much others smoke. The final variable identified is outcome behaviors. This includes smoking behaviors, which includes both self-reported intentional smoking (whether or not the preteen thinks he/she will smoke before the end of the current school year) and self-reported actual smoking (frequency and amount of smoking). Figure 10-2 depicts the theoretical model.

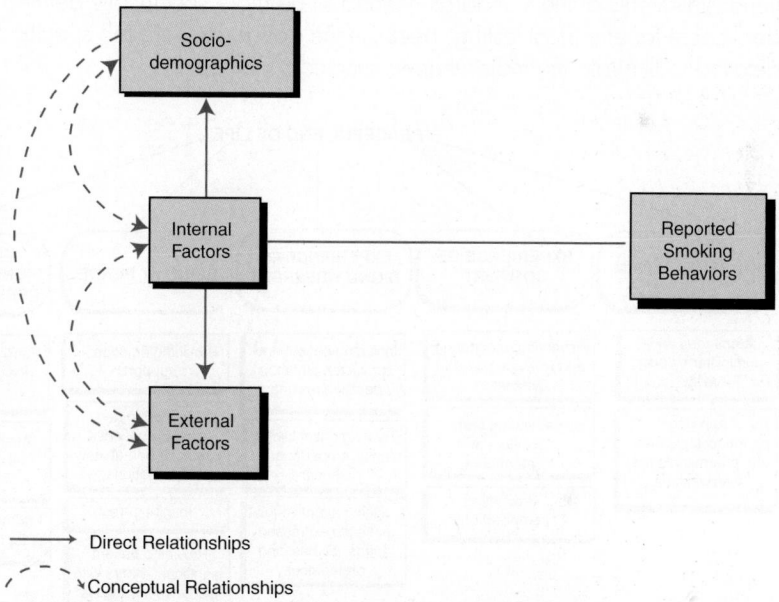

Figure 10-2 Theoretical model of influences on smoking behaviors.
Note: The solid lines indicate direct relationships that can be tested. The broken lines represent conceptual relationships that are supported by the literature. (McGahee, T. W., Kemp, V., & Tingen, M. (2000). A theoretical model for smoking prevention studies in preteen children. *Pediatric Nursing, 26*(2), 137. Reprinted with permission of the publisher, Janetti Publications, Inc. East Holly Avenue/Box 56, Pitman, NJ 08071-0056; (856)256-2300; FAX 589-7463; Web site: www.pediatricnursing.net; For a sample copy of the journal, please contact the publisher.)

Middle Range Theory Derived From Practice Guidelines or Standard of Care

Practice guidelines or standards of care appear to be the least common source for middle range theory development, as only a few examples could be found. In one example, the Public Health Nursing Practice Model (Smith & Bazini-Barakat, 2003) was developed by "melding of nationally recognized components" (p. 44) of public health nursing (PHN) practice. The identified components were the Standards of PHN practice, the 10 Essential Services of Public Health, *Healthy People 2010's* 10 Leading Health Indicators, and Minnesota's Public Health Interventions Model. In other examples, Good (1998) used clinical guidelines for management of postoperative pain to develop a middle range theory of acute pain management, and Huth and Moore (1998) used practice standards to develop a theory of acute pain management in infants and children. Finally, Ruland and Moore (1998) used standards of care to develop the Theory of the Peaceful End of Life from standards of care for terminally ill patients.

NURSING EXEMPLAR 5: MIDDLE RANGE THEORY DERIVED FROM PRACTICE GUIDELINES OR STANDARD OF CARE

Ruland and Moore (1998) developed the Theory of the Peaceful End of Life from standards of care for terminally ill patients. In this work, the theorists observed that relational statements of the standards needed to be more specifically defined to make them applicable for empirical testing. Because the standards were too specific, they were too detailed to illustrate the major themes succinctly.

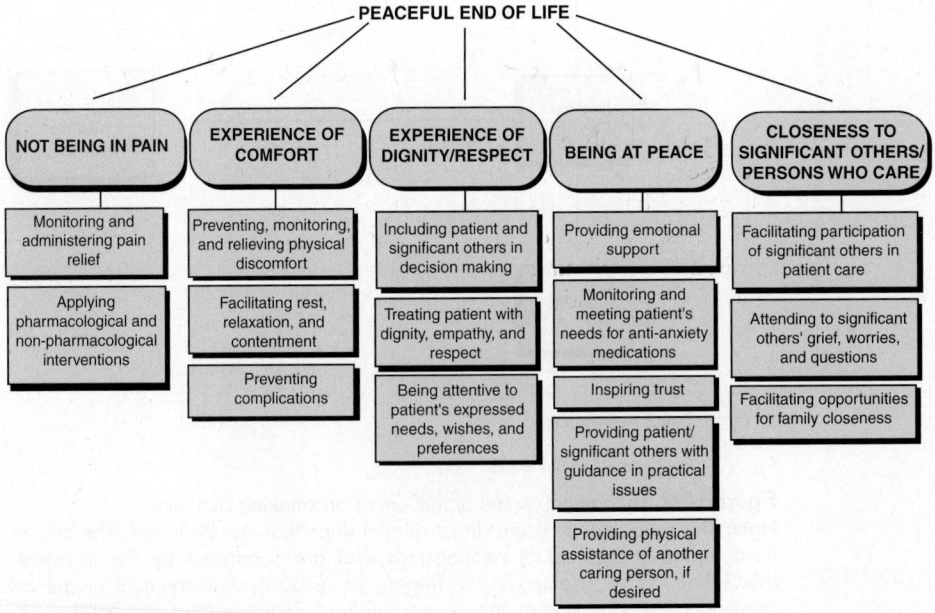

Figure 10-3 Theory of peaceful end of life: Relationships between the concepts of the theory. (Reprinted from Ruland, C. M., & Moore, S. M. (1998). Theory construction based on standards of care: A proposed theory of the peaceful end of life. *Nursing Outlook, 46,* 174.) Used with permission from Elsevier.

Theory Development Process: The first step of the theory development process was to define the theory's assumptions based on the standards of care. The second step was to perform a "statement synthesis," whereby five outcome criteria were developed that contributed to a peaceful end of life (not being in pain, experiencing comfort, experiencing dignity and respect, being at peace, and experiencing closeness to significant others or another caring person). For the third step, conceptual definitions for each of the outcome indicators were determined, and the fourth step involved defining relational statements between the outcome indicators and the nursing interventions. In this step, all process criteria from the standard were examined and combined into "prescriptors" to facilitate the desired outcome. The process of theory synthesis was then used to combine the relational statements into an integrated structure or theory. The final step was to draw a diagram of the relationships as a model (Figure 10-3).

Final Thoughts on Middle Range Theory Development

Middle range theories should be "user friendly" in language and style. They need to be described with practice implications in journals that practicing nurses are likely to read, and the theorists need to identify implications and specific interventions suggested by the theory (Lenz, 1996). Liehr and Smith's (1999) specific recommendations to enhance development and use of middle range theory include:

- Clearly articulate the theory name.
- Succinctly describe approaches used for generating the theory.
- Clarify the conceptual linkages of the theory in a diagrammed model.
- Elucidate the research–practice links of the theory.
- Explain the association between the theory and the discipline of nursing.

Analysis and Evaluation of Middle Range Theory

The move to enhance middle range theory development and use in nursing practice and research necessitates corresponding analysis and critique. Like grand theories and conceptual frameworks, middle range theories should be subject to evaluation. In addition, research guided by middle range theory should be congruent with the philosophical underpinnings of the theory and should be critiqued with regard to more than just the statistical significance of the findings.

Whall (2005) specifically addressed analysis and evaluation of middle range theory. Her criteria modified the guidelines she used for analysis and evaluation of grand nursing theories. The modifications removed explicit review of the metaparadigm concepts, which are assumed to be more implicit than explicit in middle range theory, and added questions regarding the "fit of the middle range theory with the existing nursing perspective and domains" (p. 14). Further, Whall explained that middle range theories should provide specific empirical referents for defined concepts. The ability to operationalize and measure aspects of the theory is extremely important in middle range theory, and operational definitions should be evaluated. Finally, she suggested analysis of middle range theories to assess their congruence with grand theories.

Smith (2013) also proposed a format for evaluation of middle range theories. She suggested evaluation based on three categories: substantive foundations, structural integrity, and functional adequacy. When evaluating substantive foundations, one would determine whether the theory was within the focus of nursing; whether assumptions are specified and congruent with the focus; whether the theory provides substantive description, explanation, or interpretation of a phenomenon that would be considered middle range; and whether the theory is rooted in practice or research experience. Evaluation of structural integrity would determine whether concepts are clearly defined and at the middle range of abstraction, whether the number of concepts is appropriate, and whether the concepts and relationship are logically represented with a model. Evaluation of functional adequacy examines whether the theory can be applied in practice or with various client groups, if empirical indicators have been identified for theoretical concepts, and if there are published examples of use of the theory in practice or research.

Chapter 5 includes a more detailed discussion of analysis and evaluation of middle range theories. In addition, the synthesized method for theory evaluation (see Box 5-3) can be used as a guide for analysis and evaluation of middle range theory.

Summary

This chapter has described the current emphasis of nursing theory development, which focuses on efforts to construct, test, refine, and evaluate middle range theories. To help advance the discipline, nurses should be encouraged to write and publish papers that describe middle range theories and report research studies in which a middle range theory has been used. This process of middle range theory generation and refinement will further develop the discipline's substantive knowledge base.

Annette Cohen, the graduate student in the opening case study who was working toward development of a theory of spiritual health, related it to the practice of hospice nursing. Like Annette, nurses in all settings should strive to learn about existing or emerging middle range theories or seek to develop and describe theories that will explain phenomena they observe in practice.

Nursing has the knowledge, skills, manpower, and resources to move beyond delineation of conceptual models and domain concepts to emphasize development and application of middle range theory. Middle range theory holds much promise for the evolution of the discipline's science and practice. But, as Liehr and Smith (1999) pointed out, the challenge is to develop middle range theories that are empirically sound, coherent, meaningful, useful, and illuminating.

Key Points

- Middle range nursing theories were first introduced into nursing in the mid-1970s; their number and use have grown dramatically in the last decade.
- Middle range theories are more specific, have fewer concepts, and encompass a more limited aspect of the real world compared with grand nursing theories; they are also more readily testable in research.
- Middle range theories may be developed through research, practice, or literature synthesis; they may be derived from grand nursing theories or non-nursing theories; or they may be derived from practice guidelines and standards.
- Before being used in a research study or applied in practice, middle range nursing theories should be analyzed or evaluated.

Learning Activities

1. Search current nursing journals for examples of the development, analysis, or use of middle range theories in the discipline of nursing. Can any trends be identified?
2. Select one of the middle range theories derived from a grand nursing theory and one derived from a non-nursing theory. Analyze both for ease of application to research and practice.

REFERENCES

Ajzen, I., & Fishbein, M. (1980). *Understanding attitudes and predicting social behavior.* Englewood Cliffs, NJ: Prentice-Hall.

Alligood, M. R. (2010). State of the art and science of nursing. In A. M. Tomey & M. R. Alligood (Eds.), *Nursing theorists and their work* (7th ed., pp. 765–772). St. Louis: Mosby/Elsevier.

Bandura, A. (1977). *Social learning theory.* Englewood Cliffs, NJ: Prentice-Hall.

Bandura, A. (1986). *Social foundations of thought and action: A social cognitive theory.* Englewood Cliffs, NJ: Prentice-Hall.

Becker, M. H., & Maiman, L. A. (1975). Sociobehavioral determinates of compliance with health and medical care recommendations. *Medical Care, 13,* 10–24.

Benner, P. (2001). *From novice to expert: Excellence and power in clinical nursing practice* (commemorative edition). Englewood Cliffs, NJ: Prentice-Hall.

Benoit, R., & Mion, L. (2012). Risk factors for pressure ulcer development in critically ill patients: A conceptual model to guide research. *Research in Nursing & Health, 35*(4), 340–362.

Blegen, M. A., & Tripp-Reimer, T. (1997). Implications of nursing taxonomies for middle range theory development. *Advances in Nursing Science, 19*(3), 37–50.

Cazzell, M. (2008). Linking theory, evidence, and practice in assessment of adolescent inhalant use. *Journal of Addictions Nursing, 19,* 17–25.

Chinn, P. L., & Kramer, M. K. (2011). *Theory and nursing: Integrated knowledge development* (8th ed.). St. Louis: Mosby.

Cody, W. K. (1999). Middle range theories: Do they foster the development of nursing science? *Nursing Science Quarterly, 12*(1), 9–14.

Covell, C. L. (2008). The middle-range theory of nursing intellectual capital. *Journal of Advanced Nursing, 63*(1), 94–103.

Cox, C. (1985). The self-determinism index. *Nursing Research, 34,* 177–183.

Davidson, J. E. (2010). Facilitated sensemaking: A strategy and new middle-range theory to support families of intensive care unit patients. *Critical Care Nurse, 30*(6), 28–39.

Dobratz, M. C. (2011). Toward development of a middle-range theory of psychological adaptation in death and dying. *Nursing Science Quarterly, 24*(4), 370–376.

Dunn, K. S. (2004). Toward a middle range theory of adaptation to chronic pain. *Nursing Science Quarterly, 17*(1), 78–84.

Dyess, S. M., & Chase, S. K. (2012). Sustaining health in faith community nursing practice: Emerging processes that support the development of a middle-range theory. *Holistic Nursing Practice, 26*(4), 221–227.

Eakes, G., Burke, M. L., & Hainsworth, M. A. (1998). Middle range theory of chronic sorrow. *Image: Journal of Nursing Scholarship, 30*(2), 179–185.

Fawcett, J., & DeSanto-Madeya, S. (2013). *Contemporary nursing knowledge: Analysis and evaluation of nursing models and theories* (3rd ed.). Philadelphia: F. A. Davis.

Fitzpatrick, J. J. (2003). Foreword. In M. J. Smith & P. R. Liehr (Eds.), *Middle range theory for nursing* (pp. ix–x). New York: Springer.

Good, M. (1998). A middle range theory of acute pain management: Use in research. *Nursing Outlook, 46*(3), 120–124.

Hamilton, R. J., & Bowers, B. J. (2007). The theory of genetic vulnerability: A Roy model exemplar. *Nursing Science Quarterly, 20*(3), 254–264.

Hastings-Tolsma, M. (2006). Toward a theory of diversity of human field pattern. *Visions: The Journal of Rogerian Nursing Science, 14*(2), 34–46.

Higgins, P. A., & Moore, S. M. (2000). Levels of theoretical thinking in nursing. *Nursing Outlook, 48*(4), 179–183.

Hodges, H. F., Troyan, P. J., & Keeley, A. C. (2010). Career persistence in baccalaureate-prepared acute care nurses. *Journal of Nursing Scholarship, 42*(1), 83–91.

Holland, B. E., Gray, J., & Pierce, T. B. (2011). The client experience model: Synthesis and application to African American with multiple sclerosis. *The Journal of Theory Construction & Testing, 15*(2), 36–40.

Huth, M. M., & Moore, S. M. (1998). Prescriptive theory of acute pain management in infants and children. *Journal of the Society of Pediatric Nurses, 3*(1), 23–32.

Johnson, M. J. (2002). The medication adherence model: A guide for assessing medication taking. *Research and Theory for Nursing Practice, 16*(3), 179–192.

Kelly, C. W. (2008). Commitment to health theory. *Research and Theory for Nursing Practice: An International Journal, 22*(2), 148–158.

Kim, H. S. (2010). *The nature of theoretical thinking in nursing* (3rd ed.). New York: Springer.

Kolcaba, K. (1994). A theory of holistic comfort for nursing. *Journal of Advanced Nursing, 19,* 1178–1184.

Lauver, D. (1992). A theory of care-seeking behavior. *Image: Journal of Nursing Scholarship, 24*(4), 281–287.

Lazarus, R. S., & Folkman, S. (1984). *Stress, appraisal and coping.* New York: Springer.

Lenz, E. R. (1996, May). *Middle range theory: Role in research and practice.* Paper presented at the Sixth Rosemary Ellis Scholar's Retreat, Cleveland, OH.

Lenz, E. R., Pugh, L. C., Milligan, R. A., Gift, A., & Suppe, F. (1997). The middle range. *Advances in Nursing Science, 19*(3), 14–27.

Lenz, E. R., & Shortridge-Baggett, L. (Eds.). (2002). *Self-efficacy and nursing.* New York: Springer.

Lenz, E. R., Suppe, F., Gift, A. G., Pugh, L. C., & Milligan, R. A. (1995). Collaborative development of middle range nursing theories: Toward a theory of unpleasant symptoms. *Advances in Nursing Science, 17*(3), 1–13.

Liehr, P., & Smith, M. J. (1999). Middle range theory: Spinning research and practice to create knowledge for the new millennium. *Advances in Nursing Science, 21*(4), 81–91.

Martin, K. S. (2005). *The Omaha system: A key to practice, documentation, and information management.* St. Louis: Elsevier.

McCreaddie, M., & Wiggins, S. (2009). Reconciling the good patient persona with problematic and non-problematic humour: A grounded theory. *International Journal of Nursing Studies, 46,* 1079–1091.

McGahee, T. W., Kemp, V., & Tingen, M. (2000). A theoretical model for smoking prevention studies in preteen children. *Pediatric Nursing, 26*(2), 135–140.

Mefford, L. C. (2004). A theory of health promotion for preterm infants based on Levine's Conservation Model of Nursing. *Nursing Science Quarterly, 17*(3), 260–266.

Meleis, A. I. (2012). *Theoretical nursing: Development and progress* (5th ed.). Philadelphia: Lippincott Williams & Wilkins.

Melzak, R., & Wall, P. D. (1992). Psychophysiology of pain. In D. C. Turk & R. Melzak (Eds.), *Handbook of pain and assessment* (pp. 3–25). New York: Guilford Press.

Mercer, R. T. (1985). The process of maternal role attainment over the first year. *Nursing Research, 34*(4), 198–204.

Mishel, M. H., & Clayton, M. F. (2003). Theories of uncertainty in illness. In M. J. Smith & P. R. Liehr (Eds.), *Middle range theory for nursing* (pp. 25–48). New York: Springer.

Morris, D. L. (1996, May). *Middle range theory: Role in education.* Paper presented at the Sixth Rosemary Ellis Scholar's Retreat, Cleveland, OH.

Murrock, C. J., & Higgins, P. A. (2009). The theory of music, mood and movement to improve health outcomes. *Journal of Advanced Nursing, 65*(10), 2249–2257.

Nivens, A. S., Herman, J., Weinrich, S. P., & Weinrich, M. C. (2001). Cues to participation in prostate cancer screening: A theory for practice. *Oncology Nursing Forum, 28*(9), 1449–1456.

Olson, J., & Hanchett, E. (1997). Nurse-expressed empathy, patient outcomes and development of a middle range theory. *Image: Journal of Nursing Scholarship, 29*(1), 71–76.

Parker, M. E., & Smith, M. C. (2010). *Nursing theories & nursing practice* (3rd ed.). Philadelphia: F. A. Davis.

Pender, N. J., Murdaugh, C., & Parsons, M. A. (2011). *Health promotion in nursing practice* (6th ed.). Upper Saddle River, NJ: Pearson.

Peterson, S. J. (2013). Introduction to the nature of nursing knowledge. In S. J. Peterson & T. S. Bredow (Eds.), *Middle range theories: Application to nursing research* (3rd ed., pp. 1–37). Philadelphia: Lippincott Williams & Wilkins.

Polk, L. V. (1997). Toward a middle range theory of resilience. *Advances in Nursing Science, 19*(3), 1–13.

Poss, J. E. (2001). Developing a new model for cross-cultural research: Synthesizing the health belief model and the theory of reasoned action. *Advances in Nursing Science, 23*(4), 1–15.

Purnell, L. (2000). A description of the Purnell model for cultural competence. *Journal of Transcultural Nursing, 11*(1), 40–46.

Reed, P. G. (1991). Toward a nursing theory of self-transcendence: Deductive reformulation using developmental theories. *Advances in Nursing Science, 13*(4), 64–77.

Rew, L. (2003). A theory of taking care of oneself grounded in experiences of homeless youth. *Nursing Research, 52*(4), 234–241.

Riegel, B., Jaarsma, T., & Stromberg, A. (2012). A middle-range theory of self-care of chronic illness. *Advances in Nursing Science, 35*(3), 194–204.

Rogers, B. (1994). *Occupational health nursing: Concepts and practice.* Philadelphia: Saunders.

Rosenstock, I. (1990). The health belief model: Explaining health behavior through expectancies. In K. Glanz, F. Lewis, & B. Rimer (Eds.), *Health behavior and health education* (pp. 39–62). San Francisco, CA: Jossey-Bass.

Ruland, C. M., & Moore, S. M. (1998). Theory construction based on standards of care: A proposed theory of the peaceful end of life. *Nursing Outlook, 46*(4), 169–175.

Shanley, E., & Jubb-Shanley, M. (2007). The recovery alliance theory of mental health nursing. *Journal of Psychiatric and Mental Health Nursing, 14*(8), 734–743.

Smith, C. E., Pace, K., Kochinda, C., Kleinbeck, S. V. M., Koehler, J., & Popkess-Vawter, S. (2002). Caregiving effectiveness model evaluation to a midrange theory of home care: A process for critique and replication. *Advances in Nursing Science, 25*(1), 50–64.

Smith, K., & Bazini-Barakat, N. (2003). A public health nursing practice model: Melding public health principles with the nursing process. *Public Health Nursing, 20*(1), 42–48.

Smith, M. C. (2013). Evaluation of middle range theories for the discipline of nursing. In M. J. Smith & P. R. Liehr (Eds.), *Middle range theory for nursing* (3rd ed., pp. 35–50). New York: Springer.

Smith, M. J. & Liehr, P. R. (Eds.). (2013). *Middle range theory for nursing* (3rd ed.). New York: Springer.

Sousa, V. D., & Zauszniewski, J. A. (2005). Toward a theory of diabetes self-care management. *Journal of Theory Construction and Testing, 9*(2), 61–67.

Sun, F. K., Long, A., Boore, J., & Tsao, L. I. (2006). A theory for the nursing care of patients at risk of suicide. *Journal of Advanced Nursing, 53*(6), 680–690.

Suppe, F. (1996, May). *Middle range theory: Nursing theory and knowledge development.* Paper presented at the Sixth Rosemary Ellis Scholar's Retreat, Cleveland, OH.

Swanson, K. M. (1991). Empirical development of a middle range theory of caring. *Nursing Research, 40*(3), 161–166.

Tsai, P. F. (2003). A middle range theory of caregiver stress. *Nursing Science Quarterly, 16*(2), 137–145.

Ulbrich, S. L. (1999). Nursing practice theory of exercise as self-care. *Image: The Journal of Nursing Scholarship, 31*(1), 65–70.

Wallace, R., Benson, H., & Wilson, A. F. (1971). A wakeful hypometabolic physiologic state. *American Journal of Physiology, 221*(3), 795–799.

Watson, J. (2005). *Caring science as sacred science.* Philadelphia: F. A. Davis.

Weiss, J. A., Jampol, M. L., Lievano, J. A., Smith, S. M., & Wurster, J. L. (2008). Normalizing risky sexual behaviors: A grounded theory study. *Pediatric Nursing, 34*(2), 163–169.

Whall, A. L. (2005). The structure of nursing knowledge: Analysis and evaluation of practice, middle range and grand theory. In J. J. Fitzpatrick & A. L. Whall (Eds.), *Conceptual models of nursing: Analysis and application* (4th ed., pp. 5–20). Upper Saddle River, NJ: Prentice-Hall.

Whittemore, R., & Roy, C. (2002). Adapting to diabetes mellitus: A theory synthesis. *Nursing Science Quarterly, 15*(4), 311–317.

CHAPTER 11

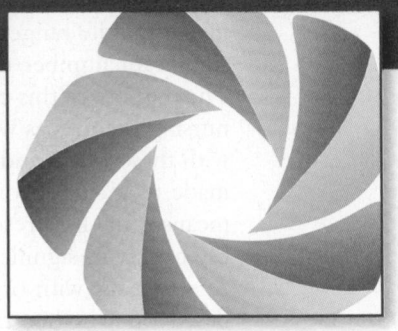

Overview of Selected Middle Range Nursing Theories

Melanie McEwen

Elaine Chavez is employed as a nurse at a public health clinic in an urban area. She is also in her second semester of a graduate nursing program preparing to become a mental health nurse practitioner. In her practice, Elaine has worked with a number of women who have been abused by their partners, and she has observed a pattern of comorbidities in these women, including depression, alcoholism, substance abuse, and suicide attempts. Over the last few months, Elaine has reviewed the nursing literature and identified several intervention strategies that have been effective in working with women who have been victims of domestic violence. Using this information, she would like to implement a program to promote early identification of abuse and multiple-level interventions. This is a project that will work well with one of her master's portfolio assignments.

From her literature review, Elaine identified several theories related to her study. She was particularly interested in examining the set of circumstances that would cause the women to seek help. For this, she performed a more detailed literature review and identified Kolcaba's (1994, 2003, 2013) Theory of Comfort, which helped her conceptualize many of the issues that the women faced. Indeed, the theory described individual characteristics that contributed to health-seeking behavior. These were stimulus situations, which can cause negative tension. By providing comfort measures, the nurse can help decrease negative tensions and promote positive tension. Elaine wanted to continue to identify comfort measures that would encourage the women to seek care for their problems.

For the next phase of her project, Elaine collected all of the information she could find on Kolcaba's theory. This included studies that had used the model as a conceptual framework and studies that had tested the model. From that information and the articles she had gathered previously about issues related to domestic violence, she was able to draft a set of interventions that she hoped to implement at the clinic following approval by her supervisor.

Previous chapters have described the growing emphasis on the development and testing of middle range theories in nursing. As a result, during the past two decades, a significant number of these theories have been presented in the nursing literature. The purpose of this chapter is to introduce some of the commonly used middle range nursing theories as well as some of the recently published ones to familiarize readers with these works and direct them to resources for more information. An attempt was made to include works from a variety of areas and from many scholars, but by no means is the list presented here exhaustive. Nor does inclusion or exclusion relate to the quality or significance of the theory or its usefulness in research or practice.

To assist with organization of the chapter, the theories are divided into sections based on whether they appear to be "high," "middle," or "low" middle range theories. As explained in Chapter 10, the high/middle/low distinction relates to the level of abstraction as posed by Liehr and Smith (1999), with the "high" middle range theories being the most abstract and nearest to the grand theories. The "low" middle range theories, on the other hand, are the least abstract, and they are similar to practice or situation-specific theories. It is noted that these designations are arguably arbitrary and that one theory that is listed here as "high middle" may be considered by others to be a grand theory. Likewise, another theory listed here as "middle middle" might be considered by others to be a high middle range theory, and so forth.

Elements of theory description and theory analysis as explained in Chapter 5 serve as the basis for the more detailed discussions of selected theories. Each will include a brief overview, an outline of the purpose and major concepts of the theory, and context for use and nursing implications. Finally, evidence of empirical testing and application in practice are described.

High Middle Range Theories

The high middle range theories presented here are some of the more well known and most widely used theories in nursing. Included are the works of Benner, Leininger, Pender, and Meleis. These theories may be considered grand theories or conceptual frameworks by other nursing scholars and possibly by the author of the theory. These theories, however, do not totally fit with the criteria for grand theories as outlined in this text and therefore are not covered in the chapters dealing with that content. In addition, the Synergy Model, a nursing model that is widely used in research and practice, particularly in critical care, will be discussed. Table 11-1 lists other high middle range theories or conceptual models, their purposes, and major concepts.

Benner's Model of Skill Acquisition in Nursing

Patricia Benner's theoretical model was first published in 1984. The model, which applies the Dreyfus model of skill acquisition to nursing, outlines five stages of skill acquisition: novice, advanced beginner, competent, proficient, and expert. Although her work is much more encompassing in regard to nursing domains and specific functions and interventions, it is the five stages of skill acquisition that has received the most attention with regard to application in administration, education, practice, and research.

Purpose and Major Concepts

Benner's model delineates the importance of retaining and rewarding nurse clinicians for their clinical expertise in practice settings because it describes the evolution of "excellent caring practices." She notes that research demonstrates that practice

Table 11-1 High Middle Range Nursing Theories

Theory/Model	Purpose	Major Concepts
Tidal model (psychiatric and mental health nursing) (Barker, 2001a, 2001b)	Describes psychiatric nursing practice focusing on three care processes; emphasizes the fluid nature of human experience characterized by change and unpredictability	Personhood (dimensions—world, self, others), discrete holistic (exploratory) assessment; focused (risk) assessment, empowerment, narrative as the medium of self
Parish nursing (Bergquist & King, 1994)	Describes the integration of physical, emotional, and spiritual components in provision of holistic health care in a faith community	Client (spiritual, physical, emotional components), parish nurse (spiritual maturity, pastoral team member, autonomy, caring, effective communication), health (physical, emotional, and spiritual wellness and wholeness), environment (faith community)
Parish nursing (Miller, 1997)	Integrates the concepts of evangelical Christianity with application of parish nursing interventions	Person/parishioner, health, nurse/parish nurse, community/parish, the triune God
Neal theory of home health nursing (Neal, 1999a, 1999b)	Describes the practice of home health nurses as they use process of adaptation to attain autonomy	Autonomy, three stages (dependence, moderate dependence, and autonomy), logistics, client's home, client's resources, client's needs, and learning capacity
Occupational health nursing (Rogers, 1994)	Shows how the occupational health nurse works to improve, protect, maintain, and restore the health of the worker/workforce and depicts how practice is affected by both external and internal work setting influences	Work setting influences (corporate culture/mission, resources, work hazards, workforce characteristics), external factors (economics, population/health trends, legislation/politics, technology), occupational health nursing practice (health promotion, workplace hazard detection, case management/primary care, counseling, management, research, legal/ethical monitoring, community orientation)
Omaha System (Martin, 2005)	Comprehensive classification system that promotes documentation of client care, generally in community and home health nursing practice	Depicts the nursing process as circular rather than linear; steps are: collect and assess data, state problems, identify admission problem rating, plan and intervene, identify interim/dismissal problem rating, and evaluate problem outcomes.
Schuler Nurse Practitioner Practice Model (Schuler & Davis, 1993).	Integrates essential nursing and medical orientations to provide a framework for holistic practice for nurse practitioners (NP)	Patient and NP inputs (noted as episodic and comprehensive with and without health problem); data gathering/role modeling; patient and NP throughputs include identification of problems and diagnosing, contracting, and planning and implementing of the plan of care. Outputs involve comprehensive evaluation of patient and NP outcomes.
Public health nursing practice (Smith & Bazini-Barakat, 2003)	Guides public health nurses to improve the health of communities and target populations	Interdisciplinary public health team, standards of public health nursing practice, essential public health services, health indicators, population-based practice (systems, community, individual, and family focus), healthy people in health communities
Rural nursing (Weinert & Long, 1991)	Guides rural nursing practice, research, and education by understanding and addressing the unique health care needs and preferences of rural persons	Health (health as ability to work), environment (distance and isolation), person (self-reliance and independence), nursing (lack of anonymity, outsider/insider, and old-timer/newcomer)

grows "through experiential learning and through transmitting that learning in practical settings" (Benner, 2001, p. vi). Expertise develops when the clinician tests and refines propositions, hypotheses, and principle-based expectations in actual practice situations. Finally, the model seeks to describe clinical expertise including six areas of practical knowledge (graded qualitative distinctions; common meanings; assumptions, expectations, and sets; paradigm cases and personal knowledge; maxims; and unplanned practices) (Benner, Tanner, & Chesla, 2009).

The central concepts of Benner's model are those of competence, skill acquisition, experience, clinical knowledge, and practical knowledge. She also identifies the following seven domains of nursing practice:

- Helping role
- Teaching or coaching function
- Diagnostic client-monitoring function
- Effective management of rapidly changing situations
- Administering and monitoring therapeutic interventions and regimens
- Monitoring and ensuring quality of health care practices
- Organizational and work-role competencies (Benner, 2001)

Context for Use and Nursing Implications

The Benner model has been used extensively as rationale for career development and continuing education in nursing. Areas specifically cited for utilization include nursing management, career enhancement, clinical specialization, staff development programs, staffing, evaluation, clinical internships, and precepting students and novice nurses (Benner, 2001; Benner et al., 2009).

Evidence of Empirical Testing and Application in Practice

Over the previous decade, dozens of articles have been written based on Benner's model, and a number of these were research-based studies. For example, Keilman and Dunn (2010) used Benner's work as a conceptual framework in a study examining advanced practice nurses' effectiveness in diagnosing, treating, and managing urinary incontinence. In other research, Meretoja and Koponen (2011) used Benner's model to compare nurses' optimal and actual competencies in clinical settings, and Abraham (2011) reported on a study to evaluate a program based on Benner's model, which was designed to develop leadership skills and professionalism. In qualitative studies, Lyneham, Parkinson, and Denholm (2008) used Benner's model to examine the notion of "intuition" among expert Emergency Department (ED) nurses, and Uhrenfeldt and Hall (2009) examined how "proficient" nursing leaders worked with their staff to improve high-quality care for patients.

Non–research-based articles included a report by Cathcart (2008), which explained the role of the chief nursing officer based on tenets of Benner's work, and a personal account of a nurse describing her orientation experiences as she transitioned from an experienced and expert nurse in a medical-surgical unit into her new role in the ED of a trauma teaching hospital (Hatfield, 2011). A fairly common theme was noted as several writers discussed Benner's applicability in development of procedures and protocols for orientation of new nurses and new graduates into specialty areas. For example, Coyle (2011) presented an internship program in home health for new graduates, Dumchin (2010) described a method for using online learning experiences to develop perioperative nurses, Brixey and Mahon (2010) described an evaluation tool to assess the practice of oncology nurses, and Wilson, Harwood, Oudshoorn, and Thompson (2010) examined the practice of hemodialysis nurses and observed a theme of "perpetual novice." Finally, Benner's work was used in several articles (e.g., Haag-Heitman, 2012; Owens & Cleaves, 2012; Vuorinen, Heino, & Meretoja, 2009) to discuss the development or updating of career enhancement or clinical ladder programs.

Leininger's Cultural Care Diversity and Universality Theory

Madeleine Leininger was instrumental in demonstrating to nurses the importance of considering the impact of culture on health and healing (Leininger, 2002). Prior to her death in 2012, she was a prolific nursing researcher and scholar, and she is credited with starting the specialty of transcultural nursing. In addition, she was a leading proponent of the idea that nursing is synonymous with caring.

Leininger reported that she conceptualized transcultural nursing as a distinct area of nursing practice in the late 1950s during her doctoral work in anthropology; she continued to study and develop a transcultural nursing conceptual framework throughout the 1960s. In the mid-1970s, she presented a "transcultural health model" that was expanded in 1978 and 1980. The Leininger Sunrise Model was first described as such in 1984 and depicts the transcultural dimensions of culturologic interviews, assessments, and therapies (Leininger & McFarland, 2006; McFarland, 2010).

Purpose and Major Concepts

The purpose of Leininger's theory is to generate knowledge related to the nursing care of people who value their cultural heritage and lifeways. Major concepts of the model are culture, culture care, and culture care differences (diversities) and similarities (universals) pertaining to transcultural human care. Other major concepts are care and caring, emic view (language expressions, perceptions, beliefs, and practice of individuals or groups of a particular culture in regard to certain phenomena), etic view (universal language expression beliefs and practices in regard to certain phenomena that pertain to several cultures or groups), lay system of health care, professional system of health care, and culturally congruent nursing care (Leininger, 2007; McFarland, 2010).

Context for Use and Nursing Implications

The goal for application of Leininger's theory is to provide culturally congruent nursing care to persons of diverse cultures. A central tenet of the theory is that it is important for the nurse to understand the individual's view of illness. Also, the focus is on recognizing and understanding cultural similarities and differences and using this information to positively influence nursing care and health (Leininger & McFarland, 2006). The theory has been widely used for research, and findings are appropriate for nurses in any setting who work with individuals, families, and groups from a cultural background different from the nurse's.

Evidence of Empirical Testing and Application in Practice

Leininger (2007) explained that her theory was derived and refined through a number of years of study. Over the past two decades, research on various groups was conducted, and she listed cultural values and culture care meanings and action modes for 23 cultural groups in her book. Many graduate students and nursing scholars have used Leininger's theory as a basis for research, and as a result, hundreds of examples of articles can be located in the literature. Many of these used Leininger's work as a conceptual framework to study cultural implications of a variety of health problems. For example, Long and colleagues (2012) examined health beliefs among four different Latino subgroups specifically related to type 2 diabetes; Gillum and colleagues

(2011) researched cardiovascular disease in the Amish; and Vogler, Altmann, and Zoucha (2010) studied the attitudes and perceptions of native Hawaiians regarding cultural sensitivity of health care providers.

Leininger's model has also been used by many authors to identify variables or characteristics of cultural groups or subcultures that might influence health. For example, Hallas, Fernandez, Lim, and Carobene (2011) examined strategies to reduce early childhood caries in culturally diverse populations, and Lee (2012) used Leininger-inspired "ethnonursing research methods" to discover care meanings and expression among Appalachian mothers living with their children in a homeless shelter.

A number of non-research articles describing aspects of transcultural nursing and focusing on Leininger's works have also been published in recent years. These include a review of cultural education in nursing (Campesino, 2008), a report on how to enhance awareness of diversity and racism in nursing education (Lancellotti, 2008), and an article describing the "evolution of the African American family" (Revell & McGhee, 2012). Other examples of research studies using Leininger's model are listed in Box 11-1.

Pender's Health Promotion Model

Nola Pender began studying health-promoting behavior in the mid-1970s and first published the Health Promotion Model (HPM) in 1982. She reported that the model was constructed from expectancy-value theory and social cognitive theory using a nursing perspective. The model was modified slightly in the late 1980s and again in 1996 (Pender, 1996; Pender, Murdaugh, & Parsons, 2011).

Purpose and Major Concepts

The HPM was proposed as a framework for integrating nursing and behavioral science perspectives on factors that influence health behaviors. The model is to be used as a guide to explore the biopsychosocial processes that motivate individuals to engage

Box 11-1 Research Studies Using Leininger's Theory of Cultural Care Diversity and Universality

Coleman, J. (2009). Culture care meanings of African American parents related to infant mortality and health care. *Journal of Cultural Diversity, 16*(3), 109–119.

Evans, J., Bell, J. L., Sweeney, A. E., Morgan, J. I., & Kelly, H. M. (2010). Confidence in critical care nursing. *Nursing Science Quarterly, 23*(4), 334–340.

Lange, J., Evans-Benard, S., Cooper, J., Fahey, E., Kalapos, M., Tice, D., et al. (2009). Puerto Rican women's perceptions of heart disease risk. *Clinical Nursing Research, 18*(4), 291–306.

Lewallen, L. P., & Street, D. J. (2010). Initiating and sustaining breastfeeding in African American women. *JOGNN: Journal of Obstetric, Gynecologic & Neonatal Nursing, 39*(6), 667–674.

Millender, E. (2012). Acculturation stress among Maya in the United States. *Journal of Cultural Diversity, 19*(2), 58–70.

Morris, E. J. (2012). Respect, protection, faith and love: Major care constructs identified within the subculture of selected urban African American adolescent gang members. *Journal of Transcultural Nursing, 23*(3), 262–269.

Wagner, J. (2009). Barriers for Hispanic women in receiving the human papillomavirus vaccine: A nursing challenge. *Clinical Journal of Oncology Nursing, 13*(6), 671–675.

in behaviors directed toward health enhancement (Pender et al., 2011). The model has been used extensively as a framework for research aimed at predicting health-promoting lifestyles as well as specific behaviors.

Major concepts of the HPM are individual characteristics and experiences (prior related behavior and personal factors), behavior-specific cognitions and affect (perceived benefits of action, perceived barriers to action, perceived self-efficacy, activity-related affect, interpersonal influences, and situational influences), and behavioral outcomes (commitment to a plan of action, immediate competing demands and preferences, and health-promoting behavior). Figure 11-1 shows the HPM.

Context for Use and Nursing Implications

Health promotion interventions are essential for improving the health of populations everywhere. It is noted that people of all ages can benefit from health promotion care, which should be delivered at sites where people spend much of their time (e.g., schools and workplaces). Nurses can develop and execute health-promoting interventions to individuals, groups, and families in schools, nursing centers, occupational health settings,

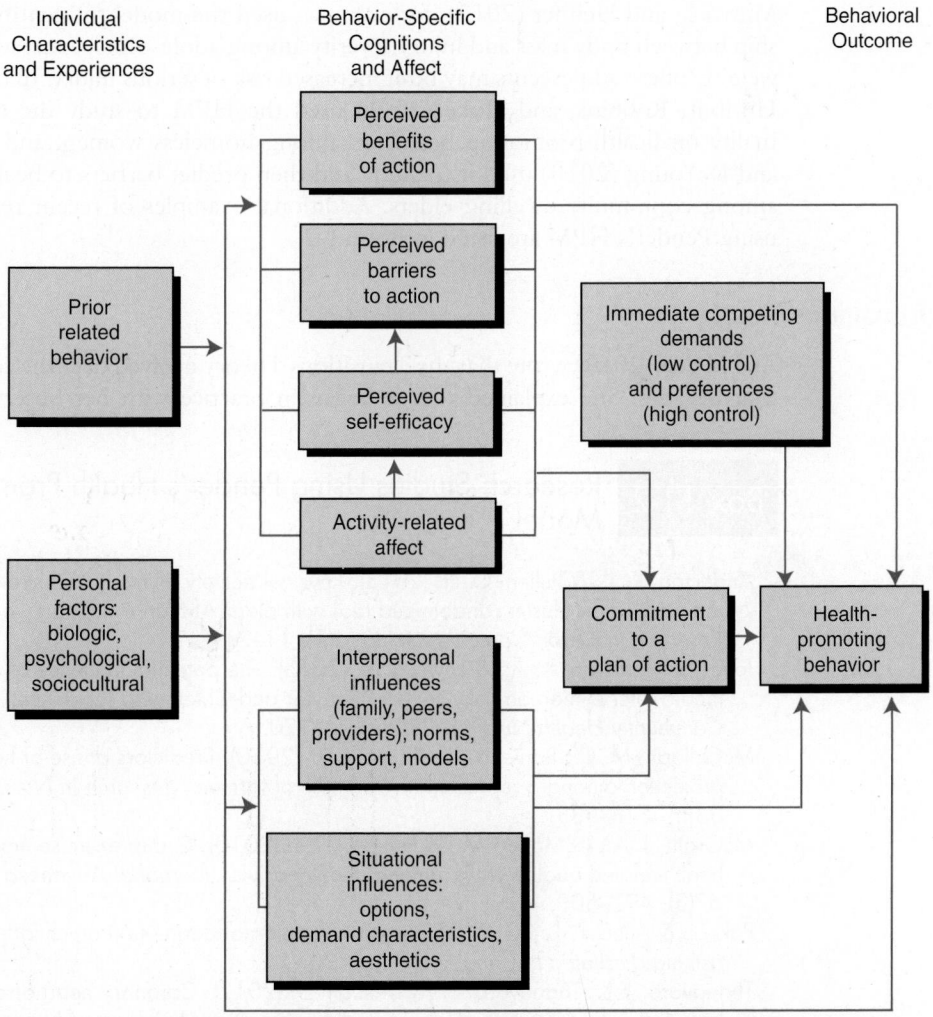

Figure 11-1 Health promotion model. (Adapted from Pender, N. J., Murdaugh, C. L., & Parsons, M. A. (2011). *Health promotion in nursing practice* (6th ed.). Reprinted by permission of Pearson Education, Inc., Upper Saddle River, NJ.)

and the community at large. Nurses should work toward empowerment for self-care and enhancing the client's capacity for self-care through education and personal development.

Evidence of Empirical Testing and Application in Practice

Pender and colleagues (2011) wrote that the model has been used by a very significant number of nursing scholars and researchers and has been useful in explaining and predicting specific health behaviors. Indeed, in the last decade, more than 250 English language articles that reported using or applying Pender's HPM have been published.

Most research studies used Pender's work as one component of a conceptual framework for study. For example, Wise and Arcamone (2011) used the HPM to study food choices of adolescents during pregnancy, and Maglione and Hayman (2009) used the model to explain how social support, self-efficacy and a commitment plan influenced physical activity in college students. Also focusing on physical activity, Esposito and Fitzpatrick (2011) examined the relationship between nurses' beliefs about the benefits of exercise, their personal exercise behavior, and their recommendation of exercise to their patients.

Other studies use health promotion as an outcome or to predict behaviors. Burns, Murrock, and Heifner (2012), for example, used the model to identify the relationship between body mass and injury severity among adolescents, concluding that overweight/obese adolescents may be at increased risk of serious injury. In other research, Hurlbut, Robbins, and Hoke (2011) used the HPM to study the effect of spirituality on health-promoting behaviors among homeless women, and Stark, Chase, and DeYoung (2010) used it to study and then predict barriers to health promotion among community-dwelling elders. Additional examples of recent research studies using Pender's HPM are listed in Box 11-2.

Transitions Theory

Afaf Meleis (2010) wrote that the Transitions Theory evolved over the course of about four decades. She explained that it began in practice with her observations of the

Box 11-2 Research Studies Using Pender's Health Promotion Model

Anderson, K. J., & Pullen, C. H. (2013). Physical activity with spiritual strategies intervention: A cluster randomized trial with older African American women. *Research in Gerontological Nursing, 6*(1), 11–21.

Jones, K., Baldwin, K. A., & Lewis, P. R. (2012). The potential influence of a social media intervention on risky sexual behavior and Chlamydia incidence. *Journal of Community Health Nursing, 29*(2), 106–120.

McCullagh, M. C., Ronis, D. L., & Lusk, S. L. (2010). Predictors of use of hearing protection among a representative sample of farmers. *Research in Nursing & Health, 33*(6), 528–538.

McGrath, J. A., O'Malley, M., & Hendrix, T. J. (2010). Group exercise mode and health-related quality of life among healthy adults. *Journal of Advanced Nursing, 67*(3), 491–500.

Pak, L., & Allen, P. J. (2012). The impact of maternal depression on children with asthma. *Pediatric Nursing, 38*(1), 11–30.

Thanavaro, J. L., Thanavaro, S., & Delicath, T. (2012). Coronary heart disease knowledge tool for women. *Journal of the American Academy of Nurse Practitioners, 22*(2), 62–69.

experiences that humans face as they deal with changes relating to health, well-being, and their ability to care for themselves. Meleis' work moved through multiple steps, including concept analysis and several comprehensive literature reviews. The result was a conclusion that "transitions" is a central concept in nursing (Schumacher & Meleis, 1994). More focused attention through observation and research has contributed to formal development, testing, and application of the theory (Meleis, 2010).

Purpose and Major Concepts

Transitions Theory attempts to describe and attend to the interactions between nurses and patients, suggesting that nurses are concerned with the experiences of people as they undergo transitions whenever health and well-being are the desired outcome. The goal of "nursing therapeutics," then, is to conceptualize and address the potential problems that individuals encounter during transitional experiences and develop preventative and therapeutic interventions to support the patient during these occasions (George & Hickman, 2011; Im, 2010; Meleis, 2010).

Meleis (2010) defined transitions as "a passage from one fairly stable state to another fairly stable state, and it is a process triggered by a change" (p. 11). Further, transitions are characterized by different stages, milestones, and turning points. These changes, or transitions, can be assisted or managed by nurse as they care for patients.

Numerous years of research and analysis into transitions led Meleis and her colleagues to the identification "of four major categories of transitions that nurses tend to be involved in" (Meleis, 2010, p. 3). These transitions and representative examples are:

- Developmental transitions—birth, adolescence, menopause, aging, death
- Situational transitions—changes in educational and professional roles, changes in family situations (e.g., divorce, widowhood) or living arrangements (e.g., move to a nursing home, homelessness)
- Health–illness transitions—recovery process, hospital discharge, diagnosis of chronic illness
- Organizational transition—changing environmental conditions that affect the lives of clients; may be social, political, or economic (Im, 2010).

Other key concepts include "patterns" and "properties" of the transitions. Patterns denote whether the transitions are single, multiple, sequential, simultaneous, related, or unrelated. Properties of the transition experience are often interrelated in a complex way and refer to awareness, engagement, change/difference, time span, and critical points and events (Im, 2010).

In Transitions Theory, the nurse must consider the "facilitators" and "inhibitors" of the transition conditions. These include personal meanings, cultural beliefs and attitudes, socioeconomic status, preparation, and knowledge. Community conditions and societal conditions may also facilitate or inhibit transitions (Im, 2010).

"Nursing therapeutics" are those activities and actions that nurses may take during times of transitions (Schumacher & Meleis, 1994). These include assessment of readiness (assessment of each of the transition's conditions), preparation for transition (typically involves education to enhance optimal conditions to prepare for transition), and role supplementation (use of education and practice to facilitate the transitional process) (George & Hickman, 2011). The outcomes of transitions, and potential for nursing therapeutics, include the "patterns of response" of the patient. These are designated as process indicators (feeling connected, interacting, locating and being situated, developing confidence, and coping) and outcome indicators (mastery and "fluid integrative identities") (Im, 2010). Figure 11-2 shows the interaction of the major constructs of the theory.

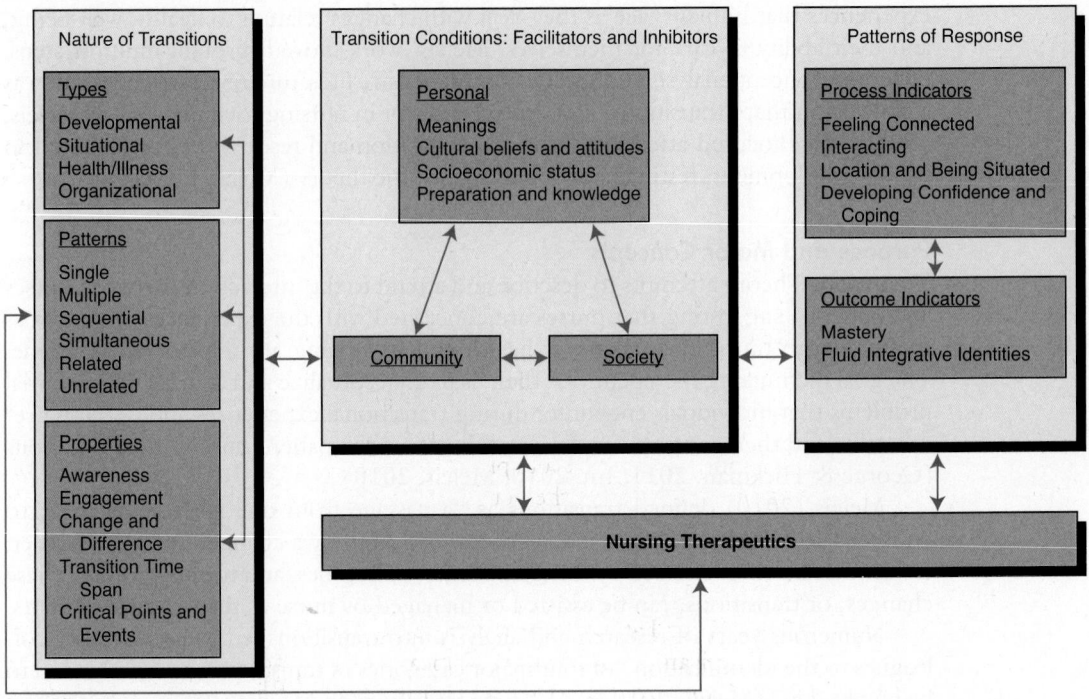

Figure 11-2 Transitions Theory. (From Meleis, A. I., Sawyer, L. M., Im., E. O., Messias, D. K. H., & Schumacher, K. (2000). Experiencing transitions: An emerging middle range theory. *Advances in Nursing Science, 23*(10), 12–28. Used with permission.)

Context for Use and Nursing Implications

According to Meleis (2010), most nursing care occurs during a transition that the patient is experiencing, and the goal of nursing care is to promote or encourage health outcomes during these occasions. Indeed, Meleis and Trangenstein (1994) defined nursing as the art and science of facilitation of the transitions of health and well-being and noted that nurses are concerned "with the processes and experiences of human beings undergoing transitions where health and perceived well-being is the outcome" (p. 257).

Transitions Theory is widely applicable and provides a comprehensive guide that considers cultural and social diversity. It was developed from multiple research studies among very diverse groups of people, during many types of transitions. Additionally, it has been shown repeatedly to be able to direct nursing practice, research, and education.

Evidence of Empirical Testing and Application in Practice

Transitions Theory has been based both in research and generated research (George & Hickman, 2011; Meleis, 2010). Meleis (2010) recently compiled and published a history of the development of the theory along with multiple examples of research and application in practice. Additional examples are becoming increasingly evident in the literature. Some of these focus on research examining patient transitions encountered by nurses in various specialty areas. For example, Reedy and Blum (2010) addressed patients experiencing transitions following bariatric surgery; Rew, Tyler, Fredland, and Hannah (2012) examined adolescents' concerns as they transition through high school; Halding and Heggdal (2011) looked at patients' experiences of health transitions during pulmonary rehabilitation; and Haggstrom, Asplund, and Kristiansen (2012) researched patients' transition from the intensive care unit (ICU).

Several research studies using Transitions Theory focused on the experience of caregivers. One (Blum & Sherman, 2010) was an extensive review of the literature to examine the transitions encountered by patients with cancer and their caregivers. The intent was to develop more focused interventions and allocation of resources to assist the caregivers during this change. In another example, Dossa, Bokhour, and Hoenig (2012) performed a grounded theory study that examined the transitions from hospital to home for patients with mobility impairments and their family caregivers; they concluded that health care providers need to improve systems to address patient concerns after discharge, focusing on improving communication and coordination to facilitate recovery and prevent complications.

Finally, Geary and Schumacher (2012) presented an interesting look at the integration of Transitions Theory with concepts from complexity science. They argued that the complexity of many of the transition situations encountered by nurses today is better described when the theories are integrated, concluding that the integration encourages recognition that transitions affect many, including the patients, their caregivers, health care providers, and the health care system. Integration of the theories should enhance dialogue and promote better understanding of the situations through changing outcomes for the better.

The Synergy Model

The Synergy Model for Patient Care was developed in the mid-1990s by a panel of nurses of the American Association of Critical-Care Nurses (AACN) Certification Corporation as a framework for certified practice. The initial model was revised somewhat, and the revised version was then used as the basis for the AACN's certification examination (Curley, 2007; Hardin, 2013).

Purpose and Major Concepts

The purpose of the Synergy Model is to articulate nurses' contributions, activities, and outcomes with regard to caring for critically ill patients. The model identifies eight patient needs or characteristics and eight competencies of nurses in critical care situations (AACN, 2013). "According to the model, each patient brings a unique set of characteristics to the health care situation" (Hardin, 2005, p. 4). Of the many unique characteristics nurses assess, the eight most consistently observed are listed in Box 11-3. The nursing competencies denote how knowledge, skills, and experience are integrated within nursing care.

Box 11-3 The Synergy Model: Patient Characteristics and Nurse Competencies

Patient Characteristics	Nurse Competencies
Resiliency	Clinical judgment
Vulnerability	Clinical inquiry
Stability	Facilitation of learning
Complexity	Collaboration
Resource availability	Systems thinking
Participation in care	Advocacy and moral agency
Participation in decision-making	Caring practices
Predictability	Response to diversity

Source: AACN (2013).

The Synergy Model also describes three levels of outcomes—those relating to the patient, the nurse, and the system. Patient outcomes include functional and behavioral change, trust, satisfaction, comfort, and quality of life. Nurse outcomes include physiologic changes, presence or absence of complications, and extent to which care objectives were attained. System outcomes include recidivism, costs, and resource utilization (Curley, 1998; 2007). Figure 11-3 depicts the Synergy Model.

Context for Use and Nursing Implications

As mentioned, the Synergy Model was originally developed to structure the AACN's certification examination by identifying nursing competencies that are essential for those providing care to the critically ill. In 2002, assumptions of the model were expanded to establish it as a conceptual framework for designing practice and developing competencies required to care for critically ill patients. Use of the Synergy Model in practice is designed to optimize patient outcomes. When patient characteristics and nurse competencies match and synergize, outcomes for the patient are optimal (Curley, 2007; Hardin, 2013). In addition, the model can be used for developing nursing curricula and for conducting research (Curley, 2007; Hardin, 2013).

Evidence of Empirical Testing and Application in Practice

Although the Synergy Model is relatively new, a significant number of articles have been published describing its use in practice and education. Identified were two articles that

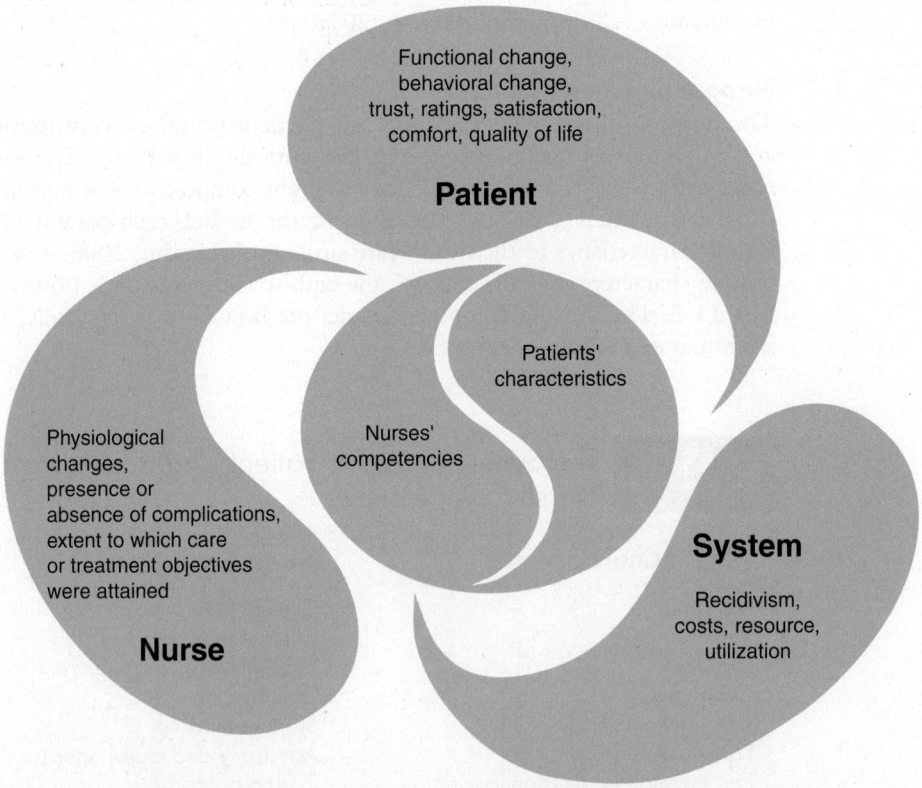

Figure 11-3 The Synergy Model delineates three levels of outcomes: Those derived from the patient, those derived from the nurse, and those derived from the health care system. (From Curley, M. A. Q. (1998). Patient–nurse synergy: Optimizing patients' outcomes. *American Journal of Critical Care, 7*(1), 69. Used with permission of American Association of Critical-Care Nurses.)

Box 11-4 The Synergy Model in Practice and Education

Durkin, G. (2010). Development and implementation of an independence rating scale and evaluation process for nursing orientation of new graduates. *Journal of Nurses in Staff Development, 26*(2), 64–72.

Freyling, M. E., Kesten, K. S., & Heath, J. (2008). The Synergy Model at work in a military ICU in Iraq. *Critical Care Nursing Clinics of North America, 20*(1), 23–29.

Goran, S. F. (2011). A new view: Tele-intensive care unit competencies. *Critical Care Nurse, 31*(5), 17–29.

Gralton, K. S., & Brett, S. A. (2012). Integrating the Synergy Model for patient care at Children's Hospital of Wisconsin. *Journal of Pediatric Nursing, 27*(1), 74–81.

Hardin, S. R. (2012). Engaging families to participate in care of older critical care patients. *Critical Care Nurse, 32*(3), 35–40.

Kaplow, R., & Reed, K. D. (2008). The AACN Synergy Model for Patient Care: A nursing model as a force of magnetism. *Nursing Economics, 26*(1), 17–25.

Kohr, L. M., Hickey, P. A., & Curley, M. A. Q. (2012). Building a nursing productivity measure based on the Synergy Model: First steps. *American Journal of Critical Care, 21*(6), 420–431.

Schulman, C. S. (2010). Standards for frequency of measurement and documentation of vital signs and physical assessments. *Critical Care Nurse, 30*(3), 74–76.

tested application of the model in critical care situations. For example, Arashin (2010) described development and implementation of a guide for "Rapid Response Teams" to provide interventional care to patients experiencing acute changes in their conditions using the Synergy Model as a guide. In another work, Stacy (2011) used the Synergy Model as a framework when reporting on "progressive care units," which are increasingly being used to bridge the gap between ICUs and medical-surgical units. A few works (Hardin, 2012; Tejero, 2011; Wysong & Driver, 2009) described research studies using the Synergy Model as a framework. Box 11-4 shows several examples of articles describing the model's use in leadership/administration, practice, and education.

Middle Middle Range Theories

A number of nursing theories may be categorized as "middle middle range." Four theories that have been cited in a considerable number of nursing studies are discussed in the following sections. They are Mishel's (1984) Uncertainty in Illness Theory; Kolcaba's (1994) Theory of Comfort; Lenz and colleagues' Theory of Unpleasant Symptoms (Lenz, Suppe, Gift, Pugh, & Milligan, 1995; Lenz, Pugh, Milligan, Gift, & Suppe, 1997); and Reed's (1991a) Self-Transcendence Theory. Table 11-2 lists other middle middle range theories that have been used in nursing practice and research.

Mishel's Uncertainty in Illness Theory

Merle Mishel began studying the concept of uncertainty in illness in the early 1980s when she desired to explain the stress that results from hospitalization (Mishel, 1981, 1984). She developed the Mishel Uncertainty in Illness Scale to better examine the concept, and since that time, her model and instrument have been used in numerous nursing studies (Bailey & Stewart, 2010; Mishel, 1984, 1988). In the late 1980s, she formally developed the theory, which she then revised in the early 1990s (Mishel, 1988, 1990).

Table 11-2 Middle Middle Range Nursing Theories

Theory/Model	Purpose	Major Concepts
Self-help (Braden, 1990)	Describes a process of factors that decrease self and life quality and factors that increase learning a self-help response and thus a greater quality of life	Disease characteristics, background inducements, monitoring (level of information about illness), severity of illness, dependency, uncertainty, enabling skill, self-help, life quality
Chronic illness trajectory framework (Corbin & Strauss, 1991, 1992)	Describes a view of chronic illness with eight phases, from pretrajectory to dying, with each possessing the possibilities of reversals, plateaus, and upward or downward movement; allows for conceptualization of the course of illness to comprehensively direct care and conduct research	Trajectory, trajectory phases (pretrajectory, trajectory onset, crisis, acute, stable, unstable, downward, and dying), trajectory projection, trajectory scheme (shape illness course, control symptoms, and handle disability)
Motivation in health behavior (health behavior, self-determinism) (Cox, 1985)	Describes intrinsic motivation in health behavior	Individual's self-determined health judgments, self-determined health behavior, perceived competency in health matters, internal–external cue responsiveness
Theory of care-seeking behavior (Lauver, 1992)	Explains the probability of engaging in health behavior as a function of psychosocial variables and facilitating conditions regarding the behavior	Clinical and sociodemographic variables, affect (feelings associated with care-seeking behavior), utility (expectations and values about outcomes), normative influences, habits, care-seeking behavior
Self-efficacy (Lenz & Shortridge-Baggett, 2002)	Applies Bandura's work in nursing to assist people to be as independent as possible in managing their health	Person (perception, self-referent), behavior (initiation, effort, persistence), efficacy–expectation (magnitude, strength, generality), information sources (performance, vicarious experiences, verbal persuasion, physiologic information), and outcome expectations
Model for social support (Norbeck, 1981)	Outlines the elements and relationships that must be studied to incorporate social support into nursing practice; emphasis placed on developing the environment	Properties of the person (age, demographic characteristics, needs), properties of the situation (role demands, resources, stressors), need for social support, available social support
Theory of resilience (Polk, 1997)	Proposes interrelatedness of dispositional, relational, situational, and philosophical patterns to describe concept of resilience to guide generation of nursing interventions to assess and strengthen resilience	Dispositional pattern (pattern of physical and ego-related psychosocial attributes that contribute to manifestation of resilience), relational pattern (roles and relationships that influence resilience), situational pattern (characteristic approach to situations or stressors), philosophical pattern (personal beliefs)
Theory of caring (Swanson, 1991)	Proposes a definition of caring and the five essential categories or processes that characterize caring	Knowing, being with, doing for, enabling, and maintaining belief

Purpose and Major Concepts

According to Mishel (1988, 1999), the Uncertainty in Illn
ents cognitively process illness-related stimuli and constr
Uncertainty is seen as the inability to structure meaning an
does not form a "cognitive schema for illness events" (Mishel, 1

The early iteration of the model (Mishel, 1988) described t
"stimuli frame" (symptom pattern, event familiarity, event congruency,
nitive capacities," and "structure providers" (credible authority, social supp
education) that may lead to uncertainty. Other concepts include appraisal, inference, illusion, and opportunity, as well as coping mechanisms; these may lead to adaptation. In 1990, the process of theory derivation was used to update and revise the theory to address issues related to chronic uncertainty. Interestingly, chaos theory was used in this process (Mishel, 1990). Figure 11-4 shows the Uncertainty in Illness Theory.

Context for Use and Nursing Implications

The Uncertainty in Illness Theory explains how individuals cognitively process illness-related stimuli and how they structure meaning for those events. In the theory, adaptation is the desirable end-state achieved after coping with the uncertainty. Nurses may develop nursing interventions that attempt to influence the person's cognitive process to address the uncertainty. This, in turn, should produce positive coping and adaptation (Mishel, 1984, 1999).

Evidence of Empirical Testing and Application in Practice

During the process of theory development and refinement, Mishel developed and tested several research instruments. These are the Adult Uncertainty in Illness Scale

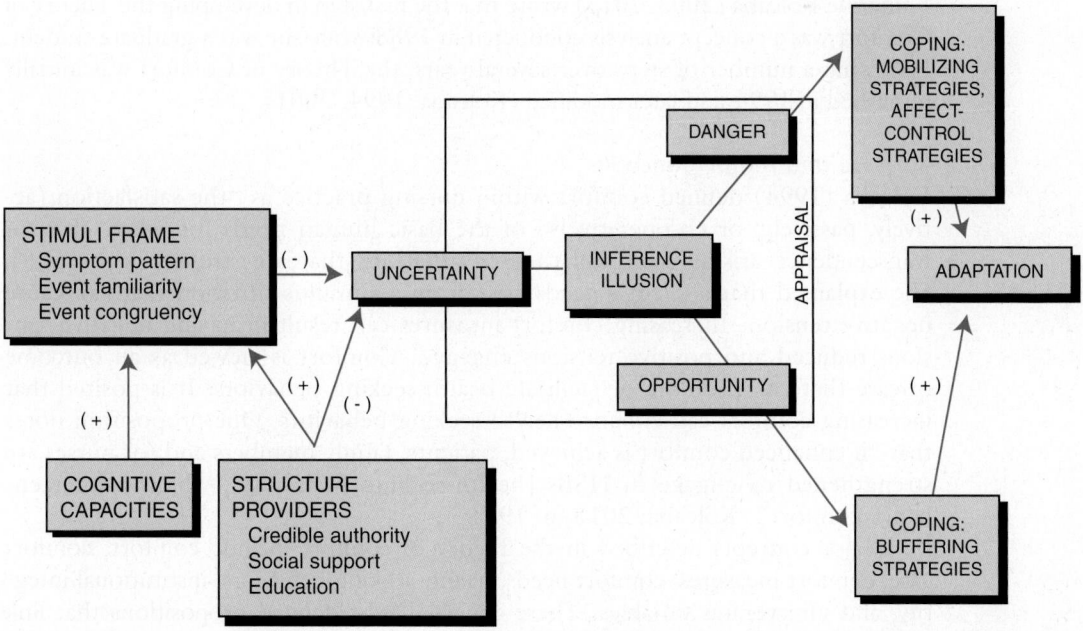

Figure 11-4 Model of perceived uncertainty in illness. (From Mishel, M. H. (1990). Reconceptualization of the uncertainty in illness theory. *Image: Journal of Nursing Scholarship, 22*(4), 256–262. Used with permission of John Wiley & Sons, Ltd.)

and the Adult Uncertainty in Illness Scale—Community Form; the Parents' Perception of Uncertainty in Illness Scale; the Parents' Perception of Uncertainty in Illness Scale—Family Member (Mishel, 2013); and the Uncertainty Scale for Kids (Stewart, Lynn, & Mishel, 2010).

The Uncertainty in Illness model is becoming increasingly recognized in nursing literature as a resource for research and practice. A significant number of articles have been published involving Mishel's work, and a number of research studies were identified using Mishel's theory or instruments or both in addressing health issues among a wide variety of groups and covering many different health problems. For example, Mishel and colleagues (2009) conducted a clinical trial to use educational prompts and communication skills training as an intervention to manage uncertainty about treatment decision making in early stage prostate cancer. In another work, a research group headed by Bailey (2010) examined uncertainty and fatigue in patients with chronic hepatitis C; Lin, Yeh, and Mishel (2010) used Mishel's theory to examine uncertainty in parents of children with cancer; and Cahill, LoBiondo-Wood, Bergstrom, and Armstrong (2012) conducted an integrative literature search to identify antecedents to uncertainty among patients with brain tumors. Interestingly, most identified research using Mishel's theory was directed at oncology patients and their families. In addition to those studies mentioned earlier, Halliday and Boughton (2011) examined uncertainty related to reproduction and motherhood after cancer in young adult women; Germino and colleagues (2013) looked at uncertainty management in breast cancer survivors; and Suzuki (2012) studied quality of life, uncertainty, and involvement in decision-making among patients with cancer of the head or neck.

Kolcaba's Theory of Comfort

Katherine Kolcaba (2003, 2013) wrote that the first step in developing the Theory of Comfort was a concept analysis conducted in 1988 while she was a graduate student. Following a number of steps over several years, the Theory of Comfort was initially published in 1994 and later modified (Kolcaba, 1994, 2001).

Purpose and Major Concepts

Kolcaba (1994) defined comfort within nursing practice as "the satisfaction (actively, passively, or co-operatively) of the basic human needs for relief, ease, or transcendence arising from health care situations that are stressful" (p. 1178). She explained that a client's needs arise from a stimulus situation that can cause negative tension. Increasing comfort measures can result in having negative tensions reduced and positive tensions engaged. Comfort is viewed as an outcome of care that can promote or facilitate health-seeking behaviors. It is posited that increasing comfort can enhance health-seeking behaviors. One proposition notes that "if enhanced comfort is achieved, patients, family members and/or nurses are strengthened to engage in HSBs [health-seeking behaviors], which further enhance comfort" (Kolcaba, 2013, p. 197).

Major concepts described in the theory of comfort include comfort, comfort care, comfort measures, comfort needs, health-seeking behaviors, institutional integrity, and intervening variables. There are also eight defined propositions that link the defined concepts (Box 11-5) (Kolcaba, 2001, 2013). Figure 11-5 presents the Theory of Comfort.

Box 11-5 Propositions of Comfort Theory

1. Nurses and members of the health care team identify comfort needs of patients and family members.
2. Nurses design and coordinate interventions to address comfort needs.
3. Intervening variables are considered when designing interventions.
4. When interventions are delivered in a caring manner and are effective, the outcome of enhanced comfort is attained.
5. Patients, nurses and other health care team members agree on desirable and realistic health-seeking behaviors.
6. If enhanced comfort is achieved, patients, family members, and/or nurses are more likely to engage in health-seeking behaviors; these further enhance comfort.
7. When patients and family members are given comfort care and engage in health-seeking behaviors, they are more satisfied with health care and have better health-related outcomes.
8. When patients, families, and nurses are satisfied with health care in an institution, public acknowledgment about that institution's contributions to health care will help the institution remain viable and flourish. Evidence-based practice or policy improvements may be guided by these propositions and the theoretical framework.

Adapted from Kolcaba (2001, 2013).

Context for Use and Nursing Implications

Comfort Theory observes that patients experience needs for comfort in stressful health care situations. Some of these needs are identified by the nurse, who then implements interventions to meet the needs (Kolcaba, 1995). Kolcaba (2013) stated that "Comfort Theory can be adapted to any health care setting or age group . . ." (p. 198). Understanding of comfort can promote nursing care that is holistic and inclusive of physical, psychospiritual, social, and environmental interventions. It is noted that any actually unhappy, unhealthy, or unwell patients can be made more comfortable (Kolcaba, 1994). Finally, outcomes of comfort can be measurable, holistic, positive, and nurse sensitive.

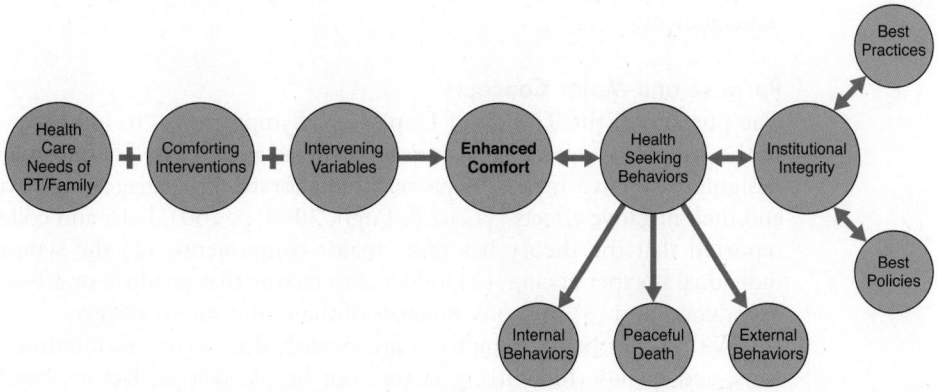

Figure 11-5 The conceptual framework for the theory of comfort. (© Kolcaba, 2007. Used with permission.) http://thecomfortline.com

Evidence of Empirical Testing and Application in Practice

The General Comfort Questionnaire (GCQ) is a 48-item, Likert-type scale that was developed to measure concepts and propositions described in the theory (Kolcaba, 2013). The GCQ has been modified to be used for different populations in a number of studies, and a shortened GCQ (28 items) is also in use (Kolcaba, 2013).

Kolcaba (2013) described development of other tools to assist in research and practice application for the Theory of Comfort. These include the Verbal Rating Scale Questionnaire, the Radiation Therapy Comfort Questionnaire, the Hospice Comfort Questionnaire, the Urinary Incontinence and Frequency Comfort Questionnaire, and the Comfort Behaviors Checklist, which was developed to measure comfort in patient who can't use traditional questionnaires or other instruments.

A number of research studies have been conducted by Kolcaba and her colleagues using the instruments listed above. For example, Whitehead, Anderson, Redican, and Stratton (2010) reported using Kolcaba's instruments to study the effects of an end-of-life nursing education program on nurses' death anxiety, knowledge of the dying process, and related concerns. Also examining nursing care at the end of life, Murray (2010) used Kolcaba's instruments to assess spiritual beliefs and practices of nurses caring for patients at the end of life, along with similarities and differences in spiritual beliefs and practices comparing hospice nurses and nurses working on oncology and other special care units.

In other examples, Doolin, Quinn, Bryant, Lyons, and Kleinpell (2010) used Kolcaba's Comfort Theory as part of a framework for implementation of formal policies and procedures for family presence during CPR, and two articles (March & McCormack, 2009; Wechter & Averill, 2010) were observed that described application of Comfort Theory as a component of quality, interdisciplinary health care.

Lenz and Colleagues' Theory of Unpleasant Symptoms

The Theory of Unpleasant Symptoms was developed by a group of nurses interested in a variety of nursing issues, including symptom management, theory development, and nursing science (Lenz, Gift, Pugh, & Milligan, 2013). The theory was initially published in the nursing literature in the mid-1990s (Lenz et al., 1995) and then updated a few years later (Lenz et al., 1997). The theory was based on the premise that there are commonalities in experiencing different symptoms among different groups and in different situations. The theory was developed to integrate existing knowledge about a variety of symptoms to better prepare nurses in symptom management.

Purpose and Major Concepts

The purpose of the Theory of Unpleasant Symptoms is "to improve understanding of the symptom experience in various contexts and to provide information useful for designing effective means to prevent, ameliorate, or manage unpleasant symptoms and their negative effects" (Lenz & Pugh, 2008, p. 160). Lenz and colleagues (1997) reported that the theory has three major components: (1) the symptoms that the individual is experiencing, (2) influencing factors that produce or affect the symptom experience, and (3) the consequences of the symptom experience.

Within the theory, symptoms are described in terms of duration, intensity, distress, and quality. Influencing factors can be physiologic factors, psychological factors, and/or situational factors. Performance is described in terms of functional status, cognitive functioning, or physical performance (Lenz et al., 2013). Figure 11-6 depicts the Theory of Unpleasant Symptoms.

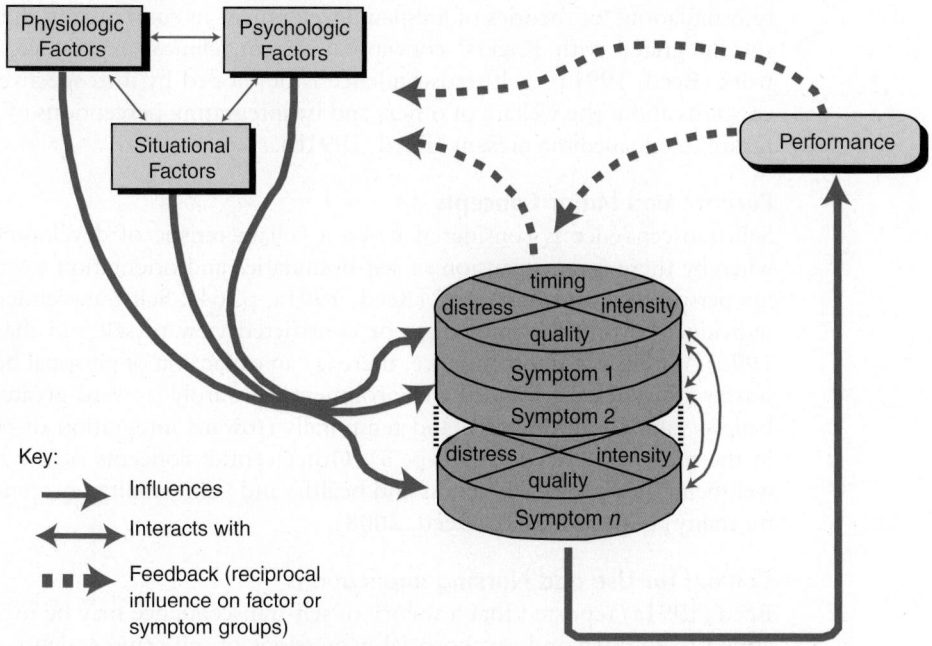

Figure 11-6 Updated version of the middle range theory of unpleasant symptoms. (From Lenz, E. R., Pugh, L. C., Milligan, R. A., Gift, A., & Suppe, F. (1997). The middle range Theory of Unpleasant Symptoms: An update. *Advances in Nursing Science, 19*(3), 14–27.) Used with permission.

Context for Use and Nursing Implications

The Theory of Unpleasant Symptoms helps nurses recognize the need to assess multiple aspects of symptoms, including characteristics of the symptom(s) itself; the underlying disease or other cause; as well as the frequency, intensity, duration, quality, and distress felt by the patient due to the symptom(s) (Lenz et al., 2013). The developers of the Theory of Unpleasant Symptoms note that it is clinically applicable to multiple client situations because it should stimulate nurses to consider factors that might influence more than one symptom and the ways in which symptoms interact with each other (Lenz et al., 1997). The theory's developers noted that it has been used in an emergency department to develop a symptom assessment scale for cardiac patients and has been useful in predicting the need for hospitalization among patients with chronic obstructive pulmonary disease (COPD).

Evidence of Empirical Testing and Application in Practice

A growing number of research studies using the Theory of Unpleasant Symptoms as a conceptual or organizing framework have been conducted. One study by Motl and McAuley (2009) used the theory to examine symptom clusters of fatigue, pain, and depression as a predictor of physical activity in patients with multiple sclerosis. Other works applied the Theory of Unpleasant Symptoms in caring for patients undergoing bariatric surgery (Tyler & Pugh, 2009), patients with heart failure (Jurgens et al., 2009), and patients with inflammatory bowel disease (Farrell & Savage, 2010).

Reed's Self-Transcendence Theory

Pamela Reed first wrote about the concept of self-transcendence in 1983 and formally outlined her theory in 1991 (Reed, 1991a). She reported that she used "deductive reformulation" of theories of lifespan development in constructing the theory. These she integrated with Rogers' conceptual system, clinical experience, and empirical work (Reed, 1991a). Self-transcendence is developed by introspective activities and concerns about the welfare of others and by integrating perceptions of one's past and future to enhance the present (Reed, 1991b).

Purpose and Major Concepts

Self-transcendence is considered to be a "characteristic of developmental maturity whereby there is an expansion of self-boundaries and orientation toward broadened life perspectives and purposes" (Reed, 1991a, p. 64). Self-transcendence moves the individual beyond the immediate or constricted view of self and the world (Reed, 1996). Within self-transcendence, there is "an expansion of personal boundaries outwardly (toward others and the environment), inwardly (toward greater awareness of beliefs, values, and dreams), and temporally (toward integration of past and future in the present)" (Reed, 1996, p. 3). Other central concepts of the theory include well-being (a sense of wholeness and health) and vulnerability (awareness of personal mortality) (Coward, 2010; Reed, 2008).

Context for Use and Nursing Implications

Reed (1991a) reported that a theory of self-transcendence may be used by nurses to attend to spiritual and psychosocial expressions of self-transcendence in clients who are confronted with end-of-life issues. To promote self-transcendence, nurses may use interventions such as meditation, self-reflection, visualization, religious expression, counseling, and journaling to expand the individual's boundaries.

Evidence of Empirical Testing and Application in Practice

A number of nursing research studies have used the theory of self-transcendence. In an early work, Reed (1991b) found support for the theory in an examination of the mental health of elders. In the study, she identified a relationship between self-transcendence and mental health and an inverse relationship between self-transcendence and depression. More recently, Coward and Kahn (2005) reported on efforts to facilitate self-transcendence among breast cancer patients.

Several current projects have looked at self-transcendence among nurses and/or nursing students. For example, Hunnibell, Reed, Quinn-Griffin, and Fitzpatrick (2008) studied differences in self-transcendence between hospice and oncology nurses, analyzing how it influenced burnout in those groups. In similar works, Palmer, Quinn-Griffin, Reed, and Fitzpatrick (2010) studied self-transcendence and engagement in acute care RNs, and Walsh, Chen, Hacker, and Broschard (2008) examined whether student nurses' self-transcendence could positively influence their attitudes toward caring for elders. Finally, Reed (2009) discussed how self-transcendence is important in mental health nursing practice and described how the self-transcendence scale can be used in practice and research for this nursing specialty area.

Low Middle Range Theories

The number of low middle range theories appears to be growing as nursing researchers and nursing scholars describe phenomena directly related to practice. Three theories are examined in the following sections. They are Eakes, Burke, and Hainsworth's (1998) Theory of Chronic Sorrow; Beck's (1993) Postpartum Depression Theory; and Mercer's (1983) Conceptualization of Maternal Role Attainment/Becoming a Mother. Table 11-3 lists other low middle range theories.

Table 11-3 Low Middle Range Nursing Theories

Theory/Model	Purpose	Major Concepts
Theory of adaptation to chronic pain (Dunn, 2004)	Describes the process and outcome of adaptation to chronic pain through use of religious and nonreligious coping to create human and environmental integration that promotes survival, growth, and integrity	Stimuli (background contextual variables, total pain intensity), compensatory life process (religious and nonreligious coping), adaptive modes (functional ability, psychological and spiritual well-being)
Acute pain management (Good, 1998; Good & Moore, 1996)	Proposes prescriptions for nursing activities to reduce pain after surgery or trauma to ensure that clients have less intense pain with minimal side effects of medications	Potent pain medication, pharmacologic adjuvant, nonpharmacologic adjuvant, assessment of pain and side effects, goal setting, and balance between analgesia and side effects
Theory of suffering (Morse, 2001)	Describes phases of suffering and relationship between states of enduring suffering and caregiver response	Enduring (emotional suppression) and emotional suffering, outcomes (recognition, acknowledgments, acceptance)
Theory of the peaceful end of life (Ruland & Moore, 1998)	Directs care necessary for terminally ill clients, enhances nursing care by combining the dimensions that are important to dying in a unifying whole	Not being in pain, experience of comfort, experience of dignity and respect, being at peace, closeness to significant others and people who care
Caregiving effectiveness model (Smith et al., 2002)	Explains and predicts outcomes of technology-based home caregiving provided by family members	Caregiving context (caregiving characteristics, caregiving/care-receiving interactions, patient education), adaptive context (family economic stability, caregiver health status, family adaptation, reactions to caregiving), caregiving effectiveness outcomes (patient quality of life, caregiver quality of life, patient condition, technologic side effects)
Theory of caregiver stress (Tsai, 2003)	Predicts caregiver stress and its outcomes from demographic characteristics, burden in care giving, stressful life events, social support, and social roles	Caregiver adaptation, input (objective burden, stressful life events, social support, social roles, demographic information), control process (perceived caregiver stress and depression), output (physical function, self-esteem, role enjoyment, marital satisfaction)
Theory of keeping the spirit alive: the spirit within children with cancer and their families (Woodgate & Degner, 2003)	Describes how children and their families use the core process of keeping the spirit alive in response to cancer	Core phenomenon: "keeping the spirit alive" (basic psychosocial process), "getting through all the rough spots" (basic psychosocial phenomenon), "way of being in the world" (living through it, sense of self, sense of well-being)

Eakes, Burke, and Hainsworth's Theory of Chronic Sorrow

The concept of chronic sorrow was introduced in the early 1960s to describe grief observed in the parents of children with mental deficiencies. Subsequent research indicated similar patterns of chronic sorrow in parents of mentally or physically disabled children. The Nursing Consortium for Research on Chronic Sorrow expanded the concept to include individuals who experience a variety of loss situations and to their family caregivers (Eakes, 2013; Eakes et al., 1998).

The middle range Theory of Chronic Sorrow was formalized in 1998. The theory was inductively derived and validated through a series of studies and a critical review of the existing research. Chronic sorrow is defined as the "periodic recurrence of permanent, pervasive sadness or other grief related feelings associated with a significant loss" (Eakes et al., 1998, p. 179), which was described as a normal response to ongoing disparity associated with loss.

Purpose and Major Concepts

The Theory of Chronic Sorrow was developed to help analyze individual responses of people experiencing ongoing disparity due to chronic illness, caregiving responsibilities, loss of the "perfect" child, or bereavement. Chronic sorrow was characterized as pervasive, permanent, periodic, and potentially progressive in nature. The person has a perception of sadness or sorrow over time in a situation with no predictable end. The sadness or sorrow is cyclic or recurrent and brings to mind a person's losses, disappointments, or fears (Eakes, 2013).

The primary antecedent to chronic sorrow is involvement in an experience of significant loss. The loss is often ongoing with no predictable end. Disparity is a second antecedent and is created by loss experiences when the individual's current reality differs from the idealized. Trigger events (e.g., milestones, circumstances, situations, and conditions that create negative disparity resulting from the loss experience) focus or exacerbate the experience of disparity. The "lack of closure associated with ongoing disparity sets the stage for chronic sorrow, with the loss experienced in bits and pieces over time" (Eakes, 2013, p. 98).

Context for Use and Nursing Implications

Chronic sorrow is commonly experienced by individuals across the lifespan who have encountered significant loss or experience ongoing loss. The theory's developers suggest that nurses need to view chronic sorrow as a normal response to loss and provide support by fostering positive coping strategies and encouraging activities that increase comfort.

Interventions that demonstrate an empathic presence and a caring professional are helpful. These include taking time to listen, offering support and reassurance, recognizing and focusing on feelings, and appreciating the uniqueness of each individual. Other interventions include providing information in a manner that can be understood and offering practical tips for dealing with the challenges of caregiving.

Evidence of Empirical Testing and Application in Practice

Eakes and colleagues (1998) reported that a number of research studies were used to develop and support the theory. Several recent research studies were identified using the Theory of Chronic Sorrow as a conceptual framework. These include Isaksson and Ahlstrom's (2008) examination of the experiences of patients with multiple sclerosis; Bowes, Lowes, Warner, and Gregory's (2009) study of chronic sorrow in parents of children with type 1 diabetes, and Smith's (2009) research on the association of chronic sorrow and substance abuse among female victims of child abuse.

Other works focused on how to care for those experiencing chronic sorrow. Among them, Gordon (2009) provided a nicely explained, evidence-based approach for supporting parents with chronically ill children. Also, Joseph (2012) described the importance of emergency department (ED) nurses recognizing chronic sorrow among family member of patients seen in the ED.

Beck's Postpartum Depression Theory

Building on a background of research on postpartum depression (Beck, Reynolds, & Rutowski, 1992), Cheryl Beck (1993) developed a theory regarding postpartum depression. A grounded theory approach was used to formulate the theory, which she described as a four-stage process of "teetering on the edge" into postpartum depression.

Purpose and Major Concepts

The purpose of the theory was to provide insight into the experience of postpartum depression. The concepts or stages in Beck's (1993) theory were defined as encountering terror (horrifying anxiety attacks, obsessive thinking, and enveloping fogginess), dying of self (alarming "unrealness," isolation of self, and contemplation of self-destruction), struggling to survive (battling the system, praying for relief, and seeking solace), and regaining control (making transitions, mounting lost time, and attaining a guarded recovery). A meta-synthesis of postpartum depression by Beck (2002a) produced a list of predictors or risk factors, including prenatal depression, child care stress, life stress, social support, prenatal anxiety, marital satisfaction, history of depression, infant temperament, maternity blues, self-esteem, socioeconomic status, marital status, and whether the pregnancy was planned. Distillation of predictors and risk factors of postpartum depression added these stressors/potential consequences: sleeping and eating disturbances, anxiety and insecurity, emotional lability, mental confusion, loss of self, guilt and shame, and suicidal thoughts (Maeve, 2010).

Context for Use and Nursing Implications

The model proposed nursing interventions to alert nurses to the incidence and impact of postpartum depression. Beck stressed the importance of identifying new mothers who might be suffering from postpartum depression and suggested interventions such as referral to postpartum depression support groups (Beck et al., 1992).

Evidence of Empirical Testing and Application in Practice

Beck's theory is fairly new, but it has been used in a significant number of nursing studies. To further examine the concept of postpartum depression, Beck (1995, 1998) performed a meta-analysis to document its effects. Based on the information from a meta-analysis, Beck and Gable (2000) developed the Postpartum Depression Screening Scale (PDSS) to improve detection of the disorder. The tool was revised in 2002 (Beck, 2002b), translated into Spanish (Beck & Gable, 2003), and revised further in 2006 (Beck, Records, & Rice, 2006). These tools have been validated (Beck et al., 2006; Clemmens, Driscoll, & Beck, 2004) and used by nurses in a growing list of research studies in many countries and in additional languages (Maeve, 2010).

In one example, Le, Perry, and Sheng (2009) used the PDSS to examine the feasibility of using the Internet to screen for postpartum depressive symptoms, concluding that it is viable and feasible tool to screen for postpartum depression. Akyuz, Severn, Devran, and Demiralp (2010) also used the PDSS as one tool to examine whether a history of infertility is a risk factor for postpartum depression among Turkish women, and Lucero, Beckstrand, Callister, and Sanchez-Brikhead (2012) used the Spanish version of the PDSS to examine the prevalence of postpartum depression among Hispanic immigrants in the United States. Lastly, Hunker, Patrick, Albrecht, and Wisner (2009) used Beck's theory and instruments to study the relationship between postpartum depression and a difficult childbirth.

Mercer's Conceptualization of Maternal Role Attainment/Becoming a Mother

Ramona Mercer first described a theoretical framework for the maternal role in the early 1980s; she expanded on the process in a subsequent publication in 1985. She reported that the theory was based on role theory, knowledge of the infant's traits, and a review of the literature to identify variables that influence or are influenced by maternal roles. She defined maternal role attainment as a process "in which the mother achieves competence in the role and integrates the mothering behaviors into her established role set so that she is comfortable with her identity as a mother" (Mercer, 1985, p. 198).

Following a review and synthesis of research related to the concept of "maternal role attainment," Mercer (2004) proposed changing the name of her theory to "Becoming a Mother." This change was later expanded upon (Mercer, 2006) and a number of related nursing interventions were identified supporting the change (Mercer & Walker, 2006).

Purpose and Major Concepts

Mercer attempted to identify the "form and strength of the relationships between key maternal and infant variables and maternal role attainment" as well as "other factors that appear to influence maternal role attainment" (Mercer, 1983, p. 73). She proposed that the variables of age, perception of the birth experience, early maternal–infant separation, social stress, support system, self-concept and personality traits, maternal illness, child-rearing attitudes, infant temperament, infant illness, culture, and socioeconomic level affect the maternal role.

In the more recent iteration of her theory, Mercer (2004) explains that the process of establishing maternal identity in becoming a mother is (1) commitment, attachment, and preparation (during pregnancy); (2) acquaintance, learning, and physical restoration (in the first 2 to 6 weeks following birth); (3) moving toward a new normal (2 weeks to 4 months); and (4) achievement of the maternal identity (around 4 months). She noted that these stages may overlap and may be highly variable due to maternal and infant variables as well as the social/environmental context. Additional key concepts and ideas identified in Mercer's works include infant temperament, infant health status, infant characteristics, and infant cues, as well as family, family functioning, father or intimate partner, mother–father relationship, and social support (Meighan, 2010).

Context for Use and Nursing Implications

Nurses in postpartum situations should recognize that competency in the maternal role toward "becoming a mother" increases with age and experience. Also, the demands on first-time mothers challenge the nurse to be active in anticipatory socialization and guidance to prepare for the realities of the maternal role. Interventions suggested in Mercer's works include promoting parenting groups to highlight maternal needs during the first months.

Evidence of Empirical Testing and Application in Practice

In early works, Mercer (1985) reported that mothering over the first year presents similar challenges for all groups, and a study by Fowles (1994) used Mercer's theory as part of her conceptual framework to examine the relationship between maternal attachment, postpartum depression, and maternal role attainment. More recently, a comprehensive study of maternal role attainment with medically fragile infants was undertaken to examine the quality of parenting (Holditch-Davis, Miles, Burchinal, & Goldman, 2010) and characteristics that influenced maternal role attachment longitudinally (Miles, Holditch-Davis, Burchinal, & Brunssen, 2011). In other works, Logsdon (2008) studied long-term maternal role functioning among adolescents, and Gaffney (2006) examined how "becoming a mother" influenced postpartum smoking relapse.

Link to Practice 11-1

Applying Multiple Middle Range Theories in Practice

How might nurses apply multiple middle range theories in their practice? Consider these situations:

1) A nurse is providing care for a woman with ovarian cancer (Theory of Unpleasant Symptoms) who recently immigrated to the United States from Somalia (Leininger's Culture Care Diversity and Universality Theory) in an ICU (Synergy Model).
2) A nurse manager is charged with developing an orientation packet (Benner's Model of Skill Acquisition) for nurses new to a hospice practice (Kolcaba's Theory of Comfort) focusing on their awareness of beliefs, values, and well-being (Reed's Self-Transcendence Theory).
3) A family nurse practitioner is working with a new mother (Mercer's Theory of Becoming a Mother) who has just given birth to a child with a severe genetic disorder (Theory of Chronic Sorrow).
4) A public health nurse is charged with teaching a group of American Indian women (Leininger's Culture Care Diversity and Universality Theory) how to develop a healthy lifestyle (Pender's Health Promotion Model).

Summary

This chapter presented a wide variety of middle range nursing theories. Because of space limitations, the descriptions are very brief and are intended to merely introduce the theories. The reader is directed to original and supporting sources for more information.

Elaine Chavez, the graduate student from the opening case study, saw how one of the numerous middle range nursing theories that have been published in recent years could be used to develop interventions in her practice. All nurses should likewise continue to review current nursing literature for new theories and ideas that are being presented to remain current and knowledgeable about nursing practice. To illustrate, Link to Practice 11-1 provides some thoughts on how nurses can apply middle range theories in their daily practice.

It must be mentioned again that the high, middle, and low range theories described here are by no means an exhaustive display of the growing number that have been presented in the nursing literature. Indeed, it was remarkable to observe the growth in middle range theory development since the first edition of this book was published more than 10 years ago, and it is anticipated that this emphasis will continue well into the future.

Key Points

- A growing number of widely used middle range theories have been proposed, applied, and tested and have been presented in the nursing literature.
- Among the "high" middle range nursing theories (theories that are relatively abstract and apply to a very broad aspect of nursing) frequently used by nurses for research and practice are the works of Benner, Pender, Leininger, Meleis, and the Synergy Model.

- "Middle" middle range nursing theories (theories that apply in a many aspects and situations) frequently used by nurses for research and practice include the Uncertainty in Illness Theory, the Theory of Comfort, the Theory of Unpleasant Symptoms, and Reed's Self-Transcendence Theory.
- "Low" middle range nursing theories (theories that are fairly concrete and apply to a narrow range of patients and situations) frequently used by nurses in research and practice include the Theory of Chronic Sorrow, Beck's Postpartum Depression Theory, and Mercer's Theory of Maternal Role Attainment.
- Many other middle range theories have been described in the nursing literature, and new ones are being developed by researchers and scholars to improve nursing care and patient outcomes.

Learning Activities

1. Select one of the middle range theories discussed in this chapter. Obtain a copy of the original work(s) and perform an analysis/evaluation using the criteria presented in Chapter 5.
2. Select one of the high middle range theories covered in this chapter and obtain a copy of the original work. Review three or four of the research studies cited for that theory that either study relationships of the theory or use it as a conceptual framework. While reviewing these works, consider the following questions: Do the studies appear to use the theory appropriately? Are the works consistent in their use of the theory? Do the studies contribute to the knowledge base of the theory? How? Write a paper describing your findings.
3. Search current nursing journals for examples of the development, analysis, or use of middle range theories in the discipline of nursing. Debate trends with classmates or develop your analysis into a paper.

REFERENCES

Abraham, P. J. (2011). Developing nurse leaders: A program enhancing staff nurse leadership skills and professionalism. *Nursing Administration Quarterly, 35*(4), 306–312.

Akyuz, A., Severn, M., Devran, A., & Demiralp, M. (2010). Infertility history: Is it a risk factor for postpartum depression in Turkish women? *Journal of Perinatal & Neonatal Nursing, 24*(2), 137–145.

American Association of Critical-Care Nurses. (2013). The AACN Model for Patient Care. Retrieved from http://www.aacn.org/WD/Certifications/Docs/SynergyModelforPatientCare.pdf

Arashin, K. A. (2010). Using the Synergy Model to guide the practice of rapid response teams. *Dimensions of Critical Care Nursing, 29*(3), 120–124.

Bailey, D. E., Barroso, J., Muir, A. J., Sloane, R., Richmond, J., McHutchison, J., et al. (2010). Patients with chronic hepatitis C undergoing watchful waiting: Exploring trajectories of illness uncertainty and fatigue. *Research in Nursing & Health, 33*(5), 465–473.

Bailey, D. E., & Stewart, J. L. (2010). Uncertainty in illness theory. In M. R. Alligood & A. M. Tomey (Eds.), *Nursing theorists and their work* (7th ed., pp. 599–617). St. Louis: Mosby.

Barker, P. (2001a). The tidal model: Developing a person-centered approach to psychiatric and mental health nursing. *Perspectives in Psychiatric Care, 37*(3), 79–87.

Barker, P. (2001b). The tidal model: Developing an empowering, person-centred approach to recovery within psychiatric and mental health nursing. *Journal of Psychiatric and Mental Health Nursing, 8*, 233–240.

Beck, C. T. (1993). Teetering on the edge: A substantive theory of postpartum depression. *Nursing Research, 42*(1), 42–48.

Beck, C. T. (1995). The effects of postpartum depression on maternal–infant interaction: A meta-analysis. *Nursing Research, 44*(5), 298–304.

Beck, C. T. (1998). The effects of postpartum depression on child development: A meta-analysis. *Archives of Psychiatric Nursing, 12*(1), 12–20.

Beck, C. T. (2002a). Mothering multiples: A meta-synthesis of qualitative research. *MCN: The American Journal of Maternal Child Nursing, 27*(4), 214–221.

Beck, C. T. (2002b). Revision of the postpartum depression predictors inventory. *Journal of Obstetric, Gynecologic, and Neonatal Nursing, 31*(4), 394–402.

Beck, C. T., & Gable, R. K. (2000). Postpartum depression screening scale: Development and psychometric testing. *Nursing Research, 49*(5), 272–281.

Beck, C. T., & Gable, R. K. (2003). Postpartum depression screening scale: Spanish version. *Nursing Research, 52*(5), 296–306.

Beck, C. T., Records, K., & Rice, M. (2006). Further development of the postpartum depression predictors inventory—revised. *AWHONN: The Association of Women's Health, Obstetrics and Neonatal Nurses, 35*(6), 735–742.

Beck, C. T., Reynolds, M. A., & Rutowski, P. (1992). Maternity blues and postpartum depression. *Journal of Obstetric, Gynecologic, and Neonatal Nursing, 21*(4), 287–293.

Benner, P. (1984). *From novice to expert: Excellence and power in clinical nursing practice*. Menlo Park, CA: Addison Wesley.

Benner, P. (2001). *From novice to expert: Excellence and power in clinical nursing practice* (commemorative edition). Englewood Cliffs, NJ: Prentice-Hall.

Benner, P., Tanner, C., & Chesla, C. (2009). *Expertise in nursing practice: Caring clinical judgment, and ethics* (2nd ed.). New York: Springer Publishing.

Bergquist, S., & King, J. (1994). Parish nursing: A conceptual framework. *Journal of Holistic Nursing, 12*(2), 155–170.

Blum, K., & Sherman, D. W. (2010). Understanding the experience of caregivers: A focus on transitions. *Seminars in Oncology Nursing, 26*(4), 243–258.

Bowes, S., Lowes, L., Warner, J., & Gregory, J. W. (2009). Chronic sorrow in parent of children with type 1 diabetes. *Journal of Advanced Nursing, 65*(5), 992–1000.

Braden, C. J. (1990). A test of the self-help model: Learned response to chronic illness experience. *Nursing Research, 39*(1), 42–47.

Brixey, M. J., & Mahon, S. M. (2010). A self-assessment tool for oncology nurses: Preliminary implementation and evaluation. *Clinical Journal of Oncology Nursing, 14*(4), 474–480.

Burns, K., Murrock, C. J., & Heifner, C. (2012). Body mass index and injury severity in adolescent males. *Journal of Pediatric Nursing, 27*(5), 508–513.

Cahill, J., LoBiondo-Wood, G., Bergstrom, N., & Armstrong, T. (2012). Brain tumor symptoms as antecedents to uncertainty: An integrative review. *Journal of Nursing Scholarship, 44*(2), 145–155.

Campesino, M. (2008). Beyond transculturalism: Critiques of cultural education in nursing. *Journal of Nursing Education, 47*(7), 298–304.

Cathcart, E. B. (2008). The role of the chief nursing officer in leading the practice: Lessons from the Benner tradition. *Nursing Administration Quarterly, 32*(2), 87–91.

Clemmens, D., Driscoll, J. W., & Beck, C. T. (2004). Postpartum depression as profiled through the postpartum depression screening scale. *MCN: The American Journal of Maternal Child Nursing, 29*(3), 180–185.

Corbin, J. M., & Strauss, A. (1991). A nursing model for chronic illness management based upon the trajectory framework. *Scholarly Inquiry for Nursing Practice, 5*(3), 155–174.

Corbin, J. M., & Strauss, A. (1992). A nursing model for chronic illness management based upon the trajectory framework. In P. Woog (Ed.), *The chronic illness trajectory framework: The Corbin and Strauss nursing model* (pp. 9–28). New York: Springer.

Coward, D. D. (2010). Pamela G. Reed: Self-transcendence theory. In M. R. Alligood and A. M. Tomey (Eds.), *Nursing theorists and their work* (7th ed., pp. 618–637). St. Louis: Mosby.

Coward, D. D., & Kahn, D. L. (2005). Transcending breast cancer: Making meaning from diagnosis and treatment. *Journal of Holistic Nursing, 23*(3), 264–283.

Cox, C. (1985). The self-determinism index. *Nursing Research, 34*(3), 177–183.

Coyle, J. S. (2011). Development of a model home health nurse internship program for new graduates: Key lessons learned. *The Journal of Continuing Education in Nursing, 42*(5), 201–214.

Curley, M. A. Q. (1998). Patient–nurse synergy: Optimizing patient's outcomes. *American Journal of Critical Care, 7*(1), 64–72.

Curley, M. A. Q. (2007). *Synergy: The unique relationship between nurses and patients*. Indianapolis, IN: Sigma Theta Tau.

Doolin, C. T., Quinn, L. D., Bryant, L. G., Lyons, A. A., & Kleinpell, R. M. (2010). Family presence during cardiopulmonary resuscitation: Using evidence-based knowledge to guide the advance practice nurse in developing formal policy and practice guidelines. *Journal of the American Academy of Nurse Practitioners, 23*(1), 8–14.

Dossa, A., Bokhour, B., & Hoenig, H. (2012). Care transitions from the hospital to home for patients with mobility impairments: Patient and family caregiver experiences. *Rehabilitation Nursing, 37*(6), 277–287.

Dumchin, M. (2010). Redefining the future of perioperative nursing education: A conceptual framework. *AORN Journal, 92*(1), 87–100.

Dunn, K. S. (2004). Toward a middle range theory of adaptation to chronic pain. *Nursing Science Quarterly, 17*(1), 78–84.

Eakes, G. (2013). Chronic sorrow. In S. J. Peterson & T. S. Bredow (Eds.), *Middle range theories: Application to nursing research* (3rd ed., pp. 96–106). Philadelphia: Lippincott Williams & Wilkins/Wolters Kluwer.

Eakes, G., Burke, M. L., & Hainsworth, M. A. (1998). Middle range theory of chronic sorrow. *Image: Journal of Nursing Scholarship, 30*(2), 179–185.

Esposito, E. M., & Fitzpatrick, J. J. (2011). Registered nurses' beliefs of the benefits of exercise, their exercise behavior and their patient teaching regarding exercise. *International Journal of Nursing Practice, 17*(4), 351–356.

Farrell, D., & Savage, E. (2010). Symptom burden in inflammatory bowel disease: Rethinking conceptual and theoretical underpinnings. *International Journal of Nursing Practice, 16*(5), 437–442.

Fowles, E. R. (1994). *The relationship between prenatal maternal attachment, postpartum depressive symptoms and maternal role attainment*. Chicago: Loyola University of Chicago.

Gaffney, K. F. (2006). Postpartum smoking relapse and becoming a mother. *Journal of Nursing Scholarship, 38*(1), 26–30.

Geary, C. R., & Schumacher, K. L. (2012). Care transitions: Integrating transition theory and complexity science concepts. *Advances in Nursing Science, 35*(3), 236–248.

George, J. B., & Hickman, J. S. (2011). Other theories of the 1980s. In J. B. George (Ed). *Nursing theories: The base for professional nursing practice* (6th ed., pp. 606–634). Upper Saddle River, NJ: Pearson Education.

Germino, B. B., Mishel, M. H., Crandell, J., Porter, L., Blyler, D., Jeanerette, C., et al. (2013). Outcomes of an uncertainty management intervention in younger African American and Caucasian breast cancer survivors. *Oncology Nursing Forum, 40*(1), 82–92.

Gillum, D. R., Staffileno, B. A., Schwartz, K. S., Coke, L., Fogg, L., & Reiling, D. (2011). Cardiovascular disease in the Amish: An exploratory study of knowledge, beliefs and health care practices. *Holistic Nursing Practice, 25*(6), 289–297.

Good, M. (1998). A middle range theory of acute pain management: Use in research. *Nursing Outlook, 46*(3), 120–124.

Good, M., & Moore, S. M. (1996). Clinical practice guidelines as a new source of middle range theory: Focus on acute pain. *Nursing Outlook, 44*(2), 74–79.

Gordon, J. (2009). An evidence-based approach for supporting parents experiencing chronic sorrow. *Pediatric Nursing, 35*(2), 115–119.

Haag-Heitman, B. (2012). Supporting transitions in clinical practice development. *Journal of Perinatal & Neonatal Nursing, 26*(1), 5–7.

Haggstrom, M., Asplund, K., & Kristiansen, L. (2012). How can nurses facilitate patient's transitions form intensive care? A grounded theory of nursing. *Intensive and Critical Care Nursing, 28*(6), 224–233.

Halding, A. G., & Heggdal, K. (2011). Patients' experiences of health transitions in pulmonary rehabilitation. *Nursing Inquiry, 119*(4), 345–356.

Hallas, D., Fernandez, J., Lim, L., & Carobene, M. (2011). Nursing strategies to reduce the incidence of early childhood caries in culturally diverse populations. *Journal of Pediatric Nursing, 26*(3), 248–256.

Halliday, L. E., & Boughton, M. A. (2011). Exploring the concept of uncertain fertility, reproduction and motherhood after cancer in young adult women. *Nursing Inquiry, 18*(2), 135–142.

Hardin, S. R. (2005). Introduction to the AACN Synergy Model for patient care. In S. R. Hardin & R. Kaplow (Eds.), *Synergy for clinical excellence: The AACN Synergy Model for patient care* (pp. 3–10). Sudbury, MA: Jones & Bartlett Publishers.

Hardin, S. R. (2012). Hearing loss in older critical care patients: Participation in decision making. *Critical Care Nurse, 32*(6), 43–50.

Hardin, S. R. (2013). The AACN Synergy Model. In S. J. Peterson & T. S. Bredow (Eds.), *Middle range theories: Application to nursing research* (3rd ed., pp. 294–305). Philadelphia: Lippincott Williams & Wilkins.

Hatfield, B. (2011). Polar shift: From expert to novice in 30 seconds. *Journal of Emergency Nursing, 37*(5), 510–511.

Holditch-Davis, D., Miles, M. S., Burchinal, M. R., & Goldman, B. D. (2010). Maternal role attainment with medically fragile infants: Part 2. Relationship to the quality of parenting. *Research in Nursing & Health, 34*(1), 35–48.

Hunker, D. F., Patrick, T. E., Albrecht, S. A., & Wisner, K. L. (2009). Is difficult childbirth related to postpartum maternal outcomes in the early postpartum period? *Archives of Women's Mental Health, 12*(4), 211–219.

Hunnibell, L. S., Reed, P. G., Quinn-Griffin, M., & Fitzpatrick, J. J. (2008). Self-transcendence and burnout in hospice and oncology nurses. *Journal of Hospice and Palliative Nursing, 10*(3), 172–179.

Hurlbut, J. M., Robbins, L. K., & Hoke, M. M. (2011). Correlations between spirituality and health-promoting behaviors among sheltered homeless women. *Journal of Community Health Nursing, 28*(2), 81–91.

Im, E. O. (2010). Afaf Ibrahim Meleis: Transition Theory. In M.R. Alligood & A.M. Tomey (Eds). *Nursing theorists and their work* (7th ed., pp. 416–433), St. Louis: Mosby.

Isaksson, A., & Ahlstrom, G. (2008). Managing chronic sorrow: Experiences of patients with multiple sclerosis. *Journal of Neuroscience Nursing, 40*(3), 180–191.

Joseph, H. A. (2012). Recognizing chronic sorrow in the habitual E.D. patient. *Journal of Emergency Nursing, 38*(6), 539–540.

Jurgens, C. Y., Moser, D. K., Armola, R., Carlson, B., Sethares, K., & Rigel, B. (2009). Symptom clusters of heart failure. *Research in Nursing & Health, 32*(5), 551–560.

Keilman, L. J., & Dunn, K. S. (2010). Knowledge, attitudes and perceptions of Advanced Practice Nurses regarding urinary incontinence in older adult women. *Research and Theory for Nursing Practice: An International Journal, 24*(4), 260–279.

Kolcaba, K. Y. (1994). A theory of holistic comfort for nursing. *Journal of Advanced Nursing, 19*(6), 1178–1184.

Kolcaba, K. Y. (1995). The art of comfort care. *Image: Journal of Nursing Scholarship, 27*(4), 287–289.

Kolcaba, K. (2001). Evolution of the middle range: Theory of Comfort for outcomes research. *Nursing Outlook, 49*(2), 86–92.

Kolcaba, K. (2003). *Comfort theory and practice: A vision for holistic health care and research.* New York: Springer.

Kolcaba, K. (2013). Comfort. In S. J. Peterson & T. S. Bredow (Eds.), *Middle range theories: Application to nursing research* (3rd., pp. 193–209). Philadelphia: Lippincott Williams & Wilkins.

Lancellotti, K. (2008). Culture care theory: A framework for expanding awareness of diversity and racism in nursing education. *Journal of Professional Nursing, 24*(3), 179–183.

Lauver, D. (1992). A theory of care-seeking behavior. *Image: Journal of Nursing Scholarship, 24*(4), 281–287.

Le, H. N., Perry, D. F., & Sheng, X. (2009). Using the internet to screen for postpartum depression. *Maternal & Child Health Journal, 13*(2), 213–221.

Lee, R. C. (2012). Family homelessness viewed through the lens of health and human rights. *Advances in Nursing Science, 35*(2), E47–E59.

Leininger, M. M. (2002). Culture care theory: A major contribution to advance transcultural nursing knowledge and practices. *Journal of Transcultural Nursing, 13*(3), 189–192.

Leininger, M. M. (2007). Theoretical questions and concerns: Response from the Theory of Culture Care Diversity and Universality perspective. *Nursing Science Quarterly, 20*(1), 9–15.

Leininger, M. M., & McFarland, M. (2006). *Culture care diversity and universality: A worldwide nursing theory* (2nd ed.). Sudbury, MA: Jones & Bartlett.

Lenz, E. R., Gift, A., Pugh, L. C., & Milligan, R. A. (2013). Unpleasant symptoms. In S. J. Peterson & T. S. Bredow (Eds.), *Middle range theories: Application to nursing research* (3rd ed., pp. 68–80). Philadelphia: Lippincott Williams & Wilkins.

Lenz, E. R., & Pugh, L. C. (2008). Theory of unpleasant symptoms. In M. J. Smith & P. R. Liehr (Eds.), *Middle range theory for nursing* (2nd ed., pp. 159–181). New York: Springer.

Lenz, E. R., Pugh, L. C., Milligan, R. A., Gift, A., & Suppe, F. (1997). The middle range theory of unpleasant symptoms: An update. *Advances in Nursing Science, 19*(3), 14–27.

Lenz, E. R., & Shortridge-Baggett, L. M. (2002). *Self-efficacy in nursing: Research and measurement perspectives.* New York: Springer.

Lenz, E. R., Suppe, F., Gift, A. G., Pugh, L. C., & Milligan R. A. (1995). Collaborative development of middle range nursing theories: Toward a theory of unpleasant symptoms. *Advance in Nursing Science, 17*(3), 1–13.

Liehr, P., & Smith, M. J. (1999). Middle range theory: Spinning research and practice to create knowledge for the new millennium. *Advances in Nursing Science, 21*(4), 81–91.

Lin, L., Yeh, C. H., & Mishel, M. H. (2010). Evaluation of a conceptual model based on Mishel's theories of uncertainty in illness in a sample of Taiwanese parents of children with cancer: A cross-sectional questionnaire survey. *International Journal of Nursing Studies, 47*(12), 1510–1524.

Logsdon, M. C. (2008). Maternal role functioning in adolescents at 12 months postpartum. *Women's Health Care: A Practical Journal for Nurse Practitioners, 7*(10), 27–32.

Long, J. M., Sowell, R., Bairan, A., Holtz, C., Curtis, A. B., & Fogarty, K. J. (2012). Exploration of commonalities and variations in health related beliefs across four Latino subgroups using focus group methodology: Implications in care for Latinos with type 2 diabetes. *Journal of Cultural Diversity, 19*(4), 133–142.

Lucero, N. B., Beckstrand, R. L., Callister, L. C., & Sanchez-Brikhead, A. C. (2012). Prevalence of postpartum depression among Hispanic immigrant women. *Journal of the American Academy of Nurse Practitioners, 24*(12), 726–734.

Lyneham, J., Parkinson, C., & Denholm, C. (2008). Explicating Benner's concept of expert practice: Intuition in emergency nursing. *Journal of Advanced Nursing, 64*(4), 380–387.

Maeve, M. K. (2010). Cheryl Tatano Beck: Postpartum depression theory. In M. R. Alligood and A.M. Tomey (Eds.), *Nursing theorists and their work* (7th ed., pp. 722–739). St. Louis: Mosby.

Maglione, J. L., & Hayman, L. L. (2009). Correlates of physical activity in low income college students. *Research in Nursing & Health, 32*(6), 634–646.

March, A., & McCormack, D. (2009). Modifying Kolcaba's Comfort Theory as an institution-wide approach. *Holistic Nursing Practice, 23*(2), 75–80.

Martin, K. S. (2005). *The Omaha System: A key to practice, documentation and information management* (2nd ed.). Philadelphia: Elsevier.

McFarland, M. (2010). Madeleine Leininger: Culture care Theory of Diversity and Universality. In M. R. Alligood & A. M. Tomey (Eds.), *Nursing theorists and their work* (7th ed., pp. 454–478). St. Louis: Mosby.

Meighan, M. (2010). Ramona T. Mercer: Maternal Role Attainment: Becoming a Mother. In M. R. Alligood & A. M. Tomey (Eds.), *Nursing theorists and their work* (7th ed., pp. 581–598). St. Louis: Mosby.

Meleis, A. I. (2010). *Transitions Theory: Middle-range and situation specific theories in nursing research and practice.* New York: Springer.

Meleis, A. I., & Trangenstein, P. A. (1994). Facilitating transitions: Redefinition of the nursing mission. *Nursing Outlook, 42*(6), 255–259.

Mercer, R. T. (1983). A theoretical framework for studying factors that impact on the maternal role. *Nursing Research, 30*(2), 73–77.

Mercer, R. T. (1985). The process of maternal role attainment over the first year. *Nursing Research, 34*(4), 198–204.

Mercer, R. T. (2004). Becoming a mother versus maternal role attainment. *Journal of Nursing Scholarship, 36*(3), 226–232.

Mercer, R. T. (2006). Nursing support of the process of becoming a mother. *AWHONN: The Association of Women's Health, Obstetrics and Neonatal Nurses, 35*(5), 649–651.

Mercer, R. T., & Walker, L. O. (2006). A review of nursing interventions to foster becoming a mother. *AWHONN: The Association of Women's Health, Obstetrics and Neonatal Nurses, 35*(5), 568–582.

Meretoja, R., & Koponen, L. (2011). A systematic model to compare nurses' optimal and actual competencies in the clinical setting. *Journal of Advanced Nursing, 68*(2), 414–422.

Miles, M. S., Holditch-Davis, D., Burchinal, M. R., & Brunssen, S. (2011). Maternal role attainment with medically fragile infants: Part 1. Measurement and correlates during the first year of life. *Research in Nursing & Health, 34*(1), 20–34.

Miller, L. W. (1997). Nursing through the lens of faith: A conceptual model. *Journal of Christian Nursing, 14*(1), 17–21.

Mishel, M. H. (1981). The measurement of uncertainty in illness. *Nursing Research, 30*(5), 258–263.

Mishel, M. H. (1984). Perceived uncertainty and stress in illness. *Research in Nursing and Health, 7,* 163–171.

Mishel, M. H. (1988). Uncertainty in illness. *Image: Journal of Nursing Scholarship, 20*(4), 225–232.

Mishel, M. H. (1990). Reconceptualization of the uncertainty in illness theory. *Image: Journal of Nursing Scholarship, 22*(4), 256–262.

Mishel, M. H. (1999). Uncertainty in chronic illness. *Annual Review of Nursing Research, 17,* 269–294.

Mishel, M. H. (2013). How to request Dr. Mishel's scales. Retrieved from http://nursing.unc.edu/people/merle-mishel/

Mishel, M., Germino, B., Lin, L., Pruthi, R., Wallen, E., Crandell, J., et al. (2009). Managing uncertainty about treatment decision making in early stage prostate cancer: A randomized clinical trial. *Patient Education & Counseling, 77*(3), 349–359.

Morse, J. (2001). Toward a praxis theory of suffering. *Advances in Nursing Science, 24*(1), 47–59.

Motl, R. W., & McAuley, E. (2009). Symptom cluster as a predictor of physical activity in multiple sclerosis: Preliminary evidence. *Journal of Pain and Symptom Management, 38*(2), 270–280.

Murray, R. P. (2010). Spiritual care beliefs and practices of special care and oncology RNs at patients' end of life. *Journal of Hospice and Palliative Nursing, 12*(1), 51–58.

Neal, L. J. (1999a). Neal theory of home health nursing practice. *Image: Journal of Nursing Scholarship, 31*(3), 251.

Neal, L. J. (1999b). The Neal theory: Implications for practice and administration. *Home Health Care Nurse, 17*(3), 181–187.

Norbeck, J. S. (1981). Social support: A model for clinical research and application. *Advances in Nursing Science, 3*(4), 43–59.

Owens, A. L., & Cleaves, J. (2012). Then and now: Updating clinical nurse advancement programs. *Nursing 2012, 42*(12), 15–17.

Palmer, B., Quinn-Griffin, M. T., Reed, P., & Fitzpatrick, J. J. (2010). Self-transcendence and work engagement in acute care staff registered nurses. *Critical Care Nursing Quarterly, 33*(2), 138–147.

Pender, N. J. (1996). *Health promotion in nursing practice* (3rd ed.). Stamford, CT: Appleton & Lange.

Pender, N. J., Murdaugh, C. L., & Parsons, M. A. (2011). *Health promotion in nursing practice* (6th ed.). Upper Saddle River, NJ: Pearson.

Polk, L. V. (1997). Toward a middle range theory of resilience. *Advances in Nursing Science, 19*(3), 1–13.

Reed, P. G. (1991a). Toward a nursing theory of self-transcendence: Deductive reformulation using developmental theories. *Advances in Nursing Science, 13*(4), 64–77.

Reed, P. G. (1991b). Self-transcendence and mental health in oldest-old adults. *Nursing Research, 40*(1), 5–11.

Reed, P. G. (1996). Transcendence: Formulating nursing perspectives. *Nursing Science Quarterly, 9*(1), 2–3.

Reed, P. G. (2008). Theory of self-transcendence. In M. J. Smith & P. R. Liehr (Eds.), *Middle range theory for nursing* (2nd ed., pp. 105–129). New York: Springer.

Reed, P. G. (2009). Demystifying self-transcendence for mental health nursing practice and research. *Archives of Psychiatric Nursing, 23*(5), 397–400.

Reedy, S. & Blum, K. (2010). Applying middle-range nursing theory to bariatric surgery patients: Experiencing transitions. *Bariatric Nursing and Surgical Patient Care, 5*(1), 35–45.

Revell, M. A., & McGhee, M. N. (2012). Evolution of the African American family. *International Journal of Childbirth Education, 27*(4), 44–48.

Rew, L., Tyler, D., Fredland, N., & Hannah, D. (2012). Adolescents' concerns as they transition through high school. *Advances in Nursing Science, 35*(3), 205–221.

Rogers, B. (1994). *Occupational health nursing: Concepts and practice.* Philadelphia: Saunders.

Ruland, C. M., & Moore, S. M. (1998). Theory construction based on standards of care: A proposed theory of the peaceful end of life. *Nursing Outlook, 46*(4), 169–175.

Schuler, P. A., & Davis, J. E. (1993). The Schuler Nurse Practitioner Model: A theoretical framework for nurse practitioner clinicians, educators and researcher. *Journal of the American Academy of Nurse Practitioners, 5*(1), 11–18.

Schumacher, K. L., & Meleis, A. I. (1994). Transititions: A central concept in nursing. *Image, Journal of Nursing Scholarship, 26*(2), 119–125.

Smith, C. S. (2009). Substance abuse, chronic sorrow and mothering loss: Relapse triggers among female victims of child abuse. *Journal of Pediatric Nursing, 24*(5), 401–412.

Smith, K., & Bazini-Barakat, N. (2003). A public health nursing practice model: Melding public health principles with the nursing process. *Public Health Nursing, 20*(1), 42–48.

Smith, C. E., Pace, K., Kochinda, C., Kleinbeck, S. V. M., Koehler, J., & Popkess-Vawter, S. (2002). Caregiving effectiveness model evolution to a midrange theory of home care: A process for critique and replication. *Advances in Nursing Science, 25*(1), 50–64.

Stacy, K. M. (2011). Progressive care units: Different but the same. *Critical Care Nurse, 31*(3), 77–83.

Stark, M. A., Chase, C., & DeYoung, A. (2010). Barriers to health promotion in community dwelling elders. *Journal of Community Health Nursing, 27*(4), 175–186.

Stewart, J. L., Lynn, M. R., & Mishel, M. H. (2010). Psychometric evaluation of a new instrument to measure uncertainty in children and adolescents with cancer. *Nursing Research, 59*(2), 119–126.

Suzuki, M. (2012). Quality of life, uncertainty and perceived involvement in decision making in patient with head and neck cancer. *Oncology Nursing Forum, 39*(6), 541–548.

Swanson, K. M. (1991). Empirical development of a middle range theory of caring. *Nursing Research, 40*(3), 161–166.

Tejero, L. M. S. (2011). The mediating role of the nurse–patient dyad bonding in bringing about patient satisfaction. *Journal of Advanced Nursing, 68*(5), 994–1002.

Tsai, P. F. (2003). A middle range theory of caregiver stress. *Nursing Science Quarterly, 16*(2), 137–145.

Tyler, R., & Pugh, L. C. (2009). Application of the theory of unpleasant symptoms in bariatric surgery. *Bariatric Nursing and Surgical Patient Care, 4*(4), 270–276.

Uhrenfeldt, L., & Hall, E. O. C. (2009). Caring for nursing staff among proficient first-line nurse leaders. *International Journal for Human Caring, 13*(2), 40–44.

Vogler, J., Altmann, T. K., & Zoucha, R. (2010). Native Hawaiian attitudes of culturally sensitive healthcare provider traits and behaviors. *Journal of Cultural Diversity, 17*(3), 90–98.

Vuorinen, R., Heino, E., & Meretoja, R. (2009). Endoscopy nurse as a patient care coordinator. *Gastroenterology Nursing, 32*(6), 410–413.

Walsh, S. M., Chen, S., Hacker, M., & Broschard, D. (2008). A creative-bonding intervention and a friendly visit approach to promote nursing students' self-transcendence and positive attitudes toward elders: A pilot study. *Nurse Education Today, 28*(3), 363–370.

Wechter, S. M., & Averill, J. B. (2010). Kolcaba's Comfort Theory: Innovation for pediatric nursing. *Communicating Nursing Research, 43,* 559.

Weinert, C., & Long, K. A. (1991). The theory and research base for rural nursing practice. In A. Bush (Ed.), *Rural nursing* (pp. 21–38). Newbury Park, CA: Sage.

Whitehead, P. B., Anderson, E. S., Redican, K. J., & Stratton, R. (2010). Studying the effects of the end-of-life nursing education consortium at the institutional level. *Journal of Hospice and Palliative Nursing, 12*(3), 184–193.

Wise, N. J., & Arcamone, A. A. (2011). Survey of adolescent views of healthy eating during pregnancy. *MCN: The American Journal of Maternal Child Nursing, 36*(6), 381–386.

Wilson, B., Harwood, L., Oudshoorn, A., & Thompson, B. (2010). The culture of vascular access cannulation among nurses in a chronic hemodialysis unit. *The CANNT Journal, 20*(3), 35–41.

Woodgate, R. L., & Degner, L. F. (2003). A substantive theory of keeping the spirit alive: The spirit within children with cancer and their families. *Journal of Pediatric Oncology Nursing, 20*(3), 103–119.

Wysong, P. R., & Driver, E. (2009). Patients' perceptions of nurses' skill. *Critical Care Nurse, 29*(4), 24–37.

CHAPTER 12

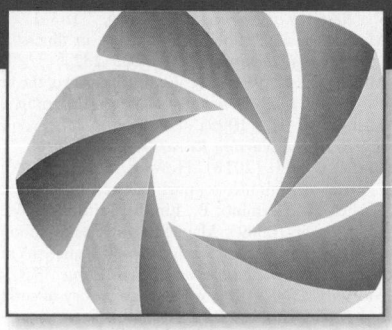

Evidence-Based Practice and Nursing Theory

Evelyn M. Wills and Melanie McEwen

Helen Soderstrom was stricken with changes in her vision, disturbances of gait, and occasional periods of severe fatigue during her senior year of nursing school. She experienced intermittent periods of normality as well as illness, and the periods when she had no symptoms lasted many months. During a time when her symptoms were unusually active, she sought medical help, and her physician determined that her symptoms were related to stress. Despite the periods of weakness and fatigue, she was able to complete the nursing program and graduated with honors.

During Helen's first year of practice, she experienced two periods of symptom exacerbation, but each was short-lived. With full insurance, she was able to see a neurologist who concluded that she was experiencing the beginning stages of a neuromuscular disease. Because there was no "cure," the neurologist worked with Helen to find interventions that helped her manage the symptoms when they became problematic.

After a few years in practice, Helen enrolled in a graduate program to work toward a career in nursing education. During her first year of graduate studies, she seldom experienced neurologic symptoms, but during her practice teaching course, they returned.

The recurrence of symptoms, along with a new understanding of evidence-based practice from her graduate courses, led Helen to make her personal health experience the topic of her final paper. To learn more, she sought resources that would help her gain better control of the neuromuscular symptoms as well as assist her in her studies. To that end, she contacted her University's neuroscience department and joined a research team. As she learned more about EBP, she considered what system she would use to develop guidelines on symptom management and selected the Iowa Model because of its extensive use in research.

The idea of evidence-based practice (EBP) was introduced in the 1970s by Dr. Archie Cochrane, an Englishman who wrote a dynamic book questioning the efficacy of non–research-based practices in medicine (Melnyk & Fineout-Overholt, 2011).

In particular, Dr. Cochrane emphasized the critical review of research, largely focusing on randomized control trials (RCTs) to support medical practice. His influence eventually led to development of the Cochrane Collaboration, an organization charged with developing, maintaining, and updating systematic reviews of health care interventions (Cochrane Collaboration, 2013). Although the notion of EBP was somewhat delayed in being recognized and implemented in nursing, over the past two decades, EBP has appeared with increasing frequency in the nursing literature and now has essentially become the standard for research-based, informed decision making for nursing care.

EBP is similar to research-based practice and has been called an approach to problem solving that conscientiously uses the current "best" evidence in the care of patients (LoBiondo-Wood & Haber, 2010). EBP involves identifying a clinical problem, searching the literature, critically evaluating the research evidence, and determining appropriate interventions. Nursing scholars note that EBP relies on integrating research, theory, and practice and is equivalent to theory-based practice as the objective of both is the highest level of safety and efficacy for patients (Fawcett & Garity, 2009).

Overview of Evidence-Based Practice

The concept of EBP is widely accepted as a requisite in health care. EBP is based on the premise that health professionals should not center practice on tradition and belief but on sound information grounded in research findings and scientific development (Melnyk & Fineout-Overholt, 2011; Schmidt & Brown, 2012). Until the early part of the 21st century, the concept of EBP was more common in Canadian and English nursing literature than in U.S. nursing literature. Over the last decade, however, the term has become ubiquitous. This is attributed in part to the guideline initiatives of the Agency for Health Care Quality, the Institute of Medicine, and the U.S. Preventative Services Task Force, among others (Hudson, Duke, Haas, & Varnell, 2008; Melnyk & Fineout-Overholt, 2011).

Many nursing scholars (DiCenso, Guyatt, & Ciliska, 2005; Ingersoll, 2000; LoBiondo-Wood & Haber, 2010; Melnyk & Fineout-Overholt, 2011; Rycroft-Malone, 2004) have pointed out that EBP and research are not synonymous. They are both scholarly processes but focus on different phases of knowledge development—application versus discovery. In general, EBP refers to the integration of individual clinical expertise with the best available external clinical evidence from systematic research. It is largely based on research studies, particularly studies using clinical trials, meta-analysis, and studies of client outcomes, and it is more likely to be applied in practice settings that value the use of new knowledge and in settings that provide resources to access that knowledge.

Definition and Characteristics of Evidence-Based Practice

In medicine, EBP has been defined as the conscientious, explicit, and judicious use of the current best evidence in making decisions about the care of individual patients (Sackett, Straus, Richardson, Rosenberg, & Haynes, 2000). It is an approach to health care practice in which the clinician is aware of the evidence that relates to clinical practice and the strength of that evidence (Jennings & Loan, 2001; Tod, Palfreyman, & Burke, 2004).

To distinguish nursing from medicine in discussing EBP, a number of definitions have been presented in the literature. Sigma Theta Tau International (2005, para. 4) defined "evidence-based nursing" as "an integration of the best evidence available, nursing expertise, and the values and preferences of the individuals, families, and communities who are served." Similarly, DiCenso and colleagues (2005) defined EBP as "the integration of best research evidence with clinical expertise and patient values to facilitate clinical decision making" (p. 4). Both of these definitions use similar terms (e.g., best evidence, expertise, patient values). Ingersoll (2000) used slightly different terms when she suggested that evidence-based nursing practice "is the conscientious, explicit, and judicious use of theory-derived, research-based information in making decisions about care delivery to individuals or groups of patients and in consideration of individual needs and preferences" (p. 152).

In nursing, EBP generally includes careful review of research findings according to guidelines that nurse scholars have used to measure the merit of a study or group of studies. Evidence-based nursing de-emphasizes ritual, isolated, and unsystematic clinical experiences; ungrounded opinions; and tradition as a basis for practice and stresses the use of research findings. Other measures or factors, including nursing expertise, health resources, patient/family preferences, quality improvement efforts, and the consensus of recognized experts, are also incorporated as appropriate (Melnyk & Fineout-Overholt, 2011; Schmidt & Brown, 2012).

In summary, EBP has several critical features. First, it is a problem-based approach and considers the context of the practitioner's current experience. In addition, EBP brings together the best available evidence and current practice by combining research with tacit knowledge and theory. Third, it incorporates values, beliefs, and desires of the patients and their families. Finally, EBP facilitates the application of research findings by incorporating first- and second-hand knowledge into practice. Link to Practice 12-1 presents information on databases that nurses and others can access to find specific information on current guidelines and other collections of "evidence" that can be used to improve health care.

Link to Practice 12-1

Key Resources for Evidence-Based Practice

Several important databases have been set up over the last 20 years to promote integration of "evidence" in health care. Information on three of the most influential are presented here.

Cochrane Collaboration - http://www.cochrane.org/

The Cochrane Collaboration is an international network that helps health care practitioners, policy makers, patients, and their advocates make informed decisions about health care. The Cochrane Library prepares, updates, and promotes the accessibility of the *Cochrane Database of Systematic Reviews.*

Joanna Briggs Institute - http://www.joannabriggs.edu.au/

The Joanna Briggs Institute is an international research and development organization from the School of Translational Science at the University of Adelaide, South Australia. The Institute and its collaborating entities promote and support the synthesis, transfer, and utilization of evidence through identifying feasible, appropriate, meaningful, and effective health care practices to assist in the improvement of health care outcomes.

Agency for Healthcare Research and Quality (U.S. Preventative Services Task Force/ National Guideline Clearinghouse) http://www.guideline.gov/

The National Guideline Clearinghouse (NGC) is a database of evidence-based clinical practice guidelines. It is intended to be used by health professionals, practitioners, patients, and others to obtain objective, detailed information on clinical practice guidelines and to further their dissemination, implementation, and use.

Concerns Related to Evidence-Based Practice in Nursing

Despite growing acceptance of application of EBP in nursing, some criticisms and concerns have been voiced in the nursing literature. For example, there is the concern that EBP is more focused on the science of nursing than on the art of nursing. Some authors have expressed concern that strict concentration on empirically based knowledge will lead to the failure to capture the uniqueness of nursing and the importance of holistic care in contemporary practice (Fawcett, Watson, Neuman, Walker, & Fitzpatrick, 2001; Hudson et al., 2008; Upton, 1999).

Another concern is that strict reliance on EBP will place nurses in the role of medical extender or medical technician, where nursing will be reduced to a technical practice. This concern was voiced as equating EBP with "cookbook care" and a disregard for individualized patient care (Finkelman & Kenner, 2013; Melnyk & Fineout-Overholt, 2011). Indeed, although evidence may provide direction for development of procedures, techniques, and protocols for nursing, it has been established that these are not the only knowledge that informs the nursing practice and that consideration of individual needs and values is essential (Hudson et al., 2008; Mitchell, 2013).

Third, because research involving humans is complex, findings may be open to interpretation and therefore should not be the sole basis for practice. Research must be considered within the context of the practice prescribed by theory, and it must integrate the values and beliefs of nursing philosophy (Chinn & Kramer, 2011; McKenna & Slevin, 2008; Walker & Avant, 2011).

A fourth concern relates to promoting a link with evidence-based medicine and its emphasis on positivist thinking and the dominance of randomized clinical trials as the major evidence. This concern is related to the absence of consideration of evidence gathered through qualitative research and theory development (Fawcett et al., 2001; Jennings & Loan, 2001; Stevens, 2001).

A fifth concern relates to the potential for linking health care reimbursement exclusively to interventions that can be substantiated by a documented body of evidence (Ingersoll, 2000). This leads to a number of ethical questions and issues that should be considered.

Finally, it is argued that not all practice in the health professions can or should be based on science. In many cases, researchers have yet to accumulate a sufficient body of knowledge. In other cases, a different frame of reference provides a different rationale for action (McKenna & Slevin, 2008). In these instances, strict reliance on EBP may result in numerous voids when developing a plan of care.

Concerns such as these have been addressed by DiCenso and colleagues (2005), who assert that a fundamental principle of EBP is that research evidence alone is not sufficient to plan care. Other ethical and pragmatic factors, such as benefits and risks, associated costs, and patient's wishes, should be considered. Further, they note that "best research evidence" can be quantitative or qualitative and does not necessarily rely on RCTs. These notions are also supported by Rycroft-Malone (2004), who maintains that well-conceived and well-conducted qualitative and quantitative research evidence, clinical experience, and patient experiences, combined with local or organizational influences, are necessary to facilitate EBP.

Evidence-Based Practice and Practice-Based Evidence

Recently, a new concept—"practice-based evidence" (PBE)—was introduced into the discussion of EBP (Horn & Gassaway, 2007). The notion of PBE addresses many of the concerns noted previously and is grounded in the recognition that frequently interventions have limited formal research support, particularly in the number or quality of RCTs.

The premise of PBE is that large databases—not just clinical research—should be reviewed or "mined" to gather data to demonstrate quality and effectiveness. This type of review can provide comprehensive information about patient characteristics, care processes, and outcomes while controlling for patient differences (Walker & Avant, 2011). PBE acknowledges the importance of the environment in determining practice recommendations and recognizes that knowledge can be generated from practice as well as from research (Chinn & Kramer, 2011).

The intent behind PBE is to determine what works best for which patients, under what circumstances, and at what costs by providing a more comprehensive picture than RCTs, which typically examine one intervention with limited populations and under strictly controlled circumstances (Huston, 2011). Additional sources beyond formal research studies that are appropriate as PBE include benchmarking data, clinical expertise, cost-effective analyses, infection control data, medical record data, national standards of care, quality improvement data, and patient and family preferences (Huston, 2011).

Horn and Gassaway (2007) concluded that use of the PBE analyses can uncover better practices more rapidly leading to improved patient outcomes. Figure 12-1 illustrates one interpretation of the interrelationships among EBP, PBE, research, and theory in nursing.

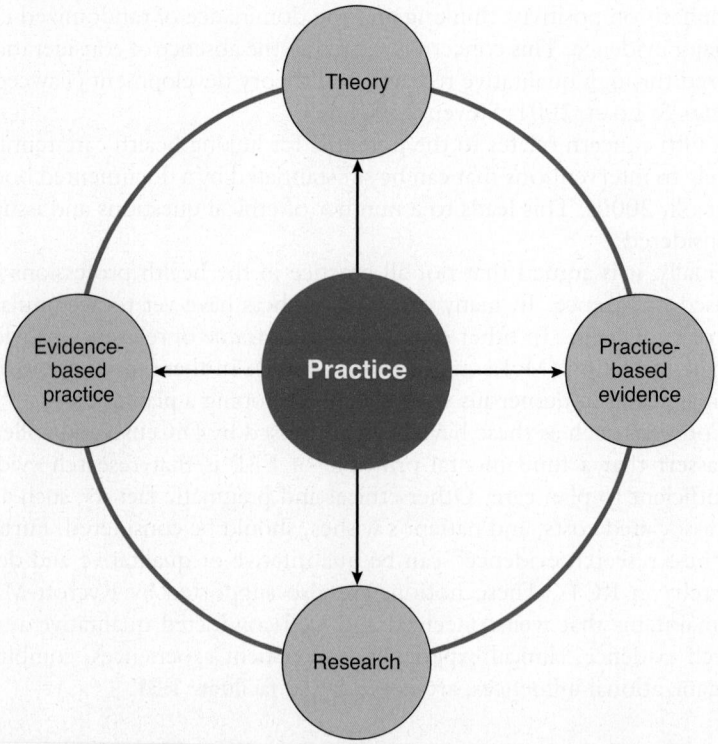

Figure 12-1 Relationships among practice, theory, research, and the PBE/EBP cycle. (From Walker, L. O., & Avant, K. C. [© 2011]. *Strategies for theory construction in nursing* [5th ed., Fig. 2-3; p. 46]. Reprinted by permission of Pearson Education, Inc., Upper Saddle River, NJ.)

Promotion of Evidence-Based Practice in Nursing

Implementation of EBP in nursing is still evolving, as often, nursing interventions are based on experience, tradition, intuition, common sense, and untested theories. While emphasis on EBP is growing rapidly, the actual incorporation of nursing research findings in practice has lagged. Melnyk and Fineout-Overholt (2011) have outlined barriers to implementation of research and EBP in nursing (Box 12-1).

There is significant support for increasing emphasis on EBP in nursing, and many organizations such as the Institute of Medicine, Sigma Theta Tau International, and the Magnet Recognition Program of the American Nurses Credentialing Center, among others, have designed initiatives to advance EBP (Finkelman & Kenner, 2013; Huston, 2011; Melnyk & Fineout-Overholt, 2011). Indeed, practitioners, researchers, and scholars should welcome it because a systematic process of EBP may assist nurses in reducing the gap between theory and practice.

Theory and Evidence-Based Practice

The growing interest and appreciation of EBP in nursing, along with its considerable interconnectedness with research, has served in some ways to de-emphasize theory. As nurses become more aware of and attuned to EBP, however, they are renewing their appreciation of the linkages among research, theory, and practice. It has been observed that nursing focus on EBP has the potential to promote and draw new attention to this connection (Chinn & Kramer, 2011).

Walker and Avant (2011) pointed out that practice is the central and core phenomenon and focus of nursing; arguably, it is the reason for nursing's existence. Thus, it is critical to remember that theory guides practice and it also generates models of testing in research through both PBE and EBP. Further, research and clinical data provide evidence for EBP or PBE and can generate practice guidelines and/or theories (e.g., situation-specific theories). This process is interactive and iterative (Walker & Avant, 2011). For nursing therefore, practice must not only be evidence-based but also theory-based, for when

Box 12-1 Barriers to Evidence-Based Practice in Nursing

- Lack of EBP knowledge and skills
- Misperceptions or negative attitudes about research and evidence-based care
- Lack of belief that EBP will result in more positive outcomes than traditional care
- Voluminous amounts of information in professional journals
- Lack of time and resources to search for and appraise evidence
- Overwhelming patient loads
- Organizational constraints (e.g., lack of administrative support or incentives)
- Demands from patients for a certain type of treatment
- Peer pressure to continue with practices that are steeped in tradition
- Resistance to change
- Lack of consequences for not implementing EBP
- Lack of autonomy over practice and incentives
- Inadequate EBP content and behavioral skills in educational programs
- Continued teaching of rigorous research methods in BSN and MSN programs instead of teaching evidence-based approach to care

Source: Melnyk and Fineout-Overholt (2011).

research validates a theory, it provides the evidence required for EBP. Finally, as more research is conduced about a specific theory, more evidence is provided to support practice (Chinn & Kramer, 2011; George, 2011).

Fawcett and colleagues (2001) wrote of a preference for the term "theory-guided, evidence-based practice," noting that theory is the reason for, and the value of, evidence. The "evidence," they stated, must extend beyond an emphasis on empirical research and RCTs to include evidence generated from theories. Indeed, the evidence itself refers to evidence about theories. Further, they contend that theory determines what counts as evidence; thus, theory and evidence are inextricably linked.

Theoretical Models of EBP

Numerous models of EBP have been developed by nurses to encourage translation of nursing research into practice. In many instances, the goal or intent is to create or establish EBP protocols, procedures, or guidelines. In some instances, universities and hospital groups have developed models to assist students or health care professionals in implementing EBP in their setting. In other instances, nurse researchers and scholars have interpreted the transfer of research evidence to nursing education and practice through processes that progressed from theory-based nursing, quality improvement, research utilization, and lately, evidence-based nursing practice. This section reviews five EBP models that are among the most frequently cited in the nursing literature. These have been widely studied and applied, many in multiple settings and for a variety of patient issues, situations, or nursing care processes. These models include:

- Academic Center for Evidence-Based Practice Star Model (ACE Star Model) (Stevens, 2004)
- Advancing Research and Clinical Practice Through Close Collaboration (ARCC Model) (Melnyk & Fineout-Overholt, 2011)
- Iowa Model (Titler et al., 2001)
- Johns Hopkins Nursing Evidence-Based Practice Model (JHNEBP) (Newhouse, Dearholt, Poe, Pugh, & White, 2007)
- Stetler Model of Evidence-Based Practice (Stetler, 2001)

These models can provide guidance for practicing nurses and advanced practice nurses to promote or enhance EBP and to develop practice guidelines, protocols, or interventions as appropriate. Each model will be described briefly and reviewed for its utility in nursing practice and education.

ACE Star Model of Knowledge Transformation

The ACE Star Model was developed by faculty at the University of Texas Health Science Center at San Antonio (UTHSCSA) (Stevens, 2004). The Star Model is depicted by five points of knowledge transformation. The five forms of knowledge transformation occur in "relative sequence" when research evidence progresses through several cycles and is combined with other knowledge and then applied in practice.

Each point of the star represents a step in a process. The step-wise depiction allows for easy comprehension and is therefore useful even for novice nurses. In order, the points are:

1. Discovery research
2. Evidence summary
3. Translation to guidelines
4. Practice integration
5. Process, outcome evaluation (UTHSCSA, 2012) (Figure 12-2)

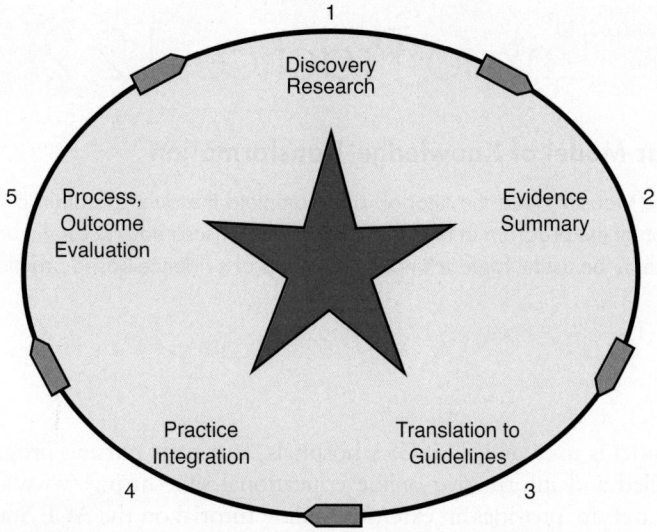

© 2012 Stevens

Figure 12-2 Diagram of the ACE star model for evidence-based practice. (Used with permission from Stevens, K. R. (2012). ACE Star Model: Knowledge transformation©. Academic Center for Evidence-Based Practice. Available at http://www.acestar.uthscsa.edu/acestar-model.asp)

This sequence allows the nurse to move research-based knowledge from one point to the next in sequence to provide a translation of evidence on which to base practice (Stevens, 2004, 2005). Knowledge transformation consists of eight premises that underlie and explain the position of the researchers who created the model. These are presented in Box 12-2. The rigor of the process the nurse or committee uses is part of the value of the knowledge transformation that occurs when using this model.

Box 12-2 ACE Star Model: Knowledge Transformation—Underlying Premises

1. Knowledge transformation (KT) is necessary prior to using research results in clinical decision making.
2. KT derives from multiple sources, including research, experience, authority, trial and error, and theoretical principles.
3. Systematic processes control bias; the research process is the most stable source of knowledge.
4. Evidence can be classified into a hierarchy of strength of evidence depending on the rigor of the science that produced the evidence.
5. Knowledge exists in a variety of forms. As research is converted through a system of steps, other knowledge is created.
6. The form in which knowledge exists can be referenced to its use.
7. The form of knowledge determines its usability.
8. Knowledge is transformed through steps, such as summarization, translation, application, integration, and evaluation.

Abstracted from Stevens, K. R. (2012). ACE Star Model, UT Health Science Center, San Antonio. http://www.acestar.uthscsa.edu/acestar-model.asp (Accessed May 29, 2013).

Link to Practice 12-2

ACE Star Model of Knowledge Transformation

Access the website, take the tutorial, and complete the quiz to obtain a certificate of completion of the program at http://www.acestar.uthscsa.edu/acestar-model.asp. This Web site may be useful for teaching the elements of evidence-based practice to nursing students.

The model is used at UTHSCSA hospitals, and their nursing program maintains a very detailed and informative online educational site (http://www.acestar.uthscsa.edu/). The website provides an extensive online tutorial on the ACE Star Model complete with detailed information, resources, instructive videos, and slides. A quiz and a certificate of attendance are available for those completing instruction in the model (see Link to Practice 12-2). The ACE Star Model is useful in teaching nurses and nursing students the process of research evidence utilization in practice (Schaffer, Sandau, & Diedrick, 2013). One concern or criticism of the ACE Star Model has been noted by White (2012), who pointed out that it does not use evidence other than research per se.

Advancing Research and Clinical Practice Through Close Collaboration Model

Melnyk and Fineout-Overholt (2002) developed the ARCC Model through their work with many health care institutions seeking to advance and sustain EBP. This development was a process that involved many iterations and empirical testing of key relationships. The framework of the ARCC Model is taken from control theory and cognitive behavioral theories, which help guide nurses' behaviors as they gain acumen in EBP (Melnyk & Fineout-Overholt, 2011). Numerous studies and examples of how the ARCC Model has been implemented in clinical practice are available in the literature (Melnyk, 2002; Melnyk, 2004; Melnyk, Feinstein, & Fairbanks, 2002; Melnyk et al., 2011).

The AARC Model relates best to clinical practice, and much of the research supporting its development and implementation was conducted in acute care, pediatric settings. The central constructs are assessment of organizational culture and readiness for EBP, identification of strengths and major barriers to EBP, and development and use of EBP mentors. These constructs are done sequentially and followed by EBP implementation. Outcomes that should be evaluated include health care provider satisfaction, cohesion, intent to leave, turnover, improved patient outcomes, and hospital costs (Melnyk & Fineout-Overholt, 2011).

In employing the ARCC Model, the authors developed several scales to measure the ability to implement EBP. These are the Organizational Culture and Readiness Scale for System-wide Integration of Evidence-based Practice (OCRSIEP) and the EBP Beliefs scale (EBPB) (Melnyk & Fineout-Overholt, 2011). Organizational readiness is first assessed, and when feasible, mentors are identified and developed. The clinical nurses are then mentored through use of the ARCC system. Melnyk and Fineout-Overholt (2011) state that measuring the key constructs along with workshops and academic offerings assist organizations to adopt and sustain EBP. Finally, Melnyk and Fineout-Overholt (2011) developed a flow chart to assist in use of the model. Box 12-3 gives examples of research that has been conducted employing the ARCC Model of EBP.

Box 12-3 Research Based on the ARCC Model of EBP

O'Haver, J., Moore, I. M., Reed, P. G., Melnyk, B. M., & Savoie, M. (2010). Parental perceptions of risk and protective factors associated with the adaptation of siblings of children with cystic fibrosis. *Pediatric Nursing, 36*(6), 284–291.

Levin, R. F., & Lewis-Holman, S. (2011). Developing guidelines for critical protocol development. *Research and Theory for Nursing Practice, 25*(4), 233–237.

Melnyk, B. M., Fineout-Overholt, E., Gallagher-Ford, L., & Kaplan, L. (2012). Critical implications for nurse leaders and educators. *Journal of Nursing Administration, 42*(9), 410–417.

Melnyk, B. M., Fineout-Overholt, E., Giggleman, M., & Cruz, R. (2010). Correlates among cognitive beliefs, EBP implementation, organizational culture, cohesion and job satisfaction in evidence-based practice mentors from a community hospital system. *Nursing Outlook, 58*(6), 301–308.

Thorsteinsson, H. S. (2013). Icelandic nurses' beliefs, skills, and resources associated with evidence-based practice and related factors: A national survey. *Worldviews on Evidence-Based Nursing, 10*(2), 116–126.

The Iowa Model of Evidence-Based Practice to Promote Quality Care

The Iowa Model of EBP was developed in 1994 to promote quality care through research utilization. It is intended to provide guidance for nurses and others in making decisions about practice that affects patient outcomes. The Iowa Model incorporates starting points, which are nursing problems that are termed "triggers." It continues through multiple decision points and feedback loops to provide for evaluation of any changes (Titler et al., 2001).

The model has been refined over time to produce the current iteration (Titler, 2004; Titler & Adams, 2010). The diagram of the model shows the starting points, decision points, and feedback loops. When implemented, it will assist in providing quality care to clients of clinics, home health agencies, and hospitals (Titler et al., 2001) (see Figure 12-3). The Iowa Model is very detailed and specific and has been applied to address a number of clinical topics. It is also one of the best researched EBP models. Box 12-4 shows some of the recent research studies that have used the Iowa model.

The Johns Hopkins Nursing Evidence-Based Practice Model

The Johns Hopkins Nursing EBP (JHNEBP) Model was developed to accelerate the transfer of research to practice and to promote nurse autonomy, leadership, and engagement with interdisciplinary colleagues (Melnyk & Fineout-Overholt, 2011). The JHNEBP Model was designed as a problem-solving approach to clinical decision making. It combines elements of the nursing process, the American Nurses Association's Standards of Practice, critical thinking, and research utilization processes (Newhouse et al., 2007). The model has numerous levels of activity, but it is based on practical teaching processes to promote use by novice nurses as well as more experienced nurses.

The JHNEBP process is based on three core elements: a practice question, evidence, and translation (PET) (Newhouse et al., 2007). As presented in Box 12-5, 18 steps are included in the model. As shown, each of the PET phases is based on several steps that clarify how the processes are to proceed.

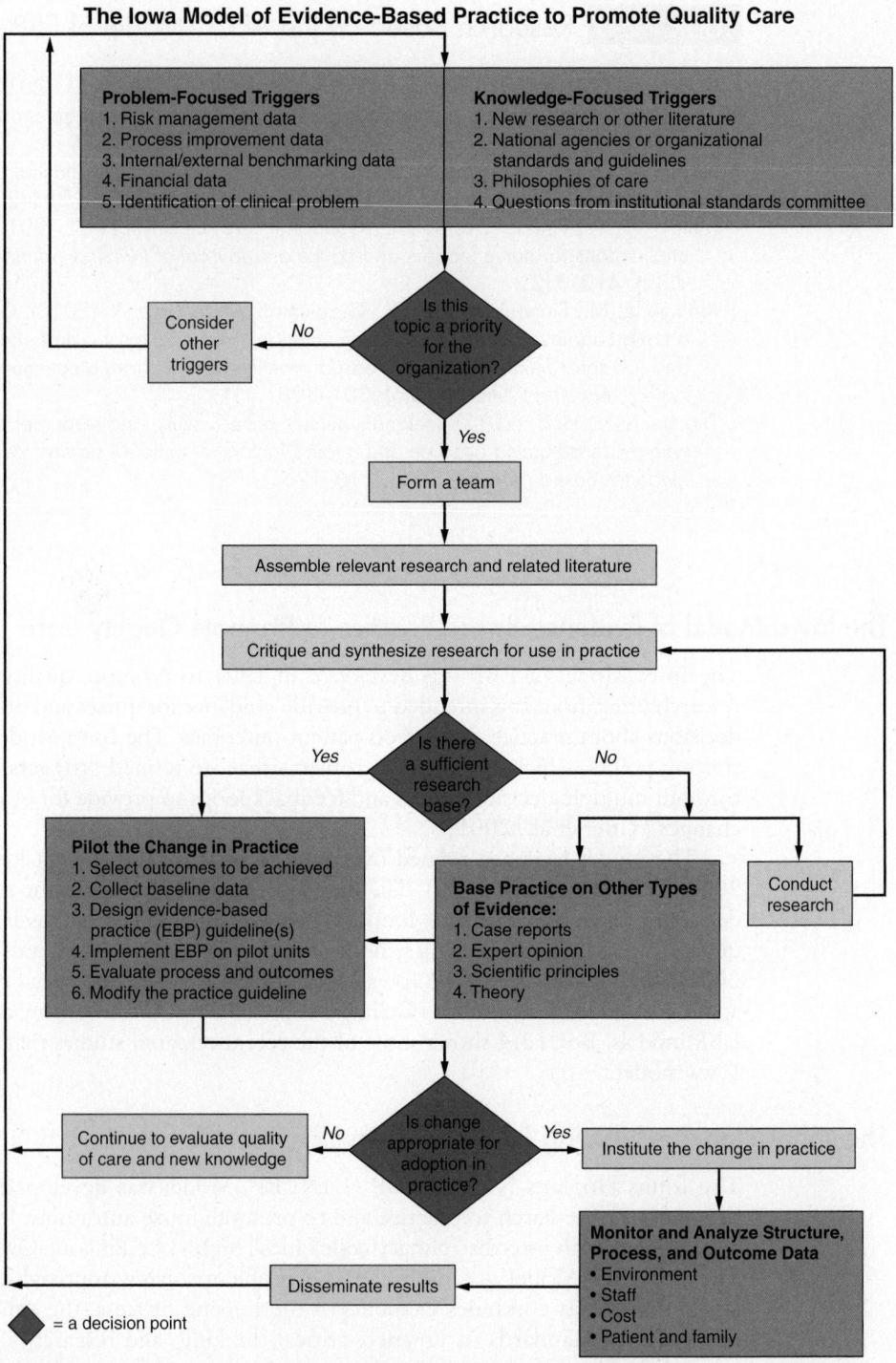

Figure 12-3 Diagram of the Iowa method of evidence-based practice. (Reprinted with permission from University of Iowa Hospitals and Clinics. © 1998. For permission to use or reproduce the model, please contact University of Iowa Hospitals and Clinics at 319-384-9098.)

Box 12-4 Research Based on the Iowa Model of Evidence-Based Practice to Promote Quality Care

Alexander, L., & Allen, D. (2011). Establishing an evidence-based inpatient medical oncology fluid balance measurement policy. *Clinical Journal of Oncology Nursing, 15*(1), 23–25.

Bergstrom, K. (2011). Development of a radiation skin care protocol and algorithm using the Iowa Model of Evidence-Based Practice. *Clinical Journal of Oncology Nursing, 15*(6), 593–597.

Chung, K., Davis, I., Moughrabi, S., & Gawlinski, A. (2011). Use of an evidence-based shift report tool to improve nurses' communication. *Medsurg Nursing, 20*(5), 255–268.

Hermes, B., Deakin, K., Lee, K., & Robinson, S. (2009). Suicide risk assessment: 6 steps to a better instrument. *Journal of Psychosocial Nursing and Mental Health Services, 47*(6), 44–49.

Kowal, C. D. (2010). Implementing the Critical Care Pain Observation Tool using the Iowa Model. *Journal of the New York State Nurses Association, 41*(1), 4–10.

Myrick, K. M. (2011). Improving follow-up after fragility fractures: An evidence-based initiative. *Orthopaedic Nursing, 30*(3), 174–181.

Popovitch, M. A., Boyd, C., Dachenhaus, T., & Kusler, D. (2012). Improving stable patient flow through the emergency department by utilizing evidence-based practice: One hospital's journey. *Journal of Emergency Nursing, 38*(5), 474–478.

Box 12-5 Steps of The Johns Hopkins Nursing Evidence-Based Practice Model (PET)

P: Practice Question Steps

1. Identify an EBP question (PICO).
2. Define the scope of the practice question.
3. Assign responsibility for leadership.
4. Recruit an interdisciplinary team.
5. Schedule a team conference.

E: Evidence Steps

6. Conduct an internal and external search for evidence.
7. Appraise all types of evidence.
8. Summarize the evidence.
9. Rate the strength of the evidence.
10. Develop recommendations for change in systems or processes of care based on the strength of the evidence.

T: Translation Method of Evidence-Based Practice Steps

11. Determine the appropriateness and feasibility of translating recommendations into the specific practice setting.
12. Create an action plan.
13. Implement the change.
14. Evaluate outcomes.
15. Report the results of the preliminary evaluation to decision makers.
16. Secure support from decision makers to implement the recommended change internally.
17. Identify the next steps.
18. Communicate the findings.

Source: Newhouse et al., 2007, pp. 42–47.

This method begins with an EBP question, and the first step is to generate an answerable **P**ractice question which includes the patient, population, and the problem. It goes on to define an **I**ntervention, makes a **C**omparison with other treatments if possible, and finally defines the desired **O**utcome (PICO) (Newhouse et al., 2007). Four other steps in the "practice question" phase include defining the scope of the question, assigning responsibility for leadership, recruiting a team, and scheduling conferences. In the evidence phase, literature searches and appraisal and recommendations come from the team (Newhouse et al., 2007).

In the third phase, translation, the team decides whether or not and how to implement the changes, evaluate any such implementation, and communicate the findings to appropriate individuals or groups (Newhouse et al., 2007). The JHNEBP Model is clearly explained and simple to apply. Related writings include the guidelines and definitions of the background, elements of the process, and the steps of the model (Newhouse et al., 2007).

Stetler Model of Evidence-Based Practice

The Stetler Model of EBP was initiated in the 1970s as a quality improvement (QI) effort using the research utilization (RU) ideals then in widespread use (Melnyk & Fineout-Overholt, 2011). Through several iterations, Stetler updated the approach and clarified the series of phases of the model such that it is readily implemented by practicing nurses and useful at the bedside (Stetler, Ritchie, Rycroft-Malone, Schultz, & Charns, 2007). Stetler and colleagues (1998) and Stetler and Caramanica (2007) argued that all research studies are not ready for use at the bedside. Further, they explained that alternative sources or evidence are necessary to fill the gaps in nursing research evidence.

The Stetler Model is similar to the nursing process; therefore, it is easily assimilated by practicing bedside nurses. The phases of the approach include preparation, validation, comparative evaluation/decision making, translation/application, and evaluation. It provides practitioners with stepwise directions for integrating research into practice. See Table 12-1 for description of the phases. The Stetler Model incorporates five steps to generate a process that takes into account the many other facets of nursing and the clinical situation prior to using research findings in the nurse's clinical practice. When implemented, the results should be systematically evaluated to track goal-oriented outcomes and proffer both formative and summative evaluation strategies. The major outcomes of RU or EBP should be improved patient results as well as enhanced professional practice (Stetler & Caramanica, 2007).

Theoretical Models: A Summary

The five EBP models described above are compared in Table 12-2 on page 272 using the following criteria:

- Groups of health care professionals affected (Groups Affected)
- Environmental factors in which the model is useful (Environment)
- Analysis of the model (Analysis)
- Implementation: barriers/facilitators (Implementation)
- Evaluation of effectiveness identified by the model (Evaluation)

As shown, there are a number of similarities among the models. Schafffer and colleagues (2013) recently compiled a review of models for organizational change based on EBP. Similar to what has been presented here, their overview examined the

Table 12-1 Phases of the Stetler Model

Phase	Content	Actions
I	Preparation (Purpose, control, and sources of research evidence)	■ Define potential issues ■ Seek sources of research evidence ■ Perceive problems ■ Focus on high-priority issues ■ Decide on need for a team ■ Consider other influential factors ■ Define desired outcomes ■ Seek systematic reviews ■ Determine need for explicit research evidence ■ Select research sources with conceptual fit
II	Validation (Credibility of findings and potential for/detailed qualifiers of application)	■ Credibility of findings ■ Critique and synthesize resources ■ Critique systematic reviews ■ Reassess fit of individual sources ■ Rate the level and quality of evidence ■ Differentiate statistical and clinical significance ■ Eliminate noncredible sources ■ End the process if there is no evidence or clearly insufficient credible research evidence
III	Comparative evaluation/decision making (Synthesis and decisions/ recommendations for criteria of applicability)	■ Synthesize the cumulative findings ■ Evaluate the degree and nature of other criteria ■ Make a decision whether/what to use ■ If decide to "not use," STOP use of the model ■ If decide to use, determine recommendations for a specific practice
IV	Translation/application (operational definition of use/actions for change)	■ Types ■ Methods ■ Levels ■ Direct instrumental use ■ Cognitive use ■ Symbolic use ■ Caution: Assess whether translation/product or use goes beyond actual findings/evidence ■ Formal dissemination and change strategies should be planned per relevant research ■ Consider need for appropriate reasoned variation
V	Evaluation (alternative types of evaluation)	■ Evaluation can be formal or informal, individual or institutional ■ Consider cost-benefit of evaluation efforts ■ Use RU as a process to enhance credibility of evaluation data ■ For both dynamic and pilot evaluations include two types of evaluative information

From Stetler, C. B. (2001). Updating the Stetler model of research utilization to facilitate evidence-based practice. *Nursing Outlook, 49*(6), p. 277. From Figure 3B. Stetler Model Part II: Additional, per phase details.

key features of six models with the view to change practice in organizations. Most of the models incorporate the steps of the research process in some way, and all the models are focused on bringing the best in safe and effective nursing care to their major focus: the patient, or recipient of nursing care. Nurses who are actively engaged in promoting EBP are encouraged to review these as well as other published models and to select the one that best fits their needs and desired outcomes.

Table 12-2 Comparison of Selected Models of EBP

	Models of Evidence-Based Practice				
Comparison Element	**ACE Star Model**	**ARCC Model**	**Iowa Model**	**Johns Hopkins Model**	**Stetler Model**
Groups of health care professionals (Users)	Instructors, students, practicing nurses	Advanced practice nurses, practicing nurses	Instructors, students, practicing nurses	Practicing nurses	Practicing nurses or groups of nurses
Environmental factors in which the model is useful (Environment)	Learning environments, hospitals	Patient care organizations	Nursing schools and patient care agencies	Learning environments, hospitals	Clinical situations
Analysis of the model (Analysis)	Five major points similar to the nursing process	Five constructs with similarity to nursing process	Six steps of the model: Identify knowledge or problem focused triggers (catalysts to critical thinking). Priority: organizational Form a team responsible for development, implementation and evaluation of EBP	PET (see Box 12-5, p. 269) 18 steps are the basis for the model. Team approach to answer *P*ractice questions, critique *E*vidence and *T*ranslate it into usable form	Five phases: (I) Preparation (II) Validation (III) Comparative evaluation/ decision making (IV) Translation/ application (V) Evaluation
Implementation: barriers/ facilitators (Implementation)	Implementation into practice is the fifth stage and involves bringing evidence to clinical decision making	Implementation is based on the mentor's determination of organizational readiness.	Determine sufficiency of evidence. If yes: Pilot recommended change.	Team determines feasibility and creates an action plan to implement the change.	Translation and application is the fourth step.
Evaluation of the effectiveness of the model (Evaluation)	Evaluation is the final stage and focuses on verification of the success EBP (Stevens, 2004).	Evaluation is the fifth of the constructs and has three levels that provide feedback. (Melnyk & Fineout-Overholt, 2002).	Evaluate pilot success and disseminate results; implement into practice. (Titler et al., 2001).	Step 14: Evaluate the outcomes, report the results, and communicate findings. (Newhouse et al., 2007).	Evaluation is the last step (Stetler, 2001).

Helen, the nurse from the opening case study, conducted a systematic review of neuromuscular illnesses and treatments using the Iowa Model of EBP. During this process, she came to better understand her illness and the treatments that would most likely forestall deterioration of her condition. The complexity and high level of information she accumulated through her review of the research guided by theories of EBP and PBE brought Helen to a level of practice where she could not only help herself but also her patients and clients. Following graduation, she based her clinical practice on the expertise she had gained through her extensive study of the research and practice in neuromuscular diseases.

Summary

There is little doubt that EBP has become one of the key tenets of quality nursing care. As described, however, it is critical to remember that EBP must go beyond research per se and emphasis on RCT but must also be theory based. Indeed, the growing attention to the concept of PBE has renewed attention to the essential role of theory in excellent nursing practice. Many authors have written about the problems and barriers to EBP, and others have written on how to strengthen the process and make it relevant to practicing nurses.

Over the last decade, a number of models have been constructed to assist nurses to learn how to proceed in the development of evidence-based guidelines and promotion of EBP, as illustrated by the work of Helen in the case study. The five models described here, along with a number of others that have been mentioned in the nursing literature, give nurses information about the steps and processes necessary to elicit the evidence that is needed to provide safe, effective interventions that are effective in nursing practice. Nurses who seek to use research in their clinical areas are advised to seek out a working model of EBP and follow it through to effect reasonable, safe, and effective changes for the benefit of their patients or clients.

Key Points

- In nursing, research, theory, and practice are integrated; EBP is a key element and outcome of that linkage.
- EBP is an approach to problem solving that uses the current best evidence in the care of patients.
- In nursing, EBP has been defined as "the conscientious, explicit, and judicious use of theory-derived, research-based information in making decisions about care delivery . . . in consideration of individual needs and preferences."
- Nursing as a profession has been relatively slow to incorporate EBP; that has changed in recent years.
- Many nurses are concerned that too much attention to EBP will draw attention away from the art of nursing care—that nursing will become lost in the science.
- Models of EBP have developed from early studies of research utilization and quality improvement. Many of these models have been developed with the impetus of hospitals or educational institutions' support.
- The major impetus for integration and implementation of research evidence—guided by EBP—should be reasonable, effective, and safe care for patients.

Learning Activities

1. Select one model of EBP presented. Using your current clinical setting and a practice problem you have noticed, determine what you would do to institute EBP into your current practice to address the problem.
2. Compare and contrast two EBP models and write a blog on which would most likely work in your agency or clinical unit. Explain why one model would work better than the other with your colleagues or your organizational culture.
3. Prepare a proposal for practice change in your agency or clinical unit using one of the models given in this chapter. Use as many of the steps of the model as possible and project the outcomes for the remaining steps.

REFERENCES

Chinn, P. L., & Kramer, M. K. (2011). *Integrated theory and knowledge development in nursing* (8th ed.). St. Louis: Elsevier.

Cochrane Collaboration (2013). *About us.* Retrieved from http://www.cochrane.org/about-us

DiCenso, A., Guyatt, G., & Ciliska, D. (2005). Introduction to evidence-based nursing. In A. DiCenso, D. Ciliska, & G. Guyatt (Eds.), *Evidence-based nursing: A guide to clinical practice* (pp. 3–19). St. Louis: Elsevier.

Fawcett, J., & Garity, J. (2009). *Evaluating research for evidence-based nursing practice.* Philadelphia: F. A. Davis.

Fawcett, J., Watson, J., Neuman, B., Walker, P. H., & Fitzpatrick, J. J. (2001). On nursing theories and evidence. *Journal of Nursing Scholarship, 33*(2), 115–119.

Finkelman, A., & Kenner, C. (2013). *Professional nursing concepts: Competencies for quality leadership.* Burlington, MA: Jones & Bartlett Learning.

George, J. B. (2011). Nursing theory and clinical practice. In J. B. George, (Ed.). *Nursing theories: The base for professional nursing practice* (6th ed.). Boston: Pearson.

Horn, S. D., & Gassaway, J. (2007). Practice-based evidence study design for comparative effectiveness research. *Medical Care, 45*(10), S50–S57.

Hudson, K., Duke, G., Haas, B., & Varnell, G. (2008). Navigating the evidence-based practice maze. *Journal of Nursing Management, 16*(6), 409–416.

Huston, C. J. (2011). *Professional issues in nursing: Challenges & opportunities* (2nd ed.). Philadelphia: Lippincott Williams & Wilkins.

Ingersoll, G. L. (2000). Evidence-based nursing: What it is and what it isn't. *Nursing Outlook, 48*(4), 151–152.

Jennings, B. M., & Loan, L. A. (2001). Misconceptions among nurses about evidence-based practice. *Journal of Nursing Scholarship, 33*(2), 121–127.

LoBiondo-Wood, G., & Haber, J. (2010). Integrating the processes of research and evidence-based practice. In G. LoBiondo-Wood & J. Haber (Eds.), *Nursing research: Methods, critical appraisal, and utilization* (7th ed., pp. 5–26). St. Louis: Mosby.

McKenna, H. P., & Slevin, O. D. (2008). *Nursing models, theories and practice.* West Sussex, United Kingdom: Blackwell Publishing.

Melnyk, B. M. (2002). Strategies for overcoming barriers in implementing evidence-based practice. *Pediatric Nursing, 28*(2), 159–161.

Melnyk, B. (2004). Sparking a change to evidence-based practice in health care organizations. *Evidence-Based Nursing, 1*(2), 83–84.

Melnyk, B. M., & Fineout-Overholt, E. (2002). Key steps in implementing evidence-based practice: Asking compelling, searchable questions and searching for the best evidence. *Pediatric Nursing, 28*(3), 262–266.

Melnyk, B. M., & Fineout-Overholt, E. (2011). Making the case for evidence-based practice and cultivating the spirit of inquiry. In B. M. Melnyk & E. Fineout-Overhold (Eds.), *Evidence-based practice in nursing and healthcare: A guide to best practice* (2nd ed., pp. 3–24). Philadelphia: Lippincott Williams & Wilkins.

Melnyk, B. M., Feinstein, N. F., & Fairbanks, E. (2002). Effectiveness of informational/behavioral interventions with parents of low birth weight (LBW) premature infants: An evidence base to guide clinical practice. *Pediatric Nursing, 28*(5), 511–516.

Melnyk, B. M., Fineout-Overholt, E., Feinstein, N. F., Li, H., Small, L., & Kraus, R. (2004). Nurses' perceived knowledge, beliefs, skills, and needs regarding evidence-based practice: Implications for accelerating the paradigm shift. *Worldviews on Evidence-Based Nursing, 1*(3), 185–193.

Mitchell, G. J. (2013). Evidence-based practice: Critique and alternative view. In W. K. Cody (Ed.), *Philosophical and theoretical perspectives for advanced nursing practice* (5th ed., pp 321–330). Burlington, MA: Jones and Bartlett.

Newhouse, R. P., Dearholt, S. Poe, S., Pugh, L. C., & White, K. (2007). Organizational change strategies for evidence-based practice. *Journal of Nursing Administration, 37*(12), 552–557.

Rycroft-Malone, J. (2004). The PARIHS framework—A framework for guiding the implementation of evidence-based practice. *Journal of Nursing Care Quality, 19*(4), 297–304.

Sackett, D. L., Straus, S. E., Richardson, W. S., Rosenberg, W., & Haynes, R. B. (2000). *Evidence-based medicine: How to practice and teach EBM.* London, United Kingdom: Churchill Livingstone.

Schaffer, M. A., Sandau, K. E., & Diedrick, L.(2013). Evidence-based practice models for organizational change: Overview and practical applications. *Journal of Advanced Nursing, 69*(5), 1197–1209.

Schmidt, N. A., & Brown, J. M. (2012). *Evidence-based practice for nurses: Appraisal and application of research* (2nd ed.). Burlington, MA: Jones & Bartlett Learning.

Sigma Theta Tau International. (2005). *Position statement on evidence based nursing.* Retrieved from http://www.nursingsociety.org/aboutus/PositionPapers/Pages/EBN_positionpaper.aspx

Stetler, C. B. (2001). Updating the Stetler Model of research utilization to facilitate evidence-based practice. *Nursing Outlook, 49*(6), 272–279.

Stetler, C. B., Brunell, M., Giuitano, K. K., Morsi, D., Prince, L., & Newell-Stokes, V. (1998). Evidence-based practice and the role of nursing leadership. *Journal of Nursing Administration, 28*(7–8), 45–53.

Stetler, C. B., & Caramanica, L. (2007). Evaluation of an evidence-based practice imitative: Outcomes, strengths and limitations of a retrospective conceptually-based approach. *Worldviews on Evidenced-Based Nursing, 4*(4), 187–199.

Stetler, C. B., Ritchie, J., Rycroft-Malone, J., Schultz, A., & Charns, M. (2007). Improving quality of care through routine, successful implementation of evidenced-based practice at the bedside: An organizational case study protocol using the Pettigrew and Whipp model of strategic change. *Implementation Science, 2*(3), 1–13. doi:10.1186/1748-5908-2-3

Stevens, K. R. (2001). The truth, the whole truth . . . about EBP and RCTs. *Journal of Nursing Administration, 32*(5), 232–233.

Stevens, K. R. (2005). *Essential competencies for evidence-based practice in nursing.* San Antonio: Academic Center for Evidence-Based Practice (ACE) of The University of Texas Health Science Center.

Stevens, K. R. (2012). *ACE star model.* San Antonio: Academic Center for Evidence-Based Practice, University of Texas Health Science Center. Retrieved from http://www.acestar.uthscsa.edu/acestar-model.asp

Titler, M. (2004). Methods in translation science. *Worldviews on Evidence-Based Nursing, 1*(1), 38–48.

Titler, M., & Adams, S. (2010). Developing an evidence-based practice. *Nursing research: Methods, critical appraisal, and utilization.* In G. LoBiondo-Wood & J. Haber (Eds.), (7th ed., pp. 385–437). St. Louis: Mosby Elsevier.

Titler, M. G., Kleiber, C., Steelman, V. J., Rakel, B. A., Budreau, G., Everett, L. Q., et al. (2001). The Iowa model of evidence-based practice to promote quality care. *Critical Care Nursing Clinics of North America, 13*(4), 497–509.

Tod, A., Palfreyman, S., & Burke, L. (2004). Evidence-based practice is a time of opportunity for nursing. *British Journal of Nursing, 13*(4), 211–216.

Upton, D. J. (1999). How can we achieve evidence-based practice if we have a theory–practice gap in nursing today? *Journal of Advanced Nursing, 29*(3), 549–555.

University of Texas Health Science Center at San Antonio. (2012). *ACE star model.* Retrieved from http://www.acestar.uthscsa.edu/acestar-model.asp

Walker, L. O., & Avant, K. C. (2011). *Strategies for theory construction in nursing* (5th ed.). Upper Saddle River, NJ: Prentice Hall.

White, K. M. (2012). Evidence-based practice. In K. M. White & S. Dudley-Brown (Eds)., *Translation of evidence into nursing and health care practice* (pp. 3–22). New York: Springer.

UNIT III

Shared Theories Used by Nurses

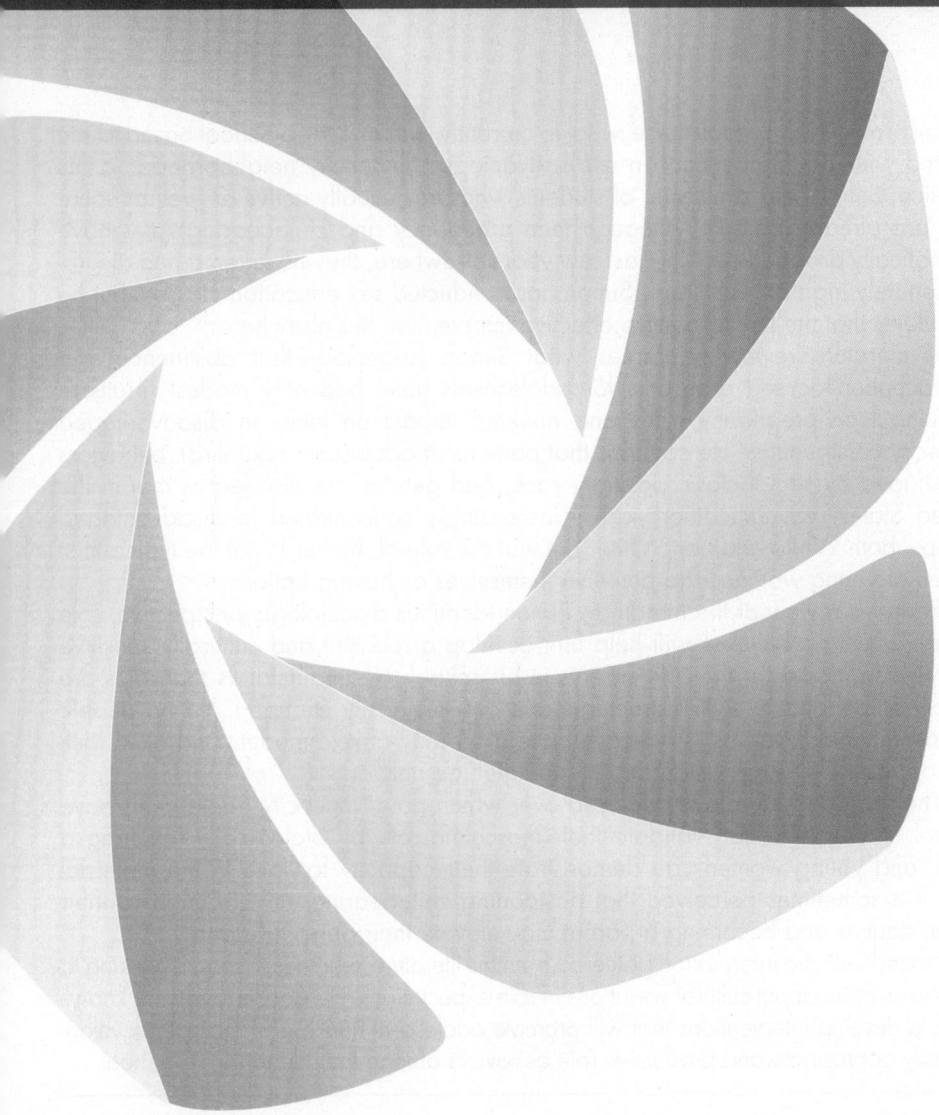

CHAPTER 13

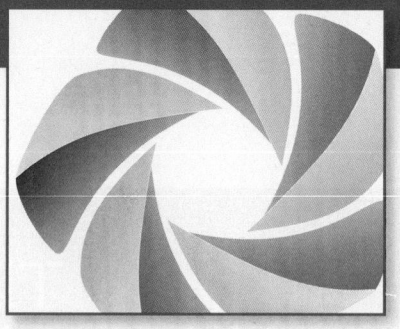

Theories From the Sociologic Sciences

Grace Bielkiewicz

Simon Brown is a school nurse who is currently working in a school-based clinic located within a high school in a disadvantaged, inner-city neighborhood. In his practice, Simon sees a number of students who are sexually active as well as some who are already parents. Although teen pregnancy and childbearing rates have dramatically dropped over the last few years elsewhere, they have remained disproportionately high at his school. Simon has conducted sex education classes, but he speculates that the key to a more effective intervention lies elsewhere.

A literature review reinforces what Simon suspected—that abstinence and contraception-focused programs for adolescents have had only modest results in reducing teen pregnancy rates and minimal impact on teens in disadvantaged inner-city communities. He confirms that patterns of adolescent sexual-risk behaviors are shaped by social class, position, race, and gender. He also learns that in the United States, young motherhood is increasingly concentrated in disadvantaged groups, both White and non-White, but that the role of mother is not the typical first choice of young women who perceive themselves as having options.

From his review of the literature, Simon identifies a sociologic perspective, role theory, which he believes will help him develop a relevant and culturally sensitive intervention model for the adolescents in his school. He understands that roles are deeply embedded in social structures and are not easily changed. Young people in inner-city neighborhoods typically have a scarcity of role models and often lack appropriate adult supervision and meaningful job networks.

The reproductive role is one area over which poor, inner-city adolescents have control. Young men can validate their masculine role by biologically fathering a child, and young women can demonstrate their capacity for love in the maternal role. It is sometimes perceived that postponing childbearing will not improve their circumstances and becoming a parent may elevate their personal status.

Armed with the information gathered from his literature searches, Simon is seeking to learn even more about cultural variations in role expectations. His goal is to use this knowledge to develop interventions that will promote adolescent health and facilitate developmentally appropriate and productive role behaviors among the students in his school.

Historically, nursing has been responsive to society's needs. Early nurse leaders such as Nightingale, Barton, Wald, Sanger, and Staupers were, to varying degrees, social activists. They observed and understood the historical and social forces that affected large aggregates of individuals. Their understanding was demonstrated through their population-focused nursing interventions. C. Wright Mills (1959) coined the term "*sociological imagination*" to refer to this process of looking at social phenomena to discover the unseen and repetitive patterns that govern individuals' social existence.

Beginning in the early 1900s, as Americans became increasingly focused on the ideology of individualism and as cures were discovered for dreaded infectious diseases, the emphasis of health care shifted from populations and social factors that affect health to the individual and personal lifestyles. Consideration of the influences of social forces became almost obsolete. An understanding of theories from sociology and related disciplines that focuses on the interaction between human society and individuals is important for nurses, however, because sociologic issues have a dramatic impact on the health and well-being of individuals, families, groups, and society. Thus, advanced nursing practice and research must consider the social factors and issues that constrain and shape health behaviors.

This chapter reviews selected sociologic concepts, theories, and frameworks for their relevance to nursing practice, research, administration, and education. Three major sections are presented: exchange theories, interaction theories, and conflict theories. These are followed by an overview of chaos and postmodern social theories. Each section begins with a brief historical overview that is followed by a discussion of basic assumptions, central concepts, and differing theoretical viewpoints. Examples of nursing practice or research application of the theory are included where available.

Exchange Theories

Theories that have become known as "exchange theories" have their basis in the philosophical perspective called *utilitarianism*. Utilitarianism developed between the late 18th century and the mid-19th century and is a legacy from both moral philosophy and classic economic theory. The moral philosophy component considers the satisfaction of an individual's desires or utility. Philosophically, maximization of each individual's satisfaction automatically leads to maximum satisfaction of the wants of all. Translated into more familiar terms, "the greatest good for the greatest number" is an underlying principle of utilitarianism.

Three basic assumptions about individuals and exchange relations are added from classic economic theory. First, individuals are purposive and motivated to maximize material benefits from exchanges with others in a free and competitive marketplace. Second, as agents in a free market, individuals have access to all the information needed to weigh alternatives and calculate costs for each alternative. Third, based on their own calculations, individuals are able to rationally choose the activities that will maximize their profits (Turner, 2013).

Modern Social Exchange Theories

The influence of utilitarianism is evident in modern exchange theories to varying degrees. Utilitarian principles were reformulated for modern exchange theories in an attempt to explain human interactions in all social contexts and without the limitations imposed by a pure economic framework, hence the label "social" exchange theory. Assumptions of social exchange theories as outlined by Turner (2013) are listed in Box 13-1.

Box 13-1 Assumptions of Social Exchange Theories

1. Humans do not seek to maximize profits but attempt to make some profit in their social transactions with others.
2. Humans are not perfectly rational, but they do engage in calculations of costs and benefits in social transactions.
3. Humans do not have perfect information on all available alternatives, but they are usually aware of at least some alternatives, which form the basis for assessment of costs and benefits.
4. Humans always act under constraints, but they still compete with one another in seeking to make a profit in their transactions.
5. Humans always seek to make a profit in their transactions, but they are limited by the resources that they have when entering an exchange relation.
6. Humans engage in economic transactions in clearly defined marketplaces in all societies, but these transactions are only special cases of more general exchange relations.
7. Humans pursue material goals in exchanges, but they also mobilize and exchange nonmaterial resources, such as sentiments, services, and symbols.

Source: Turner (2013).

The *social exchange* perspective emerged in American sociology in the 1960s with the work of Homans (1961) and Blau (1964) and later with Nye (1979) and Emerson (1981), and in social psychology with Thibaut and Kelley (1959). Modern exchange theories emphasize the social and psychological motivation of individuals. There are two major divisions of social exchange theories: the individualistic or microlevel theories and the societal/collectivist or macrolevel theories.

Within the *individualistic social exchange* framework, the central focus is motivation; human beings are motivated by self-interest to act. Relationships are deemed successful and continue when each party feels that the nature of an exchange is fair and beneficial. Beneficial or rewarding relationships require commitment to sustain them. When *reciprocity* is absent or unrewarding within the relationship, or costs exceed rewards, individuals tend to withdraw from further exchanges. This premise applies to all social groups, including the family. Divorce is an example of withdrawing from an unsatisfactory exchange relationship.

In contrast to the individualistic or microlevel perspective are the macrolevel theories. This second broad division of social exchange theories is derived from a *collectivist* tradition and gives greater weight to society. Collectivism has its roots in the perspective of French anthropologist Levi-Strauss (1969), whose work emphasized the integration of exchanges from larger social structures. In this perspective, the focus is on reciprocity from an institutional level.

Three fundamental exchange principles relate to the concept of integration as proposed by Levi-Strauss (1969). First, individuals incur costs in all exchange relations, but costs are attributed to the customs, rules, laws, and values of society, as opposed to the individual motives found in economic or psychological explanations of exchange. Second, social norms and values regulate the distribution of all scarce and valued resources. Third, the norm of reciprocity governs all exchange relations (Turner, 2013). An example of costs associated with customs is the money dance conducted at some wedding receptions in the United States. During the designated dance, currency is "pinned" on the bride and groom in exchange for a brief portion of the dance. This ritual signifies a socially sanctioned way for guests to give cash to the newlyweds and for the young couple to reciprocate.

Table 13-1 Central Concepts in Social Exchange Theories

Concept	Meaning
Agency	Individuals actively create or construct their social world, and as thinking, feeling, and acting beings, they are motivated to control or to condition the situations that affect their social lives to maximize their advantage.
Rationality	Individuals are acquisitive and success oriented, and motivated for immediate rewards. Therefore, to gain the most benefit, individuals calculate costs and the probabilities of receiving rewards or avoiding punishments in social interactions.
Structure	Social and cultural influences that constrain and shape an individual's behavior and conscious experiences are assumed to be located in the unconscious mind, in material relationships, in the symbolic relationships of myth or language, or in repetitive patterns of permanent interactions.

Source: Waters (1994).

Rational choice theory (Coleman, 1990; Hechter, 1987) is the most recently proposed exchange theory. Rational choice theory attempts to explain the macrolevel behavioral processes of both small and large social systems. Rational choice theory has a systems focus, but the psychological needs and motives of individuals are removed.

Three major sociologic concepts, *agency, rationality*, and *structure*, are evident in the assumptions and propositions of contemporary social exchange theories (Table 13-1). The individualistic perspective emphasizes agency and considers that individuals actively shape their social lives, rather than being passive recipients. Individuals affect their own lives by adapting to, negotiating with, and changing social structures.

Inherent in the concept of rationality is the assumption that every individual has control over a supply of socially valued resources, either material or psychological, that serve as bartering tools. Individuals barter these resources in the social "marketplace" to maximize rewards by enhancing the valuables they control. Homans (1961) attempted to "soften" the more utilitarian or calculative perspective by emphasizing the influence of personal values on determining what individuals view as rewarding. The last concept, *structure*, is highly abstract and not directly observable. Social structure generally refers to the enduring and recurring patterns of behavior in groups and society.

Subsumed in these concepts (agency, rationality, and structure) are related issues of *inequality, power*, and *conflict*. A generation or so prior to its appearance in exchange theorizing, Karl Marx (1977) noted that inequality exists in hierarchical class structures where those who have control of resources with high economic value also have the power to exploit those with fewer such resources. Conflict, according to Marx, is inevitable with oppression, and resolution of conflict requires emancipatory actions. Factors associated with positions of privilege and power include gender, age, ethnicity, and socioeconomic status. Conflict theories are discussed in detail later in this chapter.

Application to Nursing

Recent nursing studies that used social exchange theory as their conceptual framework were identified in the literature. For example, Hamrin, McCarthy, and Tyson (2010) used social exchange to explore initiation and adherence to psychotropic medication in children and adolescents. Picot, Youngblut, and Zeller (2011) combined social exchange theory with equity theory to develop the *Picot Caregiver Rewards Scale* (PCRS) in order to obtain a more holistic view of the caregiver experience and to plan health promotion interventions for caregivers. Similarly, Carruth (2011) found that social exchange and equity theory provided a conceptual framework for studying reciprocal intergenerational exchanges of assistance and support and for developing a caregiver reciprocity scale (CRS). Finally, Ihlenfed (2011) used the *Arizona Social Support Interview Schedule* (ASSIS) to assess nurses' perceptions of social support from their administrators.

Related Theories

There are many theories, principles, and concepts derived from, or related to, exchange theories. Exchange theories that are commonly used by nurses include systems theory and social networks.

General Systems Theory

General systems theory (GST) is one type of exchange theory. GST or, more specifically, *open systems theory* (OST) (von Bertalanffy, 1968), is regarded as a universal grand theory because of its unique relevancy and applicability (Johnson & Webber, 2010).

The GST was initially introduced in the 1930s by von Bertalanffy. In GST, systems are composed of both structural and functional components that interact within a boundary that filters the type and rate of exchange with the environment. Living systems are open because there is an ongoing exchange of matter, energy, and information. The following elements are common to systems (Figure 13-1):

- Input—matter, energy, and information received from the environment
- Throughput—matter, energy, and information that is modified or transformed within the system
- Output—matter, energy, and information that is released from the system into the environment
- Feedback—information regarding environmental responses used by the system (may be positive, negative, or neutral) (Kenney, 1995)

Basic tenets of GST are that (1) a system is composed of subsystems, each with its own function; (2) systems contain energy and matter; (3) a system may be open or closed (open systems exchange energy and closed systems have clearly defined boundaries); and (4) open and closed systems reach stationary states (Mason & Attree, 1997).

For survival, a system must achieve a balance internally and externally (equilibrium). Equilibrium depends on the system's ability to regulate input and output to achieve a balanced relationship of the interactive parts. The system uses various adaptation mechanisms to maintain equilibrium. Adaptation may occur through accepting or rejecting the matter, energy, or information or by accommodating the input and modifying the systems responses (Kenney, 1995). Several OST principles that are purported to be applicable to all systems are shown in Box 13-2.

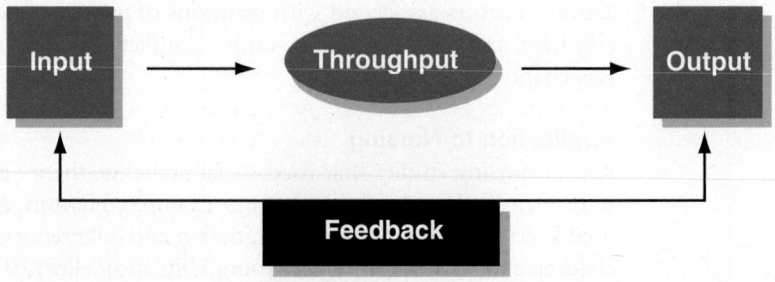

Figure 13-1 Elements of a system.

Box 13-2 Open Systems Theory Principles

1. A system is a unit that is greater than the sum of its parts (wholeness is a major premise of both GST and OST).
2. A system comprises subsystems that are themselves part of suprasystems (hierarchically "nested").
3. A system has boundaries (i.e., abstract entities such as rules, norms, and values) that permit exchange of information and resources both into (inputs) and out of (outputs) the system (boundaries can also hinder or block exchange processes).
4. Communication and feedback mechanisms between system parts are essential for system function.
5. A change in one part leads to change in the whole system (*circular causality*).
6. A system goal or end point can be reached in different ways (*equifinality*).

Application to Nursing

Systems theory has been frequently applied to nursing practice, generally in the areas of management and administration. Meyer and O'Brien-Pallas (2010) for example, applied open systems theory to large-scale organizations and from their data developed the "Nursing Services Delivery Theory." Reviewing the literature Myny and colleagues (2011) identified five categories of nondirect patient care factors related to nurses' workload in acute care hospitals. Guided by systems theory, a conceptual model was built from the data. Kitson (2009) found that to hasten the application of research and new knowledge to practice, there must be a purposeful integration of systems theory with knowledge translation theories.

In direct-care clinical research, major tenets of family systems theory, a derivative of systems theory, was applied to patients in palliative cancer care to provide optimal care to them and their families (Mehta, Cohen, & Chan, 2009) and to family members caring for adult children with mental illness (Fujino & Okamura, 2009). Finally, Jordan, Lanham, Anderson, and McDaniel (2010) suggested that complex adaptive systems theory, another derivative of systems theory, could enhance interpretations of research observations of health care organizations.

Social Networks

The study of *networks* can be a productive approach to understanding systems in nursing. In terms of the health and well-being of individuals, *social support networks*, as actual or potential resources, are especially relevant. Among members of social support networks, reciprocity and commitments are shaped by culturally mandated norms. This particularly relates to family networks (Logan & Spitze, 1996).

Social networks should examine the underlying patterns of social relationships; this is done irrespective of their content or substance (Turner, 2013). The units to be examined can range from individuals to positions, such as those found in health care organizations (e.g., nurses, physicians, pharmacists, and administrators). In *network analysis*, these units are referred to as *points*. Ties link points and represent the directional flow of resources. Figure 13-2 illustrates the exchange process in a simplistic diagram. In this figure, A, B, C, D, and E represent points, and arrows indicate ties. In the illustration, B has reciprocal ties to all other points, but A, C, D, and E have ties to only three other points. In the social world, resource exchanges can be instrumental, as in the exchange of information or materials, or *affective*, as shown by respect, approval, or an empathic ear.

Examples of techniques or tools for capturing and mapping network patterns include Moreno's (1953) *sociograms*, which plot the patterning of sentiments among

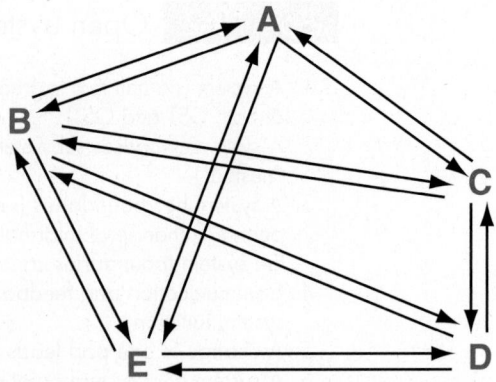

Figure 13-2 Example of resource flows in a noncomplex network.

group members; the echo-map used in family assessments to diagram exchange relations between families and their external environment; and the exchange theory and network analysis program developed by Emerson (1981). In contrast to more traditional exchange theories, Emerson's approach focuses on mapping the structure of exchange relations among *actors*, rather than the motivation of individuals. The idea of the analysis is to discover what events could influence the relational unit(s) (Turner, 2013).

Application to Nursing

Resources, both affective and instrumental, flow through network exchange processes. Variations in social networks are dependent on context and health issues, such as hepatitis B virus (HBV) infection, and are complicated, as in the case of Korean American immigrants whose networks are not geographically bounded (Lee, Hann, Yang, & Fawcett, 2011). In much the same way, lower levels of primary caregiver burden was found to be significantly associated with high levels of social support in a Taiwanese population of patients with colorectal cancer (Shieh, Tung, & Liang, 2012), and social exchange factors were found to be most influential on difficulties experienced by Mexican American family caregivers in administering daily medications to elderly family members (Kao, 2011). Additionally, patterns of social exchange behavior within stroke caregiving networks in Bangkok were identified by Sakunhongsophon, Sirapo-ngam, Tripp-Reimer, and Junda (2011).

Support from social networks is widely regarded as mediating the adverse effects of stressful events. Lee, Wang, Lin, and Kao (2012), for example, found a significant moderating effect of perceived nurses' support on fathering ability and paternal stress for Taiwanese fathers of premature infants, and lack of perceived social support was found to be significantly associated with antenatal depressive symptoms among Chinese women (Lau, 2011; Ngai & Chan, 2012). In a final example, fostering emotional functional social support from significant others in the social networks of new mothers can reduce morbidity (Leahy-Warren, McCarthy, & Corcoran, 2011). Thus, health care providers need to routinely assess the adequacy of individuals' perceived social support networks and target relevant interventions for those with inadequate support.

Interactionist Frameworks

In the late 19th century, the focus of sociology shifted from macrostructures and processes (e.g., evolution, class conflict) to social interactional processes that link individuals to each other and to society. A diverse group of interactionist theories resulted from this shift. Two of these theories, symbolic interactionism and role theory, are discussed here.

Symbolic Interactionism

The early foundation for what was later to be called symbolic interactionism by Blumer (1969) was laid in the late 1800s. Three scholars from the philosophical tradition called *pragmatism* are credited with the seminal ideas from which symbolic interactionism sprang. From James' (1890) typology of selves came the concept of the "self." The concept of self was refined by Cooley (1902) a few years later to include the notion of "the looking glass self," or the self that comes from the process of symbolic communication with others in the "primary group." Dewey (1922) contributed his idea of "mind" as a process that emerges from, and is sustained through, interactions with others.

Mead (1934), the acknowledged father of symbolic interactionism, synthesized the concepts of self, mind, and society or social environment, which he perceived to be inseparable. Central to Mead's work is the notion that humans adapt to, and survive in, their environment by sharing common symbols, both verbal and nonverbal. A distinctive feature of this symbolic interaction is that humans can imagine themselves in other social roles, a concept termed "role-taking," and internalize the attitudes, values, and norms of the "generalized other" or social group. Mead outlined stages of interactional learning by which he believed humans acquire social understanding. For Mead, the self is nonexistent at birth and emerges as the result of social experience. Mead's basic assumptions are listed in Box 13-3.

"What humans define as real has real consequences" (Thomas & Thomas, 1928, p. 572) is a basic principle from social psychology. This principle is referred to as the *definition of the situation* and links how individuals perceive their environment and how they respond or act in that environment. Mead stressed that this environmental perception and response is in actuality a problem-solving interaction. From these interactions comes the phenomenon Mead viewed as society because it is through the processes of mind and self that society is both altered and maintained (Turner, 2013).

The focus for symbolic interactionism is on the connection between *symbols* (shared meanings) and *interactions.* Mead emphasized the process of role-taking as a basic mechanism by which interactions occur. Role-taking refers to the ability to not only put yourself in the role of another person but also to anticipate how that person will think, feel, or respond (Mead, 1934; Stryker & Statham, 1985). Although they are sometimes used interchangeably, role-taking and empathy are not synonymous. Role-taking is a cognitive process, whereas empathy emphasizes the affective.

Box 13-3 Assumptions of Symbolic Interactionist Theories

1. Human beings have the capacity to create and use symbols.
2. Through the capacity to create and use symbols, humans have freed themselves from most of their instinctual and biologic programming.
3. Human beings adapt and survive in the social world.
4. Humans use words and language symbols to communicate, and they also use nonverbal gestures that have common meanings.
5. Humans can effectively communicate because of their ability to read symbols produced by others and to take on the position or point of view of another person.
6. Humans acquire a mind and self from interactions with others.
7. Human interactions form the basis of society.

Sources: Turner (2013); Lindesmith & Strauss (1968).

The concept of role was extended to include the expectations attached to structural positions in society, and the concept of *self* became associated with the multiple roles played within these positions.

Application to Nursing

Several qualitative research studies in nursing were found that used symbolic interaction as a conceptual framework. For example, Martsolf, Draucker, and Bednarz (2011) explored how adolescents make sense of their troubled dating relationships (i.e., verbal, emotional, sexual, or physical abuse). In another study, symbolic interactionism provided part of the theoretical framework in exploring young gay and bisexual men's definition of being healthy as well as their fears and concerns. Findings from this study can assist nurses in identifying culturally appropriate ways for interacting/intervening with this population (Guarnero, 2011). In another example rooted in symbolic interactionism, Horton and Dworkin (2013) explored the notion of gender-based power imbalances in HIV risk reduction and suggested moving beyond the interpersonal in HIV prevention policy solutions to include broader social inequalities and power imbalances that impact, for instance, condom negotiations.

Other studies used a grounded theory approach that derives from symbolic interactionism in which the processes of interaction between people's social roles and behaviors are explored. Mauritz and van Meijel (2009) examined the lived experience of loss and grief in persons with schizophrenia. Grounded theory was used to understand the decision-making processes that occur between persons with end-stage cancer and their family caregivers in a home setting. Implications for practice include palliative care education for nurses in all health care settings and health-promotion initiatives for advance directives education and end-stage illness management in home settings (Edwards, Koop, Northcott, & Olson, 2012).

Role Theory

The concept of "role" comes from the theater and conveys the notion that normative expectations and requirements, such as culturally defined behavioral rules, are attached to positions (status) in social organizations (e.g., family, corporation, society). Succinctly stated, an individual occupies a status but plays a role (Lindesmith & Strauss, 1968).

Through the enactment of roles, static social positions are brought to life. Roles can be assumed to carry not only certain rights and privileges but duties and obligations as well. For example, a registered nurse has the right to be paid on time and in turn has the obligation to report to work when scheduled and in a timely manner.

A status may include a number of roles, with each role appropriate to a specific social context. For instance, a woman who occupies the status of chief executive officer of a large company has multiple roles attached to that position. She may also have duties and obligations associated with other statuses, such as daughter, sister, wife, mother, Red Cross volunteer, and so on. Role behavior, in any given situation, depends on the statuses occupied by interacting individuals. Staff nurses, for example, behave one way toward their clients, another way toward their coworkers, and yet another way toward their supervisors.

Social positions are *ascribed* based on such characteristics as class (e.g., poor, middle class, wealthy), gender, and racial or ethnic group membership or are *achieved* through education, training, and so forth. There are societal constraints on all statuses. For instance, an African American male nurse occupies several relevant statuses. He is a qualified professional, but there will undoubtedly be situations in which others will expect him to enact behaviors traditionally associated with his other ascribed status(es) (i.e., male, African American, son, brother, father).

Role strain, or role stress, is a subjective experience produced by such conditions as *role ambiguity, role incongruity, role overload*, and *role conflict*. Ill-defined, vague, or unclear role expectations can result in role ambiguity (e.g., the staff nurse assigned to temporarily act as head nurse with no preparation). Role incongruity can occur when role expectations run counter to the individual's values and self-perception; for example, a staff nurse who takes pride in her caring and supportive behaviors toward clients and coworkers is promoted to supervisor and must "trim the budget." The nurse faced with an imbalance in ratio of demands (excessive) and time (inadequate) on an understaffed acute intensive care unit may experience *role overload*. Occupying more than one status at a time increases the likelihood of an individual being unable to enact the roles associated with one status without violating those of another status (e.g., administrative/supervisor-professional nurse/client advocate). The individual faced with such mutually exclusive or contradictory role expectations will likely experience *role conflict*.

The roles an individual plays have a profound effect on attitude and behavior as well as on self-perceptions. As society in general, and health care systems in particular, become increasingly more complex and resources shrink, role stress can be expected to continue and expand. Various researchers have studied various roles. Link to Practice 13-1 focuses on role changes across generations.

Link to Practice 13-1

Significant attention has recently focused on the notion of "generational differences" in nursing education and administration. The observations of the differences and subsequent implications are rooted in research and can be related to many of the theories and principles described in this chapter (e.g., culture, social exchange/social networks, role theory, conflict, transactions).

In one example, Hendricks and Cope (2013) explained that generational cohorts carry similar traits based on sharing of important life events at critical development stages. In their discussion of the commonly described "generations" (e.g., veterans or traditionals, baby boomers, generation Xers, and millennials), they explicitly discussed the "cultural" differences and distinctions of the different generations and focused on some of the variations in techniques of communication and potential sources of conflict. In another example, Sparks (2012) examined differences in "empowerment" and sentinel characteristics consistent with critical social theory in her study of job satisfaction in baby boomers and generation X nurses.

Lastly, Arhin and Cormier (2007) explicitly looked at generational differences among nursing students from a postmodern perspective, concluding that learning styles of generation Y (millennials) differs from previous generations. Indeed, they noted that the younger cohorts do not ascribe as well to the linear thinking as previous generations; as a result, the authors supported the idea of shifting educational strategies to include a "postmodern philosophy."

Arhin, A. O., & Cormier, E. (2007). Using deconstruction to educate generation Y nursing students. *Journal of Nursing Education, 46*(2), 562–567.

Hendricks, J. M., & Cope, V. C. (2013). Generational diversity: What nurse managers need to know. *Journal of Advanced Nursing, 69*(3), 717–725.

Sparks, A. M. (2012). Psychological empowerment and job satisfaction among baby boomer and generation X nurses. *Journal of Nursing Management, 20,* 451–460.

Structural Role Theory

No one scholar is credited with *structural role theory*; contributions came from many sources. A descriptive analogy for understanding the overall assumptions of this approach comes from a passage in William Shakespeare's *As You Like It*:

> *All the world's a stage,*
> *And all the men and women merely players:*
> *They have their exits and their entrances;*
> *And one man in his time plays many parts.* (Act II, Scene VII)

Human interaction is viewed as being similarly structured; individual actors adhere to societal norms or "scripts" attached to statuses or positions they occupy. Role directives come from those with power, and actors adjust their responses or "performances" to others with whom they interact, as well as their reference group or "audience." Through self-concepts and role-playing, individuals develop their own unique interactional styles (Turner, 2013).

Structural role theorists de-emphasize the creative aspects of mind and self and place more emphasis on the impact of social structure on interaction. Structural role theorists posit that individuals spend a great deal of time in groups of one kind or another and are shaped or socialized by the groups to which they belong. An individual uses groups to help define personal beliefs, attitudes, and values; these are called *reference groups*. The influence of reference groups continues even when that individual is away from the group members because the group's norms and values have been internalized. The internalized norms and values are continually used as a measuring stick by which the behaviors of one's self and others are evaluated. An example of a reference group for student nurses would be professional nurses. Reference groups can be positive or negative; the former have individuals that are desirable to emulate, whereas the latter provide a model to avoid.

Process Role Theory

Role theory focuses on the impact of behavior on self-conceptions and is viewed by some as being too structured and deterministic (Turner, 2013). *Process role theory* proposes a different perspective. There are three dominant characteristics of process role theory: (1) individuals negotiate their roles in most social contexts; (2) roles are general configurations about conduct; and (3) roles are not fixed and predetermined. In most social encounters (including highly structural situations), individuals actively make roles and negotiate with others their right to enact a given role.

Application to Nursing

In recent years, a significant amount of research on role strain and related concepts has been performed. For example, Brown and Oyetunde (2012) examined professional accountability within the theoretical framework of role theory for primary nursing practice. Elements for a framework to help clarify psychiatric nurse practice roles and eliminate professional stress were identified by Machin and Stevenson (2011).

Caregiver roles have been examined by a number of researchers. Wang, Shu, Chen, & Yang (2011), for example, examined the effects of work demands on role strain and depressive symptoms of adult–child family caregivers of Taiwanese elders with dementia and, in a related work, studied the moderating effects of work conditions and interactive family caregiving (i.e., mutuality and preparedness) (Wang et al., 2013). In a final example, Hansen, Archbold, Stewart, and Westfall (2011) explored the concepts of role strain and satisfaction with family caregivers making life-sustaining treatment decisions within the context of ongoing care for elderly ill relatives in a variety of settings.

Conflict Theories

Society is generally regarded as a system, composed of interdependent and essentially harmonious parts that are linked together into a boundary-maintaining whole. Social integration results from the mixing of parts and consensus on societal goals and cultural values. With cooperation being the primary social process, change is gradual and adaptive, and society remains stable (Eitzen, Baca-Zinn, & Smith, 2010).

But individuals' perceptions of the water glass as being either half empty or half full are similar to how society can be viewed. The same social phenomenon can be seen as maintaining system balance and integrity (a functionalistic perspective), or it can be seen as generating divisiveness and conflict.

The conflict perspective sees conflict as endemic to social organizations. This is due to the existence of structural constraints, which result in the unequal distribution of power. These imbalances of power may result in competitive interactions among and between groups. Social problems (e.g., gender, class, and racial/ethnic inequality; poverty, violence, and health disparities) are in actuality societally induced conditions (Eitzen et al., 2010).

How the causes, consequences, and interventions of social problems are addressed depends on the theoretical perspective of either conflict or order. The order perspective tends to "blame the victim" (Ryan, 1976) or label the "deviant." Rehabilitating individuals is the remedy. From the conflict perspective, rehabilitation of individuals is like treating symptoms and ignoring the root cause(s). What needs to be fixed is society because society has failed to meet the needs of individuals and needs restructuring.

Eitzen and colleagues (2010) explain that social problems are typically found within the institutional framework of society rather than being an exclusive function of individual pathologies. They propose a synthesis of the order and conflict models. Assumptions of their proposed synthesis model are summarized in Box 13-4.

Conflict theories share common ground in the elements analyzed in human societies: inequality, power/authority, domination/subjugation, interests, and conflict. Modern conflict theories have their roots in the writings of Karl Marx, the most famous conflict theorist, with later influences from Max Weber (1958) and Georg Simmel (1956). Marx argued that economic-based class conflict is the most basic and influential source of all social change. He viewed class conflict as inevitable because of the unequal allocation of goods and services in capitalist societies. Marx's model of

Box 13-4 Assumptions of the Order and Conflict Synthesis Model

1. Processes of stability and change are properties of all societies. Human societies are paradoxical—they are always ordered and always changing.
2. Societies are organized, but the process of organization generates conflict. Conflict is generated by the unequal distribution of power in decision-making processes over scarce resources in a system of social stratification.
3. Society is a social system. Parts of the system may have complementary and consensual as well as exclusive and incompatible interests and goals.
4. Societies are held together by complementary interests, by consensus on cultural values, and also by coercion.
5. Social change is common to all societies; it may be gradual or abrupt, reforming or revolutionary.

Source: Eitzen, Baca-Zinn, & Smith (2010).

conflict was shaped by Europe's transition from a feudal to a capitalistic society, and to him, capitalism is an economic system that perpetuates inequality. Marx believed that the only means for emancipatory social change within a capitalist society was violent revolution, with the workers fighting against the capitalists. He argued that the ideology of any society is always the ideology of the ruling class or the powerful people, as those in power use ideology to ensure their value system reigns (Eitzen et al., 2010).

Weber (1958) rejected Marx's dichotomous model of the relationships between conflict and power. He believed that the potential for conflict decreases as societies moved from traditional authoritarian relationships to relationships organized around rational/legal authority in industrial/bureaucratic societies.

Simmel (1956) shared Marx's and Weber's view that conflict was an "inevitable and ubiquitous feature" of society resulting from divergent interests but believed that conflict also came from the innate aggressive instincts of humans. He perceived conflict to be necessary for adaptation and growth of humans and society; without conflict, there could be no adaptation and growth. It was from these conflict-driven processes that solidarity was promoted, both within and between human groups. Conflict was therefore functionally necessary.

Modern conflict theories have modified Marx's model. Dahrendorf (1958), a contemporary conflict theorist, regards Marx's theory of class conflict and social change as too simplistic because other social groups (e.g., political groups) also experience conflict. Implicit in his perspective is the notion that conflict meets systems' functional need for change. Society is characterized by struggles between social classes and between powerful and less powerful groups because of the inequality embedded in hierarchical social structures. The potential for conflict is then inherent in the majority of human relationships because social organization means, among other things, the unequal distribution of power resulting in the "haves" and the "have-nots" (Eitzen et al., 2010).

Lewis Coser (1956) was critical of the failure of Marx and Dahrendorf to acknowledge the integrative and adaptive functions of societies. In his view, conflict acts to alert social systems of problems. Through the process of addressing problems, a system adapts and structurally becomes better suited to remediate future problems. According to Coser, an inverse relationship exists between goals and level of conflict.

Three perspectives or types of conflict theory, feminism, critical social theory, and cultural bias are examined frequently by nurses in research and are applicable in practice. They are described here.

Feminist Theory

Gender differences and subordination have traditionally been viewed as both natural and inevitable, but some believe that gender is socially constructed and tends to justify the subordination and exploitation of women. A core assumption in feminist theories is that women are oppressed. This perspective has been determined to be too simplistic, however, and beginning in the 1960s, new views of feminism were presented (Eitzen et al., 2010; Waters, 1994).

A rather wide range of perspectives fall under the rubric of feminist theory. Feminist theory has been described as an analysis of women's subordination for the purpose of figuring out how to change it (Eitzen et al., 2010). There are many issues, themes, and assumptions that are common in feminism. Osmond and Thorne (1993) discuss relevant themes in feminist theory; some of these are summarized in Box 13-5.

Variations of Feminist Theory

There is considerable variation among feminist perspectives. A few of the most commonly encountered are described in this section.

Box 13-5 Themes in Feminist Theories

1. Women's experiences are central, normal, and valuable; experiences open new ways of knowing the world.
2. Gender is a basic organizing concept. The concept of *gender* involves two interrelated elements: (a) the social construction and exaggeration of differences between women and men (i.e., there is a fundamental basis of inequality, or social stratification, similar to social class and race), and (b) gender distinctions are used to legitimize and perpetuate power relations between women and men (i.e., compared with men, women are devalued and socially, economically, politically, and legally subordinated).
3. Gender distinctions occur in daily processes of constructing and reconstructing differences between women and men and devalues women. However, rather than passive victims, women participate in gendering processes as active agents, actors, and creators of culture.
4. Gender relations must be analyzed within specific sociocultural and historical contexts.
5. Monolithic, bounded notions (e.g., "the family") contribute to an ideology that contains class, cultural, and heterosexual biases and supports the oppression of women.

Source: Osmond & Thorne (1993).

Liberal feminism is concerned with the political life and well-being of women. Friedan (1963) is probably the most well-known liberal feminist. She argued against the entrapment of women by the *feminine mystique*, an ideology that claims women are separate but special by extolling the virtues of women's traditional roles of wife and mother. Especially noteworthy is Freidan's examination of differences in women's pathologies (e.g., married women compared to unmarried women are more susceptible to diseases/disorders).

Socialist (Marxist) feminism is exemplified by Millet's (1971) work describing the impact of patriarchy on the social structure, which she saw as a masculine system of political domination. She questioned the persistence of patriarchal beliefs and attitudes into an era where women are educated and free yet continue to be subordinate and devalued. She determined that because patriarchal domination is socially constructed, women can take emancipatory actions and reconstruct gender relations.

Firestone's *The Dialectic of Sex* (1970) is perhaps the epitome of *radical feminism*. She refuted Marx's notion of economic class and argued instead that "sex class divisions" are at the root of women's oppression. "[T]o assure the elimination of sexual classes requires the revolt of the underclass (women) and the seizure of control of *reproduction*" (Waters, 1994, p. 267).

Brownmiller (1975), another radical feminist, argued that it is not women's biologic constraints but sexual relationships that subordinate women. She focused on violence against women and believed that rape is possible because human sexual behavior is unique. According to Brownmiller, rape is about power and control and therefore about domination and power over women.

A branch of radical feminism is *cultural feminism*, which focuses on women's differences. Cultural feminism condones separatism and suggests that rather than striving to be like men, women should work toward reorganizing society around a female-dominated community—"womanculture."

Psychoanalytic feminism takes the male-centered and sexist assumptions of Freudian theory and reworks them. Chodorow (1989) refuted the notions of the Oedipal complex and penis envy by connecting the role of mothering to the construction of gendered personalities. Gilligan (1982) addressed the "different voice" of moral reasoning. These two theorists, as well as others, have helped to bridge the gap to consider the internal psyches of girls and women (Osmond & Thorne, 1993).

Application of Feminist Theory to Nursing

Feminist theory and philosophy have been frequently cited in the nursing literature. Beginning in the late 19th century, Florence Nightingale wrote on gender roles. Examples of Nightingale's feminist views included her efforts to obtain women's right to education, self-development, and occupations and her criticism of the double sexual standard of the times (Chinn, 1999; Pfettscher, 2010).

In more contemporary writings, feminist theory, as an interpretive perspective situated within a nonoppressive process, begins with the narratives of women from widely varied populations. For example, from an Afrocentric feminist perspective, Fouquier (2011) explored the experiences of three generations of African American women in their transition to motherhood. Preterm labor was examined from two perspectives, the woman's perspective and physician's perspective, and alternative approaches were identified that placed the lives of women at the center of the treatment process (Williams & Mackey, 2011). Women's lived experiences with electroshock therapy (ECT) were explored and compared with nurses perceptions of ECT. Whereas nurses saw the treatment as beneficial, the women associated ECT with damage and devastating loss. It was suggested that nurses need to carefully consider this disconnect (van Daalen-Smith, 2011). In another work, Merritt-Gray and West (2011) provided a model that frames the actions of women leaving abusive conjugal relationships in geographically isolated areas within a survivor framework.

Critical Social Theory

The early foundation for *critical social theory* can be found in Marx's argument that oppressive arrangements require revolutionary action. The concept of emancipatory alternatives has replaced Marx's revolutionary (and more violent) action in contemporary critical social theories. To identify and address oppressive social arrangements, individuals cannot simply accept that how they perceive the social world is indeed factual. Rather, they must question their assumptions to identify oppressive social arrangements. This is made possible through the unique capacity for self-reflection that humans possess.

Critical social theory uses societal awareness to expose social inequalities that keep people from reaching their full potential. It is derived from the belief that social meanings structure life through social domination. Proponents of critical social theory maintain that social exchanges that are not distorted by power imbalances will stimulate the evolution of a more just society. Furthermore, critical theory assumes that truth is socially determined (Martins, 2011).

Habermas (1991) is perhaps the best-known contemporary critical social theorist. In opposition to Marx's revolutionary action, Habermas argued that emancipation from domination is possible through "[rational] communicative [inter-]action." He supported employment of negotiation as integral to communicative action, realizing that negotiation must be conducted without the use of power or coercion by either of the interacting parties. With his emphasis on interaction through communication, Habermas discounted the importance of both material and structural constraints on changing social systems.

In the health care industry, health maintenance organizations provide an example of purposive and rational social structures that are not designed with "communicative action" between client and health care providers in mind. Authority relationships are maintained within these agencies, and negotiation is often not a possibility.

Critical social theory or critical theory is both theoretical and philosophical and has increasingly been used in nursing research to address sociopolitical conditions that affect health and health care. Perhaps the most significant contribution to nursing science may be achieved by challenging the fundamental ideologies upon which nursing knowledge is developed.

Application to Nursing

Concepts from critical social theory or critical theory have been examined in recent nursing literature, typically within the context of working with disadvantaged or marginalized groups. For example, one study examined the lived experiences of minority women with HIV within the social context of disease stigma, poverty, sexism, and racism (Lyon, 2011). Critical theory and feminism were combined to frame exploration of women's perceptions of their interactions with primary care nurse practitioners. The women valued caring clinicians that they defined as treating them with some degree of equality and respect for their knowledge and life experiences. Dole, Dole, and Shambley-Ebron (2009) used a conceptual framework integrating critical social theory, critical feminist theory, and critical race theory to explore adolescent mothering through socially constructed concepts of gender, race, and class. In a fourth example, data from an exploratory study of adolescents with diabetes indicated paternalistic care delivery approaches from health care professionals. It was suggested that nurses can not only advocate for these adolescents but can assist them to become advocates for themselves (Dickinson, 2011).

Researchers also used a critical social theory perspective to discuss other aspects of nursing. For instance, the definition of needs, as defined in nursing literature, was determined to be inadequate in fundamental ways (Holmes & Warelow, 2011). Sumner, Scott, and Arndt (2011) illuminated a different paradigm—caring in nursing—and advanced an egalitarian model for nursing practice. The account of nurses' participation in the Nazi euthanasia program was analyzed from a critical-feminist perspective and its epistemologic salience for contemporary nursing discussed (Benedict & Georges, 2009). Hall and Fields (2012) explored how subtle racism or "microaggression" is embedded in nursing practice and education and suggested that this may be one means by which marginalization and health disparities occur. Finally, a critical social theory lens was used to examine the expansive influence of power upon attempts to integrate patient-centered care into health care organizations; viable solutions were discussed (Beanlands et al., 2012).

Cultural Diversity and Cultural Bias

An interest in cultural diversity and cultural bias is not a phenomenon peculiar to the social sciences or sociology in particular. Culture, as socially patterned human thought and behavior (Bodley, 2011), is an integral and highly influential component of the interface between humans and their social environment. The word *culture* comes from the Latin root *colere*, to inhabit, cultivate, or honor. In general, it refers to human activity; different definitions of culture reflect different theories for understanding, or criteria for valuing, human activity. The interest in and the study of culture in the United States has been steadily pushing its way to the forefront since the mid-1980s (Alexander & Smith, 2009). It was also during this time that a shift occurred in U.S. population demographics and the corresponding increase in diverse ethnic groups became more pronounced, resulting in the concepts of culture and cultural diversity becoming an increasingly relevant topic.

Box 13-6 Sociologic Definitions of Culture

- A way of life, a system of ideas, values, beliefs, knowledge, and customs passed on from generation to generation
- All the learned and shared products of a society
- The entire complex of ideas and material objects that people of a society (or group) have created and adopted for carrying out the necessary tasks of collective life

Source: Ferrante (2012).

There is little consensus among sociologists in this specialized area of study as to just what the concept of culture means. From a sociologic perspective, culture can be broadly conceived as the symbolic/expressive dimension of social life. Examples of three different sociologic definitions are listed in Box 13-6 with an anthropologic comparison in Table 13-2.

Despite the disagreement on definition, sociologists do agree on the essential principles of culture. These principles are that (1) culture consists of tangible (material) and intangible (nonmaterial) components; (2) people inherit and learn a culture; (3) biologic, environmental, and historical forces shape and change culture; and (4) culture is a tool that people use to evaluate other societies and adapt to problems of living (Ferrante, 2012).

The word *bias* refers to an inclination for or against some phenomenon that inhibits impartial and objective judgment and that can, in the extreme, constitute prejudice. *Cultural bias*, interpreting and judging phenomena in relation to one's own culture, is an ever-present danger and central to social and human societies. A multitude of historical and contemporary examples of cultural biases deal with the "isms": racism, sexism, classism, and ageism. An alternate perspective views cultural bias as a normative response to safeguard that which is known and familiar to the individual—ethnocentrism. Any normative belief about human beings can be reasonably isolated as a cultural belief and consequently lead to a biased perspective.

Table 13-2 Anthropologic Definitions of Culture

Topical	Culture consists of everything on a list of topics or categories, such as social organization, religion, or economy.
Historical	Culture is social heritage, or tradition, that is passed on to future generations.
Behavioral	Culture is shared, learned human behavior, a way of life.
Normative	Culture is ideals, values, or rules for living.
Functional	Culture is the way humans solve problems of adapting to the environment or living together.
Mental	Culture is a complex of ideas, or learned habits, that inhibit impulses and distinguish people from animals.
Structural	Culture consists of patterned and interrelated ideas, symbols, or behaviors.
Symbolic	Culture is based on arbitrarily assigned meanings that are shared by a society.

Source: Bodley (2011).

Application to Nursing

To be effective, nursing interventions must be derived from culturally embedded theories, as one size does *not* fit all. For example, hindrances to information about spontaneous abortion prevention for southern Sudanese women included belief in a family curse related to husbands' failure to follow the cultural rules of bridewealth payment (Onyango & Mott, 2011). Montalvo-Liendo, Wardell, Engebretson, and Reininger (2009) described cultural factors that deterred disclosure of intimate partner violence by women of Mexican descent, and, traditions, cultural rules, and lack of means of empowerment were found to be critical factors underlying Jordanian women staying with abusive husbands (Gharaibeh & Oweis, 2009).

To promote development and well-being of children, clinicians need to understand how Jordanian Muslim parents perceive parenting and incorporate this understanding into the design and delivery of services to enhance parental roles (Oweis, Gharaibeh, Maaitah, Gharaibeh, & Obeisat, 2012). To effectively measure the health and well-being of Korean older adults living alone in the community, a three-stage translation process was used to obtain a culturally and linguistically sensitive method for the population (You et al., 2009). Finally, in a review of the nursing literature for publications concerning lesbian, gay, bisexual, and transgender health, a notable "silence" was found in the United States; the impact of this bias was discussed in a study by DeJoseph, Dibble, and Eliason (2010).

Current methods of research, practice, and training are challenged by multiculturalism. Results from these and other culturally based studies have implications for health care professionals to provide culture-specific and evidence-based care regardless of geographic location. Box 13-7 gives guidelines on how to avoid cultural bias in research and thereby improve health care for all.

Chaos Theory

Problematic with explaining chaos theory is that the word *chaos* immediately brings to mind the common meaning of "a condition or place of great disorder or confusion" or of randomness—"having no specific pattern." When used in the scientific context, chaos, as will be explained, means something very different. A second problem lies in

Box 13-7 Recommendations for Avoidance of Cultural Biases in Research

- Acknowledge your own cultural beliefs and values through ongoing self-assessments.
- Question the value, purpose, cultural origins, and relevance of current practices wherever they are found.
- Critically examine any cross-cultural research in literature reviews for potential bias and pretension and be prepared for anti-intuitive findings and rejection of assumptions.
- Engage persons culturally similar to the study sample at each step of the research process.
- Promote cultural diversity in scientific nursing communities (local, state, national, and international) to provide checks and balances for individual biases.
- Create environments for egalitarian and pluralistic dialogue.
- Collaborate (or consult) with a multicultural interdisciplinary research group.
- Consider a qualitative ethnographic study for exploring differences.

simplifying the somewhat exotic and strange terminology (Ward, 1995). Application poses an additional problem because much of the argument of the theory has been developed through complex mathematical formulae (Weigel & Murray, 2000). The last problem is that large data sets with long time sequences are necessary for chaos to become evident (Shelley & Wagner, 1998). This section discusses concepts related to chaos theory and their application.

The modernist or Newtonian-type theories of Western science emerging from the Enlightenment period (e.g., general systems theory) focus on linearity, homeostasis, order, equilibrium, predictability, and control (e.g., causal models). These concepts form a sort of invisible template that constrains many scientists from examining the "noise" or variation in their data (e.g., outliers); thus, they are unable to "look outside the box." An emerging postmodern science of nonlinear dynamic systems, in particular chaos theory, takes science "outside that box."

Chaos theory has its origins in meteorology in the 1960s (Johnson & Webber, 2010) and is part of an emerging postmodern science. The interdisciplinary application of chaos theory has steadily gained momentum since the 1990s. Chaos theory is the study of unstable, aperiodic behavior in deterministic (nonrandom) nonlinear dynamical systems. Dynamical refers to the time-varying behavior of a system and aperiodic is the nonrepetitive but continuous behavior that results from the effects of any small disturbance.

More simply stated, chaos theory is about finding the underlying order in the apparent disorder of natural and social systems and understanding how change occurs in nonlinear dynamical systems over time (Hayles, 1999) (Box 13-8). According to Young (1992), chaos theory provides "insight and guidance into the delicate and shifting relationship between order and disorder in ways not permitted in modern science nor imagined in more traditional knowledge processes" (p. 446). Based on chaos theory, therefore, natural and social systems survive precisely because of their nonlinear behavior. Examples of dynamical instability in the real world include disease, political unrest, and families and communities in trouble. Chaos may also be found in the physical body in heart rhythms, electrical brain activity, and chemical reactions (e.g., neurotransmitters).

Concepts From Chaos Theory

Sociology (and nursing), as well as other social science disciplines, have much to gain in the way of useful knowledge by adopting the concepts and logics of chaotic dynamics (Young, 1991). This section presents four of those concepts.

Sensitive dependence on initial conditions, the hallmark of chaotic systems, is where even small differences can cause dramatically divergent paths. Because equilibrium is never reached in a dynamical system, trajectories that start from "arbitrarily close" points will ultimately diverge exponentially (Robinson, 1982, cited in Mark, 1994). This sensitivity to initial conditions is commonly referred to

Box 13-8 Principles of Chaos Theory

- Systems, no matter their level of complexity, rely on an underlying order, seek stability, and survive precisely because of their nonlinear behavior or *orderly disorder*.
- Simple events can result in very complex behaviors or events.

as the "butterfly effect"—where hypothetically, a butterfly flapping its wings on one side of the world can cause a tornado the next month on the other side of the world. This concept was dramatized in the 2004 release of the movie *The Butterfly Effect*, but it has been at least intuitively known for centuries, as written in the well-known proverb:

> *For want of a nail, the shoe was lost;*
> *For want of a shoe, the horse was lost;*
> *For want of a horse, the rider was lost;*
> *For want of a rider, a message was lost;*
> *For want of a message, the battle was lost;*
> *For want of a battle, the kingdom was lost!*

A small change—no nail—resulted in the huge concluding event of a lost kingdom.

This effect was illustrated by Heaton & Call (1995). They examined the relationship between age at time of marriage for a large sample of couples in two age groups: 23 to 26 and 27 to 29 years of age. The marriage survival rates were almost identical at 5 years, but divergent trajectories became increasingly evident at 10 and 15 years. At 20 years, the marital survival rates were significantly higher for the 27- to 29-year-olds. The age difference between the two groups was small, yet those differences caused two groups of nonlinear dynamical systems to take divergent paths.

A *strange attractor* (strange because its appearance was unexpected) is similar to a magnet that exerts its pull on objects to return them to their original starting point. With this controlling action, an attractor provides a boundary (Shelley & Wagner, 1998). For example, an attractor in relationships is "the behavioral pattern that underlies the period of stability" (p. 435). In a clinical example, Gottman (1991) identifies a sense of "we-ness" as an attractor in stable marriages. An attractor can be visualized (with appropriate software) by graphing the changing behavior of an attribute(s) of a system. Figure 13-3 is an example of a strange attractor showing chaotic motion from a simple three-dimensional model; note the butterfly resemblance.

A *bifurcation* "indicates the transition from a steady state to a state characterized by periodicity . . . [the system shows] an abrupt qualitative change in behavior" (Mark, 1994). This change occurs when a system is pushed so far from its steady state that it is unable to recover; a chaos or crisis state is reached. At this point, the system arrives at a "fork in the road"—a choice of two or more alternative steady states, each different from the first (Prigogine & Stengers, 1984). The history of the system is influential as to which choice is made. When stressors again impact the system, the process is repeated. At each crisis point, the system reaches a bifurcation with choices. With successive bifurcations, choices become increasingly limited. A diagram of bifurcations would resemble a decision tree (Ward, 1995) or, with a more familiar analogy, the human vascular system.

Dissipative structures refers to the capacity of systems that are far from equilibrium, to change to higher or more complex levels of orderliness. Dissipative, or self-organizing systems, arise spontaneously out of conditions that look chaotic but in fact have a hidden order (Mark, 1994). The reasons for calling these structures

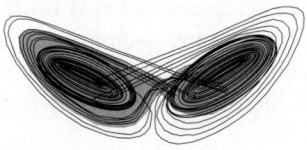

Figure 13-3 Three-dimensional model of a strange attractor.

Box 13-9 Dissipative Structures

Structures are called dissipative for the following reasons:
- The definition recognizes the constructive role of dissipative processes in their creation.
- Dissipative systems require more energy to maintain because they incorporate adaptive structures profoundly different from those existing previously.

Source: Mark (1994).

dissipative are listed in Box 13-9. Such systems "maintain their ability to continue their activities over prolonged periods of time by importing physical or social energy from the environment and exporting used energy in the form of waste" (Ward, 1995). Paraphrasing Ward's example, a toddler is an open system who draws energy from his or her environment—food, parents' time and attention, as well as information. He or she also exports waste (e.g., bodily, disorder or mess, and parental exhaustion) to the environment. Needless to say, the toddler is affected by and in turn affects the larger system in which he or she is embedded.

Chaos is natural and universal and can be found in such diverse phenomena as the human heartbeat and the world economy (Lorenz, 1999) and in "human systems as disease, dis-ease, dilemmas, crises, or need" (Ray, 1994). While chaos may cause uncertainty, it also offers opportunities that can create hope and bring about change; both are integral components of nursing practice.

Application to Nursing

The application of the science of chaos theory in nursing is quite diverse. One example was found that had a distinct direct clinical focus. Fisher & Wineman (2009) presented the possibilities for chaos theory and nonlinear methods for conceptualizing and exploring complex physiologic patterns that occur in response to aging, disease, and treatment. Two indirect clinical applications were identified. Chaos theory provided the framework for action to promote a holistic multidisciplinary team approach to patient assessment (Carbonu, 2011); Barker (2011) explored how chaos might contribute to a metaparadigm of nursing, and Benham-Hutchins and Clancy (2010) discussed how social networks are complex adaptive systems and explained how understanding social networks can lead to improved communication patterns in health care organizations.

Postmodern Social Theory

Postmodernity is generally regarded as a new social and political epoch that supposedly succeeded the "modern era" or "modernity." It is a broad and wide-ranging term that first emerged in the 1950s but as a movement dates back to the 1920s. *Postmodernism* refers to cultural products (e.g., art, architecture) that are viewed as different from modern cultural products (Ritzer, 1996a).

Postmodern theory is a term applicable to a variety of fields both academic and nonacademic that includes literature, art, philosophy, sociology, architecture, and culture, among others. It is basically a philosophical reaction to the underlying assumptions and universalizing tendency of the doctrine of positivism and scientific objectivity characterized by modernity.

Difference Between Postmodern and Modern

Postmodern social theory, a type of social theory that is distinctly different from modern social theory, relies on concrete experience over abstract principles and is highly sceptical of explanations that claim to be valid for all groups, cultures, traditions, or races, and instead focuses on the relative truths of each person.

When discussing social theory, the "modern" reflects the belief that the hidden processes of society can be revealed and perhaps even manipulated to bring about a new and better society. Postmodern social theory, on the other hand, is *opposed* to or *after* this dream of transparent, better society (Ritzer & Goodman, 2006). Postmodern social theory poses new ways of thinking qualitatively, and postmodern social theorists are inclined to be more interested in focusing on the more peripheral aspects of society as opposed to looking at the core beliefs and tenets of society (e.g., rationalism or capitalism) (Ritzer, 1996b).

As with modern social theory, not all postmodern social theories are the same. Ritzer and Goodman (2006) discuss three fundamental positions taken by postmodern social theorists: (1) the *extreme postmodernists,* who believe that there has been a radical rupture and modern society has been replaced by a postmodern society; (2) *moderate postmodernists,* who hold that although society has changed, postmodernity grows out of, and is continuous with, modernity; and (3) theorists who see *modernity and postmodernity as engaged in a long-running relationship with one another,* with postmodernity continually pointing out the limitations of modernity.

Postmodern social theories have been criticized for being untestable, unsystematic, overly abstract, and relativistic. Also, they are criticized for being too strongly linked to politics. Ritzer and Goodman (2006) explained that characteristics of postmodern social theory can be related to a contingency focus (Box 13-10). The authors argued that these characteristics are connected to an attempt to reveal that things could be different. In addition, there is a belief that the objective of theory is not showing why things are as they are but to open up alternatives and create new possibilities. With a focus on contingency, postmodern social theory structures the types of questions that can be asked and the key controversies that should be addressed by society.

While postmodernity has many critics, Ritzer, Zhao, and Murphy (2006) view postmodern social theories as offering a useful set of new ideas and tools. Some forms of social theory, for example, symbolic interactionism and critical theory, have been receptive to postmodern ideas. And although controversial, postmodern social theories have helped lead the way for other theoretical orientations and viewpoints

Box 13-10 Characteristics of Postmodern Social Theories

- Skepticism toward grand narratives
- Abandonment of any basis for claiming certainty
- Rejection of universal standards
- Playful rhetoric
- A subversive approach
- An emphasis on the irrational

Source: Ritzer and Goodman (2006).

that have become meaningful and academically institutionalized. These include feminist and gender studies and multicultural studies (Ritzer & Goodman, 2006).

Application to Nursing

Two concepts from postmodern social theory are especially relevant for nursing, the questioning of traditional foundational theories or explanations and the use of therapeutic narratives. For example, Mitchell (2011) examined the impact of the fabrication of health, illness, and patient subjectivity and suggested that nurses need to resist the discursive practices that both disempower and reduce choice. Drawing on ideas from both poststructuralism and postmodernism, Nosek, Kennedy, and Gudmundsdottir (2010) conducted a narrative analysis of women's distress during menopause; the postmodern feminist framework and methodology supported the interpretations of personal narratives and the role of social dialogue in the women's lives. Similarly, Clark and Standard (2011) explored the use of narrative to inform and transform caregiver burden for elderly female caregivers.

In other examples, Kirkham and Anderson (2010) used a postcolonial feminism framework, drawn from postmodern schools of thought, to explore how nurse researchers negotiate the dialectic of analysis and advocacy to address social justice for marginalized groups, and O'Mahony and Donnelly (2010) advocated for use of a postmodern perspective to shed light on the embedded social structures and discourses that impact immigrant women's mental health experiences. Lastly, Huntington and Gilmour (2011) critiqued modernism and postmodernism and underscored the impact of both on nurses' practice.

Summary

Theories from the sociologic sciences are integral to the discipline of nursing. Indeed, nurses in virtually all settings, caring for all types of clients, use concepts and principles from social theories daily because social forces have a strong impact on health. Simon, the nurse in the opening case study, recognized that in dealing with the problem of teenage pregnancy, it was essential to move beyond the logical intervention of providing more information on sexuality. Because he recognized that teen pregnancy is a social problem, he knew that it must be addressed using social science concepts and principles.

Sociologic theories are rich and substantively diverse. Because of this richness and diversity, it was impossible to include all theories and perspectives that are relevant to the discipline of nursing in this chapter. It is hoped, however, that the reader has gained an appreciation of the sociologic perspective and understands its significance to professional nursing.

Developing a sociologic perspective is not always comfortable because it calls for confronting and questioning existing ideologies and assumptions regarding social arrangements. It is important to do this, however, and the knowledge gained can benefit not only clients but the health care system and professional nurses as well.

Key Points

- Theories from the sociologic sciences have greatly influenced nursing; indeed, many early nursing leaders (e.g., Nightingale, Barton, Wald, Sanger) were social activists.

- Exchange theories are based on the philosophical perspective termed "utilitarianism," which supports the notion of "the greatest good for the greatest number." Exchange theories apply to human interactions in social context; general systems theory and social networks are examples.
- Interactions frameworks, such as symbolic interactionism and role theory, describe how humans relate to each other (e.g., using language, gestures, and symbols to communicate) and in roles they take or are ascribed to them.
- Conflict theories present the social processes of stability and change and explain how conflict is endemic to all social organizations because of unequal distribution of power. Critical social theory, feminist theory, and cultural diversity/cultural bias are examples of conflict theories and perspectives used by nurses.
- Chaos theory explains the interrelatedness and dependence of nonlinear dynamics and seeks to find underlying order in apparent disorder of natural and social systems. It also attempts to explain how changes occur in nonlinear systems over time.
- Postmodern theory is a philosophical reaction to the underlying assumptions and universalizing tendencies of "modernity." It supports abstract principles and is highly sceptical of explanations that claim to be valid for all groups, cultures, traditions, or races. Postmodernity focuses on the relative truths of each person and supports the belief that the objective of theory is to open up alternatives and create new possibilities.

Learning Activities

1. Select one of the theories presented in this chapter and obtain copies of the theorist's work(s). Read the work and consider ways to apply the concepts and principles in nursing. Are the concepts and principles more applicable in some settings than in others? Are the concepts and principles more applicable with some groups or aggregates than others?
2. Select a theory presented in this chapter. Review the nursing literature and identify nursing articles and studies describing how/when the theory is used in nursing. Present the findings in a paper or share them with colleagues.
3. Select one of the grand nursing theorists and review her work. Identify any concepts, principles, and theories drawn from the social sciences. Share findings with colleagues.

REFERENCES

Alexander, J. C., & Smith, P. (2009). The strong program in cultural sociology. In J. Turner (Ed.), *The handbook of sociological theory* (2nd ed., pp. 135–150). New York: Springer.

Barker, P. (2011). *Chaos and the way of Zen: Psychiatric nursing and the 'uncertainty principle.'* Paper presented at a Sigma Theta Tau Research Conference. Retrieved from http://hdl.handle.net/10755/166683

Beanlands, H., Fredericks, S., Lapum, J., McCay, E., Romaniuk, D., & Schwind, J. (2012). Discussion of patient-centered care in health care organizations. *Quality Management in Health Care, 21*(3), 127–134.

Benedict, S., & Georges, J. M. (2009). Nurses in the Nazi "euthanasia" program: A critical feminist analysis. *Advances in Nursing Science, 32*(1), 63–74.

Benham-Hutchins, M., & Clancy, T. R. (2010). Managing organizational complexity: Social networks as embedded complex adaptive systems. *Journal of Nursing Administration, 40*(9), 352–356.

Blau, P. (1964). *Exchange and power in social life.* New York: Wiley.

Blumer, H. (1969). *Symbolic interactionism.* Englewood Cliffs, NJ: Prentice Hall.

Bodley, J. H. (2011). *Cultural anthropology: Tribes, states, and the global system.* Plymouth, United Kingdom: Alta Mira Press.

Brown, V. B., & Oyetunde, M. O. (2012). Professional accountability: Implications for primary healthcare nursing practice. *JONA'S Healthcare Law, Ethics and Regulation, 14*(4), 109–114.

Brownmiller, S. (1975). *Against our will.* New York: Simon & Schuster.

Carbonu, D. M. (2011). *Promoting a holistic multidisciplinary team approach to patient assessment and reassessment: Challenges and outcomes.* Paper presented at a Sigma Theta Tau International Research Conference. Retrieved from http://hdl.handle.net/10755/151372

Carruth, A. (2011). *Development and testing of the caregiver reciprocity scale.* Paper presented at a Sigma Theta Tau International Research Conference. Retrieved from http://hdl.handle.net/10755/174589

Chinn, P. L. (1999). Gender and nursing science. In E. C. Polifroni & M. Welch (Eds.), *Perspectives on philosophy of science in nursing: An historical and contemporary anthology* (pp. 462–466). Philadelphia: Lippincott Williams & Wilkins.

Chodorow, N. (1989). *Feminism and psychoanalytic theory.* New Haven, CT: Yale University Press.

Clark, M., & Standard, P. L. (2011). The caregiving story: How the narrative approach informs caregiving burden. Paper presented at a Sigma Theta Tau International Research Conference. Retrieved from http://hdl.handle.net/10755/180429

Coleman, J. (1990). *Foundations of social theory.* Cambridge, MA: Belknap Press.

Cooley, C. H. (1902). *Human nature and the social order.* New York: Charles Scribner's Sons.

Coser, L. A. (1956). *The functions of social conflict.* London, United Kingdom: Free Press of Glencoe.

Dahrendorf, R. (1958). Toward a theory of social conflict. *Journal of Conflict Resolution, 2,* 170–183.

DeJoseph, J., Dibble, S., & Eliason, M. J. (2010). Nursing's silence on lesbian, gay, bisexual, and transgender issues: The need for emancipatory efforts. *Advances in Nursing Science, 33*(3), 206–218.

Dewey, D. (1922). *Human nature and human conduct.* New York: Henry Holt.

Dickinson, J. (2011). *A critical social theory approach to nursing care of adolescents with diabetes.* Paper presented at a Sigma Theta Tau International Research Conference. Retrieved from http://hdl.handle.net/10755/167261

Dole, D., Dole, D. M., & Shambley-Ebron, D. (2009). *Cultural meanings of mothering in African American adolescent mothers: Through their own eyes.* Paper presented at a Sigma Theta Tau International Research Conference. Retrieved from http://hdl.handle.net/10755/158948

Eitzen, D. S., Baca-Zinn, M., & Smith, K. E. (2010). *In conflict and order: Understanding society* (12th ed.). Boston: Allyn & Bacon.

Edwards, S. B., Koop, P. M., Northcott, H. C., & Olson, K. (2012). Patient and family caregiver decision making in the context of advanced cancer. *Cancer Nursing, 35*(3), 178–186.

Emerson, R. (1981). Social exchange theory. In M. Rosenberg & R. Turner (Eds.), *Social psychology* (pp. 30–65). New York: Basic Books.

Ferrante, J. (2012). *Sociology: A global perspective* (8th ed.). Belmont, CA: Wadsworth.

Firestone, S. (1970). *The dialectic of sex.* London, United Kingdom: Paladin.

Fisher, E. M., & Wineman, N. M. (2009). Conceptualizing compensatory responses: Implications for treatment and research. *Biological Research for Nursing, 10*(4), 400–408.

Fouquier, K. F. (2011). The concept of motherhood among three generations of African American women. *Journal of Nursing Scholarship, 43*(2), 145–153.

Friedan, B. (1963). *The feminine mystique.* London, United Kingdom: Gollancz.

Fujino, N., & Okamura, H. (2009). Factors affecting the sense of burden felt by family members caring for patients with mental illness. *Archives of Psychiatric Nursing, 23*(2), 128–137.

Gharaibeh, M., & Oweis, A. (2009). Why do Jordanian women stay in an abusive relationship: Implications for health and social well-being. *Journal of Nursing Scholarship, 41*(4), 376–384.

Gilligan, D. (1982). *In a different voice: Psychological theory and women's development.* Cambridge, MA: Harvard University Press.

Gottman, J. M. (1991). Chaos and regulated change in families: A metaphor for the study of transitions. In P. A. Cowan & M. Hetherton (Eds.), *Family transitions* (pp. 247–272). Hillsdale, NJ: Lawrence Erlbaum.

Guarnero, P. (2011). *Health promotion behaviors among a group of 18–29 year old gay and bisexual.* Paper presented at a Sigma Theta Tau International Research Conference. Retrieved from http://hdl.handle.net//10755/158057

Habermas, J. (1991). The critical theory of Jurgen Habermas. In J. Turner (Ed.), *The structure of sociological theory* (pp. 254–281). Belmont, CA: Wadsworth.

Hall, J., & Fields, B. (2012). Race and microaggression in nursing knowledge development. *Advances in Nursing Science, 35*(1), 25–38.

Hamrin, V., McCarthy, E. M., & Tyson, V. (2010). Pediatric psychotropic medication initiation and adherence: A literature review based on social exchange theory. *Journal of Child and Adolescent Psychiatric Nursing, 23*(3), 151–172.

Hansen, L., Archbold, P. G., Stewart, B., & Westfall, U. B. (2011). *Role theory and life-sustaining treatment decisions.* Paper presented at a Sigma Theta Tau International Research Conference. Retrieved from http://hdl.handle.net//10755/175122

Hayles, N. K. (1999). From chaos to complexity: Moving through metaphor to practice. *Chaos and Complexity in Nursing,* 4. Retrieved from http://www.southernct.edu/chaos-nursing/chaos4.htm

Heaton, T. B., & Call, V. R. A. (1995). Modelling family dynamics with event history techniques. *Journal of Marriage and the Family, 57*(4), 1078–1090.

Hechter, M. (1987). *Principles of group solidarity.* Berkeley, CA: University of California Press.

Holmes, C., & Warelow, P. J. (2011). *Culture, needs and nursing: A critical theory approach.* Paper presented at a Sigma Theta Tau International Research Conference. Retrieved from http://hdl.handle.net/10755/178370

Homans, G. (1961). *Social behavior.* London, United Kingdom: Routledge.

Horton, K. L., & Dworkin, S. L. (2013). Redefining gender-based power to move beyond interpersonal approaches to HIV prevention. *Advances in Nursing Science, 36*(1), 42–50.

Huntington, A., & Gilmour, J. (2011). *Reforming the practice of nurses: Decolonization or getting out from under.* Paper presented at a Sigma Theta Tau International Research Conference. Retrieved from http://10755/178713

Ihlenfed, J. (2011). *Nurses' perceptions of administrative social support.* Paper presented at a Sigma Theta Tau International Research Conference. Retrieved from http://hdl.handle.net/10755/176357

James, W. (1890). *The principles of psychology.* New York: Henry Holt.

Johnson, B. M., & Webber, P. B. (2010). *An introduction to theory and reasoning in nursing* (3rd ed.). Philadelphia: Lippincott Williams & Wilkins.

Jordan, M., Lanham, H. J., Anderson, R. A., & McDaniel, R. R., Jr. (2010). Implications of complex adaptive systems theory for interpreting research about health care organizations. *Journal of Evaluation in Clinical Practice, 16*(1), 228–231.

Kao, H. F. S. (2011). Medication administration hassles for Mexican American family caregivers of older adult. *Nursing and Health Sciences, 13*(2), 133–140.

Kenney, J. W. (1995). Relevance of theory-based nursing practice. In P. J. Christensen & J. W. Kenney (Eds.), *Nursing process: Application of conceptual models* (4th ed., pp. 3–17). St. Louis: Mosby.

Kirkham, S. R., & Anderson, M. (2010). The advocate-analyst dialectic in critical and postcolonial feminist research: Reconciling tensions around scientific integrity. *Advances in Nursing Science, 33*(3), 196–205.

Kitson, A. L. (2009). The need for systems change: Reflections on knowledge translation and organizational change. *Journal of Advanced Nursing, 65*(1), 217–228.

Lau, Y. (2011). A longitudinal study of family conflicts, social support, and antenatal depressive symptoms among Chinese women. *Archives of Psychiatric Nursing, 25*(3), 206–219.

Leahy-Warren, P., McCarthy, G., & Corcoran, P. (2011). Postnatal depression in first-time mothers: Prevalence and relationships between functional and structural social support at 6 and 12 weeks postpartum. *Archives of Psychiatric Nursing, 25*(3), 174–184.

Lee, H., Hann, H. W., Yang, J., & Fawcett, J. (2011). Recognition and management of HBV infection in a social context. *Journal of Cancer Education, 26,* 516–521.

Lee, T. Y., Wang, M. M., Lin, K. C., & Kao, C. H. (2012). The effectiveness of early intervention on paternal stress for fathers of premature infants admitted to a neonatal intensive care unit. *Journal of Advanced Nursing, 69*(5), 1085–1095.

Levi-Strauss, C. (1969). *The elementary structures of kinship.* Boston: Beacon Press.

Lindesmith, A., & Strauss, A. (1968). *Social psychology.* New York: Holt, Rinehart & Winston.

Logan, J. R, & Spitze, G. (1996). *Family ties: Enduring relations between parents and their grown children.* Philadelphia: Temple University Press.

Lorenz, E. N. (1999). Lorenz: An auspicious salutation. *Chaos and Complexity in Nursing*, 4. Retrieved from http://www.southernct.edu/chaos-nursing/chaos4.htm

Lyon, D. (2011). *Critical social theory: Amplifying the voices of HIV-infected minority women.* Paper presented at a Sigma Theta Tau International Research Conference. Retrieved from http://hdl.handle.net/10755/176701

Machin, T., & Stevenson, C. (2011). *Towards a framework for clarifying psychiatric nursing roles.* Paper presented at a Sigma Theta Tau International Research Conference. Retrieved from http://hdl.handle.net/10755/177527

Mark, B. A. (1994). Chaos theory and nursing systems research. *Theoretic and Applied Chaos in Nursing, 1*(1). Retrieved from http://www.southernct.edu/chaos-nursing/volume1.htm

Martins, D. C. (2011). Thinking upstream: Nursing theories and population-focused nursing practice. In M. A. Nies & M. McEwen (Eds.), *Community/public health nursing: Promoting the health of populations* (4th ed., pp. 37–49). Philadelphia: Elsevier/Saunders.

Martsolf, D., Draucker, C. B., & Bednarz, J. L. (2011). *Listening to the voices: How adolescents make sense of troubled dating relationships.* Paper presented at a Sigma Theta Tau International Research Conference. Retrieved from http://hd.handle.net/10755/158884

Marx, K. (1977). *Capital: A critical analysis of political economy* (Vol. 1). (B. Folkes, Trans.). New York: Vintage Books.

Mason, G., & Attree, M. (1997). The relationship between research and the nursing process in clinical practice. *Journal of Advanced Nursing, 26*(5), 1045–1049.

Mauritz, M., & van Meijel, B. (2009). Loss and grief in patients with schizophrenia: On living in another world. *Archives of Psychiatric Nursing, 23*(3), 251–260.

Mead, K. (1934). *Mind, self, and society: From the standpoint of a social behaviorist.* (C. W. Morris, Ed.). Chicago: University of Chicago Press.

Mehta, A., Cohen, S. R., & Chan, L. S. (2009). Palliative care: A need for a family systems approach. *Palliative and Supportive Care, 7*(2), 235–243.

Merritt-Gray, M., & West, J. (2011). *Reclaiming self: A feminist grounded theory of the leaving process in abusive conjugal relationships.* Paper presented at a Sigma Theta Tau International Research Conference. Retrieved from http://hdl.handle.net/10755/176899

Meyer, R. M., & O'Brien-Pallas, L. L. (2010). Nursing services delivery theory: An open system approach. *Journal of Advanced Nursing, 66*(12), 2828–2838.

Millet, K. (1971). *Sexual politics.* New York: Avon/Equinox.

Mills, C. W. (1959). *The sociological imagination.* New York: Oxford University Press.

Mitchell, D. (2011). *Postmodernism, health and illness.* Paper presented at a Sigma Theta Tau International Research Conference. Retrieved from http://hdl.handle.net/10755/177435

Montalvo-Liendo, N., Wardell, D. W., Engebretson, J., & Reininger, B. M. (2009). Factors influencing disclosure of abuse by women of Mexican descent. *Journal of Nursing Scholarship, 41*(4), 359–367.

Moreno, J. (1953). *Who shall survive?* New York: Beacon Press.

Myny, D., Goubergen, D. V., Gobert, M., Vanderwee, K., Hecke, A. V., & Defloor, T. (2011). Non-direct patient care factors influencing nursing workload: A review of the literature. *Journal of Advanced Nursing, 67*(10), 2109–2129.

Ngai, F., & Chan, S. (2012). Stress, maternal role competence and satisfaction among Chinese women in the perinatal period. *Research in Nursing & Health, 35*(1), 30–39.

Nosek, M., Kennedy, H. P., & Gudmundsdottir, M. (2010). Silence, stigma, and shame: A postmodern analysis of distress during menopause. *Advances in Nursing Science, 33*(3), 24–36.

Nye, F. I. (1979). Choice, exchange, and the family. In W. R. Burr, R. Hill, F. I. Nye, & I. I. Reiss (Eds.), *Contemporary theories about the family* (pp. 1–41). New York: Free Press.

O'Mahony, J. M., & Donnelly, T. T. (2010). A postcolonial feminist perspective inquiry into immigrant women's mental health care experiences. *Issues in Mental Health Nursing, 31*(7), 440–449.

Onyango, M. A., & Mott, S. (2011). The nexus between bridewealth, family curse, and spontaneous abortion among southern Sudanese women. *Journal of Nursing Scholarship, 43*(4), 376–384.

Osmond, M. W., & Thorne, B. (1993). Feminist theories: The social construction of gender in families and society. In P. G. Boss, W. J. Doherty, R. LaRossa, W. R. Schumm, & S. K. Steinmetz (Eds.), *Sourcebook of family theories and methods: A contextual approach* (pp. 591–623). New York: Plenum Press.

Oweis, A., Gharaibeh, M., Maaitah, R., Gharaibeh, H., & Obeisat, S. (2012). Parenting from a Jordanian perspective: Findings from a qualitative study. *Journal of Nursing Scholarship, 44*(3), 242–248.

Pfettscher, S. A. (2010). Florence Nightingale. In A. M. Tomey & M. R. Alligood (Eds.), *Nursing theorists and their work* (6th ed., pp. 71-89). St. Louis: Mosby.

Picot, S., Youngblut, J., & Zeller, R. (2011). *Development and testing of a measure of perceived caregiver rewards in adults.* Paper presented at a Sigma Theta Tau International Research Conference. Retrieved from http://hdl.handle.net/10755/180623

Prigogine, I., & Stengers, I. (1984). *Order out of chaos, Man's new dialogue with nature.* New York: Bantam.

Ray, M. A. (1994). Complex caring dynamics: A unifying model of nursing inquiry. *Theoretic and Applied Chaos in Nursing*, 3. Retrieved from http://www.southernct.edu/chaos-nursing/volume1.htm

Ritzer, G. (1996a). *Postmodern social theory.* New York: McGraw-Hill.

Ritzer, G. (1996b). *Classical sociological theory.* New York: McGraw-Hill.

Ritzer, G., & Goodman, D. (2006). Postmodern social theory. In J. H. Turner (Ed.), *Handbook of sociological theory* (2nd ed., pp. 151–170). New York: Springer.

Ritzer, G., Zhao, S., & Murphy, J. (2006). Metatheorizing in sociology: The basic parameters and the potential contributions of postmodernism. In J. H. Turner (Ed.), *Handbook of sociological theory* (2nd ed., pp. 113–131). New York: Springer.

Ryan, W. (1976). *Blaming the victim.* New York: Pantheon.

Sakunhongsophon, S., Sirapo-ngam, Y., Tripp-Reimer, T., & Junda, T. (2011). Stroke caregiving networks in Bangkok: Patterns of social exchange behaviour. *Pacific Rim International Journal of Nursing Research, 15*(2), 152–164.

Shieh, S. C., Tung, H. S., & Liang, S. Y. (2012). Social support as influencing primary family caregiver burden in Taiwanese patients with colorectal cancer. *Journal of Nursing Scholarship, 44*(30), 223–231.

Shelley, R. K., & Wagner, D. (1998). Chaos in social theory: Explaining complex events with simple ideas. *Sociological Focus, 31*(4), 357–372.

Simmel, G. (1956). *Conflict and the web of group affiliations.* (K. H. Wolff, Trans.). Glencoe, IL: Free Press.

Stryker, S., & Statham, A. (1985). Symbolic interaction and role theory. In G. Lindzey & E. Aronson (Eds.), *The handbook of social psychology* (3rd ed., pp. 311–378). New York: Random House.

Sumner, J., Scott, A, & Arndt, M. (2011). Caring in nursing: A critical theory study. Paper presented at a Sigma Theta Tau International Research Conference. Retrieved from http://hdl.handle.net/10755/174095

Thibaut, J. W., & Kelley, H. M. (1959). *The social psychology of groups.* New York: Wiley.

Thomas, W. I., & Thomas, D. S. (1928). *The child in America: Behavior problems and programs.* New York: Knopf.

Turner, J. H. (2013). *Contemporary sociological theory.* Los Angeles: Sage.

van Daalen-Smith, C. (2011). Waiting for oblivion: Women's experiences with electroshock. *Issues in Mental Health Nursing, 32*(7), 457–472.

von Bertalanffy, L. (1968). *General system theory: Foundation, development, and applications.* New York: Braziller.

Wang, Y. N., Shu, Y. I. L., Chen, M. C., & Yang, P. S. (2011). Reconciling work and family caregiving among adult-child family caregivers of older people with dementia: Effects on role strain and depressive symptoms. *Journal of Advanced Nursing, 67*(4), 829–240.

Wang, Y. N., Shu, Y. I. L., Chen, M. C., Tsai, W. C., Yang, P. S., & Yao, G. (2013). Exploring conflict between caregiving and work for caregivers of elders with dementia: A cross-sectional, correlational study. *Journal of Advanced Nursing, 69*(5), 1051–1062.

Ward, M. (1995). Butterflies and bifurcations: Can chaos theory contribute to our understanding of family systems? *Journal of Marriage and the Family, 57*(3), 629–638.

Waters, M. (1994). *Modern sociological theory.* Thousand Oaks, CA: Sage.

Weber, M. (1958). *The Protestant ethic and the spirit of capitalism.* New York: Charles Scribner's Sons.

Weigel, D., & Murray, C. (2000). The paradox of stability and change in relationships: What does chaos theory offer for the study of romantic relationships? *Journal of Social and Personal Relationships, 17*(3), 425–449.

Williams, S., & Mackey, M. C. (2011). *Women's experiences of preterm labor: A feminist critique.* Paper presented at a Sigma Theta Tau International Research Conference. Retrieved from http://hdl.handle.net//10755/177298

You, K. S., Lee, H. O., Fitzpatrick, J. J., Kim, S., Marui, E., Lee, J. S., et al. (2009). Spirituality, depression, living alone, and perceived health among Korean older adults in the community. *Archives of Psychiatric Nursing, 23*(4), 309–322.

Young, T. R. (1991). Chaos theory and symbolic interaction theory: Poetics for the postmodern sociologist. *Symbolic Interaction, 14*(3), 321–334.

Young, T. R. (1992). Chaos theory and human agency: Humanistic sociology in a postmodern era. *Humanity and Society, 16*(4), 441–460.

CHAPTER 14

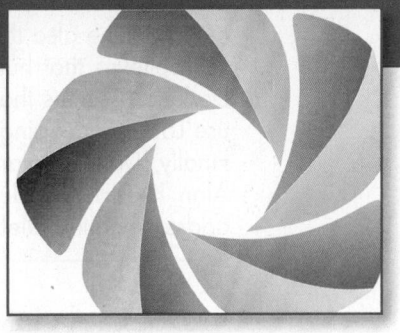

Theories From the Behavioral Sciences

Debra Brossett Garner

Darlene Williams is in a master's degree program that will allow her to become an adult psychiatric/mental health nurse practitioner. In a course on the application of theory in nursing, one of her assignments is to write a paper describing how she has applied a theory in providing care for a client. Although Darlene has been working as a nurse in a psychiatric hospital for the past 10 years, she is finding this assignment difficult because, thus far in the course, the instructor has focused primarily on grand nursing theories. Darlene knows little about these theories because in her practice, she uses a broad, eclectic approach, predominantly applying theories from the behavioral sciences.

Darlene discusses her dilemma with her professor and learns that she can use any theory or set of theories for the assignment; it is not necessary to rely strictly on nursing theories. The discussion with her professor enlightens Darlene about the necessity of applying non-nursing theories to nursing practice. With the realization of the importance of theories from other disciplines to nursing, Darlene's interest in the many psychologically based theories is piqued, and she conducts a literature review.

The person that Darlene chooses for her assignment is Alan, a 41-year-old Caucasian male, who is married and the father of two adolescents. Alan was admitted to the hospital with diagnoses of major depression, substance dependence with physiologic dependency, and hepatitis C. Assessments revealed that he had problems with his primary support group, problems related to the social environment, occupational problems, and problems related to interaction with the legal system.

Although this is Alan's first hospitalization, he has had a long history of alcohol abuse. He also admits to using cocaine or marijuana occasionally on the weekends. His father was an alcoholic who died at the age of 44 years with cirrhosis of the liver. Although not actively suicidal, Alan expresses passive death wishes. Alan is a well-known member of the community and owns a large software business, which is on the verge of bankruptcy. His motivation for entering treatment is that his wife threatened to divorce him unless he stops using alcohol and drugs.

In reviewing Alan's care, Darlene plans to use a holistic approach, incorporating principles and concepts from various theories. The first theory that Darlene chooses is Freud's psychoanalytic theory because of Alan's denial. This theory is relevant because Freud discussed how an individual uses defense mechanisms to decrease anxiety, and Darlene knows that a major defense mechanism of alcoholism is denial. Darlene also thinks the cognitive-behavioral theories are appropriate because she believes that humans need to change cognition to change behavior. Because Darlene assumes that drinking and using drugs are means of coping, she plans to use Lazarus's coping theory to help Alan develop more effective coping strategies. Finally, Darlene plans to apply humanistic psychology because she believes that Alan, like all individuals, has the potential to change, and social psychology theories address health beliefs and intent to change.

As discussed in Chapter 1, nursing is a practice discipline, and practice disciplines are considered to be applied sciences rather than pure or basic sciences (Johnson, 1959). The object of both pure and applied sciences is the same (to achieve knowledge), but according to Folta (1968), the difference between the two is their emphasis. In pure science, the emphasis is on basic research, which focuses on the application of the scientific method to add abstract knowledge. In contrast, the emphasis in applied science is on research related to the application and testing of the abstract concepts. Thus, applied sciences use the scientific method to apply and test fundamental knowledge or principles in practice. Historically, nursing science has drawn much of its knowledge from the basic sciences and then applied that knowledge to the discipline of nursing.

In learning about theories used in nursing, it is important to remember that nursing has evolved over decades and that the knowledge base for the discipline is a compilation of phenomena from many different disciplines. In the case study, Darlene discovered the notion of "shared" or "borrowed" versus "unique" theory. Johnson (1968) has defined borrowed theories as knowledge that has been identified in other disciplines and is used in nursing. According to Johnson, knowledge does not belong to any discipline but is shared across many disciplines; thus, nursing science draws on the knowledge of other disciplines to enhance the knowledge required for nursing practice.

One of the areas from which nurses draw theoretical understanding are the psychological sciences, sometimes referred to as the behavioral sciences. The contribution of the behavioral sciences to knowledge in nursing science and nursing practice cannot be denied. Even though the basic theories, concepts, and frameworks are derived from another discipline, they are applied in nursing practice. Additionally, they are frequently applied in nursing research as well as nursing education and administration.

There are many psychological theories, and it would be impossible to cover all of them in this chapter. Major theories were chosen to illustrate concepts that are used in nursing. For the purposes of this chapter, the psychological theories will be viewed in four categories: psychodynamic theories, behavioral and cognitive-behavioral theories, humanistic theories, and stress-adaptation theories. These theories look at an individual and how an individual responds to stimuli. In psychology, there is also a special field known as social psychology, which examines how society or groups of individuals respond to various stimuli. This chapter will examine two theories of social psychology commonly used in nursing: the Health Belief Model and the Theory of Reasoned Action.

Psychodynamic Theories

The late 1800s saw the creation of a new discipline, psychology/psychiatry, with a new body of knowledge. Before Sigmund Freud presented his radical works describing human thoughts and behaviors, people were considered to be either "good" or "bad," "normal" or "crazy." His work led to a major paradigm shift as scientists began to consider the thought processes of "man" and to speculate about human personality. From this paradigm shift came a number of psychological theories.

Freud's thinking was considered radical in the early 1900s. Even now in the early 21st century, many people still consider his work radical, yet others believe it to be antiquated. Despite this, his basic ideas and concepts have been used and modified extensively in the development of numerous theories about human thought and behavior.

Psychodynamic theories attempt to explain the multidimensional nature of behavior and understand how an individual's personality and behavior interface. They also provide a systematic way of identifying and understanding behavior. This section describes three psychodynamic theories—the works of Freud, Erikson, and Sullivan. These three theories are also called "stage theories," meaning that they describe clearly defined stages at which new behaviors appear based on social and motivational influences. Table 14-1 compares the developmental stages of the three theories.

Psychoanalytic Theory: Freud

According to Freudian theory, behavior is nearly always the product of an interaction among the three major systems of the personality: the id, ego, and superego. Even though each of these systems has its own functions, properties, and components, they

Table 14-1 Stages of Development

Theorist	Developmental Emphasis	Stages
Sigmund Freud	Psychosexual	1. Oral
		2. Anal
		3. Phallic
		4. Latency
		5. Genital
Erik E. Erikson	Psychosocial	1. Trust versus mistrust
		2. Autonomy versus shame and doubt
		3. Initiative versus guilt
		4. Industry versus inferiority
		5. Identity versus identity confusion
		6. Intimacy versus isolation
		7. Generativity versus stagnation
		8. Integrity versus despair
Harry S. Sullivan	Interpersonal	1. Infancy
		2. Childhood
		3. Juvenile
		4. Preadolescence
		5. Early adolescence
		6. Late adolescence

interact so closely that it is difficult to distinguish their effects on behavior. Behavior is generally an interaction among these three systems; rarely does one system operate to the exclusion of the other two (Freud, 1960).

According to Freud, the id is the original system of the personality, and it is the matrix in which the ego and superego differentiate. The id is unable to tolerate an increase in energy, which is experienced as an uncomfortable state of tension. This increased tension can be perceived either internally or externally. The id discharges the tension to return the body to a state of equilibrium. This tension release is known as the pleasure principle (Freud, 1960).

The ego distinguishes between things in the mind and things in the external world. The ego is said to follow the reality principle with the aim of preventing tension until an appropriate object is found to satisfy the need. The ego has control over all cognitive and intellectual functions and is considered to be the executive of the personality because it controls behavior. It does this by mediating the conflicting demands of the id, superego, and external environment (Freud, 1960).

The third system is the superego. The main functions of the superego are to (1) inhibit the impulses of the id, (2) encourage the ego to substitute moralistic goals for realistic goals, and (3) strive for perfection. The focus of the superego is on moral issues: "what is right" and "what is wrong" (Freud, 1960).

Freud based his theory on the scientific view of the late 19th century, which regarded the human body as an energy system. He proposed that because the body derives its energy from the work of the body (e.g., respiration, digestion), then memory and thinking are also defined by the work they perform. He labeled this concept *psychic energy* and stated that an instinct is an inborn state of somatic excitement. Furthermore, an instinct is a quantum of psychic energy or, as Freud said, "a measure of the demand made upon the mind for work" (1960, p. 168). All the instincts together yield the sum total of psychic energy (Freud, 1953).

The four characteristics of an instinct are source, aim, object, and impetus. Whereas source is the need, the aim is the removal of the tension. Object is what will satisfy the need and also includes all behaviors that occur to obtain the necessary object. The impetus of an instinct is the force or strength, which is determined by the intensity of the underlying need. Thus, psychic energy is displaced to the object to satisfy the instinctual need. Freud believed that instincts are the sole energy source for human behavior (Freud, 1953).

The environment plays two roles with regard to instinct. It either satisfies or threatens the development of the person. The individual responds with increased tension; an increase in tension is known as anxiety. The function of anxiety is to warn the person of impending danger. Anxiety motivates the person to do something; thus, a behavior is seen. As a result of increased tension or anxiety, an individual is forced to learn new methods of reducing the tension. According to Freud, these new methods are called *ego defense mechanisms* (Freud, 1956). "All defense mechanisms have two characteristics in common: (1) They deny, falsify, or distort reality and (2) they operate unconsciously so that the person is not aware of what is taking place" (Hall & Lindzey, 1978, pp. 91–92).

Freud was one of the first theorists to emphasize the developmental aspect of personality. He believed that the personality was developed within the first five years of life. Each of his stages of development, excepting latency, during which focus lies outside of one's own body, is defined as a mode of reaction to a particular zone of the body. Freud's stages were related to psychosexual development and included oral, anal, phallic, latency, and genital stages (Freud, 1953).

Application to Nursing

Although nursing theories are not based on Freud's theory, many of his ideas and concepts are relevant to nursing practice. These concepts include anxiety, developmental stages, defense mechanisms, and the identity of self.

Freud's theory helps to explain the complex nature of a person and how a person's past influences his or her personality. The complex processes of the past, which are found in the unconscious mind, suggest an explanation for the diversity in a person's behaviors. Even though the emphasis in much of nursing is on the "here and now," understanding the person's relevant past experiences can help the nurse identify underlying themes and improve care.

The id, ego, and superego are the components of the self. When there is an imbalance among these concepts, the self becomes lost and must be reconstructed. Nurses can help clients who have undergone a loss of self to discover a more active sense of self, put the self into action, and use the enhanced self as a refuge. Furthermore, an understanding of the concepts of id, ego, and superego helps the nurse understand the needs of the client and helps the nurse respond more appropriately to the behaviors.

In Alan's situation from the opening case study, the domination of the id would lead to increased substance use because of the pleasure principles. When Alan sobered, the superego would cause him to have feelings of shame and guilt. Darlene can now help Alan choose acceptable ways of behaving, thus causing an equilibrium among the id, ego, and superego. This equilibrium would help to relieve Alan's feelings of anxiety.

A behavior is the way an individual responds to increased tension or anxiety, and, in this case, Alan responded to increased tension by abusing substances (e.g., alcohol, cocaine, marijuana). Alan denied that he used substances inappropriately; he stated that he used alcohol "socially," and the drugs were only done on weekends and therefore "no big deal." Alan also stated that he had no marital problems when, in fact, his wife was going to divorce him. Alan was demonstrating Freud's concept of defense mechanisms, specifically denial. Defense mechanisms are used to help reduce anxiety and tension. Denial describes a client's behavior, and the main two definitions range from adaptive to maladaptive responses. In this case study, Alan uses denial as a maladaptive response. By using denial, Alan was able to decrease the feelings of rejection from his wife and the shame and guilt associated with abusing substances. Because Darlene recognized and understood the use of this maladaptive defense mechanism, she was able to develop a plan of care to help Alan develop more adaptive defense mechanisms to relieve anxiety.

Although denial is used in the case study to explain substance abuse, nurses encounter the use of denial with clients in almost all areas of nursing. Examples include those with obesity, cancer, hypertension, diabetes, and cardiac problems, just to mention a few. The use of denial is a way of protecting the self from a threat that could harm the person physically and decrease self-concept. When denial is used, the individual does not believe that he or she has a problem, and this can lead to noncompliant behavior. Noncompliance is one of the biggest challenges facing nursing today.

Recent nursing literature that reports on application of psychoanalytic theory covers a variety of issues. For example, Steinberg and Cochrane (2013) examined the incorporation of psychodynamic theory in managing psychiatric mental health patients on an inpatient unit, and Thomas and Hynes (2007) used a psychoanalytic perspective to describe interaction and cohesion among therapeutic group members. Other authors have used psychoanalytical theory to examine such concepts as emotional boundaries in fertility nursing (Allan & Barber, 2005), acceptance and denial-related chronic illness (Telford, Kralik, & Koch, 2006), and transference and countertransference in nursing care of patients with anorexia nervosa (Swatton, 2011).

Developmental (or Ego Developmental) Theory: Erikson

Erikson's Psychosocial Developmental Theory emerged as an expansion of Freud's concept of ego. In Erikson's theory, specific stages of a person's life from birth to death are formed by social influences that interact with the physical/psychological, maturing organism. Erikson described this as a "mutual fit of individual and environment" (Erikson, 1975, p. 102). He is the only developmental theorist who extends development through adulthood; the other theorists stop with adolescence.

Erikson's theory lists eight stages of development: the first four stages occur in infancy and childhood, the fifth stage occurs in adolescence, and the last three stages occur during the adult years. In his work, Erikson emphasized the adolescent stage, that time in an individual's life when the person makes the transition from a child to an adult. This transitional period has the greatest influence on the adult personality. Erikson believed that each stage of development builds on the next, thus contributing to the formation of the total person. Also, even though Erikson gave a chronologic timetable, it is not strict because he believed that each person has his or her own timetable for development (Erikson, 1963).

Erikson further developed the concept of ego to incorporate qualities that expanded the Freudian concept. He believed the ego is the most powerful of the three parts of the personality (id, ego, and superego) and described the ego as being robust and resilient. According to Erikson, the ego uses a combination of inner readiness and outer opportunities, with a sense of vigor and joy, to find creative solutions at each stage of development. This concentration of the potential strength of the ego empowers people to deal effectively with their problems (Erikson, 1968).

Application to Nursing

Developmental theory is often a foundational element in nursing theories, and it is important in nursing practice (Wadensten & Carlsson, 2003). For example, an essential part of the assessment process is to determine age appropriateness or arrested development. Although developmental issues are generally thought to be associated only with pediatrics, this is not the case. By assessing the developmental stage of the adult and elderly person, data can be collected about interpersonal skills and behaviors because behavioral manifestations are clues to issues that need to be addressed in client care. Furthermore, individual responsibility and the capacity to improve one's functioning are issues to be addressed by nurses.

Erikson's theory identified the degree of mastery with regard to a person's chronologic age. This mastery is known as ego strength. Bjorklund (2000) believed that promoting assessment from the perspective of ego strengths, instead of ego deficits, is a valuable skill for nurses, who then can use the data for assessment and treatment outcomes. Early and GlenMaye (2000) also proposed that nurses work with clients from an ego strength perspective, particularly when including the family in the plan of care. Besides using ego strengths for assessment and interventions, the nurse can also use them to empower the client to take control of his or her life and to deal effectively with problems.

Identifying and assessing Alan's ego strengths helped Darlene locate where Alan falls on the developmental continuum, thus providing data to develop therapeutic goals. When Darlene graduates and becomes a clinical nurse specialist, she can conduct family therapy, and Erikson's theory would be helpful in working with Alan's children, especially from the perspective of ego strength.

Developmental theory is not only used in psychiatric nursing but also in other specialty areas of nursing, and it is integral to holistic nursing practice (Reed, 1998). Nursing researchers and scholars commonly employ developmental theory in research studies or in describing practice guidelines for various groups. For example, Seal and Seal (2011) used developmental theory as the basis for interventions to promote self-competence in children to enhance their health behaviors while at a summer camp. Nurses have commonly used developmental theory to improve nursing care among elders. For example, Giblin (2011) discussed the importance of nurses supporting older adults in "successful aging," and Ehlman and Ligon (2012) used a model based on Erikson's generative process to research the developmental issue of generativity versus stagnation in older adults who shared life stories with gerontology students.

In other examples, Bailey (2012) wrote about vulnerability of adolescent girls and Handley and Ward-Smith (2005) described issues faced by young and middle-aged adults who are addicted to alcohol. These examples demonstrate that developmental theory is used throughout the life continuum (i.e., children, adolescents, adults, and elderly) and is used in pediatric, psychiatric, geriatric, and medical-surgical nursing. Further examination of these research studies suggests that both ego strengths and ego deficits are being studied by nurses.

Interpersonal Theory: Sullivan

Harry Stack Sullivan based his developmental theory on the premise that an individual does not, and cannot, exist apart from his or her relations with other people. He stated that from the first day of life, a baby is dependent on interpersonal situations and that this dependence continues throughout the person's life. Even if the person becomes a recluse and withdraws from society, the person carries the memories of interpersonal relationships, which continue to influence behavior and thinking. Sullivan stated that it is a "relatively enduring pattern of recurrent interpersonal relationships which characterize a human life" (Sullivan, 1953, p. 111).

To explain this phenomenon, the term *dynamism* must be understood. Dynamism, as defined by Sullivan, is "the relatively enduring pattern of energy transformation which recurrently characterizes the organism in its duration as a living organism" (Sullivan, 1953, p. 105). The individual's dynamisms characterize interpersonal relations. Although all people have the same dynamisms, the mode of expression varies with the situation and life experience of the individual. Although most dynamisms satisfy the basic needs of the individual, an important dynamism develops as a result of anxiety; this is known as the dynamism of self or the self-system (Sullivan, 1953). Anxiety is a product of interpersonal relationships. Anxiety may produce a threat to the security of the self, thus causing the person to use various types of protective and behavioral control measures. This, in turn, reduces anxiety but may interfere with being able to live constructively with others (Sullivan, 1953).

Sullivan also described the concept of personification, which is the image that a person has of himself or herself. Personification is a combination of feelings, attitudes, and conceptions that grow out of experiences with need satisfaction and anxiety. If interpersonal experiences are rewarding, it is known as the "good me" personification. On the other hand, if interpersonal experiences are anxiety arousing, it is known as the "bad me" personification. A synonym for personification is self-concept; thus, the "good me" personification is a high self-concept, and the "bad me" personification is a low self-concept (Sullivan, 1953).

Sullivan viewed the individual as an energy or tension system. The goal of the tension system is to reduce anxiety. According to Sullivan, the two main sources of anxiety are the tensions that arise from the needs of the organism and tensions that result from anxiety (Sullivan, 1953).

Sullivan believed that "tensions can be regarded as needs for particular energy transformations that will dissipate the tension of awareness with an accompanying change of 'mental' state, a change of awareness" (Sullivan, 1953, p. 85). Anxiety is the experience of tension that results from real or imagined threats to one's security. High levels of anxiety produce a reduction in the efficacy of satisfying needs, disturbance of interpersonal relationships, and confusion in thinking. Thus, Sullivan hypothesized that an individual learns to behave in a certain way related to the resolution or exacerbation of tension (Sullivan, 1953).

Sullivan took his theory further and described the sequence of interpersonal events to which a person is exposed from infancy to adulthood and ways in which these situations contribute to the development of that individual. Besides the six stages of interpersonal development, Sullivan also developed a three-fold classification system of cognitions: prototaxic, parataxic, and syntaxic. Although Sullivan formally rejected the importance of instinct with regard to development, he acknowledged the importance of heredity. Furthermore, he did not believe that personality is set at an early age but that it may change at any given time because new interpersonal situations arise and the human organism is malleable (Sullivan, 1953).

From Sullivan's theory, a new paradigm developed; this was the conception of participant–observer. Prior to this conception, the therapist observed only what was occurring. Now the therapist becomes an active part of the treatment. Another concept developed from Sullivan's interpersonal theory was that the environment plays an important role in treatment, thus creating the concept of a therapeutic milieu (Sullivan, 1953).

Application to Nursing

Peplau (1952, 1963) based her nursing theory, Interpersonal Relations in Nursing, on Sullivan's theory, Interpersonal Theory of Psychiatry. Orlando (1961) based her nursing theory on Peplau's theory and Sullivan's theory. Thus, it is clear that Sullivan's theory has been important to nursing.

From Sullivan's concept of degree of anxiety, Peplau developed the four levels of anxiety (mild, moderate, severe, and panic levels) that are the standards nurses use in assessing anxiety. Peplau believed that nurses play an important role in helping clients reduce their anxiety and in converting it into constructive action. Peplau also believed that the nurse's role is to help the client decrease insecurity and improve functioning through interpersonal relationships. These interpersonal relationships can be seen as microcosms of the way the person functions in his or her relationships (Thompson, 1986). This is very similar to Sullivan's concepts of the development of interpersonal relationships.

To educate the client and assist the person in gaining personal insight, Peplau (1963) elaborated on Sullivan's concept of participant–observer. According to her, nurses cannot be isolated from the therapeutic milieu if they want to be effective. Peplau's belief was that the nurse must interact with the client as a human being, with respect, empathy, and acceptance.

A major focus of Orlando's theory is client participation, which correlates with both Sullivan's and Peplau's concept of participant–observer. The formation, development, use, and termination of the nurse–client relationship is a phenomenon that is studied in nursing because it is a vital component of care and helps to determine the efficacy of treatment outcomes (Abraham, 2011; Erci, Sezgin, & Kacmaz, 2008; Senn, 2013; Sheldon & Ellington, 2008).

Another important concept of Sullivan's theory is the therapeutic milieu (i.e., a therapeutic environment). Almost all facilities today support the concept of a therapeutic environment that aids in facilitating all interactions. The therapeutic milieu is an important component of nursing practice, especially in the psychiatric setting as discussed by Mahoney, Palyo, Napier, and Giordano (2009). This concept was studied by Southard and colleagues (2012) in relation to renovation of nursing stations in adult care psychiatric units and by O'Neill, Moore, and Ryan (2008) when examining psychosocial interventions used by mental health nurse practitioners.

Sullivan also acknowledged the importance of heredity in development. Even though the heredity concept is a biologic perspective, psychologists, such as Sullivan, acknowledge the importance of heredity in personality development. In the case study, Darlene thought consideration of hereditable influences was important in working with Alan because Alan's father was an alcoholic.

Behavioral and Cognitive-Behavioral Theories

The psychodynamic theories grew from the beliefs that (1) personality is based on how the person develops, (2) development stops at a certain age, and (3) behaviors associated with development cannot be changed. In other words, a person's destiny is set at an early age. Finding these theories problematic, the behavioral theorists postulated that personality consists of learned behaviors. More explicitly, personality is synonymous with behavior, and if the behavior is changed, the personality is changed.

Initially, behavioral studies focused on human actions without much attention to the internal thinking processes. When the complexity of behaviors could not be accounted for by strictly behavioral explanations, a new component was added: a component of cognitions or thought processes. The cognitive approach is an outgrowth of behavioral and psychodynamic theories and attempts to link thought processes with behaviors. Cognitive-behavioral theory, then, focuses on thinking and behaving rather than on feelings.

One of the best known behavioral theorists is B. F. Skinner. Additional cognitive-behavioral theories discussed in this section are those proposed by Beck and Ellis.

Operant Conditioning: Skinner

Like Freud, Skinner believed that all behavior is determined, but the two have different theories regarding the origin of the behavior. Although Skinner followed the ideologies of Pavlov and Watson (two early behaviorists), he expanded the notion of stimulus–response behavioral approaches of learning to include the concept of reinforcement. The Pavlovian theory, basically a biologic theory, states that a stimulus elicits a response. Skinner took this theoretical principle further and applied it to the psychological sciences. He held that it is possible to predict and control the behaviors of others through a contingency of human reinforcers, and he expanded on Pavlovian thinking by adding motivation and reinforcement to the principles of learning (Skinner, 1969).

Operant conditioning was the term coined by Skinner to label his theory. Operant conditioning refers to the manipulation of selected reinforcers to elicit and strengthen desired behavioral reinforcers. According to Skinner, an individual performs a behavior (discharges an operant) and receives a consequence (reinforcer) as a result of performing the behavior. The consequence is either positive or negative, and the consequence will most likely determine whether the behavior will be repeated. Thus, although negative consequences have a deterrent effect on the behavior, positive consequences generally result in repetition of the behavior. Absence of reinforcement generally decreases the behavior. Skinner's premise was that reinforcement ultimately determines the existence of behavior (Skinner, 1969).

Skinner defined a reinforcer as anything that increases the occurrence of a behavior. It is important to note that the value of the reinforcer depends on its meaning to a particular individual, and the same reinforcer may have different effects on different people. According to Skinner, there are two types of reinforcers: primary and secondary. Primary reinforcers are important to survival (e.g., food, water, and sex) and secondary reinforcers are conditioned reinforcers (e.g., money, material goods, and praise) (Skinner, 1969).

Behaviors are generally multidimensional, and complex behaviors need to be broken down into smaller steps. This allows for the shaping of behavior, which consists of progressively reinforcing the smaller steps needed to achieve a certain behavior (Skinner, 1987).

Cognitive Theory: Beck

Aaron Beck based his cognitive theory on the work he did with depressed persons. He posited that biased cognitions are faulty, and he labeled these thoughts as *cognitive distortions.* Cognitive distortions are habitual errors in thinking that Beck stated are verbal or pictorial events that are formed in the conscious mind. When cognitions are distorted, an individual incorrectly interprets life events, jumps to inaccurate conclusions, and judges himself or herself too harshly. These distorted cognitions create a false basis for beliefs, particularly regarding the self, and influence one's basic attitude about the self. Thought distortions are the catalysts for how an individual perceives events in his or her life; they may keep the individual from reaching a desired goal. The process of changing cognitive distortions is called *cognitive restructuring* (Beck, 1976).

Although cognitive distortions are in the conscious mind, Beck believed that they are influenced by an automatic thinking schema that originates in the unconscious mind. The automatic thinking schemata are themes that have developed in childhood and have been reinforced throughout life. The automatic thinking schemata influence cognitions and can cause them to be faulty. Beck stated that an individual expresses illness through thoughts and attitudes. In other words, thoughts influence emotions, and behavior is controlled by thoughts. If thoughts are distorted, then illness occurs. To treat the illness, the cognitive distortions must be changed (Beck, 1976).

Rational Emotive Theory: Ellis

Another cognitive theorist was Albert Ellis, who described Rational Emotive Theory, which focuses on an interconnectedness between thoughts, feelings, and actions. An individual will think and act based on his or her perception of life events. The underlying premise is that an individual has the cognitive ability to think, decide, analyze, and do and that he or she thinks either rationally or irrationally. The repetition of irrational thoughts reinforces dysfunctional beliefs, which, in turn, produce dysfunctional behaviors. These dysfunctional beliefs lead to self-defeating behaviors, and the person experiences self-blame. Ellis stated that the individual learns these self-defeating behaviors and that the individual is capable of understanding his or her limitations. Ellis further posited that if behaviors are learned, they can be unlearned. A person can change beliefs by changing thoughts and thinking rationally. If this occurs, then the behavior is changed (Ellis & MacLaren, 2008).

Application of Behavioral and Cognitive-Behavioral Theories to Nursing

The behavioral approach is a concrete method of monitoring or managing behavior. Nurses often use it with children or adolescents and people with chronic illness because it is often successful in changing targeted behaviors.

By combining behavioral theory with cognitive theory, the nurse can help alter behaviors by encouraging the individual to change irrational beliefs through problem solving. An individual who is ill may express feelings of worthlessness, anger, and self-blame. The nurse using a cognitive-behavioral approach can point out specific positive qualities of the individual. This helps reduce self-blame and the person gradually begins to feel better about himself or herself because the belief system is changing. In essence, the nurse has changed behavior by presenting positive (secondary) reinforcement to the person, thus helping to change self-cognitions. This, in turn, changes the individual's belief system.

A cognitive-behavioral approach also helps the nurse point out the use of maladaptive defense mechanisms (e.g., projection). Projection is an unconscious process in which the individual can ascribe undesirable thoughts, impulses, ideas, and/or feelings to another person in order to externalize what he or she feels are unacceptable attributes or traits. Through projection, the individual is able to decrease anxiety and deal with the situation as a detached entity (Sadock, 2009).

People sometimes blame others for their problems. This is particularly true for those who are addicted to drugs and alcohol (like Alan); addicts frequently do not take responsibility for their substance use, misuse, and abuse. Using a cognitive approach, specifically Ellis's, the nurse teaches the person to take responsibility for his or her own behaviors. While Ellis's approach is used more with substance abuse because of the confrontational approach, Beck's is used more with depressed persons because it focuses on an empathic approach. In the case study, Alan has a dual diagnosis of depression and substance abuse, and Darlene would most likely use a cognitive-behavioral approach in planning his nursing care.

In nursing, cognitive behavioral therapies have been used to help manage multiple sclerosis (Askey-Jones, Shaw, & Silber, 2012) and to treat women with postpartum depression (Scope, Booth, & Sutcliffe, 2012). Additionally, cognitive-behavioral approaches have also been used to treat anxiety in children and adolescents with asthma (Marriage & Henderson, 2012) and adolescents with suicidality (Spirito, Esposito-Smythers, Wolff, & Uhl, 2011).

Humanistic Theories

Humanistic theories developed in response to the psychoanalytic thought that a person's destiny was determined early in life. Proponents of humanistic psychology believed that psychoanalytic theories explicitly exclude human potential. In other words, there was no hope for a person. Humanistic theories emphasize a person's capacity for self-actualization; thus, they present a relatively hopeful and optimistic perspective about humans. Humanists believe that the person contains within himself or herself the potential for healthy and creative growth. The theories of Maslow and Rogers are discussed in the following sections on humanistic theories.

Human Needs Theory: Maslow

Abraham Maslow, known as the father of humanistic psychology, believed that psychology takes a pessimistic, negative, and limited conception of humans. He charged the discipline to examine human strengths and to stress human virtue instead of human frailties, and he proposed that human science should explore individuals who realize their full potential. Furthermore, he believed that the inner core of the person is the self, which is a unique individual who possesses both characteristics similar to others and characteristics uniquely distinct to the person (Maslow, 1963).

Motivation is the key to Maslow's theory because he assumed that instead of being passive, an individual is an active participant who strives for self-actualization. Maslow's theory is basically a hierarchy of dynamic processes that are critical for development and growth of the total person. There are six incremental stages of Maslow's theory: physiologic needs, safety needs, love and belonging needs, self-esteem needs, self-actualizing needs, and self-transcendent needs. The goal of Maslow's theory is to attain the sixth level or stage: self-transcendent needs (Maslow, 1963).

In Maslow's scheme, needs are divided into "D" motives and "B" motives. "D" motives are deficiency needs. This means that these needs are basic and have the greatest strength because they are essential to human survival. "D" motive needs must be satisfied for a person to turn his or her attention to the satisfaction of the higher-level needs. These higher-level needs are called "B" motive needs and include self-esteem and self-actualization. Such needs are reflective of growth potential (Maslow, 1963).

Until basic deficiency needs are met, the individual does not pursue personal growth needs to develop his or her fullest potential as a human being. Maslow postulated an optimistic assessment by focusing on the individual's strengths instead of personal deficits. According to Maslow (1963), when a person strives for personal growth, it leads the person to her or his fullest potential. In other words, it is the person at her or his best. This means that the person develops a problem-solving approach to life, identifies with humankind, and transcends the environment. The person is able to look realistically at life and make rational decisions; this brings about inner peace. When a person accomplishes this, Maslow referred to the person as being self-actualized. Box 14-1 lists characteristics of a self-actualized person. This philosophical perspective helps a person get in touch with who he or she is and what he or she can become (Maslow, 1963).

Application to Nursing

Maslow's theory can be applied to nursing practice in three ways:

1. It allows the nurse to emphasize the person's strengths instead of focusing on the individual's deficits.
2. It focuses on human potential, thus giving the person hope.
3. It provides a blueprint for prioritizing client care according to a hierarchy of needs.

By focusing on a person's strengths, the nurse empowers the individual. In the case study, when Darlene began planning Alan's care, she followed Maslow's hierarchy by giving priority to his "D" needs (i.e., physical and safety needs that help the individual

Box 14-1 Characteristics of a Self-Actualized Person

- Realistic orientation
- Spontaneity
- Acceptance of self
- Acceptance of others
- Close relationships with others
- Autonomous thinking
- Appreciation of life
- Reactivity to others
- Consideration of others
- Respect for others

feel safe and secure). She helped him withdraw safely from the addictive substances and treated active symptoms of hepatitis C. She knew that his physical needs must be met before she could address the "B" needs (i.e., his potential for personal growth, self-esteem, and self-actualization).

Considerable nursing research has been done in humanistic psychology, largely using Maslow's theory. One research study, for example, focused on identifying the needs of hemodialysis patients in order to improve quality of life (Bayoumi, 2012), another studied the development of a fall risk assessment for hospitalized patients (Abraham, 2011), and a third evaluated concepts to enhance retention rates of registered nurses in South Africa (Mokoka, Ehlers, & Oosthuizen, 2011). Additionally, Duncan & Blugis (2011) used Maslow's theory to serve as a conceptual framework for evaluating and redefining a pediatric hospitality house to better meet the needs of patients and families utilizing this service.

Person-Centered Theory: Rogers

Carl Rogers developed a person-centered model of psychotherapy that emphasizes the uniqueness of the individual. He believed that every individual has the potential to develop his or her talents to the maximum potential; he called this the *actualizing tendency*. Furthermore, each individual possesses everything that is needed for self-understanding and for changing attitude and behavior (Rogers, 1959).

Two constructs are fundamental to Rogers' theory: organism and the self. Organism is the locus of all experience. Experience includes the awareness of everything potentially available that is going on within the organism at any given time. This totality of experience constitutes the phenomenal field, which has several components. The first component is that an individual's frame of reference can only be known by that person. The second component is that a person's behavior depends on the phenomenal field and is not dependent on stimulating conditions. The third component of a phenomenal field is that it is made up of conscious and unconscious experiences (Rogers, 1959).

A portion of the phenomenal field gradually differentiates; this is known as the self or self-concept. Self or self-concept denotes the "organized, consistent conceptual gestalt composed of perceptions of the characteristics of 'I' or 'me' and the perceptions of the relationship of the 'I' or 'me' to others and to various aspects of life with the values attached to these perceptions" (Rogers, 1959, p. 200). In addition to the self, there is an ideal self, which is what the person would like to be (Rogers, 1959).

The basic significance of the structural concepts organism and self is directly related to congruence and incongruence. These terms represent the acceptance or nonacceptance of the organism with the self. Congruence is when the self accepts the organismic experience without threat or anxiety; thus, the person is able to think realistically. Incongruence between self and organism makes an individual feel threatened and anxious, thus causing defensiveness and constricted and rigid thinking. This results in behavioral problems (Rogers, 1959).

According to Rogers, "behavior is basically the goal-oriented attempt of the organism to satisfy its needs as experienced" (Rogers, 1951, p. 491). Behaviors occur for the organism to maintain and enhance itself. Rogers believed that an individual has two learned needs, positive-regard and self-regard. Rogers stated, "If an individual should experience only unconditional positive regard, then no conditions of worth would develop, self-regard would be unconditional, the needs for positive regard and self-regard would never be at variance with organismic evaluation, and the individual would continue to be psychologically adjusted, and would be fully functioning"

(Rogers, 1959, p. 224). This is not the case when an individual receives both positive and negative evaluations by others, causing an individual to learn to differentiate between actions and feelings that are worthy or unworthy.

Organism and self are subject to strong influences from the environment, especially from the social environment. Rogers did not provide a timetable of significant changes through which an individual passes; instead, he focused on ways in which evaluation of an individual by others tends to influence the experience of the organism and the experience of the self (Rogers, 1951).

Application to Nursing

The major contribution that Rogers added to nursing practice is the understanding that each client is a unique individual who is basically good, with an inherent potential for self-actualization. He introduced the concept of a person-centered approach, which is easily adapted to nursing. Not only does this approach view the individual as unique, but there is equal collaboration between the nurse and the client in the individual's care.

Darlene followed Rogers' philosophy that each individual is unique. Even though Alan had characteristics that were similar to others, he was an individual who had characteristics that were unique to him. Darlene collaborated with Alan to develop his plan of care. This is important in all areas of nursing because clients need to feel they are special and unique and that they have a say in their care. Their input into their treatment will motivate them to accomplish their goals; thus, treatment outcomes will be enhanced.

Rogers also identified the conditions that are needed for an effective nurse–client relationship: unconditional positive regard, empathic understanding, and genuineness. An effective nurse–client relationship will help to facilitate change in the person and produce a positive outcome of treatment.

Stress Theories

Although the previous theories have dealt with the development of personality and mental illness, the stress theories deal with normal human functioning. Stress, adaptation, and coping are all natural parts of life. Stress is inevitable in everyone's life, and people must deal with stress by adapting through coping. The stress theories provide nursing with a framework to understand the effects that stress has on the individual and how the individual responds to stressful situations or life events. Although the ability to successfully adapt to stress leads to the equilibrium of the individual, the inability to adapt successfully leads to disequilibrium. The disequilibrium may result in physiologic or psychological disorders. The important thing to remember with stress theories is that stress is different for everyone. The following sections discuss Selye's general adaptation syndrome in relation to Peplau's levels of anxiety and Lazarus' Stress Coping Adaptation Theory.

General Adaptation Syndrome: Selye

Hans Selye pioneered research into stress and proposed the general adaptation syndrome (GAS). Because Selye defined stress as wear and tear on the body, the GAS explains the physiologic responses to stress. An explanation of the GAS is presented in Chapter 15, but it will be discussed here briefly because Selye's GAS is also discussed in psychological literature.

The GAS has three stages: alarm, resistance, and exhaustion. The first stage is the alarm reaction. This stage mobilizes the body's defense forces and activates the fight-or-flight syndrome, which puts the body in a state of disequilibrium. The second stage is resistance and focuses on the body's physiologic responses to regain homeostasis. The final stage is exhaustion. In this stage, the body has exhausted all its resources and a diseased state can occur (Selye, 1956).

Selye concentrated on the physiologic changes in the body and did not elaborate on the psychological changes. Kneisl and Ames (1986) correlated the three levels of the GAS with Peplau's levels of anxiety. Table 14-2 compares the stages of Selye's syndrome with Peplau's levels of anxiety. In the alarm stage, there is an increased level of alertness and anxiety is found at levels 1 (mild) and 2 (moderate). The individual focuses on the immediate task, which is to reduce the stressor. If the threat is eliminated, the person has adapted successfully. If the threat is not effectively resolved, the individual advances to the next stage (Kneisl & Ames, 1986).

In the resistance stage, the individual experiences levels 2 (moderate) or 3 (severe) of anxiety. This is the stage when the individual increases the use of coping mechanisms to adapt to the stressor. Psychosomatic symptoms may appear in this stage.

Table 14-2 Selye's and Peplau's Anxiety States

Selye's Stages of the General Adaptation Syndrome	Peplau's Levels of Anxiety	Characteristics of Levels of Anxiety
Alarm alert	Level 1 (mild)	Increased alertness
	Level 2 (moderate)	Increased awareness
		Increased efforts to reduce anxiety
		Narrowing of perceptual field
		Problem solving is present
		Coping is increased
Resistance	Level 2 (moderate)	Feels threatened
		Feels overloaded
	Level 3 (severe)	Problem-solving difficulties
		Selective inattention
		Depressed
		Irritable
		Psychosomatic symptoms
Exhaustion	Level 3 (severe)	Feels helpless
	Level 4 (panic)	Feelings of awe, dread, and terror
		Loss of control
		Personality disorganization
		Loss of rational thoughts
		Decreased ability to relate rationally to others
		Out of touch with reality
		Dissociation
		Disease process (physical and emotional)

If the individual is unable to adapt to the stressor, the individual becomes overwhelmed with the stressor and advances to the next stage (Kneisl & Ames, 1986).

The stage of exhaustion results when the stressor is not or cannot be neutralized. This occurs because the stress may have lasted too long, the person is totally overwhelmed by the stressor, or the individual's normal coping mechanisms have been exhausted. At this stage, the individual experiences anxiety at levels 3 (severe) or 4 (panic) of Peplau's levels of anxiety. The person becomes dysfunctional, and a multitude of psychopathologic symptoms can occur: disorganized thinking, disorganized personality, delusions, hallucinations, stupor, or violence (Kneisl & Ames, 1986).

Stress, Coping, and Adaptation Theory: Lazarus

Lazarus' theory deals with how a person copes with stressful situations. Whereas Selye's focus is on the body's physiologic responses, Lazarus focused on the person's psychological responses. He viewed these responses as a process and stated that a process-oriented approach is directed toward what an individual actually thinks and does within the context of a specific encounter and includes how these thoughts and actions change as the encounter unfolds. "Coping, when considered as a process, is characterized by dynamics and changes that are functions of continuous appraisals and reappraisals of the shifting person environmental relationship" (Folkman & Lazarus, 1988, p. 3).

The two major factors that are precedents to stress are the person–environment relationship and appraisals. The person–environment relationship includes such factors as personality, values, beliefs, commitments, social networks, social supports, demands and constraints, sociocultural factors, and life events. The three cognitive appraisals are primary, secondary, and reappraisal. Primary appraisal refers to the judgment that an individual makes about a particular event or stressor. Secondary appraisal is the evaluation of how an individual responds to an event. Reappraisal is simply appraisal after new or additional information has been received (Lazarus & Folkman, 1984).

Lazarus posited that stress is much more complicated than just stimulus and response. He focused on the idea that coping is not due to anxiety itself but how the person perceives the threat. Lazarus identified this perception as an appraisal and explained that a person's evaluation of a stressor or events is classified as a cognitive appraisal. He defined stress as "a particular relationship between the person and the environment that is appraised by the person as taxing or exceeding his/her resources" (Lazarus & Folkman, 1984, p. 18).

To manage the demands and emotions generated by the appraised stress, coping occurs. Coping is the process by which a person manages the appraisal. The two types are problem-focused and emotion-focused coping. Problem-focused coping actually changes the person–environment relationship, and emotion-focused coping changes the meaning of the situation. Once the person has successfully coped with a situation, reappraisal occurs. Reappraisal allows for feedback about the outcome and allows for adjustment to new information (Lazarus & Folkman, 1984).

Successful coping results in adaptation. Adaptation is "the capacity of a person to survive and flourish" (Lazarus & Folkman, 1984, p. 182). Adaptation affects three important areas: health, psychological well-being, and social functioning. These three areas are interdependent, and when one area is affected, all three areas are affected. For example, if a person develops an illness, it can cause problems in work performance, which in turn elicits a negative self-concept.

Application of Stress Theories to Nursing

Stress and adaptation are the basis of Roy's Adaptation Model (Roy, 2009) and Neuman's System Model (Neuman, 1995). Roy (2009) stated that the goal of nursing is the promotion of adaptive responses through the mode of coping. Neuman's theory deals with a person's responses to stress (Neuman, 1995).

The application of stress theories to nursing is important. Indeed, they provide a framework for nurses to assess the effects of stress, both physical and psychological, on the individual and the coping processes that the individual uses. When assessing a client's stressors, it is important for the nurse to also consider the meaning of the stressor to the individual and the resources and support that the person has in coping with the stressors. The nurse can help with problem solving or cognitive restructuring to facilitate effective coping and adaptation. This can also lead to the development of new coping strategies for the individual.

Stress theories are very important in nursing practice, and nurses using them as research frameworks have done considerable research. For example, Thomsen, Rydahl-Hansen, and Wagner (2010) utilized Lazarus and Folkman's theory of coping to research the concept of coping and associated issues from the perspective of cancer patients. The relationship between community financial hardship and the perception of stress in African American adolescents was examined by Brenner, Zimmerman, Bauermeister, and Caldwell (2013), and Graungaard, Anderson, and Skov (2011) studied and identified coping strategies that are used by parents caring for children with severe disabilities. Finally, an experimental study was conducted by Padden, Connors, and Agazio (2011) on perceived stress and coping by female spouses during their husband's active military deployment.

Social Psychology

Health professionals use many different models for understanding behavior change because it is a complex process. Further, behavior change is often difficult to achieve and sustain. When health professionals attempt to encourage healthy behaviors, they are competing against powerful influences. These powerful influences involve social, psychological, and environmental conditioning. In order for change to occur, the benefits of behavior must be desired and perceived to be beneficial to the person. Although education is an important factor in facilitating change, information is frequently not enough. The benefits of behavior change must be compelling. When implementing change, a multilevel, interactive perspective clearly shows the advantages of incorporating behavioral and environmental components. Social psychology helps to predict health behavior and is widely used in health-promoting activities.

Two models that address this issue are the Health Belief Model (HBM) and the Theory of Reasoned Action/Theory of Planned Behavior. The HBM addresses a person's perceptions of the threat of a health problem and the accompanying appraisal of a recommended behavior for preventing or managing the problem, which is manifested as a behavior. The Theory of Reasoned Action assumes that people are rational and make decisions based on the information available to them. The important determinant of a person's behavior is intent. Both of these theories will be discussed in more detail in the following sections. For more information, see Link to Practice 14-1.

Health Belief Model

The HBM was one of the first models that adapted theories from the behavioral sciences to predict health behaviors. This was done by focusing on the attitudes and beliefs of individuals. The HBM was originally developed in the 1950s by a group of social psychologists working for the U.S. Public Health Service who wanted to

Link to Practice 14-1

Recently, a team headed by Plotnikoff (2013) conducted a systematic literature review examining how several social cognitive theories—specifically the Health Belief Model, Theory of Planned Behavior, Protection Motivation Theory, Social Cognitive Theory/Self-Efficacy Theory, Transtheoretical Model, and Health Promotion Model—explained physical activity intention and behaviors in adolescents. Meta-analysis of the published research describing how these theories were supported (or not) revealed that the theories/models were more effective in explaining intention than behavior. The researchers concluded that very few studies have actually tested the predictive capacity of social cognitive theories for adolescent behavior related to physical activity and that more specific theoretical research is needed on these theories.

Based on these findings, what evidence-based interventions might nurses propose using the Health Belief Model to promote physical activity in this cohort? Using the Theory of Planned Behavior? Social Cognitive Theory (see Chapter 13)? The Health Promotion Model (see Chapter 11)? Which theory might be best for explaining/researching/enhancing intention? Which might be best for explaining/researching/enhancing behavior?

Plotnikoff, R. C., Costigan, S. A., Karunamuni, N., & Lubans, D. R. (2013). Social cognitive theories used to explain physical activity behavior in adolescents: A systematic review and meta-analysis. *Preventive Medicine, 56*(5), 245–253.

improve the public's use of preventive services (Rosenstock, 1974). Their assumption was that people fear disease and that health actions were motivated in relation to the degree of the fear and the benefits obtained. The HBM explained health behavior in terms of several constructs: perceived susceptibility of the health problem, perceived severity, perceived benefits, perceived barriers, and cues to action (Rosenstock, 1990).

Perceived susceptibility refers to one's opinion of chances of getting a condition, whereas perceived severity is one's opinion of how serious a condition and its sequelae are. One's opinion of the efficacy of the advised action to reduce risk or seriousness of impact is known as perceived benefits. Perceived barriers are one's opinion of the tangible and psychological cost of the advised action (Rosenstock, 1974). These four concepts were proposed as accounting for people's readiness to action. Thus, another concept was identified as "cues to action." These cues to action would activate the readiness to act and stimulate overt behaviors (Rosenstock, 1990) (Figure 14-1).

In 1988, Rosenstock added another concept to the HBM, which he identified as self-efficacy. Self-efficacy is one's confidence in the ability to successfully perform an action. This concept was used to help the HBM better fit the challenges of changing habitual, unhealthy behaviors such as smoking, overeating, and being sedentary (Rosenstock, 1990). Table 14-3 summarizes the major concepts of the HBM.

Theory of Reasoned Action (Theory of Planned Behavior)

The Theory of Reasoned Action (TRA) was initially developed in the late 1960s by social psychologists Icek Ajzen and Martin Fishbein (Fishbein & Ajzen, 1975). The TRA explains the relationship among beliefs, attitudes, intentions, and behavior. It

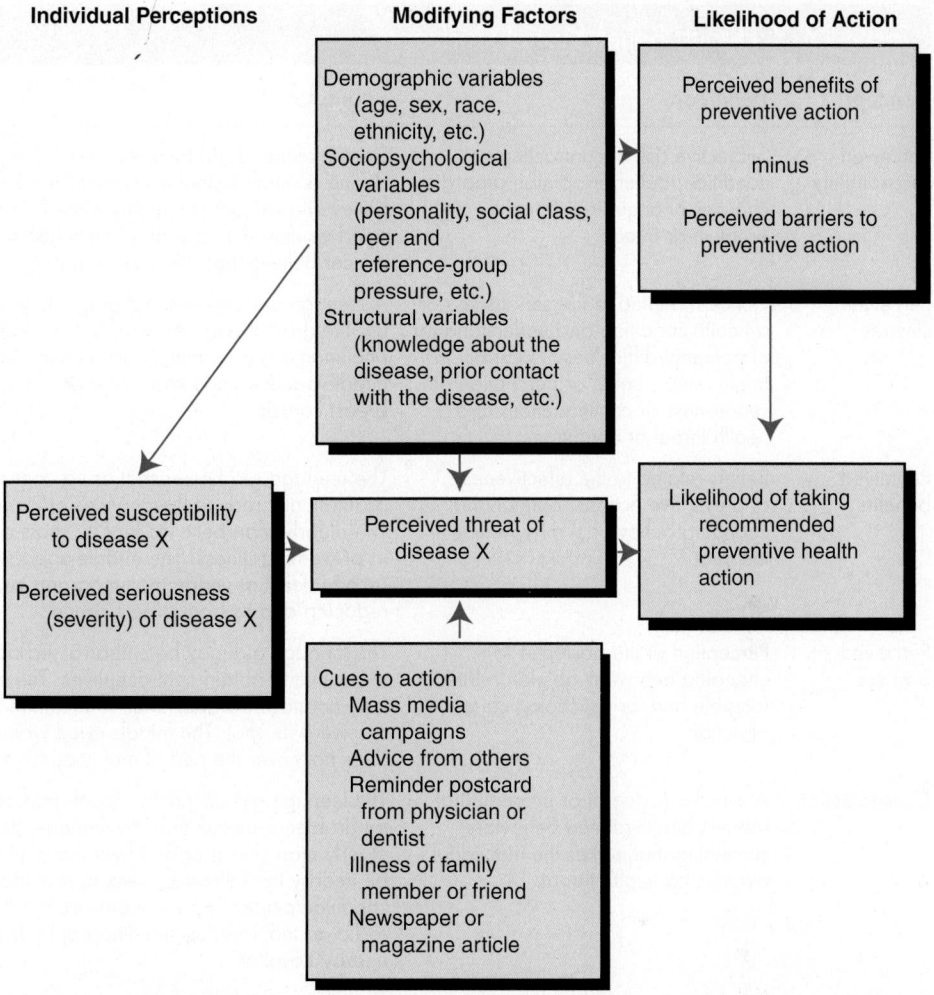

Figure 14-1 The health belief model. (From Becker, M. H., Haefner, D. P., Kasl, S. V., et al. (1977). Selected psychosocial models and correlates of individual health-related behaviors. *Medical Care, 15,* 27–46, with permission.)

assumes that people are rational and make decisions based on the information available to them. The goal of the TRA, therefore, is to understand and predict behaviors that are largely under the individual's control (Poss, 2001). The TRA was later modified to the Theory of Planned Behavior (TPB) (Montano & Kasprzyk, 2008).

According to the TPB, the most important determinant of a person's behavior(s) is intention. Intention is the cognitive representation of the individual's readiness to perform a behavior and is determined by (1) attitude toward the behavior, (2) subjective norms, and (3) perceived behavioral control.

Attitude, or behavioral beliefs, refers to the individual's positive or negative evaluation of performing the behavior; it is concerned with his or her beliefs about the consequences of performing the behavior. Attitude has been viewed as a combination of feelings, beliefs, intentions, and perceptions. Combined with knowledge, these factors analyze the acceptability of performing a behavior in relation to a bipolar scale of positive/negative or yes/no. The determinant of attitude component is called "salient belief." A person's attitude toward a behavior can be predicted by multiplying the evaluation of each of the behavior's consequences by the strength of the belief. Beliefs are

Table 14-3 Health Belief Model Concepts

Concept	Definition	Examples
Perceived susceptibility	Subjective risk of contracting a condition; belief or opinion regarding chances of acquiring a health problem or threat	Does a teenage girl believe she will get pregnant during a single sexual encounter? Does an elderly man believe he will get the flu this winter? Does a middle-aged woman with a strong family history of breast cancer believe that she is vulnerable?
Perceived severity	Concern related to the seriousness of a health condition and understanding of potential difficulties the condition might cause; belief or perception of seriousness or consequences of a health threat or condition	A teenage girl believes that pregnancy would change her life dramatically. An elderly man understands that pneumonia is a potential complication of the flu. A middle-aged woman knows her grandmother died of breast cancer.
Perceived benefits	Beliefs related to the effectiveness of preventive actions; opinion that changing behavior(s) may reduce the treat	The teenage girl knows that using contraception will dramatically reduce the chances of a pregnancy. The elderly man believes that flu shots are effective in preventing illness. The middle-aged woman recognizes that yearly mammograms are effective in reducing deaths from breast cancer.
Perceived barriers	Perception of the obstacles to changing behavior; opinion related to tangible and/or psychological costs of action	The teenage girl may be embarrassed about going to a clinic to obtain contraceptives. The elderly man may not have transportation to take him to the clinic to receive a flu shot. The middle-aged woman's insurance does not cover the cost of mammograms.
Cues to action	A stimulus (external or internal) that triggers health-related behaviors; something that makes the individual aware of a health threat	The teenage girl attends a school-sponsored program on problems encountered by teenage mothers. The elderly man sees a posted flyer that a mobile van will be nearby the following week to provide free flu shots. The middle-aged woman learns from a public service radio ad that low-cost mammography is available at a nearby hospital.
Self-efficacy	Belief that one has the ability to change one's behaviors; recognition that personal health practices and choices can positively influence health	The teenage girl decides to postpone intercourse. The elderly man attends the shot clinic provided by the mobile van. The middle-aged woman makes an appointment for a mammogram.

formed about an issue/object by associating it with all kinds of characteristics, qualities, and attributes. This leads to the development of an attitude (Ajzen & Fishbein, 1980).

Subjective norm, or normative beliefs, is seen as the social pressure upon a person to perform or not to perform a behavior. In deciding whether to perform an action or behavior, an individual may consider what his or her parents, friends, or others will think about the behavior, as well as how important it is to comply with the wishes of others. It involves both one's beliefs about the opinions of others and the person's motivation to conform to the wishes of those others. Thus, people often behave as they believe others expect them to behave.

Control beliefs, or perceived behavioral control, refer to the perceived power of factors that may facilitate or impede the behavior. In general, the more favorable the attitude and subjective norm, the greater the perceived control and the stronger would be the person's intention to perform the behavior. According to the TPB, behavioral intention is the most immediate determinant of any social

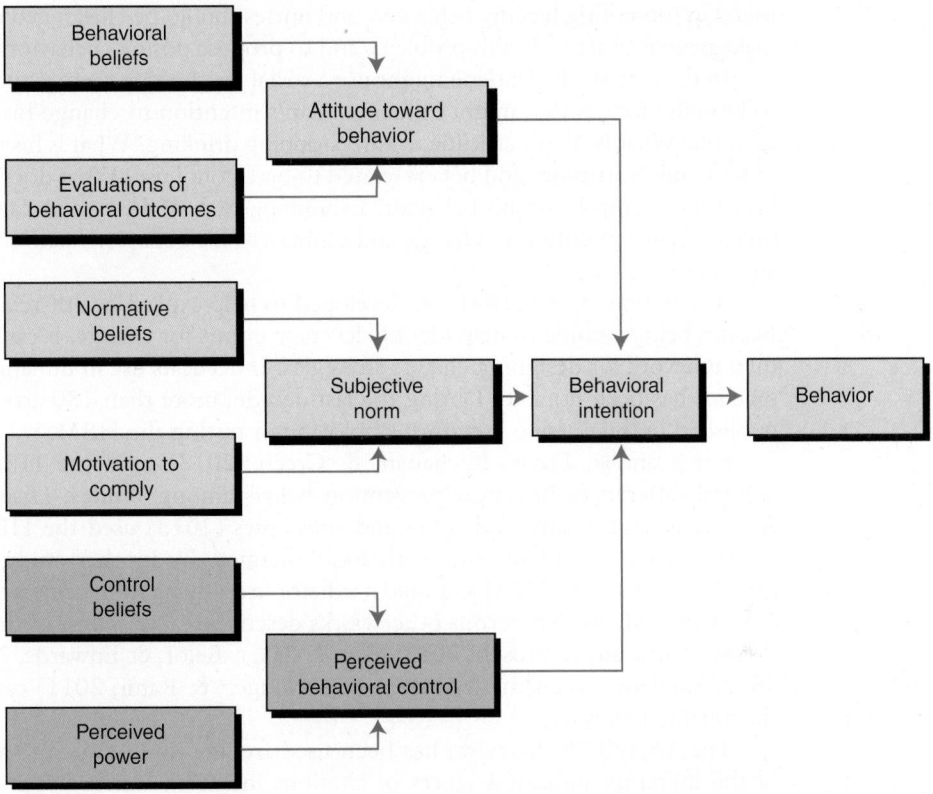

Figure 14-2 Theory of reasoned action and theory of planned behavior. (From Ajzen, I., & Fishbein, M. (1980, p. 8). *Understanding attitudes and predicting social behavior.* Reproduced by permission of Pearson Education, Inc. Upper Saddle River, NJ.) The lighter-shaded upper section shows the theory of reasoned action; the entire figure shows the theory of planned behavior.

behavior, but only under conditions where the behavior in question is under volitional control.

The TPB proposes that an individual's intention is determined in turn by his or her attitude and subjective norm regarding the performance of the behavior. Furthermore, attitude to the behavior is accounted for by beliefs about the outcomes of the behavior and evaluations of those outcomes. Subjective norm is determined by perceived pressure from specified significant others to carry out the behavior and motivation to comply with the wishes of significant others. Figure 14-2 depicts the components of the TPB.

Application of Social Psychology Theories to Nursing

The application of social psychology theories in nursing typically relates to the area of health promotion. Nurses can propose strategies and develop programs to make people aware of health problems. They can then implement these programs using the social theories to change unhealthy behaviors to healthy behaviors. That is the reason that nurses must advocate health promotion for patients using a multidimensional approach: organizational change efforts, policy development, economic supports, and environmental change. In today's society, disseminating the message is much easier. It can be delivered through printed educational material, electronic mass media, or directly in one-to-one counseling (Glanz, Rimer, & Lewis, 2008). Social psychology theories are useful in promoting healthy behaviors, and nurses should be challenged to use them to make people aware of health problems and to propose positive behavioral change.

In the case study, Darlene might use a social psychology theory, such as the TPB, to examine factors that might influence Alan's intention to change his behavior. For example: What is Alan's attitude toward stopping drinking? What is his understanding of his family's attitudes and beliefs related to his alcohol use? What does he perceive as his level of control over his behavior? Examining each of these areas can help Darlene predict Alan's intention to change and ultimately, his behavior relative to alcohol use and abuse.

As mentioned, the HBM was developed to help explain health-related behaviors. Besides being a guide to help identify leverage points for change, it can also be a useful framework for designing change strategies. Indeed, its use in nursing research and practice has been notable. During the last decade, more than 130 articles have been published in the nursing literature employing or testing the HBM.

For example, Davis, Buchanan, & Green (2013) used the HBM to explore cultural differences in cancer prevention beliefs among Whites, Hispanics, African Americans, and Asians, and Jones and colleagues (2013) used the HBM to explain self-compliance in adolescents with food allergies. In another study, Lin & Fang (2012) identified the HBM as a valid predictor in studying flu vaccine behavior among elderly individuals. Numerous other works describing application of the HBM (e.g., Brown, Patrician, & Brosch, 2012; Morris, Baker, Belot, & Edwards, 2011; Purtzer, 2012; Singleton, Bienemy, Hutchinson, Dellinger, & Rami, 2011) can be found in the nursing literature.

The TRA/TPB, likewise, has been used frequently in nursing studies. Review of the literature indicated scores of citations in recent nursing journals. Research examining the beliefs, attitudes, and intentions of health care providers was identified covering various topics. For example, Ward (2012) looked at infection control actions/behaviors among nursing and midwifery students; Pielak and team (2010) studied attitudes, beliefs, and practices of nurses and doctors as immunization providers; and Zhou, Stoltzfus, Houldin, Parks, and Swan (2010) examined knowledge, attitudes, and practices of oncology nurses regarding advanced care planning for their patients.

Other researchers have used the TRA to look at health behaviors in diverse areas, including intention to become an organ donor (Ford & Steele-Moses, 2011), to understand perceptions and beliefs of college students related to waterpipe smoking (Noonan, 2013), and to understand the reasoning and thoughts associated with the use of illegal performance-enhancing substances (Dodge, Stock, & Litt, 2012). Finally, Othman, Kiviniemi, Wu, and Lally (2012) used both the HBM and the TRA as the conceptual framework for their study of how demographic factors, knowledge, and beliefs influence women's intention to undergo mammography screening.

Summary

This chapter has presented five families of theories that attempt to explain human behavior. Although each theory emphasizes a different concept or viewpoint, no one theory best explains the complexity of human behavior. The psychodynamic theories attempt to explain an individual's behavior in terms related to the development of the self that is formed by adulthood. The behavioral theorists believe that behavior is learned by reinforcement, whereas the cognitive theorists believe that the reinforcements are related to an individual's thought patterns. Humanistic theories propose that individuals have within themselves the capacity to change. This potential for healthy and creative growth occurs throughout the individual's life span; thus, the behavior of an individual is a dynamic process. The stress-adaptation theories are associated with behaviors identified with the way a person adapts to stress through individual coping mechanisms. Finally, the social psychology theories look at how a person changes and explores ways to incorporate change through the promotion of health. Table 14-4 offers a brief comparison of these theories.

Darlene, in the opening case scenario, understands the complexity of humans and that using a single theory will not fully explain all of the variables that are associated with behavior and its impact on health. Therefore, most nurses adopt an eclectic approach to theory utilization in providing care. This means that the nurse chooses concepts from

Table 14-4 Comparison of Behavioral Theories

Theory	Theorist	Emphasis	Key Concepts
Psychodynamic	Freud	The study of unconscious mental processes of the psychodynamics of behavior	Personality structure: id, ego, superego; libido, pleasure principle, reality principle, instincts, stages of psychosexual development
	Erikson	Psychosocial factors that influence development	Id, ego, superego; conscious, preconscious, unconscious; developmental tasks; eight stages of biopsychosocial development
	Sullivan	Interpersonal experiences that influence development	Self-system, anxiety, security operations, personifications, modes of experience; stages of interpersonal growth and development
Cognitive-behavioral	Skinner	Analysis of human behavior observed in the current situation	Operant conditioning; positive and negative reinforcement
	Beck	Cognitive distortions	Arbitrary inference, overgeneralization, selective abstraction, magnification and minimization, underlying assumptions, entitlement, perfection, automatic thoughts
	Ellis	The values and assumptions that govern much of people's lives	ABC theory of rational emotive theory
Humanistic	Maslow	Fulfilling human potential	Hierarchy of needs, self-actualization
	Rogers	Person-centered	Organism and the self; congruence and incongruence; positive regard and self-regard
Stress-adaptation	Selye	Analysis of stress at the physiologic and biochemical levels of functioning	Stressor, general adaptation syndrome, alarm reaction, stages of resistance, stages of exhaustion
	Lazarus	Cognitive model of stress	Appraisal, coping, outcome
Social psychology	Rosenstock	Perceived threat and net benefits	Perceived susceptibility, perceived severity, perceived benefits, perceived barriers, cues of action, self-efficacy
	Ajzen and Fishbein	People make rational decisions based on the information they have	Intent, attitude, subjective norms

various theories that best explain the behaviors of the person. Due to the interrelatedness of the concepts in the theories (e.g., the self, anxiety, hope, development, cognitions, reinforcements, empowerment, health promotion), concepts from multiple theories can be used. The concepts from the various theories chosen for the individual will depend on the patient's particular behavior, needs, or problems. By knowing how behavior is formed, the nurse can better plan effective care to change behaviors to improve health.

Key Points

- Theories from behavioral sciences are very widely used by nurses in practice and research.
- Psychodynamic theories and theories that focus on development stages that are studied and used by nurses include the works of Freud, Erikson, and Sullivan.
- Commonly used behavior and cognitive-behavior theories include the works of Skinner, Beck, and Ellis.
- Human needs theories (e.g., Maslow and Rogers) and stress theories (e.g., Selye and Lazarus) are among the most commonly applied behavioral theories in nursing practice.
- The Health Belief Model and the Theory or Reasoned Action (Theory of Planned Behavior) are social psychology theories widely used by nurse researchers.

Learning Activities

1. Consider the case of a school nurse who is working with a 14-year-old student suspected of being addicted to alcohol. Discuss with classmates what concepts from the various theories described could be used in planning nursing interventions. Using the theories from social psychology, how could the nurse set up a health-promotion campaign for a teenage drug and alcohol program?

2. Consider the following case: A 30-year-old woman arrives in the emergency department. She is diagnosed with a drug overdose. Assessment data reveal the following information: she has three children (18 months, 4 years old, and 14 years old); she is in the process of her second divorce; she took 25 diazepam (Valium) tablets (2 mg/tablet), which her doctor had given her for stress; she is unemployed; and she did not graduate from high school. Which theory (or theories) should be used to direct her care? What concepts from other theories could be used to enhance her care?

3. Consider the following case: A 65-year-old woman is being admitted for a mastectomy due to cancer. She expresses fear and depression during the nursing assessment. What concepts from the various theories could be used in planning her care? How might her care be changed if the woman were 25 years old or 45 years old? How have the social psychology theories been used in promoting breast cancer awareness?

4. Consider the following case: A 52-year-old man is admitted to the hospital for hypertension for the third time in the past year. Each time, he stopped taking his medications because he was "feeling good." What concepts from the various theories could be used to change his behavior? How could the nurse set up a health-promotion program for managing hypertension in the hospital? In the community?

REFERENCES

Abraham, S. (2011). Fall prevention conceptual framework. *The Health Care Manager, 30*(2), 179–184.

Ajzen, I., & Fishbein, M. (1980). *Understanding attitudes and predicting social behavior.* Englewood Cliffs, NJ: Prentice-Hall.

Allan, H., & Barber, D. (2005). Emotional boundary work in advance fertility nursing roles. *Nursing Ethics, 12*(4), 391–399.

Askey-Jones, S., Shaw, P., & Silber, E. (2012). Working together: multiple sclerosis and mental health nurses. *British Journal of Neuroscience Nursing, 7*(6), 696–703.

Bailey, L. D. (2012). Adolescent girls: A vulnerable population. *Advances in Neonatal Care, 12*(2), 102–106.

Bayoumi, M. (2012). Identification of the needs of haemodialysis patients using the concept of Maslow's Hierarchy of Needs. *Journal of Renal Care, 38*(1), 43–49.

Beck, A. T. (1976). *Cognitive therapies and the emotional disorders.* New York: International University Press.

Bjorklund, P. (2000). Assessing ego strengths: Spinning straw into goals. *Perspectives in Psychiatric Care, 36*(1), 14–23.

Brenner, A., Zimmerman, M., Bauermeister, J., & Caldwell, C. (2013). Neighborhood context and perceptions of stress over time: An ecological model of neighborhood stressors and intrapersonal and interpersonal resources. *American Journal of Community Psychology, 51*(3–4), 544–556. doi:10.1007/s10464-013-9571-9.

Brown, C. G., Patrician, P. A., & Brosch, L. R. (2012). Increasing testicular self-examination in active duty soldiers: An intervention study. *MedSurg Nursing, 21*(2), 97–10.

Davis, J., Buchanan, K., & Green, B. (2013). Racial/ethnic differences in cancer prevention beliefs: Applying the Health Belief Model framework. *American Journal of Health Promotion, 27*(6), 384–389. doi:10.4278/ajhp.120113-QUAN-15.

Dodge, T., Stock, M., & Litt, D. (2012). Judgments about illegal performance-enhancing substances: Reasoned, reactive, or both? *Journal of Health Psychology, 18*(7), 962–971. doi:10.1177/1359105312445079

Duncan, M., & Blugis, A. (2011). Maslow's needs hierarchy as a framework for evaluating hospitality houses' resources and services. *Journal of Pediatric Nursing, 26*(4), 325–331.

Early, T. J., & GlenMaye, L. F. (2000). Valuing families: Social work practice with families from a strengths perspective. *Social Work, 45*(2), 118–130.

Ehlman, K., & Ligon, M. (2012). The application of a generativity model for older adults. *The International Journal of Aging and Human Development, 74*(4), 331–344.

Ellis, A., & MacLaren, C. (2008). *Rational emotive behavior therapy: A therapist's guide* (2nd ed.). Atascadero, CA: Impact.

Erci, B., Sezgin, S., & Kacmaz, Z. (2008). The impact of therapeutic relationship on preoperative and postoperative patient anxiety. *Australian Journal of Advanced Nursing, 26*(1), 59–66.

Erikson, E. H. (1963). *Childhood and society.* New York: Norton.

Erikson, E. H. (1968). *Identity: Youth and crisis.* New York: Norton.

Erikson, E. H. (1975). *Life history and the historical movement.* New York: Norton.

Fishbein, M., & Ajzen, I. (1975). *Belief, attitude, intention and behavior: An introduction to theory and research.* Reading, MA: Addison-Wesley.

Folkman, S., & Lazarus, R. S. (1988). *Manual for the ways of coping questionnaire.* Palo Alto, CA: Consulting Psychologist Press.

Folta, J. R. (1968). Perspectives of an applied science. *Nursing Research, 17*(6), 502–507.

Ford, D., & Steele-Moses, S. (2011). Predictors of African Americans' willingness to donate organs: A literature review. *Nephrology Nursing Journal, 38*(5), 405–409.

Freud, S. (1953). Three essays on sexuality. In *Standard edition of the complete psychological works of Sigmund Freud* (Vol. 7). London, United Kingdom: Hogarth (First German edition, 1905).

Freud, S. (1956). Inhibitions, symptoms and anxiety. In *Standard edition of the complete psychological works of Sigmund Freud* (Vol. 20). London, United Kingdom: Hogarth (First German edition, 1926).

Freud, S. (1960). *The ego and the id.* (J. Strachey, Trans.). New York: Norton.

Giblin, J. C. (2011). Successful aging: Choosing wisdom over despair. *Journal of Psychosocial Nursing, 49*(3), 23–27.

Glanz, K., Rimer, B. K., & Lewis, F. M. (2008). *Health behavior and health education: Theory, research and practice* (4th ed.). San Francisco, CA: Jossey-Bass.

Graungaard, A., Anderson, J., & Skov, L. (2011). When resources get sparse: A longitudinal, qualitative study of emotions, coping and resource-creation when parenting a young child with severe disabilities. *Health (London), 15*(2), 115–136.

Hall, C. S., & Lindzey, G. (1978). *Theories of personality.* New York: Wiley.

Handley, S. M., & Ward-Smith, P. (2005). Alcohol misuse, abuse and addiction in young and middle adulthood. *Annual Review of Nursing Research, 23*(1), 213–244.

Johnson, D. E. (1959). The nature of nursing science. *Nursing Outlook, 7*(5), 291–294.

Johnson, D. E. (1968). Theory in nursing: Borrowed and unique. *Nursing Research, 17*(3), 206–209.

Jones, C., Smith, H., Frew, A., Du Toit, G., Mukhopadhyay, S., & Llewellyn, C. (2013). Explaining adherence to self –care behaviours amongst adolescents with food allergy: A comparison of the health belief model and the common sense-regulation model. *British Journal of Health Psychology.* Advance online publication. doi:10.1111/bjhp.12033.

Kneisl, C. R., & Ames, S. W. (1986). *Adult health nursing: A biopsychosocial approach.* Menlo Park, CA: Addison-Wesley.

Lazarus, R. S., & Folkman, S. (1984). *Stress appraisal and coping.* New York: Springer.

Lin, M., & Fang, Y. (2012). Factors associated with receiving influenza vaccine among community-dwelling elderly in non-metropolitan area. *Sigma Theta Tau International, Virginia Henderson International Nursing Library. Retrieved from: http://hdl.handle.net/10755/243227.*

Mahoney, J. S., Palyo, N., Napier, G., & Giordano, J. (2009). The therapeutic milieu reconceptualized for the 21st century. *Archives of Psychiatric Nursing, 23*(6), 423–429.

Marriage, D., & Henderson, J. (2012). Cognitive behavior therapy for anxiety in children with asthma. *Nursing Children & Young People, 24*(9), 30–34.

Maslow, A. H. (1963). *Towards a psychology of being* (2nd ed.). Princeton, NJ: Van Nostrand.

Mokoka, K., Ehlers, V., & Oosthuizen, M. (2011). Factors influencing the retention of registered nurses in the Gauteng Province of South Africa. *Curationis, 34*(1), E1–E9.

Montano, D. E., & Kasprzyk, D. (2008). The theory of reasoned action and the theory of planned behavior. In K. Glanz, B. K. Rimer, & F. M. Lewis (Eds.), *Health behavior and health education: Theory, research and practice* (4th ed., pp. 67–99). San Francisco: Jossey-Bass.

Morris, P., Baker, D., Belot, C., & Edwards, A. (2011). Preparedness of students and staff with anaphylaxis, *Journal of School Health, 81*(8), 471–476.

Neuman, B. (1995). *The Neuman systems model* (3rd ed.). East Norwalk, CT: Appleton & Lange.

Noonan, D. A. (2013). Descriptive study of waterpipe smoking among college students. *Journal of the American Academy of Nurse Practitioners, 25*(1), 11–15.

O'Neill, M., Moore, K., & Ryan, A. (2008). Exploring the role and perspectives of mental health nurse practitioners following psychosocial interventions training. *Journal of Psychiatric and Mental Health Nursing, 15*(7), 582–587.

Orlando, I. (1961). *The dynamic nurse–patient relationship.* New York: Putnam.

Othman, A. K., Kiviniemi, M. T., Wu, Y. W, & Lally, R. M. (2012). Influence of demographic factors, knowledge and beliefs on Jordanian women's intention to undergo mammography screening. *Journal of Nursing Scholarship, 44*(1), 19–26.

Padden, O., Connors, R., & Agazio, J. (2011). Stress, coping, and well-being in military spouses during deployment separation. *Western Journal of Nursing Research, 33*(2), 247–267.

Peplau, H. E. (1952). *Interpersonal relations in nursing.* New York: Putnam.

Peplau, H. E. (1963). A working definition of anxiety. In S. F. Burd & M. A. Marshall (Eds.), *Some clinical approaches of psychiatric nursing* (pp. 323–327). Toronto: Macmillan.

Pielak, K. L., McIntyre, C., Tu, A. W., Remple, V. P., Halperin, B., & Buxton, J. A. (2010). Identifying attitudes, beliefs and reported practice of nurses and doctors as immunization providers. *Journal of Advanced Nursing, 66*(7), 1602–1611.

Poss, J. E. (2001). Developing a new model for cross-cultural research: Synthesizing the Health Belief Model and the Theory of Reasoned Action. *Advances in Nursing Science, 23*(4), 1–15.

Purtzer, M. A. (2012). A transformative decision-making process for mammography screening among rural, low-income women. *Public Health Nursing, 29*(3), 247–255.

Reed, P. G. (1998). A holistic view of nursing concepts and theories in practice. *Journal of Holistic Nursing, 16*(4), 415–419.

Rogers, C. R. (1951). *Client-centered therapy: Its current practice, implications, and theory.* Boston: Houghton Mifflin.

Rogers, C. R. (1959). A theory of therapy, personality, and interpersonal relationships as developed in the client-centered framework. In S. Koch (Ed.), *Psychology: A study of science* (Vol. 3, pp. 184–256). New York: McGraw-Hill.

Rosenstock, I. M. (1974). The health belief model and preventive health behavior. *Health Education Monographs, 2,* 354–436.

Rosenstock, I. M. (1990). The Health Belief Model: Explaining health behavior through expectancies. In K. Glanz, F. M. Lewis, & B. K. Rimer (Eds.), *Health behavior and health education: Theory, research and practice* (pp. 39–62). San Francisco: Jossey-Bass.

Roy, C. (2009). *The Roy Adaptation Model* (3rd ed.). Upper Saddle River, NJ: Pearson.

Sadock, B. (2009). Signs and symptoms in psychiatry. In B. Sadock, V. Sadock, & P. Ruiz (Eds.), *Kaplan & Sadock's comprehensive textbook of psychiatry* (pp. 918–928). Philadelphia: Lippincott Williams & Wilkins.

Scope, A., Booth, A., & Sutcliffe, P. (2012). Women's perceptions and experiences of group cognitive behaviour therapy and other group interventions for postnatal depression: A qualitative synthesis. *Journal of Advanced Nursing, 68*(9), 1909–1919.

Seal, N., & Seal, J. (2011). Developing healthy childhood behavior: Outcomes of a summer camp experience, *International Journal of Nursing Practice, 17*(4), 428–434.

Selye, H. (1956). *The stress of life.* St. Louis: McGraw-Hill.

Senn, J. F. (2013). Peplau's Theory of Interpersonal Relations: Application in emergency and rural nursing. *Nursing Science Quarterly, 26*(1), 31–35.

Sheldon, L. K., & Ellington, L. (2008). Application of a model of social information processing to nursing theory: How nurses respond to patients. *Journal of Advanced Nursing, 64*(4), 388–398.

Singleton, E. K., Bienemy, C., Hutchinson, S. W., Dellinger, A., & Rami, J. S. (2011). A pilot study: A descriptive correlational study of factors associated with weight in college nursing students. *ABNF Journal, 22*(4), 89–95.

Skinner, B. F. (1969). *Contingency of reinforcement: A theoretical analysis.* New York: Appleton-Century-Crofts.

Skinner, B. F. (1987). Whatever happened to psychology as the science of behavior? *American Psychologist, 42,* 780–786.

Southard, K., Jarrell, A., Shattell, M. M., McCoy, T. P., Bartlett, R., & Judge, C. A. (2012). Enclosed versus open nursing stations in adult acute care psychiatric settings: Does the sign affect the therapeutic milieu? *Journal of Psychosocial Nursing and Mental Health Services, 50*(5), 28–34.

Spirito, A., Esposito-Smythers, C., Wolff, J., & Uhl, K. (2011). Cognitive-behavioral therapy for adolescent depression and suicidality. *Child and Adolescent Psychiatric Clinics of North America, 20*(2), 191–204.

Steinberg, P., & Cochrane, D. (2013). Integration of psychoanalytic concepts in the formulation and management of hospitalized psychiatric patients. *Bulletin of the Menninger Clinic, 77*(1), 23–40.

Sullivan, H. S. (1953). *The interpersonal theory of psychiatry.* New York: Norton.

Swatton, A. (2011). Transference and countertransference in anorexia nervosa care. *Gastrointestinal Nursing, 9*(3), 38–43.

Telford, K., Kralik, D., & Koch, T. (2006). Acceptance and denial: Implications for people adapting to chronic illness: Literature review. *Journal of Advanced Nursing, 55*(4), 457–464.

Thomas, M., & Hynes, C. (2007). The darker side of groups. *Journal of Nursing Management, 15*(3), 375–385.

Thompson, L. (1986). Peplau's theory: An application to short term therapy. *Journal of Psychosocial Nursing and Mental Health Services, 24*(8), 26.

Thomsen, T., Rydahl-Hansen, S., & Wagner, L. (2010). A review of potential factors relevant to coping in patients with advanced cancer. *Journal of Clinical Nursing, 19*(23–24), 3410–3426.

Wadensten, B., & Carlsson, M. (2003). Nursing theory views on how to support the process of ageing. *Journal of Advanced Nursing, 42*(2), 118–124.

Ward, D. J. (2012). The application of the Theory of Planned Behaviour to infection control research with nursing and midwifery students. *Journal of Clinical Nursing, 22*(2), 296–298.

Zhou, G., Stoltzfus, J. C., Houldin, A. D., Parks, S. M., & Swan, B. A. (2010). Knowledge, attitudes, and practiced behaviors of oncology advanced practice nurses regarding advanced care planning for patient with cancer. *Oncology Nursing Forum, 37*(6), 400–410.

CHAPTER 15

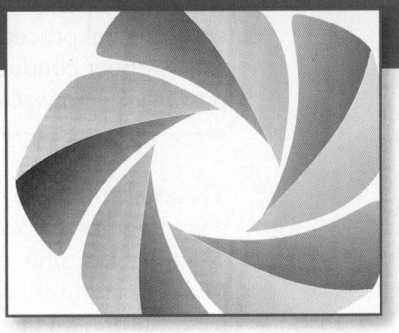

Theories From the Biomedical Sciences

Melanie McEwen

Maria Leon is in her final year of a graduate program preparing to become a certified registered nurse anesthetist (CRNA). During the course of her graduate education, Maria observed that most people reported a burning sensation as propofol (a drug used to induce general anesthesia) was administered intravenously (IV). In conducting a review of the literature and discussing her observations with other CRNAs, Maria found several techniques used to minimize the injection pain. Based on this information, Maria decided that she would like to conduct a research study to examine the effectiveness of using lidocaine to reduce the injection pain of propofol. This project would fulfill the capstone requirement for her master's degree.

A literature review of pain management led Maria to the gate control theory, which posits that there is a gating mechanism in the spinal cord. When pain impulses are transmitted from the periphery of the body by nerve fibers, the impulses travel to the dorsal horns of the spinal cord, specifically to the area of the cord called the *substantia gelatinosa*. According to the theory, when the gate is open, pain impulses ascend to the brain; when the gate is partially open, only some of the pain impulses can pass through. Pain medication has an effect on the gate, and if pain medication is administered before the onset of pain, it will help keep the gate closed, allowing fewer pain impulses to pass through.

In planning her research project, Maria used the gate control theory to guide the design and structure of the study. For the study, she decided to compare two techniques for pain prevention. One technique involved mixing 20 ml of a 1% propofol solution with 5 ml of a 2% lidocaine solution and injecting 1 ml of the mixture immediately before administration of the propofol. The second technique involved the placement of a tourniquet inflated to 50 mmHg on the arm in which the IV access device was placed. Then, 5 ml of 2% lidocaine would be injected and the tourniquet would be removed 1 minute later; propofol would then be injected. A time frame of 20 seconds would allow the clients to report pain in the arm before the propofol took effect. Maria also planned to have a control group that did not have either of the pain prevention interventions.

If the theory was correct, Maria hypothesized that both experimental groups would have less pain from the injection because the gate that allowed pain sensations would not open or would only partially open. She did not know which of the two experimental procedures would be more effective in preventing pain but was enthusiastic about conducting the study and adding to the body of knowledge on pain prevention in anesthesia.

Theories from the biomedical sciences (e.g., biology, medicine, public health, physiology, pharmacology) have had a tremendous impact on nursing practice since Nightingale's time. Indeed, many of these theories are so integral to nursing practice that they are overlooked or taken for granted. For example, at the beginning of the 21st century, the germ theory seems almost too elemental to mention because even kindergarten children are taught the basic concept of germs and how to prevent infection. But nurses should recognize the relatively recent discovery of this revolutionary theory (late 1800s) and understand that a significant amount of nursing care is based on it. Other theories, concepts, and principles are similarly ingrained within nursing practice.

Biomedical theories have been the basis for research efforts of physiologists, physicians, and laboratory-based scientists for many years. Nurses have also been involved in research of this type and are increasingly directing studies that have a physiologic or biologic basis. As with any study, the underlying theories or conceptual frameworks may be broad (e.g., germ theory) or very narrow (e.g., gate control theory).

This chapter presents some of the most commonly used theories and principles from the biomedical sciences to illustrate how they are being used in studies conducted by nurses and applied in nursing practice. The number of these theories is staggering; thus, space allows for discussion of only a few. Although there is some overlap, the theories will be grouped into two large categories: theories of disease causation (e.g., germ theory, natural history of disease) and theories related to physiology (e.g., stress and adaptation, cancer causation, pain).

Theories and Models of Disease Causation

On a day-to-day, moment-to-moment basis, nurses in practice use any one of a number of concepts, principles, and theories from biology and public health. These theories are often related to disease causation and progression. This includes pathogenesis and infection, as well as multiple epidemiologic concepts and principles (e.g., risk factor, exposure, prevention). This section provides a review of a few of these principles, theories, and models and shows how they are used in nursing practice and nursing research.

Evolution of Theories of Disease Causation

Disease refers to any condition that disturbs the normal functioning of an organism, whether it affects one organ or several systems. The term has also been defined as the failure of an organism to respond or adapt to its environment. The concept has changed dramatically over the course of time, however, and ideas about the cause of disease have been influenced by the prevailing culture and scientific thought.

In ancient times, disease was frequently viewed as a divine intervention or punishment. Early human beings attributed diseases to the influence of demons or spirits, and magic was a large part of treatment and prevention. As time passed, other interventions or treatments, such as the use of plant extracts, became more common.

As humans formed into societies and distinct cultural groups, two trends, or approaches, to medicine evolved. Sorcerers and priests embraced a magico-religious approach, whereas early physicians and scientists developed an empirico-rational approach. The empirico-rational approach was based on experience and observation and was practiced at first by priests but was adapted by nonclerical physicians. Modern medicine arose primarily from the empirico-rational approach as the human body and its functions became better known and as science led medical practice away from superstition and focus on the spiritual realm to include scientific processes and reasoning.

In the 17th century, William Harvey, an English physician and anatomist, demonstrated the dynamics of blood circulation (Donahue, 2011). Detailed studies of the organs, diseases, and processes, such as physiology and respiration, quickly followed, conducted by eminent physicians and scientists of the time. Medical debates focused on minute features of the body and how to treat particular diseases. Philosophies and theories developed that were largely reductionistic and deductive, focusing on cause and effect; the medical model quickly evolved.

In the latter part of the 19th century, scientists began to unravel the basic causes of infectious disease. Modern medicine began with the advent of Pasteur's germ theory, which posited that a specific microorganism was capable of causing an infectious disease (Black & Hawks, 2009). The focus on single-agent or single-organism cause for disease persisted for a number of decades and resulted in multiple successes in both treating and preventing communicable diseases. Today, however, the predominant general model of disease causation is multicausal, involving invasive agents, immune responses, genetics, environment, and behavior.

A number of theories and models describe disease causation and the properties that relate to disease processes and prevention. Some of the most frequently encountered models in nursing practice and research are discussed in the following sections.

Germ Theory and Principles of Infection

Louis Pasteur first proposed the germ theory in 1858. He theorized that a specific organism (i.e., a germ) was capable of causing an infectious disease (Kalisch & Kalisch, 2004). Today, this seems like a simple theory, but it is one that was critical to the development of modern medical care. Its impact has been phenomenal and has helped to radically reduce the number of deaths from infection.

At the beginning of the 21st century, theories of infection are most often applied to prevent infection (e.g., practicing strict hand washing, cleansing a scrape and applying antibiotic ointment, or prophylactically treating a surgery client with antibiotics) or to describe the process that seeks to identify, understand, and manage infectious diseases. This process initiates the search for the causative agent of an infection and method(s) of transmission. Once this has been accomplished, the focus can shift to the development of ways to prevent and treat the disease.

One of the most recent and dramatic examples of this process was the outbreak of AIDS. The syndrome was first identified by the Centers for Disease Control and Prevention in September of 1982, but months passed before it was determined that the causative agent was a retrovirus, later termed *HIV* (Shi & Singh, 2012). Early in the process, even before the virus was isolated, methods of transmission (e.g., sexual, transplacental, via blood products) were recognized and interventions for prevention proposed. Research on treatment has produced somewhat successful results in recent years and is ongoing.

Another example involves bovine spongiform encephalopathy (BSE), or mad cow disease, and its relationship with Creutzfeldt–Jakob disease (CJD). It has been hypothesized that the causative agent of BSE is a *prion,* which is not truly a germ, but a protein that is transmitted through ingestion of contaminated meat; the principles of infection, however, are similar (Secker, Hervé, & Keevil, 2011). Much additional work will be necessary to support this theory and to enhance preventive efforts. Ultimately, it is hoped that effective treatments for CJD will be found.

Application to Nursing

Research studies use the germ theory to identify the causes or agents of infection. For an infection to occur, the host must be susceptible to the invasive organism. This susceptibility may be termed *risk.* For example, a person who has experienced severe burns is at higher risk of infection because one of the first lines of defense, the skin, is damaged. Many nursing articles that present practice guidelines and nursing research studies have focused on prevention and management of infection as well as identifying factors that place an individual at risk for developing infections. These studies and guidelines use principles from the germ theory, although this is rarely acknowledged.

Examples from recent literature that detail aspects of nursing practice related to prevention of infection include interventions to promote hand hygiene (Ardizzone, Smolowitz, Kline, Thom, & Larson, 2012; Buet et al., 2013; KuKanich, Kaur, Freeman, & Powell, 2013), guidelines for prevention of infections related to urinary catheters (Chen et al., 2013; Seckel, 2013), and strategies to prevent ventilator-associated pneumonia in pediatric patients (Morinec, Icaboni, & McNett, 2012). Upshaw-Owens and Bailey (2012) and Millar, Loughrey, Bill, and Moore (2011) described efforts nurses can use to prevent methicillin-resistant *Staphylococcus aureus* (MRSA) infection in hospitals and primary care settings, respectively. With respect to the previous discussion of CJD, strategies to prevent prion infection were presented by Rentz (2008) and Stride, Hunter, and Bailey (2009).

The Epidemiologic Triangle

The classic epidemiologic model, particularly useful in the depiction of communicable disease, is the epidemiologic triangle (Figure 15-1). This model is often used to illustrate the interrelationships among the three essential components of host, agent, and environment with regard to disease causation. A change in any of the three components can result in the disease process. For example, exposure at school (environment) of a child who has not been immunized (host) to the measles virus (agent) will probably result in a case of measles.

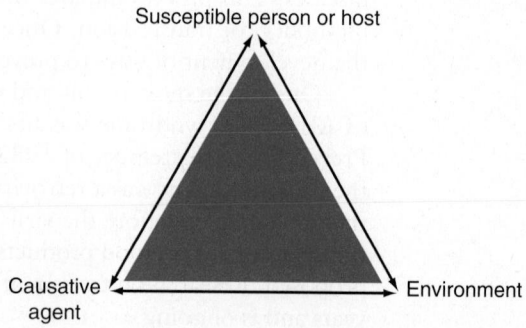

Figure 15-1 Epidemiologic triangle.

Within the epidemiologic triangle, prevention of disease lies in averting exposure to the agent, enhancing the physical attributes of the host to resist the disease, and minimizing any environmental factors that might contribute to disease development. Host, agent, and environmental factors that affect health can also influence progression of the disease process. Host factors include age, gender, race/ethnicity, marital status, economic status, state of immunity, and lifestyle factors (e.g., diet, exercise patterns, hygiene, occupation, sexual health). Agent factors include presence or absence of biologic organisms (e.g., bacteria, fungi, viruses), exposure to physical factors (e.g., radiation, extremes of temperature, noise), and exposure to chemical agents (e.g., poisons, allergens, gases). Last, environmental factors include such things as physical elements or properties (e.g., climate, seasons, geology), biologic entities (e.g., animals, insects, food, drugs), or social/economic considerations (e.g., family, public policy, occupation, culture) (McEwen & Pullis, 2009).

The Web of Causation

To explain disease and disability caused by multiple factors, MacMahon and Pugh (1970) developed the concept of "chain of causation," later termed the "web of causation." Prior to that time, it had been observed that chronic diseases (i.e., coronary artery disease and most types of cancer) are not attributable to one or two factors or causative agents. Rather, they result from the interaction of multiple factors. An example of the application of the web of causation to the development of coronary heart disease is presented in Figure 15-2.

The web of causation can also be applied to many health-related threats and conditions. The problem of teenage pregnancy, for example, is attributable to a complex interaction among a number of causative and contributing factors, including lack of knowledge about sexuality and pregnancy prevention, lack of easily accessible contraception, peer pressure, low self-esteem, social patterns in which teen mothers are more likely to be children of teen mothers, use of alcohol or other drugs, and so on. Family violence, cocaine use, and gang membership are examples of other threats to health and well-being that can be more accurately explained through a model of multiple causations.

Recognition that many health problems have multiple causes leads to the recognition that there are rarely simple solutions to these health problems. When trying to manage teen pregnancy, for example, the solution is not as simple as addressing a knowledge deficit regarding sexuality and contraception. Many (if not most) teens are well informed about contraception and the mechanics of how one gets pregnant, and they still fail to take preventive measures. To prevent heart disease in an individual at risk, interventions include health education addressing a number of areas, including smoking cessation, weight loss, cholesterol reduction, and exercise. Likewise, to prevent teen pregnancy, interventions should include health teaching on improving self-esteem, participating in role-playing exercises on how to say "no," encouraging orientation toward the future, enhancing parental supervision, and providing recreational alternatives (sports and other after-school activities), as well as giving information on sexuality, the mechanics of reproduction, and methods of contraception.

Application to Nursing

Nurses have developed interventions and proposed strategies to address complex health problems with multifactorial etiologies. For example, from a large-scale study, Nonnemacher and colleagues (2008) outlined risk factors for development of pressure ulcers among hospitalized individuals. These included previous occurrence of pressure ulcers, limited mobility, skin problems, insufficient nutrition, and friction/shearing movement.

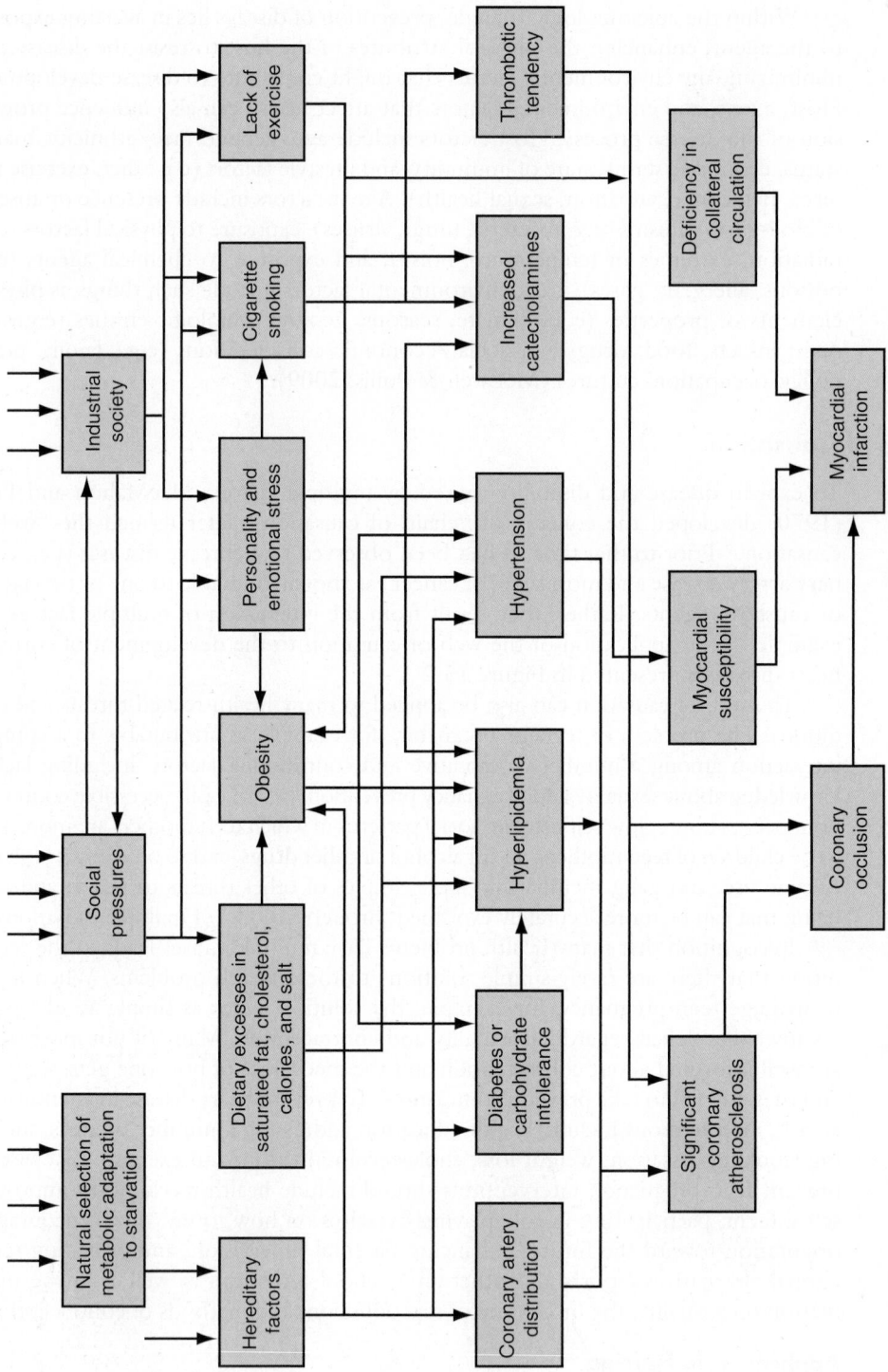

Figure 15-2 Web of causation. (Adapted with permission from Friedman, G. D. [1994]. *Primer of epidemiology* [4th ed.]. New York: McGraw-Hill.)

In another study, Johnson, Giarelli, Lewis, and Rice (2013) provided an overview of the correlational factors that are believed to contribute to development of autism spectrum disorder (ASD). These were broadly grouped into environmental factors (e.g., exposure to high levels of pollutants, viral infection during pregnancy, use of assisted reproductive therapies) and genetic factors (i.e., "genetic susceptibility" and "de novo mutations" [new, spontaneous mutations]). The researchers also described nursing implications including promotion of knowledge and skills to assess genetic risk, advocacy for families, and encouragement to assess for possible ASD in encounters with children.

In other works, Matthews and Moore (2013) examined the risk factors associated with sudden unexplained infant death (SUID)/sudden infant death syndrome (SIDS), and D'Alonzo, Johnson, and Fanfan (2012) reported on the risk factors leading to development of obesity and related illnesses among Latino immigrants in the United States. Siegel (2007) used the web of causation as the theoretical framework in her examination of the predictors of overweight in children in 6th, 7th, and 8th grades, and Van Dyke (2005) used the web of causation to explain the complex interrelationships explaining domestic violence.

Natural History of Disease

The natural history of a disease refers to the progress of a disease process in an individual over time. In their classic model, Leavell and Clark (1965) described two periods in the natural history of disease, prepathogenesis and pathogenesis. In this model, the prepathogenesis stage occurs prior to interaction of the disease agent and human host when the individual is susceptible. For example, an adult male smokes, a teenage girl considers becoming sexually active, or a preschooler attends a party also attended by a sick child. After exposure or interaction, the period of prepathogenesis proceeds to early pathogenesis (i.e., alterations in lung tissue, pregnancy, chicken pox) and on through the disease course to resolution—either death, disability, or recovery (i.e., lung cancer, teen motherhood, immunity to chicken pox).

In addition to the description of the natural history of disease progression, Leavell and Clark (1965) also outlined three levels of prevention—primary prevention, secondary prevention, and tertiary prevention—that correlate with the stages of disease progression (Box 15-1). Each of the three levels of prevention is applied at the appropriate stage of pathogenesis in an attempt to halt progression (Figure 15-3). Thus, at the primary prevention stage, interventions focus on general health promotion

Box 15-1 Levels of Prevention

- *Primary prevention:* Activities that are directed at preventing a problem before it occurs. This includes altering susceptibility or reducing exposure for susceptible individuals in the period of pre-pathogenesis. Primary prevention consists of two categories: *general health promotion* (e.g., good nutrition, adequate shelter, rest, exercise) and *specific protection* (e.g., immunization, water purification).
- *Secondary prevention:* Early detection of and prompt intervention for a disease or health threat during the period of early pathogenesis. Screening for disease and prompt referral and treatment are secondary prevention.
- *Tertiary prevention:* Consists of limitation of disability and rehabilitation during the period of advanced disease and convalescence, where the disease has occurred and resulted in a degree of damage.

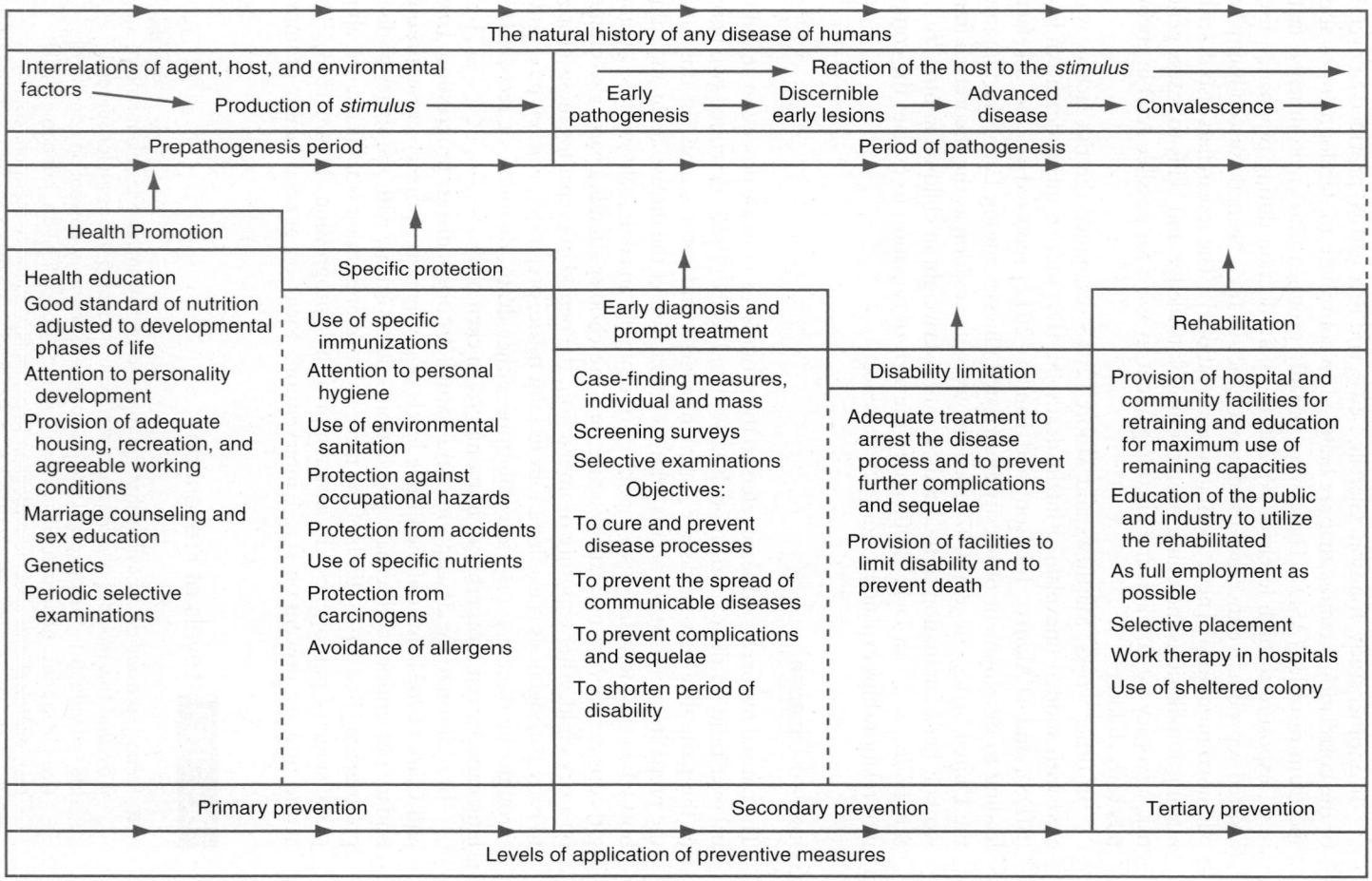

Figure 15-3 Natural history of disease. (Adapted with permission from Leavell, H. R., & Clark, E. G. [1965]. *Preventive medicine for the doctor in his community: An epidemiologic approach* [p. 18]. New York: McGraw-Hill.)

activities (e.g., encouraging a healthful diet and promoting regular exercise) and efforts to prevent specific health problems (e.g., vaccination, encouraging use of seatbelts and car seats, promoting oral hygiene).

Secondary prevention is concerned with early detection and would include any screening activity (e.g., mammography, cholesterol screening) and subsequent efforts to limit disease progression for those identified with a health condition (e.g., taking statin medications, lumpectomy with radiation/chemotherapy). Last, tertiary prevention involves efforts to enhance rehabilitation and convalescence following advanced disease.

Application to Nursing

Much of nursing practice focuses on efforts to prevent the progression of disease at the earliest period or phase using the appropriate levels of prevention. There are many examples of applying primary prevention strategies in practice. These include efforts to prevent polypharmacy among community-dwelling elders (Riker & Setter, 2012); multidrug-resistant, gram-negative infection in surgical patients (Murphy, 2012); skin cancer in children (Walker, 2012); falls among elders (Abraham, 2011), and cardiovascular disease through use of statins (Li & Zhou, 2011). Excellent examples of nursing interventions targeted to secondary prevention are also common in the nursing literature. Examples include a program to promote screening for depression among adolescents at school (Kuo, Stoep, Herting, Grupp, & McCauley, 2013), discussion of the importance of screening newborns for genetic conditions (DeLuca, Zanni, Bonhomme, & Kemper, 2013); guidelines and a screening tool for Acanthosis Nigricans (Scott & Hall, 2012), elder abuse screening (Stark, 2012), screening promotion to detect colorectal cancer among Hispanic immigrants (Gonzalez, Ziebarth, Wang, Noor, & Springer, 2012), and postpartum depression assessments for new mothers during pediatric visits (Meadows-Oliver, 2012). Tertiary prevention efforts include information to help nurses work to prevent reoccurrences and secondary malignancies among long-term survivors of cancer (Mahon, 2005). Finally, Jones-Parker (2012) presented a detailed overview examining all three levels of prevention intended to assist nurse practitioners in preventing cardiovascular disease in HIV-positive patients, and Fletcher and colleagues (2011) outlined multilevel preventive strategies for both community-based and public health initiatives for nurses to address cardiovascular disease.

Theories and Principles Related to Physiology and Physical Functioning

Many theories based on the normal physiologic functioning of the body are used in nursing practice and research. Although much of normal physiologic functioning is regarded as fact (e.g., the heart pumps blood, the lungs exchange oxygen and carbon dioxide), a great deal of research still is being conducted to uncover the mysteries of the body's physiology. Therefore, theories of physiologic functioning still need to be developed and tested.

Over the past century, scores of theories, principles, and concepts related to physiology and physical functioning of humans have been developed. Among others, these include theories and principles of aging, immunity, wound healing, cancer development, inflammation and infection, hormone action, nutrition, metabolism, and body systems (renal system, pulmonary gas exchange, cardiovascular physiology, and nervous system functioning). Space does not allow detailed explanation or presentation of multiple, similar theories on one topic. Rather, some of the most frequently cited examples from the nursing literature are discussed. These include principles or theories of homeostasis, stress and adaptation, immunity and immune function, genetics, cancer, and pain.

Homeostasis

Claude Bernard, a physiologist in the 20th century, first conceived the idea of homeostasis. He hypothesized that an organism must have the capacity to maintain its internal environment to live. A 20th century physician, Walter Canon, developed the concept of feedback mechanisms to further explain Bernard's principles of regulation. He coined the term *homeostasis,* referring to the dynamic equilibrium and flexible ongoing processes that maintain certain biologic factors within a range (Kunert, 2009). The principles of homeostasis state that all healthy cells, tissues, and organs maintain static conditions in their internal environment.

Dr. Eugene Yates introduced the related concept of homeodynamics to show that there is continuous change in physiologic processes (e.g., heart rate, blood pressure, nerve activity, hormonal secretion) based on changes within or external to the organism. Thus, to survive, the body system depends on a dynamic interplay of multiple regulatory mechanisms (Lipsitz, 2001). Homeostasis or homeodynamics includes physiologic principles often described in terms of organ-based systems (e.g., cardiovascular, respiratory, endocrine, immune, and neurologic systems). However, in reality, the body systems are integrated and are continually adapting to environmental changes. As a result, a new term, *allostasis,* has been used to recognize the complexity and variability of the levels of activity needed to reestablish or maintain homeostasis. In that regard, allostasis is a "superordinate set of systems that support homeostasis in light of environmental and life changes" (Emerson, 2010, p. 16).

Application to Nursing

There are a number of illustrations of how principles of homeostasis are applied in nursing practice. For example, Kisiel and Marsons (2009) reviewed the signs and symptoms of diabetic ketoacidosis and hyperglycemic hyperosmolar state, describing interventions to help restore homeostasis in hyperglycemic emergencies, and Yeo (2011) provided a nursing intervention to enhance cardiac homeostasis in mothers-to-be experiencing preeclampsia using low-intensity exercise. In an interesting article, Outland (2010) described homeostasis as "a cornerstone of holistic care" (p. 36) and presented the notion of "intuitive eating" to help restore and maintain "weight homeostasis" (a dynamic interaction between hormones, proteins, and neurotransmitters) to help control weight. Finally, Bellar, Kunkler, and Burkett (2009) focused on "allostasis" in their discussion of how nurses can recognize and manage "chronic critical illness syndrome."

Stress and Adaptation: General Adaptation Syndrome

In addition to the principles of homeostasis, Walter Canon also developed the concept of fight or flight to explain the body's reaction to emergencies. This fight-or-flight response prepares the body for muscular activity (i.e., running, self-defense) when reacting to a perceived or actual threat. The fight-or-flight response is a series of chemical reactions that are initiated by the adrenal medulla, which produces epinephrine (adrenaline) and norepinephrine. This reaction increases the heart rate, respiratory rate, blood pressure, and blood glucose levels. Blood is shunted to the muscles of the legs, heart, and lungs from the intestines; this prepares the body for quick response to danger (Emerson, 2010).

In the 1960s and 1970s, Hans Selye built on Canon's work by developing a framework to describe how the body responds to stress. Selye derived his theories of stress from the observations he made while caring for people who were ill. The clinical manifestations he noted were loss of appetite, weight loss, feeling and looking ill, and generalized muscle aching and pains. Selye called this response the general adaptation syndrome (GAS) because it involved generalized changes that affect the body.

Selye believed that changes in organs occur in three stages. Stage 1, the alarm phase, begins with the fight-or-flight response. In this stage, the adrenal glands enlarge and release hormones including adrenocorticotropic hormone (ACTH). This increases blood glucose and depresses the immune system. If the stress continues, the body begins to experience detrimental changes (e.g., shrinkage of the thymus, spleen, lymph nodes, and other lymphatic structures). Other physical manifestations, such as gastric and duodenal ulcers, can also develop.

Stage 2 (resistance) occurs when the body starts to react and return to homeostasis. If the stressor ends, the body should be able to return to normal. Stage 3 (exhaustion) occurs when the stressor persists and the body cannot continue to produce hormones as in stage 1, or when damage has occurred to other organs (Table 15-1) (Selye, 1976).

Selye thought that the body's response to stress is nonspecific; that is, the body reacts as a whole organism. Also, it is not just bad things that cause stress but good things as well. Health conditions thought to be related to stress include cancer, hypertension, heart disease, cerebrovascular accident, peripheral vascular disease, asthma, tuberculosis, emphysema, irritable bowel syndrome, sexual dysfunction, obesity, anorexia, bulimia, connective tissue disease, ulcerative colitis, Crohn disease, infections, and allergic and hypersensitivity diseases.

Selye's syndrome theory has been the basis of many studies. Holmes and Rahe (1967) conducted one classic study. They proposed that a large number of life changes cause stress, which in turn may cause disease. The researchers asked individuals of

Table 15-1 Selye's Stages of Stress

Stage	Characteristics	Physical Responses
Alarm	Begins with alarm; body prepares for survival (fight or flight); physiologic changes are coordinated by the central nervous system (CNS) and the sympathetic nervous system (SNS), which stimulates the adrenal medulla to secrete norepinephrine and epinephrine; the adrenal cortex is stimulated by the pituitary gland's release of ACTH.	CNS involuntary responses include secretion of specific hormones and metabolism and fluid regulation. SNS responses include increased heart rate, contraction of the spleen, release of glucose, increase in respiratory rate, decrease in clotting time, dilation of pupils, increased perspiration, and piloerection (hairs standing on end).
Resistance	The body recognizes a continued threat and physiologic forces adapt to maintain increased resistance to stressors; begins with a decrease in ACTH, and the body concentrates on organs that are most involved in the specific stress responses.	Adaptation implies return or improvement in physical health. Ineffective resistance leads to a state of maladaptation in which there is deterioration in the level of physical functioning. Chronic resistance eventually causes damage to the involved systems.
Exhaustion	The body enters exhaustion when all energy for adaptation has been used; ACTH secretion increases and the organ or organ systems show evidence of deterioration.	Symptoms include hypertrophy of the adrenal glands, ulceration in the gastrointestinal tract, and atrophy of the thymus gland.

various socioeconomic and cultural groups to rank a number of life changes according to the amount of energy needed to adapt to change. These events were ranked, and a certain number of life change units (LCUs) were assigned to each one. This scale was named the Social Readjustment Rating Scale (SRRS). The total number of LCUs experienced by a person accumulates over time and theoretically indicates the amount of stress a person has experienced. A significant accumulation of stress increases the likelihood of an incidence of major illness.

Application to Nursing

A number of nurses have used the SRRS in recent research studies. One study (Staniute, Brozaitiene, & Bunevicius, 2013) used the SRRS to examine the effects of social support and stressful life events on health-related quality of life among coronary artery disease patients. Another work (Welsh, 2009) used the SRRS to study the correlation between stress and depression in medical-surgical hospital nurses, and a third used the SRRS to examine compassion fatigue among health care providers who care for children in intensive care units. In a similar way, Ganz (2012) studied stress among ICU nurses, using the GAS as a framework.

In a discussion relative to nursing practice, Okonta (2012) conducted an integrative research review to examine whether yoga is effective in reducing high blood pressure using Selye's model as a framework. Mulvihill (2005) also used Selye's model to review the long-term impact of childhood trauma on the victim's psychological health.

Theories of Immunity and Immune Function

The immune system comprises a complex, coordinated group of systems that produces physiologic responses to injury or infection. The purpose of the immune system is to neutralize, eliminate, or destroy microorganisms that invade the body. Extensive interactions affect the manufacture of products that alter the structure and function of cells.

Immunity involves specific recognition of what is designated as an antigen, memory for particular antigens, and responsiveness on reexposure. The immune system is related to other systems involved in inflammation and healing. Each system is involved in the response of inflammation and has two characteristics: (1) recognition of a stimulating structure by specific receptors and (2) response by one or more effector elements that aims to alter or eliminate the stimulating structure.

The immune system contains a large variety of cells, called *leukocytes*, that protect the body against foreign invasion. The five classes of leukocytes are neutrophils, eosinophils, basophils, monocytes, and lymphocytes; each has a specific function in the immune response. The granulocytes (neutrophils, eosinophils, and basophils) are short-lived phagocytic cells. They search out bacteria or cell debris and destroy them through phagocytosis (Workman, 2012).

Monocytes mature into macrophages in tissues and defend against tumor cells. They secrete monokines (i.e., interleukin-1) that assist in immune and inflammatory responses. Lymphocytes originate from stem cells in the bone marrow and mature into either B or T cells. The T cells differentiate in the thymus gland, and the B cells mature in the bone marrow. Both T and B lymphocytes continually recirculate between blood, lymph, and lymph nodes. The surface of B lymphocytes is coated with immunoglobulin, and when the appropriately matched antigen is detected by a B cell, the surface immunoglobulin will bind with it. The T lymphocytes play a role in cell-mediated immunity. There are a variety of T cell subsets; some are regulatory T cells, which include helper T cells and suppressor T cells (Black & Hawks, 2009).

The complement system consists of around 20 plasma proteins found in serum and on cells. The complement system participates in inflammation by coordinating elements of the inflammatory response to microorganisms and tissue injury through generation of peptides that initiate effects such as leukocyte activation, chemotaxis, and mast cell degranulation. The system facilitates phagocytic function by coating the target particle with biologically active peptides and fragments of molecules activating the system. A series of proenzymes and other molecules initiate an attack on the cell membranes of microorganisms (Banasik, 2010a).

Antibody-mediated immunity involves antigen–antibody actions to neutralize, eliminate, or destroy foreign proteins. Antibodies for these actions are produced by B lymphocytes. The B lymphocytes become sensitized to a specific foreign protein (antigen) and synthesize an antibody directed specifically against that protein. The antibody (rather than the actual B lymphocyte) participates in action to neutralize, eliminate, or destroy that antigen. Cell-mediated immunity involves many leukocytic actions, reactions, and interactions. Lymphocyte stem cells and lymphoid tissues regulate activities and inflammation by producing and releasing cytokines. T lymphocytes can be natural killer cells or helper cells (T_4 or Th cells) (Workman, 2012).

Application to Nursing

Principles of immune function can be used as a theoretical framework for research. A number of recent nursing research studies can be identified that look at factors related to immune status. For example, a study by Hughes, Ladas, Rooney, and Kelly (2008) concluded that as an adjunct intervention, massage therapy helps reduce side effects of treatment and may boost immune function in children with cancer. In another example, Kang, McArdle, Weaver, Smith, and Carpenter (2011) concluded that persistent practice of relaxation techniques might positively influence immune responses in women diagnosed with breast cancer. Finally, in a correlational study, Starkweather (2013) examined the relationship among fatigue, pain, psychosocial factors, and immune activation in patients with persistent sciatica. She determined that immune activation associated with chronic pain affects fatigue severity and may also affect other behavioral responses.

The interrelatedness of the nervous, endocrine, and immune systems were described in two works on psychoimmunology. In one report, Ruiz and Avant (2005) examined the literature and found that maternal prenatal stress may prove to be detrimental to the immune system of both mother and developing infant. Another work (Starkweather, Witek-Janusek, & Mathews, 2005) presented an overview of the interaction of cytokines and hormones at the cellular level and discussed how they might affect immune functioning; their review was intended to serve as a framework for conducting nursing research.

Genetic Principles and Theories

Although genetic principles and theories date back to Gregor Mendel's work in the 1860s, advances in molecular biology have only recently begun to transform health care delivery. The Human Genome Project is an organized effort initiated in 1990 and completed in 2003 to create a biologically and medically useful database of the genome structure and sequence in humans. (The term *human genome* refers to the entire complement of genetic material contained on the 46 chromosomes.) It is anticipated that information gained from the Human Genome Project will increase understanding of inherited conditions, both single-gene and complex diseases as well as responses to treatment (Beery, 2008; Carroll, 2009).

A gene is the fundamental and functional unit of heredity. It is composed of a double strand of DNA, and each of the strands has thousands to millions of bases. The order of the bases codes information that directs the manufacture of a specific protein (Banasik, 2010b). A gene mutation is an alteration in DNA coding that results in a change in the protein product. Mutations in some genes cause clinical disease because of the absence of the normal protein. Sickle cell anemia, for example, results when one base is substituted with another.

Gene discoveries have provided information on genetic disorders that cause symptoms in a large proportion of persons who have abnormal genotypes. Successes include the isolation of genes for cystic fibrosis, neurofibromatosis, muscular dystrophy, Huntington disease, and some types of breast cancer (Banasik, 2010b; Porth, 2009). Many other diseases have a genetic susceptibility component that results from the interaction of multiple genes with environmental factors. Because these diseases involve many genes and many possible mutations, an enormous number of combinations of genotypes are possible. Determining the molecular pathophysiology of human disease will provide opportunities for diagnosis, prevention, and treatment.

Application to Nursing

Genetics will greatly affect the way health care is practiced in the future, and nurses will need to incorporate genetic technology and discovery into practice and research at the individual, family, and community levels. Nurses familiar with genetics and who are able to "think genetically" can ask appropriate questions of patients to assess genetic risk factors, communicate with patients and their families about inherited risks, make referrals to genetic counselors, reinforce counseling, and administer gene therapy or genetically specific drugs (See Link to Practice 15-1) (Calzone et al., 2012;

Link to Practice 15-1

Calzone and Jenkins (2013) recently discussed the expanding importance of genomics to nursing practice. They reviewed how genomics provides information that enhances understanding of the biology of disease and has resulted in new and more personalized therapies that can greatly influence health care decisions. They explained that nurses have a responsibility to be informed about the potential benefits and challenges of genomics and to use that knowledge to inform other health care professionals, individuals, families, and communities.

Several ways that nurses can integrate genomic information into clinical practice were presented. These are:

- Preconception and prenatal testing
- Newborn screening
- Disease susceptibility
- Screening and diagnosis
- Prognosis and therapeutic decisions
- Monitoring disease burden and recurrence

Calzone and Jenkins asserted that timely and effective translation of genomics into health care will require that currently practicing nurses be educated in genomics and future nurses must be taught essential genetic and genomic competencies.

From Calzone, K. A., & Jenkins, J. (2013). Relevance of genomics to healthcare and nursing practice. *Journal of Nursing Scholarship, 45*(1), 1–2.

Table 15-2 A Nursing Model for Genetics in Health Care

	Nursing Science	Genetic Education	Ecogenetic Nursing
Individual	Caring behavior and support role	Predictive genetic testing	Educating patients on genetic testing
	Care across the life span	Gene discoveries for diseases	Assisting patients to determine need for testing
	Patient counseling	Genes in pedigrees	Genetic consulting
	Medication	Pharmacogenetics	Educating about individualized medication therapy
Family	Pedigrees	Genetic role in disease	Interpreting and sharing genetic risk and health promotion
	Health promotion	Molecular pathology	Individualizing genetic testing and health promotion
	Multidisciplinary practice	Genetic specialist on the health care team	Referring to and interfacing with genetic specialists
	Informed consent	Genetic research concerns	Explaining risks and benefits of genetic study
	Teaching and counseling families	Genetic risks	Assessing and counseling families—reproductive risks and prenatal diagnosis
Community	Community assessment	Population-based screening	Community readiness for genetic screening and intervention
	Design and implement screening programs and follow-up service	Genetic testing	Availability and voluntary access to genetic information, testing, and assurance of follow-up services
Population	Clinical trials	New technology	Coordinating genetically focused research
	Nursing research	Genetic research	Collaborative research: focusing on ecogenetics, ethics, and psychosocial issues
	Patient advocacy	Ethical issues surrounding genetic tests	Ensuring that patients remain the priority of clinical treatment and research

Garcia, Greco, & Loescher, 2011; Kirk, Lea, & Skirton, 2008). Table 15-2 suggests a nursing model for application of genetics in health care illustrating how and where genetics education can be added to basic nursing science. The result is preparation of the nurses for "ecogenetic nursing."

A practicing nurse must be sensitive to issues of ethics and confidentiality related to genetic testing and genetic information. Indeed, genetics is one area of health care where technology precedes the ethical framework for dealing with issues and creates problems previously unknown; nurses must be prepared to deal with these problems (Beery, 2008; Kirk et al., 2008). Nurses knowledgeable in genetics can ensure that patients and families make informed and voluntary decisions about genetic information. Nurses can also serve as patient advocates as they obtain informed consent to participate in genetic clinical trials or to undergo genetic tests.

Nurses knowledgeable in genetics can have an important role in counseling patients at risk for complex diseases. Because complex diseases occur much more frequently than single-gene disorders, and because the number of diseases found to have genetic determinates is increasing rapidly, there will not be enough genetic counselors to serve all who are at risk (Beery, 2008; Skirton, O'Connor, & Humphreys, 2012).

Nurses must use their knowledge of genetics to identify and differentiate genetic risks in patients with complex disorders and refer these patients to a genetic counselor whenever appropriate (Prows, Hopkin, Barnoy, & Van Riper, 2013; Santos et al., 2013; Skirton et al., 2012).

Nurses are becoming more involved with managing genetic information because it is often collected and recorded when the nurse takes a family history and obtains certain blood tests (e.g., screening for breast cancer, sickle cell trait). Genetic testing and counseling combines the provision of genetic information with psychosocial counseling. It is nondirective, voluntary, and personal and should precede testing to allow informed decision making. Counseling should include an explanation of risk factors, exploration of the person's perception of the condition, and discussion of childbearing options. Potential outcomes of decisions are examined to facilitate decision making, and follow-up counseling is recommended. Goals of genetic counseling are to help clients and family members comprehend the medical genetic information, appreciate the genetic contribution to health and illness, understand health options and alternatives, and make informed health choices (i.e., whether to pursue further testing, evaluation, and treatment). Genetic counseling frequently includes referral and follow-up for family members to gain more information and possible treatment.

Nurses have also studied specific genetically based illnesses. For example, Frazier, Johnson, and Sparks (2005) reported on a review of research on the genetic basis for developing cardiovascular disease (CVD). They determined that understanding genes and genetic pathways can improve clinical practice and development of strategies to prevent CVD and reduce related mortality. Snow and Lu (2012) examined genetic "inheritability" of risk for addiction and described how understanding genetic predisposition to addiction to substances including nicotine, alcohol, or illicit drugs can help nurses develop better and more directed educational materials as well as treatment protocols.

Cancer Theories

The altered behavior of cancer cells is thought to result from several factors, including exposure to chronic irritants, chemicals, radiation, infectious agents, and genetic aberrations. Cancer cells are similar to normal cells in their basic biology and biochemistry, but regulation of their proliferation and differentiation is defective. Cells taken from malignant tumors typically differ from normal tissue cells in several ways. They are less sensitive to differentiation-inducing factors, and they can divide indefinitely. Also, key regulatory factors (i.e., oncogenes, tumor suppressor genes, and cyclins) are altered in cancer cells (Merkle, 2010).

Cancer presents as a complex series of diseases involving multiple steps. In addition, there is often an interaction among multiple risk factors (e.g., genetics, hormonal factors, immunologic mechanisms, radiation, or cancer-causing viruses) or repeated exposure to a single carcinogenic agent (e.g., asbestos, nicotine). It is thought to begin with an event that leaves a cell premalignant; this is followed by a number of promotional steps that increase the potential for an initiated cell to become malignant. The strong age correlation (i.e., incidence increases with age) supports the concept that most cancers result from the cumulative impact of multiple exposures over the lifetime (Merkle, 2010).

One theory of cancer development suggests that cancer arises as a series of genetic errors (Cavence & White, 1995). In this theory, there are three stages of cancer development: (1) initiation (referred to as the original genetic error), (2) promotion (genetic changes that continue and favor uncontrolled growth and metastasis), and (3) progression or latency (uncontrolled growth and full-blown malignant activity) (Figure 15-4).

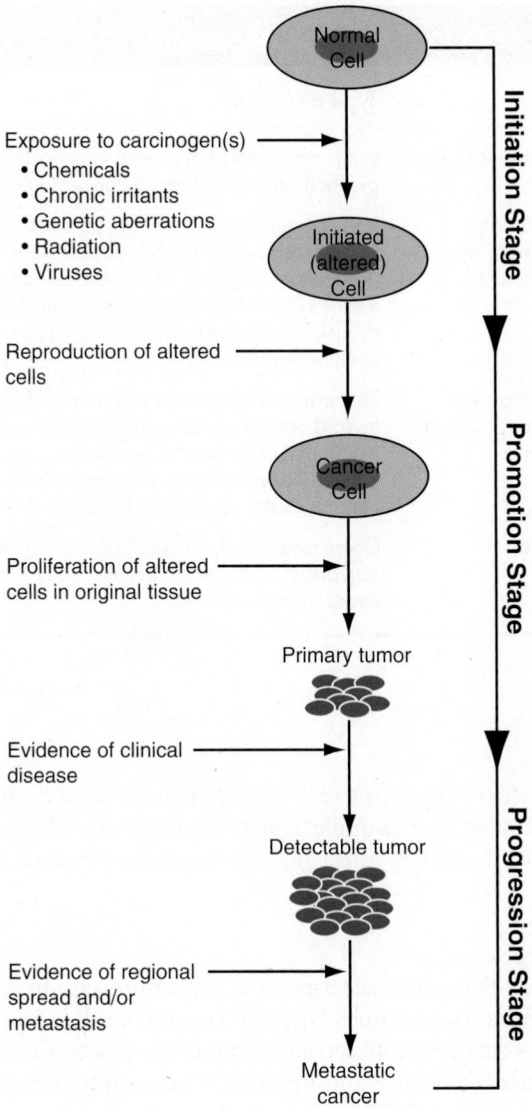

Figure 15-4 Process of cancer development.

This theory of cancer development states that cancer begins with one change in a normal cell. That change may alter cell production or cell function. This initiated cell may undergo additional malignant changes, especially if the environment supports the malignant activity. The cancer process can be stopped during the initiation stage, and even in the promotion stage, if the cellular environment is enabled to repair or control the carcinogenic genetic alteration (Banasik, 2010c).

Between 30% and 40% of all cancer deaths are preventable by modifying lifestyle factors, such as tobacco and alcohol use and diet. For example, it is thought that combined exposure to alcohol and smoking accounts for approximately 75% of all oral and pharyngeal cancers. Alcohol alone contributes to about 3% of all instances of colon, colorectal, esophageal, pancreatic, prostate, and breast cancers (Blattner, 2000). Table 15-3 lists some of the lifestyle, therapeutic, environmental, and host factors that appear to affect the development of cancer.

Theories dealing with cancer have been tested in a multitude of studies, with a goal of identifying the cause(s) of cancer, improving care, and ultimately finding

Table 15-3 Factors That Contribute to Cancer Development

Factor	Examples	Type of Cancer
Lifestyle factors	Use of tobacco and alcohol, diet	Lung, oral, and pharyngeal cancers (smoking and alcohol); colon and rectal cancer (alcohol, diet)
Therapeutic factors	Medically prescribed drugs (hormones, anticancer drugs, immunosuppressive agents)	Vaginal and cervical cancer (in *utero* exposure to diethylstilbestrol [DES]), endometrial cancer (synthetic estrogens), breast cancer (possible link to use of synthetic estrogens), leukemia (some anticancer drugs), non-Hodgkin lymphoma (drug-induced immunosuppression)
Environmental factors	Ionizing radiation, ultraviolet radiation, occupation, pollution, some infectious agents	Skin cancers (ultraviolet radiation), leukemia and thyroid cancer (ionizing radiation), lung cancer (some occupations and pollutants), cervical cancer (some subtypes of human papillomavirus), hepatocellular carcinoma (hepatitis B and C viruses)
Host factors	Inherent sensitivities to carcinogenesis	Colon and rectal cancers (familial adenomatous polyposis), site-specific breast cancers, cancer of the ovary, retinoblastoma

Source: Blattner (2000).

cures. Studies that provided a basis for a relationship between lifestyle and cancer prevention have been conducted. For example, a growing body of evidence suggests that food choices may have a protective effect on carcinogenesis (Causey & Greenwald, 2011; Kushi et al., 2012).

Application to Nursing

Several works were found that addressed aspects of cancer prevention and how nurses can promote these activities. For example, Nguyen-Truong, Lee-Lin, and Gedaly-Duff (2013) looked at factors that promote secondary prevention activities related to cancer (e.g., colorectal cancer screening and hepatitis B screening) among Vietnamese Americans. Gonzalez and team (2012) also looked at interventions to promote colorectal screening, this time among Hispanics, and another work examined nursing interventions to increase women's intention to get Pap smears (Guvenc, Akyuz, & Yenen, 2013). Lastly, Jacobson (2013) reviewed protocols and recommnedations to give nurses more information on how to assist men to determine whether and when to be screened for prostate cancer.

An example of primary prevention for cancer was presented by Chan, Chan, Ng, and Wong (2012), who performed a systematic literature review on women's knowledge and attitudes toward human papillomavirus (HPV) vaccination; they determined that women were quite knowledgeable and positively predisposed toward obtaining HPV vaccination. Another interesting look at primary prevention of cancer by nurses was presented by Rosenberg (2013) as she reviewed evidence of the relationship between cell phone use and brain cancer. Citing a number of recent studies, she summarized interventions to reduce exposure of children to radio frequency radiation and thereby potentially preventing associated brain cancer. Finally, Jablonski and Duke (2012) presented a tertiary prevention look at how to best manage pain in cancer patients living in rural areas.

Pain Management

Pain is a phenomenon that has received a great deal of attention in health care. Early pain theories emphasized the specific pathways of pain transmission. Later theories attempted to uncover the complexity of central processing of pain in specific areas of the brain. The specificity theory of pain, for example, was proposed in the early 1800s. The theory was based on the recognition that free nerve endings exist in the periphery of the body and suggested that there are highly specific structures and pathways responsible for pain transmission. These nerve endings act as pain receptors that are capable of accepting sensory input and transmitting this information along specific nerve fibers. This theory set the stage for further studies on pain and pain management (Keene, McMenamin, & Polomano, 2002).

A biochemical theory of pain perception was proposed in the 1970s following identification of endorphins and opioid receptors. This theory postulates that morphine-like substances attach to pain receptors to modulate or decrease pain. Endorphin, which is synthesized in the pituitary and basal hypothalamus, is released into the bloodstream from the pituitary gland and mediates pain at the spinal cord level through circulating spinal fluid. Opioid receptors modulate pain by binding endogenous opioid peptides. When acute pain is elicited, endogenous opioids are released and are associated with the stress response to modulate or decrease pain. If pain-relieving medications are administered, they will attach to specified sites and result in pain relief. Pain can be controlled with drugs that bind to receptors (Litwack, 2009).

Gate Control Theory

The gate control theory (GCT) was proposed in 1965 to explain the relationship between pain and emotion. Melzack and Wall (1982) concluded that pain is not just a physiologic response but that psychological variables (i.e., behavioral and emotional responses) influence the perception of pain. According to the GCT, a gating mechanism occurs in the spinal cord. Pain impulses are transmitted from the periphery of the body by nerve fibers (A, delta, and C fibers). The impulses travel to the dorsal horns of the spinal cord, specifically to the area of the cord called the *substantia gelatinosa*. The cells of the *substantia gelatinosa* can inhibit or facilitate pain impulses that are conducted by the transmission cells. If the activity of the transmission cells is inhibited, the gate is closed and impulses are less likely to be conducted to the brain. When the gate is opened, pain impulses ascend to the brain. Similar gating mechanisms exist in the descending nerve fibers from the thalamus and cerebral cortex. A person's thoughts and emotions can influence whether pain impulses reach the level of conscious awareness (Helms & Barone, 2008; Litwack, 2009).

The gate control model (Figure 15-5) differentiates the excitatory (white circle) and inhibitory (black circle) links from the *substantia gelatinosa* to the transmission cells as well as descending inhibitory control from brain stem systems. The round knob at the end of the inhibitor link implies that its action may be presynaptic, postsynaptic, or both. All connections are excitatory, except the inhibitory link from *substantia gelatinosa* to the transmission cell (Melzack & Wall, 1982).

As mentioned in the case study, it is believed that pain medication has an effect on the gating mechanism. If pain medication is administered before the onset of pain (i.e., before the gate is opened), it will help keep the gate closed longer and fewer pain impulses will be allowed to pass through. The greater the degree of pain, the greater the number of pain impulses passing through the gate. If fewer pain impulses are allowed through the gate, the person will experience less pain. If the gate is allowed to open completely, a higher dosage of pain medication is required to close the gate. Therefore, in theory, prevention and management of pain are linked to keeping the gate closed.

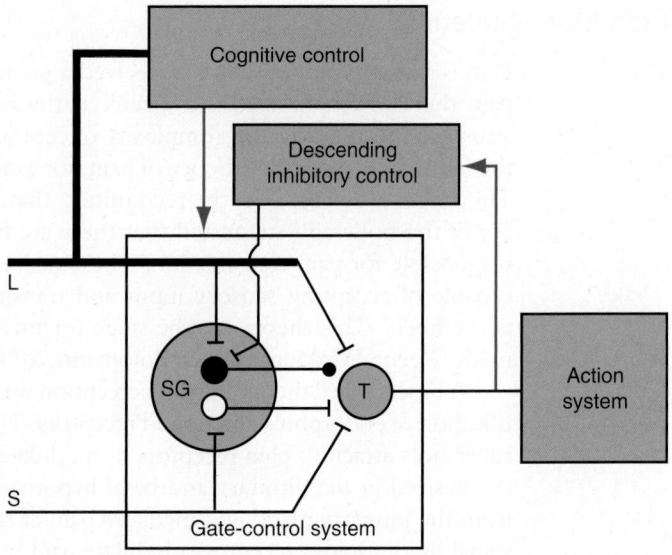

Figure 15-5 Gate control theory. ***L***, large-diameter fibers; ***S***, small-diameter fibers; ***SG***, *substantia gelatinosa;* ***T***, transmission. (Adapted with permission from Watt-Watson, J. H., & Donovan, M. I. (1992). *Pain management* (p. 20). St. Louis: Mosby.)

Application to Nursing

The GCT has also been the model for several reports related to pain management. Lane and Latham (2009), for example, presented aspects of the GCT in use of heat and cold therapy as nonpharmacologic interventions to reduce pain in hospitalized children. Tansky and Lindberg (2010) performed a comprehensive literature review on the use of breastfeeding as a intervention to reduce pain caused by immunization using the GCT as a framework. They found that there is considerable evidence that it is an effective pain management technique.

In nursing research, one study (Ngamkham, Holdern, & Wilkie, 2011) used the GCT to examine pain pattern responses in location, intensity, and quality among outpatients with cancer. Friesner, Curry, and Moddeman (2006) used GCT as the framework in a research study to compare two strategies for removal of chest tubes. They determined that encouraging slow, deep-breathing relaxation helps manage pain during chest tube removal. Finally, another experimental study, Hatfield (2008) showed that administration of an oral sucrose solution prior to immunization is effective in helping relieve pain in infants receiving routine vaccinations.

Summary

Nurses continually use concepts and principles from multiple biomedical theories in practice and in research. Indeed, these concepts, principles, and theories are so integral to nursing that they are difficult to differentiate and set aside for detailed inspection.

The biomedical theories used by nurses include theories of disease and disease causation, as well as theories related to physiology and physical functioning. Nurses, particularly advanced practice nurses such as Maria from the case study, should study these theories. They should understand their relevance to nursing practice and recognize how they are used and supported in nursing research.

Because of length constraints, only a few concepts and theories were described in this chapter. But it is hoped that these discussions will lead the reader to recognize the importance of understanding theory and to apply theory to guide practice and research. Ultimately, this will improve the care of clients.

Key Points

- Theories from the biomedical sciences have greatly influenced nursing since Nightingale's time.
- Biomedical science theories used by nurses include theories from biology, medicine, public health, physiology, and pharmacology.
- Theories and models of disease causation commonly used by nurses include the "germ theory" (principles of infection) and public health theories, such as the epidemiologic triangle and the web of causation.
- The Natural History of Disease model outlines the concepts of health promotion as well as primary, secondary, and tertiary prevention; these principles are used by nurses in all areas of practice and research.
- Theories and principles of physiology and physical functioning include homeostasis and theories of stress and adaptation; both are commonly used by nurses in practice and research.
- Theories and principles related to immunity and immune function are widely used in nursing practice and are increasingly being studied in nursing research.
- Nursing knowledge regarding genetics, genetic principles, and genetic counseling is growing, and nurses are recognizing the importance of genetic factors on health.
- Cancer theories, particularly related to prevention and early detection, are very important to nurses and a source for study for nursing research and review for nursing practice.
- Pain management is a vital part of nursing practice; nurses are continually researching how to improve pain management.

Learning Activities

1. Search current nursing journals for research studies that use epidemiologic, biologic, or physiologic theories as a framework. What theories are being tested?
2. Review the original work of one of the grand nursing theorists. Identify the epidemiologic, biologic, or physiologic concepts that are components of the theory.
3. Outline a potential research study using one of the theories or models presented in this chapter as a framework as depicted in the opening case study. Show how the model or theory can be used to generate testable hypotheses.

REFERENCES

Abraham, S. (2011). Fall prevention conceptal framework. *The Health Care Manager, 30*(2), 179–184.

Ardizzone, L. L., Smolowitz, J., Kline, N., Thom, B., & Larson, E. L. (2012). Patient hand hygiene practices in surgical patients. *American Journal of Infection Control, 41*(6), 487–491.

Banasik, J. L. (2010a). Inflammation and immunity. In L. C. Copstead & J. L. Banasik (Eds.), *Pathophysiology* (4th ed., pp. 181–221). Philadelphia: Saunders/Elsevier.

Banasik, J. L. (2010b). Genetics. In L. C. Copstead & J. L. Banasik (Eds.), *Pathophysiology* (4th ed., pp. 128–157). Philadelphia: Saunders/Elsevier.

Banasik, J. L. (2010c). Neoplasia. In L. C. Copstead & J. L. Banasik (Eds.), *Pathophysiology* (4th ed., pp. 128–157). Philadelphia: Saunders/Elsevier.

Beery, T. (2008). Genetics for advanced nursing practice. *The Nurse Practitioner, 33*(11), 10–18.

Bellar, A., Kunkler, K., & Burkett, M. (2009). Understanding, recognizing and managing chronic critical illness syndrome. *Journal of the American Academy of Nurse Practitioners, 21*(11), 571–578.

Black, J. M., & Hawks, J. H. (2009). *Medical surgical nursing: Clinical management for positive outcomes* (8th ed.). Philadelphia: Elsevier.

Blattner, W. A. (2000). Etiology of malignant disease. In H. D. Humes (Ed.), *Kelley's textbook of internal medicine* (4th ed., pp. 141–147). Philadelphia: Lippincott Williams & Wilkins.

Buet, A., Cohen, B., Marine, M., Scully, F., Alper, P., Simpser, E., et al. (2013). Hand hygiene opportunities in pediatric extended care facilities. *Journal of Pediatric Nursing, 28*(1), 72–76.

Calzone, K. I. A., Jenkins, J., Yates, J., Cusack, G., Wallen, G. R., Liewehr, D. J., et al. (2012). Survey of nursing integration of genomics into nursing practice. *Journal of Nursing Scholarship, 44*(4), 428–436.

Causey, C., & Greenwald, B. (2011). Promoting community awareness of the need for colorectal cancer prevention and screening: A replication study. *Gastroenterology Nursing, 34*(1), 34–40.

Cavence, W. K., & White, R. (1995). The genetic basis of cancer. *Scientific American, 272,* 72–79.

Carroll, E. W. (2009). Genetic control of cell function and inheritance. In C. M. Porth & G. Matfin (Eds.), *Pathophysiology: Concepts of altered health states* (8th ed., pp. 112–132). Philadelphia: Lippincott Williams & Wilkins.

Chan, Z. C. Y., Chan, T. S., Ng, K. K., & Wong, M. L. (2012). A systematic review of literature about women's knowledge and attitudes toward human papillomavirus (HPV) vaccination. *Public Health Nursing, 29*(6), 481–489.

Chen, Y. Y., Chi, M. M., Chen, Y. C., Chan, Y. U., Chou, S. S., & Wang, F. D. (2013). Using a criteria-based reminder to reduce use of indwelling urinary catheters and decrease urinary tract infections. *American Journal of Critical Care, 22*(2), 105–114.

D'Alonzo, K. T., Johnson, S., & Fanfan, D. (2012). A biobehavioral approach to understanding obesity and the development of obesogenic illness among Latino immigrants in the United States. *Biological Research for Nursing, 14*(4), 364–374.

DeLuca, J., Zanni, K. L., Bonhomme, N., & Kemper, A. R. (2013). Implications of newborn screening for nurses. *Journal of Nursing Scholarship, 45*(1), 25–33.

Donahue, M. P. (2011). *Nursing: The finest art* (3rd ed.). St. Louis: Mosby.

Emerson, R. J. (2010). Homeostasis and adaptive responses to stressors. In L. C. Copstead & J. L. Banasik (Eds.), *Pathophysiology* (4th ed., pp. 14–27). Philadelphia: Saunders/Elsevier.

Fletcher, B. J., Himmelfarb, C. D., Lira, M. T., Meininger, J. C., Pradhan, S. R., & Sikkema, J. (2011). Global cardiovascular disease prevention: A call to action for nursing; community-based and public health prevention initiatives. *Journal of Cardiovascular Nursing, 26*(45), S35–S45.

Frazier, L., Johnson, R. L., & Sparks, E. (2005). Genomics and cardiovascular disease. *Journal of Nursing Scholarship, 37*(4), 315–321.

Friesner, S. T., Curry, D. M., & Moddeman, G. R. (2006). Comparison of two pain-management strategies during chest tube removal: Relaxation exercise with opioids and opioids alone. *Heart & Lung, 35*(4), 269–276.

Ganz, F. D. (2012). Tend and befriend in the intensive care unit. *Critical Care Nurse, 32*(3), 25–33.

Garcia, S. P. Q., Greco, K. E., & Loescher, L. J. (2011). Teaching strategies to incorporate genomics education into academic nursing curricula. *Journal of Nursing Education, 50*(11), 612–629.

Gonzalez, S. A., Ziebarth, T. H., Wang, J., Noor, A. B., & Springer, D. L. (2012). Interventions promoting colorectal cancer screening in the Hispanic population: A review of the literature. *Journal of Nursing Scholarship, 44*(4), 332–340.

Guvenc, G., Akyuz, A., & Yenen, M. C. (2013). Effectiveness of nursing interventions to increase pap smear test screening. *Research in Nursing & Health, 36*(2), 146–157.

Hatfield, L. A. (2008). Sucrose decreases infant biobehavioral pain response to immunizations: A randomized controlled trial. *Journal of Nursing Scholarship, 40*(3), 219–225.

Helms, J. E., & Barone, C. P. (2008). Physiology and treatment of pain. *Critical Care Nurse, 28*(6), 38–47.

Holmes, T., & Rahe, E. (1967). The social readjustment rating scale. *Journal of Psychosomatic Research, 11,* 213.

Hughes, D., Ladas, E. L., Rooney, D., & Kelly, K. (2008). Massage therapy as a supportive care intervention for children with cancer. *Oncology Nursing Forum, 35*(3), 431–436.

Jablonski, K., & Duke, G. (2012). Pain management in persons who are terminally ill in rural acute care: Barriers and facilitators. *Journal of Hospice & Palliative Nursing, 14*(8), 533–540.

Jacobson, J. (2013). Navigating the PSA screening dilemma. *AJN, 113*(1), 19–21.

Johnson, N. L., Giarelli, E., Lewis, C., & Rice, C. E. (2013). Genomics and autism spectrum disorder. *Journal of Nursing Scholarship, 45*(1), 69–78.

Jones-Parker, H. (2012). Primary, secondary, and tertiary prevention of cardiovascular disease in patients with HIV disease: A guide for nurse practitioners. *Journal of the Association of Nurses in AIDS Care, 23*(2), 124–133.

Kalisch, P. A., & Kalisch, B. J. (2004). *American nursing: A history* (4th ed.). Philadelphia: Lippincott Williams & Wilkins.

Kang, D. H., McArdle, T., Weaver, M. T., Smith, B., & Carpenter, J. (2011). Dose effects of relaxation practice on immune responses in women newly diagnosed with breast cancer: An exploratory study. *Oncology Nursing Forum, 38*(3), E240–E252.

Keene, A., McMenamin, E. M., & Polomano, R. C. (2002). Pain. In D. D. Ignatavicius & M. L. Workman (Eds.), *Medical-surgical nursing: Critical thinking for collaborative care* (4th ed., pp. 61–94). Philadelphia: Saunders.

Kirk, M., Lea, D., & Skirton, H. (2008). Genomic health care: Is the future now? *Nursing and Health Sciences, 10*(2), 85–92.

Kisiel, M., & Marsons, L. (2009). Recognizing and responding to hyperglycaemic emergencies. *British Journal of Nursing, 18*(8), 1094–1098.

KuKanich, K. S., Kaur, R., Freeman, L. C., & Powell, D. A. (2013). Evaluation of a hand hygiene campaign in outpatient health care clinics. *AJN, 113*(3), 36–43.

Kunert, M. P. (2009). Stress and adaptation. In C. M. Porth & G. Matfin (Eds). *Pathophysiology: Concepts of altered health states* (8th ed., pp. 198–212), Philadelphia: Lippincott Williams & Wilkins.

Kuo, E. S., Stoep, A. V., Herting, J. R., Grupp, K., & McCauley, E. (2013). How to identify students for school-based depression intervention: Can school record review be substituted for universal depression screening? *Journal of Child and Adolescent Psychiatric Nursing, 26*(1), 42–52.

Kushi, L. H., Doyle, C., McCullough, M., Rock, C. L., Demark-Wahnefried, W., Bandera, E. V., et al. (2012). American Cancer Society guidelines on nutrition and physical activity for cancer prevention: Reducing the risk of cancer with healthy food choices and physical activity. *CA: A Cancer Journal for Clinicians, 62*(1), 30–67.

Lane, E., & Latham, T. (2009). Managing pain using heat and cold therapy. *Paediatric Nursing, 21*(6), 14–18.

Leavell, H. R., & Clark, E. G. (1965). *Preventive medicine for the doctor in his community: An epidemiologic approach* (2nd ed.). New York: McGraw-Hill.

Li, J., & Zhou, L. (2011). Statins for the primary prevention of cardiovascular disease. *Journal of Cardiovascular Nursing, 26*(4), 288–289.

Lipsitz, L. A. (2001). Clinical physiology of aging. In H. D. Humes (Ed.), *Kelley's textbook of internal medicine* (4th ed., pp. 118–127). Philadelphia: Lippincott Williams & Wilkins.

Litwack, K. (2009). Somatosensory function, pain, and headache. In C. M. Porth & G. Matfin (Eds.), *Pathophysiology: Concepts of altered health states* (8th ed., pp. 1225–1259). Philadelphia: Lippincott Williams & Wilkins.

MacMahon, B., & Pugh, T. F. (1970). *Epidemiologic principles and methods.* Boston: Little, Brown.

Mahon, S. M. (2005). Tertiary prevention: Implications for improving the quality of life of long-term survivors of cancer. *Seminars in Oncology Nursing, 21*(4), 260–270.

Matthews, R., & Moore, A. (2013). Babies are still dying of SIDS: A safe sleep environment in child-care settings reduces risks. *AJN, 113*(2), 59–65.

McEwen, M., & Pullis, B. (2009). *Community-based nursing* (3rd ed.). Philadelphia: Saunders/Elsevier.

Meadows-Oliver, M. (2012). Screening for postpartum depression at pediatric visits. *Journal of Psychosocial Nursing, 50*(9), 4–5.

Melzack, R., & Wall, P. D. (1982). *The challenge of pain.* New York: Penguin Books.

Merkle, C. J. (2009). Neoplasia. In C. M. Porth & G. Matfin (Eds.), *Pathophysiology: Concepts of altered health states* (8th ed., pp. 156–196). Philadelphia: Lippincott Williams & Wilkins.

Millar, B. C., Loughrey, A., Bill, R., & Moore, J. E. (2011). Community-associated MRSA in primary care. *Practice Nursing, 22*(12), 662–664.

Morinec, J., Icaboni, J., & McNett, M. (2012). Risk factors and interventions for ventilator-associated pneumonia in pediatric patients. *Journal of Pediatric Nursing, 27*(5), 435–442.

Mulvihill, D. (2005). The health impact of childhood trauma: An interdisciplinary review, 1997–2003. *Issues in Comprehensive Pediatric Nursing, 28*(2), 115–136.

Murphy, R. J. (2012). Preventing multidrug-resistant gram-negative organisms in surgical patients. *AORN Journal, 96*(3), 315–329.

Ngamkham, S., Holden, J. E., & Wilkie, D. J. (2011). Differences in pain location, intensity, and quality by pain pattern in outpatients with cancer. *Cancer Nursing, 34*(3), 228–237.

Nguyen-Truong, C. K. Y., Lee-Lin, F., & Gedaly-Duff, V. (2013). Contributing factors to colorectal cancer and hepatitis B screening among Vietnamese Americans. *Oncology Nursing Forum, 40*(3), 238–251.

Nonnemacher, M., Stusberg, J., Bartoszek, G., Lottko, B., Neuhaeuser, M., & Maier, I. (2008). Predicting pressure ulcer risk: A multifactorial approach to assess risk factors in a large university hospital population. *Journal of Clinical Nursing, 18,* 99–107.

Okonta, N. R. (2012). Does yoga therapy reduce blood pressure in patient with hypertension? An integrative review. *Holistic Nursing Practice, 26*(3), 137–141.

Outland, L. (2010) Intuitive eating: A holistic approach to weight control. *Holistic Nursing Practice, 24*(1), 35–43.

Porth, C. M. (2009). Genetic and congenital disorders. In C. M. Porth & G. Matfin (Eds.), *Pathophysiology: Concepts of altered health states* (8th ed., pp. 133–155). Philadelphia: Lippincott Williams & Wilkins.

Prows, C. A., Hopkin, R. J., Barnoy, S., & Van Riper, M. (2013). An update of childhood genetic disorders. *Journal of Nursing Scholarship, 45*(1), 34–42.

Rentz, C. (2008). Nursing care of the person with sporadic Creutzfeldt–Jakob disease. *Journal of Hospice and Palliative Nursing, 10*(5), 272–284.

Riker, G. I., & Setter, S. M. (2012). Polypharmacy in older adults at home: What it is and what to do about it—Implications for home healthcare and hospice. *Home Healthcare Nurse, 30*(8), 474–485.

Rosenberg, S. (2013). Cell phones and children: Follow the precautionary road. *Pediatric Nursing, 39*(2), 65–70.

Ruiz, R. J., & Avant, K. C. (2005). Effects of maternal prenatal stress on infant outcomes: A synthesis of the literature. *Advances in Nursing Science, 28*(4), 345–355.

Santos, E. M. M., Edwards, Q. I., Floria-Santos, M., Rogatto, S. R., Achatz, M. I. W., & MacDonald, D. J. (2013). Integration of genomics in cancer care. *Journal of Nursing Scholarship, 45*(1), 43–51.

Scott, L. K, & Hall, L. M. (2012). Reliability and validity of the acanthosis nigricans screening tool for use in elementary school-age children by school nurses. *Journal of School Nursing, 28*(6), 442–447.

Seckel, M. A. (2013). Maintaining urinary catheters: What does the evidence say? *Nursing, 43*(2), 63–65.

Secker, T., Hervé, R., & Keevil, C. (2011). Adsorption of prion and tissue proteins to surgical stainless steel surfaces and the efficacy of decontamination following dry and wet storage conditions. *Journal of Hospital Infection Control, 78*(4), 251–255.

Selye, H. (1976). *Stress in health and disease.* Boston: Butterworths.

Shi, L., & Singh, D. A. (2012). *Delivering health care in American: A systems approach.* Burlington, MA: Jones & Bartlett.

Siegel, J. H. (2007). Predictors of overweight in children in grades six through eight. Doctoral dissertation, University of Miami.

Skirton, H., O'Connor, A., & Humphreys, A. (2012). Nurses' competence in genetics: A mixed method systematic review. *Journal of Advanced Nursing, 68*(11), 2387–2398.

Snow, D., & Lu, J. H. (2012). Genetics and genomics: Unraveling new opportunities for addiction treatment and education. *Journal of Addictions Nursing, 23,* 93–96.

Starkweather, A. (2013). Psychologic and biologic factors associated with fatigue in patients with persistent radiculopathy. *Pain Management Nursing, 14*(1), 41–49.

Starkweather, A., Witek-Janusek, L., & Mathews, H. L. (2005). Applying the psychoneuroimmunology framework to nursing research. *Journal of Neuroscience Nursing, 37*(1), 56–62.

Staniute, M., Brozaitiene, J., & Bunevicius, R. (2013). Effects of social support and stressful life events on health-related quality of life in coronary artery disease patients. *Journal of Cardiovascular Nursing, 28*(1), 83–89.

Stark, S. (2012). Elder abuse: Screening, intervention, and prevention. *Nursing 2012, 42*(10), 24–20.

Stride, P., Hunter, J., & Bailey, M. (2009). Nursing patients with Creutzfeldt-Jakob disease. Are you at risk? *Australian Nursing Journal, 17*(1), 30–32.

Tansky, C., & Lindberg, C. E.(2010). Breastfeeding as a pain intervention when immunizing infants. *The Journal for Nurse Practitioners–JNP, 6*(4), 287–295.

Upshaw-Owens, M., & Bailey, C. A. (2012). Preventing hospital-associated infection: MRSA. *MedSurg Nursing, 21*(2), 77–81.

Van Dyke, N. F. (2005). Domestic violence: Differences among rural, urban and suburban women. Doctoral dissertation, State University of New York at Binghamton.

Walker, D. K. (2012). Skin protection for (SPF) kids program. *Journal of Pediatric Nursing, 27*(3), 233–242.

Welsh, D. (2009). Predictors of depressive symptoms in female medical-surgical hospital nurses. *Issues in Mental Health Nursing, 30,* 320–326.

Workman, M. L. (2012). Concepts of inflammation and the immune response. In D. D. Ignatavicius & M. L. Workman (Eds.), *Medical surgical nursing: Critical thinking for collaborative care* (6th ed., pp. 307–327). Philadelphia: Saunders.

Yeo, S. A. (2011). A risk reduction model for late-onset preeclampsia: A theory for using low-intensity exercises to enhance cardiac homeostasis in nursing research and practice. *Advances in Nursing Science, 34*(1), 78–88.

CHAPTER 16

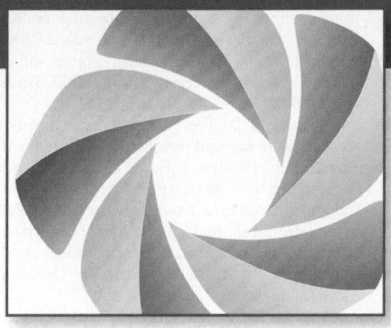

Theories, Models, and Frameworks From Leadership and Management

Melinda Granger Oberleitner

Richard Gomez, a cardiovascular clinical nurse specialist (CNS), was recently hired by a Magnet-aspiring hospital. Although he is experienced in the CNS role and is somewhat familiar with Magnet designation, he is not familiar with the expectations of the CNS practicing in a Magnet facility. As he reviews published literature related to outcomes associated with Magnet facilities, he envisions his role as that of clinical leader in performance improvement and in implementing best practices based on the latest clinical evidence. Although Richard does not consider his role to be that of an administrator or manager, he recognizes that as a clinical leader, the information he learned about leadership styles and leadership practices in graduate school (e.g., motivating people, implementing change, and leading performance improvement) will be especially helpful to him in reconceptualizing his role.

This case study illustrates a number of practical, conceptual, and theoretical issues related to administration and management. For example, is Richard considered a part of the management team? As an employee new to the unit and to the organization, how can Richard be an effective agent for change? How do performance improvement activities affect clinical care and standards of clinical care?

Nurses in management or leadership positions, regardless of role or practice setting, should have a working knowledge of theories, models, and frameworks of administration and management, which can help to guide practice. Further, even though advanced practice nurses (i.e., CNSs, nurse practitioners, and nurse midwives) are viewed primarily as clinicians, each role often has an administrative or management component. For example, the CNS, such as Richard, who is employed in a traditional acute care facility is often responsible for performance improvement activities related to a specific product or service line. A nurse practitioner in a rural clinic may have administrative responsibilities for ancillary and secretarial staff assigned to the clinic in addition to the responsibilities of a client care provider.

This chapter provides a foundation in administration for nurses in any setting. Topics presented are historical and contemporary theories and models of leadership and management, organizational theories, motivational theories, and theories related to power, change, decision-making processes, conflict management, quality control, and quality improvement (QI).

Overview of Concepts of Leadership and Management

Leadership and management are closely related and sometimes intertwined concepts. Leadership is the ability to influence followers, to inspire confidence, and to generate support among followers for the leader's direction and vision. Leadership is viewed as a component of management; however, it is not the same thing. Leaders empower others and lead others willingly; in simplistic terms, leadership usually involves one individual trying to change the behavior of others. Furthermore, leaders challenge the current or prevailing wisdom and, by doing so, create new meaning for members of an organization (Peters, 1987).

Leaders in an organization can be formal or informal. Formal leaders are appointed by official or legislative authority. Informal leaders derive power through influence and, in reality, may be more important to staff or groups than the formal, appointed, or designated leaders. Influencing followers is perhaps the most essential aspect of leadership. Leaders can influence others by utilization of their expertise, by charisma, by coercion, or, by virtue of the formal position they hold in organizations. Leaders who use expertise and charisma to influence others are the most effective in creating a sense of commitment in followers (Hellriegel, Jackson, & Slocum, 2008).

Management can be defined as the process of accomplishing work through and with other people. Effective management is often expected of a leader. In contrast to leaders, managers always have an official or appointed position within an organization through which they derive a legitimate source of power. Because of this official status, managers may direct willing and unwilling subordinates and are expected to perform specific, delineated functions, duties, and responsibilities. Effective leaders and managers are both required in today's workplace (DuBrin, 2007).

Early Leadership Theories

If one considers great historical leaders, names such as Alexander the Great, Julius Caesar, Napoleon Bonaparte, Thomas Jefferson, and Winston Churchill might come to mind. The Great Man Theory holds that leaders are born, not created. That is, certain individuals are born with the ability to lead, whereas most others are born to be led.

Trait Theories of Leadership

The Great Man Theory approach to defining leadership evolved into trait theories in the 1930s and 1940s. The trait theories assert that leaders possess certain characteristics (i.e., physical or personality traits and talents) that nonleaders do not.

Attributes, such as shyness, laziness, and aggressiveness, are considered the antithesis of characteristics a leader should possess. An example of a physical attribute associated with leadership is height (i.e., a tall person may be able to look down on others and, therefore, may cut an imposing figure of authority). The converse may be true as well. Some individuals believe if someone is born shorter than most people, the individual may have to be more assertive or aggressive and those behaviors may result in the development of a strong leader.

Personality traits or characteristics associated with leaders include intelligence, self-confidence, charisma, initiative, self-awareness, self-control, the ability to communicate effectively with individuals and in groups, goal orientation, self-directedness, the ability to assume consequences for actions and decisions, and the ability to tolerate stress. In lesser leadership positions, technical competence is important because it would be difficult to establish rapport with group members if the leader did not understand the technical details of the work (DuBrin, 2007). For example, Richard, as a CNS whose clinical area of expertise is cardiovascular nursing, would probably have a difficult time assuming the position of Director of Neuroscience Services because of the level of technical expertise required in neuroscience nursing.

Research studies designed to test trait theories of leadership have been inconsistent. The trait theories are limited by focusing only on leadership characteristics to the exclusion of the environment, the situation, and other possible confounding variables. Additionally, they focus on the attributes the leader brings to a particular situation rather than focusing on what specific actions the leader takes to address the situation.

Research attempts to identify traits consistently associated with leadership over time have been successful. Six traits have been identified that seem to best delineate the differences between leaders and nonleaders. These leader traits are the desire to lead, honesty and integrity, self-confidence, drive, intelligence, and job-relevant knowledge (Drafke, 2009).

Emotional Intelligence

An interest in the inner or personal qualities of leaders has recently reemerged, particularly with respect to ethical qualities and charisma. This interest has been fueled by the demand for leaders with vision and charisma. Personality traits and characteristics have an important influence on leader effectiveness. The traits and characteristics that are most relevant tend to vary with the situation at hand. A foundational trait for leadership effectiveness that does not vary from situation to situation is self-awareness (DuBrin, 2007).

Self-awareness is one of the four key factors in emotional intelligence (EI). According to Goleman, Boyatzis, and McKee (2001), EI is a major contributor to leader effectiveness. The concept of EI refers to managing one's self and one's relationships effectively. EI includes the abilities of self-confidence, empathy, and visionary leadership. Passion for the work and for the people who do the work is particularly important to a leader with a high degree of EI. It is difficult, if not impossible, to inspire or motivate others if the leader is not passionate about the major work activities. The leader with high EI is able to sense and articulate a group's shared, yet possibly unexpressed, feelings and is able to develop a mission that inspires others to achieve a common goal (DuBrin, 2007). EI includes understanding one's own feelings, sensitivity, and empathy for others and the regulation of emotions.

Goleman and colleagues (2001) define four key competencies of EI:

- Self-awareness—the ability to understand and modulate one's own emotions. Goleman and colleagues (2001) contend this is the most essential of the four major competencies. A self-aware individual knows his or her own strengths and weaknesses and has a high level of self-esteem. The self-aware leader seeks feedback continually to determine how well his or her actions and decisions are received by others.

- Self-management/self-control—the ability to control one's emotions; control over mood and temper. The leader who is self-controlled acts with honesty and integrity in a consistent and dependable manner.
- Social awareness—the leader has empathy for others, including subordinates, and is intuitive about organizational "political" forces. The socially aware leader shows genuine care for others in the organization.
- Social skills/relationship skills—the ability to communicate clearly and convincingly. The leader who has social and relationship skills disarms conflicts; builds strong personal and professional bonds; uses social skills to spread enthusiasm and to solve disagreements and problems; uses kindness and humor often; and constantly expands network of contacts and supporters within and outside of the organization (DuBrin, 2007; Hellriegel et al., 2008).

Goleman and colleagues (2001) discovered that the most effective leaders are alike in one essential way—they all possess a high degree of EI. Without a high degree of EI, some experts contend a leader will never become a great leader (DuBrin, 2007).

Behavioral Theories of Leadership

Movement away from trait theories to explain and define leadership began as early as the 1940s. Leadership research from the 1940s through the mid-1960s focused instead on behavioral styles that leaders demonstrated (i.e., specific behaviors of leaders that make some more effective than others) (Hitt, Black, & Porter, 2009). This set of theories is referred to as the behavioral or functional theory of leadership. The major difference between trait theories and behavioral theories is that trait theories are concerned with the leader's individual characteristics, whereas behavioral theories seek to explain specific actions taken by the leader (Wagner & Hollenbeck, 2010).

Lewin and Lippitt conducted some of the first studies of leadership behavior at the University of Iowa in the late 1930s. The researchers, using an after-school study group of 20 boys, aged 11 years, explored autocratic, democratic, and laissez-faire leadership behaviors or styles. The results of this study revealed that when the boys had a democratic leader, groups were more cohesive, the boys were more motivated, and originality of work was higher. With a democratic leader, the boys produced less work, but the work was of a higher quality than the work produced when the group leader used an authoritarian or laissez-faire leadership style. Nineteen of the 20 boys preferred the democratic style of group leadership over the other two styles (Lewin & Lippitt, 1938).

Other studies of autocratic versus democratic leadership styles concluded that democratic leadership styles produced higher performance results in some studies, whereas in other studies, performance was higher in groups with an authoritarian leader. However, what was consistent among study groups was that the level of satisfaction of group members was higher with the democratic style of leadership than with other styles.

Tannenbaum and Schmidt (1973) further explored satisfaction with leader style and developed a model known as the continuum of leader behavior. This model provides for a range of leadership behaviors from leader centered (autocratic) to employee centered (laissez-faire). In determining which leader behavior the manager should implement, the authors proposed that the manager evaluate the following three variables: characteristics of the manager (i.e., experience with a certain leadership style), characteristics of the employees (i.e., level of experience with the process/job), and characteristics of the situation (i.e., offering a new product or service for the first time). Tannenbaum and Schmidt (1973) recommended an employee-centered approach or style because this approach most often led to increased employee satisfaction, motivation, and high performance and quality of the work product.

Leader–Member Exchange Theory

Leader–Member Exchange (LMX) Theory was developed by George Graen and James Cashman. The central focus of LMX theory is the relationship and interaction between the supervisor (leader) and the subordinate (group member). The exchange between the superior and the subordinate is the unique, underlying premise of LMX. Interest in LMX has increased in recent years, leading to many field studies to test the propositions of the theory.

The theory recognizes that superiors develop unique working relationships with each subordinate or group member. According to LMX theory, leaders categorize subordinates into one of two groups: the in-group (high-quality relationship with the leader) or the out-group (low-quality relationship). Often, the leader's first impression of the subordinate's competence heavily influences the leader's assignment of the subordinate to the in- or the out-group. The theory proposes that leaders do not interact with subordinates equally because supervisors have limited time and resources (Graen & Cashman, 1975).

Members of the in-group often have attitudes and values similar to the leader and interact frequently with the leader. They have a special exchange or relationship with the leader. In-group members perform their jobs in accordance with the expectations of their employment contracts. In addition, they can be counted on by the leader to volunteer for extra work and to take on additional tasks and responsibilities. As a result, in-group members are given additional rewards (increased job latitude, extra attention from the leader, and inside information that is not available to all employees), responsibility, and trust by the supervisor in exchange for their loyalty and performance. Research on LMX in field studies reveals that members of the in-group enjoy higher degrees of autonomy, job satisfaction, and trust from the supervisor as compared to members of the out-group.

Out-group members have less in common with the leader and are detached from the leader. There is limited reciprocal trust and support in the leader–subordinate relationship. Members of the out-group receive few rewards from supervisors and are more likely to quit because of job dissatisfaction.

Supervisors who aspire to be the most effective leaders create a special exchange relationship with all of their subordinates (Graen & Uhl-Bien, 1995; Wang, Law, Hackett, Wang, & Chen, 2005). The intent is not necessarily to treat all employees the same. Those subordinates who by virtue of their position in the organization have greater responsibility or administrative authority will have a deeper level of exchange with the superior. However, it is possible and highly desirable that the leader engender relationships of mutual trust, respect, and support with all followers.

LMX theory postulates that the quality of the subordinate's relationship with the supervisor has a large impact on job behavior and performance and that the quality of that relationship has important job consequences (Bolino, 2007). Therefore, it is imperative that subordinates be evaluated based on their competencies rather than on the leader's favoritism (Graen & Uhl-Bien, 1995).

Motivational Theories of Leadership

The motivational theories expanded on the behavioral theories of leadership by focusing on factors that enhance worker/employee satisfaction and motivation and identifying factors that have a negative impact on those factors. Many of the motivational theories were based on the work of Maslow's Hierarchy of Needs Theory (1968). Maslow's work included the concepts of five basic needs (i.e., physiologic, safety, love, esteem, and self-actualization), which he described as being the driving forces or motivators of human behavior. Lower level physiologic needs, including food and rest, must be satisfied before an individual can work on accomplishing higher level needs such as self-esteem and self-actualization. Even though his theory was derived as a motivational theory, Maslow's early works were not originally applied to motivation in the workplace.

Theory X and Theory Y

Douglas McGregor first published his work on Theory X and Theory Y in an article in 1957. McGregor was influenced by the works of Maslow, Herzberg, Argyris, and Likert. McGregor believed the structure of bureaucratic organizations, as well as prevailing management philosophy and policies, resulted in a situation in which power resided exclusively with management. In this structure, the role of management was to direct workers under the assumption that all workers were unmotivated, unambitious, lazy, and preferred to be led. These assumptions were labeled by McGregor as Theory X. McGregor's theory was that workers who had no input in the performance of the job lacked interest in the job and satisfaction with the work, resulting in resistance to change.

McGregor proposed a different set of assumptions and practices for meeting organizational goals in a more effective, humanistic manner; he designated this Theory Y. Management's priorities in Theory Y are to develop worker potential, remove obstacles, create opportunities for worker growth, and provide guidance, rather than control direction, for the worker. Theory Y encourages worker responsibility and participation in decision making. McGregor believed this style of participatory management would result in greater productivity, creativity, and worker satisfaction.

Because McGregor failed to operationalize concepts in his theories, there have been few direct tests of his theories. When the theories were tested, conflicting results were obtained (Caplan, 1971; Gray, 1978; Green, 1981; Kay, 1973; Malone, 1975; Morse & Lorsch, 1970). Most recently, Kopelman, Prottas, and Davis (2008) attempted to test the substantive validity of McGregor's theory by measuring the focal construct of the central concept utilizing an investigator-developed Theory X/Y attitude measure. The researchers viewed this as a critical first step in testing the many assumptions of the theory. The new measure is content valid and has adequate reliability. Finally, although a few contemporary companies are using Theory X management, many companies subscribe to the tenets of Theory Y (Daft & Marcic, 2009).

Motivation–Hygiene Theory (Herzberg's Two-Factor Theory)

Motivation–hygiene, or two-factor theory, was established by psychologist Frederick Herzberg in 1959. Herzberg sought to describe the differences between factors that are true motivators for individuals (i.e., recognition for a job well done, opportunities for promotion or advancement, challenging and rewarding work) and hygiene or maintenance factors. Examples of hygiene or maintenance factors include salary, quality of supervision, interpersonal relationships with coworkers, and good working conditions (Herzberg, 1966).

According to Herzberg (1966), hygiene factors, although they keep workers from becoming dissatisfied, do not act as real motivators. Hygiene factors are most often extrinsic and usually cannot be changed by employee behaviors; hygiene factors do not motivate employees. Motivators are most often intrinsic factors and are correlated with increased job satisfaction. Thus, when managers want to motivate employees, motivators should be emphasized.

Contingency Theories of Leadership: Leadership and Management by Situation

As research into leadership became increasingly complex, it was recognized that leader characteristics, traits, and behaviors were not sufficient to explain the concept. The focus of research then shifted to include components of the situation or the environment into the equation as well. In other words, various external factors, such as conditions in the situation and the nature of the task to be accomplished, help to determine the leadership style that would be most effective in a particular situation.

The Fiedler Contingency Theory of Leadership

One of the earlier efforts to address contingencies in leadership situations was the Fiedler Contingency Theory of Leadership (Fiedler, 1967). Fiedler, Chemers, and Mahar (1976) state:

> *This theory holds that the effectiveness of a group or organization depends on two interacting or 'contingent' factors. The first is the personality of the leaders to determine their leadership style. The second factor is the amount of control and influence which the situation provides leaders over the group's behavior, the task, and the outcome. This factor is called situational control* (p. 3).

Fiedler (1967) developed the Least Preferred Coworker (LPC) Scale to determine and classify leadership styles. The instrument, an 18-item semantic differential scale, uses contrasting adjectives (e.g., friendly/unfriendly, open/guarded, and insincere/sincere) to direct the leader to describe an LPC. From the leader's responses on the scale, an LPC score is obtained. A leader with a high LPC score describes an LPC in a generally favorable manner. Fiedler believed this leader tends to be relationship oriented and considerate about the feelings of coworkers. Conversely, a leader with a low LPC score would be described by Fiedler as task oriented. Leaders who fall in the midrange of scores are a mix of the two types of leaders and should determine for themselves to which group they ultimately belong. Fiedler's assumption is that a leader's style is innately either relationship or task oriented and that style cannot be changed as the situation changes (Fiedler et al., 1976).

Once the leader's style has been determined by the LPC score, the next step is to match or fit the leader with the situation. Fiedler used the term "situational control" to describe three major group classifications or variables that may be used to evaluate an individual situation (Box 16-1).

Box 16-1 Group Classifications

- *Leader–member relations*: Confidence in the leader and support of the group is effective in influencing the group's performance. (This is the most important factor in determining the leader's control and influence over the group.)
- *Task structure*: Structure of the task is on a continuum from a well-defined, step-by-step procedure to a vague and undefined one.
- *Position power*: Authority is vested in the leader's position by the organization.

Leader–member relations can be classified as good or poor, task structure as high or low, and position power as strong or weak. According to Fiedler, the better the leader–member relations, the higher the task structure; the stronger the position power, the more control or influence the leader has. For example, a nurse who is in an autonomous position as the vice president of patient care services (strong position power) is highly respected (good leader–member relations) by a group of nurse practitioners (high task structure) and is employed by the hospital is influential to the nurse practitioner group.

In Fiedler's studies of more than 1,200 groups since the 1950s, the low LPC leader (task oriented) has been found to be most effective in very favorable situations (position power is strong and leader–member relations are strong) and in very unfavorable situations (position power is weak and leader–member relations are weak). Also, the low LPC leader is most effective when tasks are clear and highly structured. The high LPC leader (relationship oriented) is most effective in moderately favorable situations when position power is weak, task structure is low, and leader–member relations are good (Hitt et al., 2009).

Numerous studies have been undertaken to test the validity of the contingency model's assumptions (Chemers, Harp, Rhodewalt, & Wysocki, 1985; Fiedler, 1969; Minor, 1980). These comprehensive studies, including a meta-analysis of 125 tests of the contingency model, provide strong support for the model's validity.

Path–Goal Theory

Robert House (1971, 1996) developed the Path–Goal Theory as an extension of the earlier work of Georgopoulos, Mahoney, and Jones (1957) and from research related to the expectancy theories of motivation (Vroom, 1964). Situational factors that are examined in this theory include the nature and scope of the task to be accomplished, the employee's perceptions and expectations of the task, and the role of the leader in the work process. Expectations of the leader in this theory are to assist followers in determining and attaining goals and to provide the necessary direction and support to ensure that employee goals are compatible with those of the organization. The role of the leader is also to provide motivation and some type of reward (i.e., recognition for the employee once the task has been completed or the goal has been reached) (Podsakoff, Bommer, Podsakoff, & Mackenzie, 2005). The leader is responsible for helping the employee determine and clarify the path the worker is to take to reach the goal. An important aspect of the leader's role is to identify and remove obstacles from the path of the worker to enable him or her to successfully attain the goal.

House (1971) identified four leadership behaviors to test the assumptions of his theory. The *directive* leader provides specific guidance and direction to workers on how the task is to be accomplished; the *supportive* leader is concerned with the accomplishment of the task as well as the needs of the worker; the *participative* leader involves workers in making decisions about how the task or goal should be accomplished; and the *achievement-oriented* leader sets challenging goals and has high expectations that employees will perform at the highest level. House assumes leaders are flexible and are able to use any of these leadership behaviors as the situation warrants.

The Path–Goal Theory also proposes two sets or classes of situational or contingency variables that influence the relationship between the leadership behavior and the outcomes. These two variables are environmental variables (those outside of the control of the employee) and variables that are part of the personal attributes of the employee. Examples of environmental variables include the nature and structure of the task or the goal to be accomplished and the composition of the work group to which the employee has been assigned. Employee contingency factors include ability, locus of control, and experience. House (1971) proposed that employee performance and satisfaction are enhanced when the leader is able to compensate in some way for any shortcomings with either the employee or the work setting.

Path–goal theory remains one of the most respected approaches to understanding leadership. Research related to the path–goal model is generally supportive of the major assumptions of the model (Robbins & Coulter, 2005; Schriesheim, Castro, Zhou, & DeChurch, 2006; Vecchio, Justin, & Pearce, 2008).

Situational Leadership Theory

Situational leadership, developed by Paul Hersey and Kenneth Blanchard in the 1970s, is a contingency theory that examines the relationship among three concepts of management: task behavior, relationship behavior, and maturity level of the follower or worker. *Task behavior* is the amount of direction given by the leader to ensure that the task is accomplished. *Relationship behavior* is the amount of emotional support and energy the leader provides to the follower or worker. According to Hersey and Blanchard (1977), task behavior and relationship behavior are directly related to the *maturity level* exhibited by the employee toward the job or task.

Leaders must adjust leadership style depending on the maturity level of the employee. That is, a more directive leadership style is required with an immature worker and a less directive style is adequate for a mature worker. In this theory, a mature employee or worker is described as one who has the willingness, capacity, and initiative to set goals for himself or herself and to accomplish tasks with minimal direction. The immature employee requires more direction from the leader to accomplish the task or objective.

A worker's maturity level is not fixed or constant. Maturity levels may change when the task or objective changes; therefore, a worker's maturity level may be placed on a continuum from immature to mature. Frequent assessments of the follower or worker by the leader are necessary for the appropriate leadership style to be used.

In this theory, the leader must be able to adapt leadership styles to meet individual and situational demands. If workers in a situation are immature, the leader should provide a high level of task direction and a low level of support or relationship behavior. As the worker matures, the reverse may be true (i.e., with a mature worker, the leader's task direction decreases and relationship behavior increases). Eventually, the mature worker may need minimal task direction and relationship support from the leader (DuBrin, 2009).

Contemporary Leadership Theories

Since the late 1970s, theories of leadership have expanded the number of variables that affect effective leadership. These variables include increasing complexities of the work environment, the culture of the organization, values of the organization, leaders and followers within the organization, and the influence of the leader/manager (Vroom & Jago, 2007). Transactional and transformational leadership, authentic leadership, charismatic leadership, and visionary leadership are considered the leading, emerging contemporary leadership theories.

Transactional and Transformational Leadership

Burns (1978), a scholar in the area of leader–follower interactions, maintained that there are two types of leaders in management, the transactional leader and the transformational leader. The transactional leader is viewed as the traditional manager, a manager who is concerned with day-to-day operations. The transformational leader is a long-term visionary who can inspire and empower others with his or her vision (Avolio, Zhu, Koh, & Puja, 2004; Bass, Avolio, Jung, & Berson, 2003; Bono & Judge, 2003; Schaubroeck, Lam, & Cha, 2007; Walumbwa, Avolio, & Zhu, 2008).

Characteristics of transformational leaders include strong commitment to the profession and to the organization, the ability to help their followers look at old problems in new ways, as well as the ability to excite and motivate followers to produce extra effort to achieve group goals. The hallmark of the transformational leader is vision and the ability to communicate that vision to others so that it becomes a shared vision. This shared vision between leader and follower is translated as inspiring movement to achieve a common cause or a common goal for the organization. Research studies conducted in various settings such as in the military and business sectors support the effectiveness of transformational leadership as compared to transactional leadership in regard to employee performance and satisfaction (Robbins & Coulter, 2005).

Transformational leadership is built on transactional leadership (Judge & Piccolo, 2004). Transformational and transactional leadership should not be viewed as opposing forces (Robbins & Coulter, 2005). Contemporary management theorists caution that characteristics of both transactional and transformational leadership must be in the repertoire of the effective leader to accomplish the goals of the organization (Washington, 2007).

The concept of transformational leadership is one of the most widely researched concepts in the field of leadership (Harms & Crede, 2010). Research has validated the positive relationship between transformational leadership style and the performance and effectiveness of the leader. In addition, the impact of transformational leadership on follower satisfaction and motivation has also been extensively studied and positively validated (Judge & Piccolo, 2004).

Some contend that EI is an antecedent of transformational leadership. The concept of EI as it relates to leadership ability, especially transformational leadership, has been researched extensively in the past few years with mixed results. For example, Harms and Crede (2010) reported the results of a meta-analysis conducted to determine whether EI is related to transformational leadership and, if so, to what extent. Results indicated a moderate relationship between EI and transformational leadership and suggested that EI may contribute to successful leadership. The authors caution, however, that the results of this study also seem to suggest that commonly marketed EI assessment tools, which are often used by organizations for management screening or training, should not be overemphasized and should be used only for self-awareness and self-reflection until better screening tools are available and have been psychometrically validated and empirically tested (Harms & Crede, 2010).

The results of Lindebaum and Cartwright's (2010) research revealed that when using a strong methodologic design to evaluate the relationship between EI and transformational leadership, no relationship between EI and transformational leadership is found. Conversely, the results of another meta-analysis conducted by O'Boyle, Humphrey, Pollack, Hawver, and Story (2011) validated the relationship between EI and job performance and supported the overall validity of EI.

Authentic Leadership

Authentic leadership is a construct derived from the works of the humanistic psychologists, particularly Carl Rogers and Abraham Maslow, who focused on the human potential for achieving self-actualization. Maslow (1971) viewed the self-actualized person as someone who has full personal awareness, holds an accurate self-picture of his or her capabilities, upholds the highest ethical standards, and is not easily swayed or influenced by others. Early application of the concept of authentic leadership occurred in the disciplines of sociology and education (Avolio & Gardner, 2005).

Shamir and Eilam (2005) advance four characteristics of authentic leaders. This type of leader:

1. Does not change to meet the expectations of others; he or she remains constant in his or her convictions.
2. Is not preoccupied with attempting to achieve higher personal status or honors.
3. Makes leadership decisions based on his or her personal point of view and not based on what he or she thinks others would want him or her to do.
4. Bases actions on personal values and belief systems.

Others have extended Shamir and Eilam's definition of authentic leadership by including a positive moral perspective as another dimension or characteristic of the authentic leader (Luthans & Avolio, 2003; May, Chan, Hodges, & Avolio, 2003).

Charismatic Leadership

Charismatic leadership is an extension of attribution theory, that is, followers attribute heroic or extraordinary leadership abilities when they observe certain behaviors in their leaders (Conger & Kanungo, 1988). Several researchers, including House (1977), Bennis (1984), Conger and Kanungo (1988), and Jens and Heinitz (2007), have attempted to describe and define attributes and characteristics of the charismatic leader. These characteristics include complete and compelling self-confidence in themselves and in their abilities, strong convictions and vision, and the ability to clearly and forcefully articulate that vision to others (Jung & Sosik, 2006).

Charismatic leaders are viewed as strong agents for change rather than as caretakers or managers of the current situation or environment. They are perceived as having behavioral characteristics that are unconventional and out of the ordinary. Charismatic leaders are risk takers and often arise from areas in society or business in which there is a common or shared ideology, such as the military, religious, political, or business sectors. These leaders often emerge when the organization has undergone a crisis.

Visionary Leadership

Robbins and Judge (2009) articulated four essential skills or components of visionary leadership: the ability to explain the vision to others, the ability to express the vision, the ability to communicate the vision with performance expectations, and the ability to extend the vision by conveying a new set of values and leading by example while incorporating the new values. Followers must have a clear grasp of the vision of the leader. This vision should be compelling enough to the followers that there is enthusiasm, motivation, and commitment to actualize the vision. Leaders must be able to express the vision in ways other than verbally. That is, the vision should be expressed in the leader's behavior. Extending the vision entails making the vision meaningful to followers in different contexts and different situations (i.e., the vision should be shared by management and staff as well as across departments and levels of the organization).

Organizational/Management Theories

Frederick Taylor, a mechanical engineer in steel plants in Pennsylvania, is recognized as the father of scientific management (Williams, 2009). In 1911, Taylor published *The Principles of Scientific Management*, which revolutionized the way work was accomplished in organizations in the United States. This change led to the use of the scientific method to help determine the "one best way" for a job to be done. Taylor's work is credited with beginning modern management theory.

Scientific Management

Taylor's work evolved because of what he perceived as inefficiencies on the job by workers and management, which he believed led to only one-third of the possible output. These inefficiencies included workers applying differing techniques to get the same job done, employees working at a deliberately slow pace, management not matching worker expertise and talents to the job, and management making decisions based on hunches and intuition. Taylor (1911) devised four principles of management (Box 16-2).

As a result of implementation of Taylor's principles and ideas, profits and productivity in American organizations rose dramatically. His methods gave U.S. companies a competitive advantage over foreign companies—an advantage that lasted for approximately 50 years.

Theory of Bureaucracy/Organizational Theory

Max Weber, a political theorist and sociologist in prewar Germany, was attempting to address social and political concerns when he developed his definition of bureaucracy (Williams, 2009). Weber considered a bureaucracy to be an ideal form for an organization in which there is a clearly defined hierarchy and division of labor operating in a system of detailed rules and regulations. Weber's theory emphasized the concepts of authority, command, power, domination, and discipline. For example, in a bureaucracy, the authority for decision making depends on the individual's position in the organization (i.e., the higher the individual is ranked in the organization, the greater the level of authority of that individual) (Weber, 1970). Many of Weber's principles are still used in large health care organizations today.

Box 16-2 Taylor's Principles of Management

- Using scientific methods (i.e., time and motion studies), work can be organized to produce maximum efficiency and productivity while capitalizing on the expertise of the individual worker.
- Workers with specific attributes and qualifications should be hired and then trained and matched to the job that would make the best use of their capabilities.
- Workers should be rewarded monetarily if production exceeds established goals rather than being paid an hourly wage; workers should know where and how they fit into the organization and should be informed of the organization's mission and how they can help to accomplish the mission.
- Managers and workers should work cooperatively; however, the role of management is to plan and supervise, and the role of the worker is to get the work done.

Box 16-3 Fayol's Principles of Management

- To ensure maximum efficiency and effectiveness, there should be specialization of work regardless of whether the work is technical or administrative.
- Managers must have the right and the power to give orders; however, with authority comes responsibility. Responsibility and authority must be commensurate.
- Good discipline is essential to the organization; however, management has the responsibility to inform workers of expectations and to provide good supervision.
- When sanctions must be applied, they should be applied fairly and appropriately.
- Every employee should have only one supervisor from whom he or she receives orders and directions. Compensation for work should be judged as fair by both management and the worker.

Classic Management Theory

Henri Fayol, a French mining engineer and industrialist, successfully brought the Commentry-Fourchambault Mining Company from the brink of bankruptcy in 1888 and made it into a thriving, successful company. He accomplished this by using 14 principles of administration and management (DuBrin, 2009). These principles address areas such as division or specialization of work, authority, employee discipline, unity of direction or supervision, remuneration of workers, chain of command, equity, initiative, and esprit de corps (Fayol, 1949). Examples of Fayol's principles of management are included in Box 16-3. Many, if not most, of Fayol's principles are used in organizations today.

Motivational Theories

The ability to motivate others is a characteristic shared by leaders. Motivational theories are derived predominantly from the work of psychologist Abraham Maslow and his theory. McGregor's and Herzberg's theories were presented as evolving from Maslow's theory. The following sections discuss contemporary theories of motivation, including Achievement–Motivation or Three Needs Theory, Expectancy Theory, and Equity Theory.

Achievement–Motivation Theory

The Achievement–Motivation Theory was developed by Atkinson, McClelland, and Veroff. It focuses on aspects of personality characteristics and proposes three forms of motivation or needs in work situations (Drafke, 2009; Robbins & Judge, 2009). These three factors or motives are labeled social motives and are presented in Table 16-1.

Individuals with a high need for achievement (n-Ach) are not as concerned with the rewards of achievement as they are with the actual achievement. These individuals seek out characteristic situations in which the probability of success is neither too high nor too low, in which success can be achieved through one's own efforts, and in which personal credit can be received for a good or successful outcome. For example, if the probability of success is too high, an n-Ach individual will find motive satisfaction low—he or she perceives that there is not a sufficient challenge.

Table 16-1 Motivation Needs in Work Situations

Need	Characteristics
Achievement (n-Ach)	Need to strive for success and excellence in the work situation to accomplish what has not been accomplished before
Power (n-Pow)	Need to be influential and to control others; to be in charge or in authority
Affiliation (n-Aff)	Need to be liked, accepted, and respected by others

High n-Ach individuals are often attracted to entrepreneurial activities, such as developing their own businesses (Rue & Byars, 1977).

Research indicates that a high need to achieve is not necessarily synonymous with being a good manager. Other research has revealed that the needs for affiliation and power are closely related to managerial success. That is, the best managers appear to be those individuals who have a high need for power and a low need for affiliation (Robbins & Judge, 2009).

Expectancy Theory

Victor Vroom developed Expectancy Theory in the 1960s. Major concepts of this theory include the effects of ability and motivation on performance; they can be expressed as a mathematical statement:

$$\text{Performance} = \text{Ability} \times \text{Motivation}$$

Vroom (1960) concluded that managers should attempt to develop and motivate employees simultaneously. However, he recognized that the successful motivation of employees depends on the employee's aptitude and ability as well.

In a later work, Vroom (1964) added the concepts of expectancy, instrumentality, and valence to motivation. This premise can also be expressed as a mathematical statement:

$$\text{Motivation} = \text{Expectancy} \times \text{Instrumentality} \times \text{Valence}$$

Expectancy is defined as the association between the action and the outcome of the action. Action will lead to the achievement of a goal. *Instrumentality* describes the type of outcome derived because of an action; it is the perception that achievement of a goal will lead to a reward. *Valence* is the value placed on the desirability of the outcome by the employee (Vroom, 1964).

In short, the Expectancy Theory states that an individual will act (performance) in a certain manner because there is an expectation (motivation) that the act will result in an outcome. Employee performance is also based on the attractiveness of that outcome (reward) to the individual. Note that the attractiveness of the outcome or reward is what the *employee* perceives it to be, not what the manager perceives. An individual's own perceptions of performance and reward will determine the employee's level of effort. Therefore, it behooves managers to make certain employees understand and see the connection between performance and rewards and to determine what rewards are valued (and expected) by workers.

Equity Theory

J. Stacy Adams, a research psychologist, developed Equity Theory in 1963. This theory is based on the concepts of cognitive dissonance and distributive justice. It attempts to describe the relationship in which an individual gives something (input) and in exchange receives something (outcome) (Adams, 1965).

In a work situation, an individual expects that if he or she works hard at a job (input), he or she will receive compensation or recognition (outcome) based on what he or she has put in. The individual then compares this input–outcome ratio with relevant others in the same job situation (inside or outside of the organization). If the worker perceives the input–outcome ratio of the relevant others is equal to his or her own, then a state of equity exists. If the ratios are not equal (i.e., if the workers perceive themselves to be over- or underrewarded), a state of inequity exists, and the employee will attempt to correct the inequity (Robbins & Judge, 2009). The corrections may take several forms and include lower or higher inputs or outputs and increased absenteeism. The presence of inequity results in employee dissatisfaction.

Concepts of Power, Empowerment, and Change

In society and in organizations, the words "power" and "authority" are often used synonymously and sometimes interchangeably. However, the two concepts are not synonymous.

Power

Power is the larger concept from which authority is derived. Power can be defined as influence wielded by an individual or group of individuals to change behaviors and attitudes and to sway decisions. Power implies a dependency relationship. In other words, the more dependent an individual is on another, the more power is generated by the individual in possession of the desired attribute (e.g., wealth, information, prestige, etc.). Power can have positive or negative connotations. For example, among disenfranchised groups, power may have a negative connotation, as in abusing power or by engendering feelings of powerlessness.

Authority, on the other hand, is a formal right based on the manager's position in the organization. Authority is a source of legitimate power; however, some individuals (and organizations) are more proficient than others in using and delegating authority. Authority can be under- and overused. Usually the higher one is (by virtue of vertical position) in an organization, the greater one's authority.

French and Raven (1959) conducted early research related to the concept of power. They classified five bases or sources of power: reward, coercive, legitimate, referent, and expert power (Table 16-2). Coercive, reward, and legitimate power are considered formal bases of power; referent and expert power are personal bases of power. Two other bases of power, *informational power* and *charismatic power*, have subsequently been identified in the literature (Heineken & McCloskey, 1985). Informational power is the power held by an individual who has the information necessary for others to accomplish a task or goal. Charismatic power can be distinguished from referent power as a type of personal power rather than reflected power. Charismatic power is the power that attracts one individual to another.

Power bases can be used individually or in combination. The effect of the power bases is additive; that is, the more power bases an individual uses, the greater or broader the power that individual will exert or exercise. Research indicates that personal sources of power are most effective (Carson, Carson, & Roe, 1993).

Table 16-2 Sources of Power

Type of Power	Characteristics	Examples
Reward	The transfer of positive reinforcers from the leader to the follower	Praise, compensation, and other rewards the follower values
Coercive	The use of negative sanctions to achieve results desired by the leader	Unfavorable work assignments; unappealing work schedules
Legitimate	Power derived by virtue of the position or title held within the organization	Vice president of patient care services; chief nursing officer; charge nurse; team leader
Referent	Power that some individuals possess by virtue of their association with a more powerful individual or entity	Being on the faculty of a well-known university; working for a renowned nurse
Expert	Power derived through an individual's knowledge, experience, and expertise or skill in a certain discipline or area of specialization	A clinical nurse specialist consulting in the case of a pregnant oncology patient; a nursing professor chairing a curriculum change committee

Researchers such as McClelland (1975), Winter (1973), and Raven (2008) have determined that there are three major motivators that influence leader behavior when selecting a power strategy: need for power, need for affiliation, and need for achievement. For example, a manager with a high need for power may be more likely to operate from a base of impersonal coercive power and legitimate position power, while a supervisor with a high need for achievement may make more use of informational and expert power (Raven, 2008). Self-esteem, high or low, may also play a role in which power strategy is ultimately selected. It is theorized that individuals with low self-esteem may be more likely to utilize harsh or hard power bases such as coercion power (Kipnis, 1976). Other factors that may help to determine the choice of power strategy utilized include determining which power strategy would be more likely to influence the target individual or group and concern regarding how others may perceive and evaluate a leader or manager's choice of power strategy. For example, a manager with positive feelings toward an employee may choose to not to use a harsh base of power even when the situation justifies use of a harder power base (Raven, 2008).

Empowerment

In many organizations, including some health care organizations, power has shifted from residing exclusively with management to the worker or a group or workers, often in a team configuration. *Empowerment,* in organizational terminology, is the transfer or delegation of responsibility and authority from managers to employees; empowerment is the sharing of power. Empowerment also involves the sharing of vision, mission, knowledge, expertise, decision making, and resources necessary for employees to reach organizational goals. The concept of empowerment can be operationalized as a continuum with employees in some organizations having virtually no say in how the work is to be accomplished and employeers on the other end of the continuum having complete control over work processes (Daft & Marcic, 2009).

Empowerment is consistent with the contemporary views of leadership (e.g., transformational, visionary, etc.). In today's competitive economic environment, organizations that have been successful from an economic and quality standpoint are

Link to Practice 16-1

Most nurses today are being educated in the value of integrating evidence-based practice. However, implementing the results of research into practice by direct care providers remains inconsistent in many health care organizations.

Researchers in Canada conducted a secondary analysis of data collected from 400 Canadian nurses to determine factors that affect nurse attainment, transfer, and application of knowledge into practice. The authors were particularly interested in determining organizational factors and structures that most affect the transfer of knowledge. The study was guided by Kanter's Theory of Structural Empowerment (1977, 1993), which contends that organizational and/or structural factors within the work setting play a larger role in determining an employee's attitudes and behaviors than do personal attributes or social interactions.

The researchers hypothesized that high levels of leader–member exchange (LMX) coupled with a perception of structural empowerment by the nurse would lead to greater efforts by the nurse in personal transfer of knowledge behaviors.

The findings of this research supported the hypothesis and the main contentions of Kanter's theory. In this study, nurses with a higher perception of work environment empowerment and LMX reported increased participation in personal transfer of knowledge in the practice setting.

Davies, A., Wong, C. A., & Laschinger, H. (2011). Nurses' participation in personal knowledge transfer: The role of leader-member exchange (LMX) and structural empowerment. *Journal of Nursing Management, 19*, 632–643.

those that have empowered employees to "get the job done." This usually involves removing bureaucratic barriers to success, such as forcing workers to wait days or weeks for management approval of new work methods or for allocation of necessary resources to accomplish a task or goal. To exploit competitive marketplace advantages, decisions and changes are made rapidly and at a lower level in the organizational structure than in traditional companies. Empowered employees are often more creative and responsive to the needs of the customer or consumer. Link to Practice 16-1 illustrates one effect of workplace empowerment in nursing practice.

Change

Today, nursing and, in a broader view, health care, are arenas that seem to be in a constant state of flux or change. For most individuals, change elicits feelings of uncertainty, anxiety, and upheaval. Kurt Lewin, a German psychologist, proposed a method of planned change, which is controlled change or change by design. Theorists who have expanded the work of Lewin include Havelock, whose theories on change include six phases; Kilmann, who postulated five stages of organizational planned change; Kotter, who describes a process that includes eight stages for leading change; and Smith, who identified seven levels of change (Tomey, 2009).

Planned Change Theory

Lewin described a method in his field theory that provides a basis for considering the process of *planned* change (Lewin, 1951). Planned change occurs by design, as opposed to change that is spontaneous or that occurs by happenstance or by accident.

When Lewin's process is used correctly and in its entirety by a group or a system, effective change is implemented.

Central to Lewin's theories on planned change are the concepts of field and force. A *field* can be viewed as a system; therefore, when change occurs in one part or aspect of the system, the whole system must be examined to determine the effect of that change. *Force* is defined as a directed entity that has the characteristics of direction, focus, and strength. Lewin states that change is a move from the status quo that results in a disruption in the balance of forces or disequilibrium between opposing forces (Lewin, 1951).

According to Lewin (1951), there are two forces involved in change, *driving forces* and *restraining forces.* As the name implies, a driving force encourages or facilitates movement to a new direction, goal, or outcome. A restraining force has the opposite effect; restraining forces block or impede progress toward the goal. In planned change, driving forces should be identified and accentuated. If possible, restraining forces should also be identified and minimized to achieve the desired outcome or change. Lewin describes effective change as the return to equilibrium as a result of balancing opposing forces. If driving forces and restraining forces can be identified, it may be possible to predict if and when change would be successful. Lewin (1951) identifies three phases that must occur if planned change is to be successful: unfreezing the status quo, moving to a new state, and refreezing the change to make it permanent. In the unfreezing stage, individuals involved must be informed of the need for change and should agree that change is needed. Change, particularly in the work environment, often leads to feelings of uneasiness, uncertainty, and loss of control. Change, just for the sake of change, is viewed by most individuals as stressful and unnecessary.

Driving forces should exceed restraining forces during movement, the second phase of the planned change process. The initiator of the change, the change agent, should recognize that change takes time, should be accomplished gradually, and should be thoughtfully and comprehensively planned before implementation.

During the refreezing phase, stabilization occurs. If stabilization is successful, the change is assimilated into the system. Change disrupts the comfort of the status quo; it leads to disequilibrium. Therefore, resistance to change should always be anticipated and expected.

Kotter (1995) expanded Lewin's theory by devising a more detailed eight-step approach for implementing change that correlates to the unfreezing, movement, and refreezing phases in Lewin's model. Kotter analyzed common mistakes made when managers attempt to initiate a change. Based on these mistakes, Kotter's Eight Step Plan for Implementing Change was devised. The eight steps include:

1. Create a sense of urgency for the change.
2. Form coalitions to have enough power to lead the change.
3. Create a new vision to direct the change; strategies must be developed to achieve the new vision.
4. Communicate the new vision purposefully and effectively throughout the organization.
5. Remove barriers to change, empower others to act on the new vision, encourage an atmosphere of creativity and risk-taking.
6. Plan rewards for short-term "wins" when the organization begins to move toward the new vision.
7. Continually assess the effects of the change and make adjustments as necessary in new programs.
8. Reinforce the changes by linking new behaviors to organizational success (Robbins & Judge, 2009).

Uncertain and dynamic environments often characterize the environments of organizations today. In this environment, stability and predictability rarely exist. Disruptions in the status quo are the norm. Organizations today face constant change, often bordering on chaos. Leaders in today's environments of continual change must be prepared to efficiently and effectively adapt to change and must be able to manage all aspects of change—from both external and internal forces.

Resilience

Resilience is a concept or attribute which can be ascribed to individuals and to organizations. The word "resilience" is derived from a Latin term and refers to the ability to adapt to adversity and/or to change. Today's health care organizations, and the individuals who work in those organizations, are experiencing unprecedented periods of rapid change. Pressures placed on health care organizations from external forces such as the government, insurers, physicians, and customers, as well as from internal sources, demand organizational resilience, adaptability, and the ability to respond and react rapidly to change if the organization is to succeed and flourish.

Individuals with high levels of personal resilience are highly valued, especially in turbulent times, as they seem to be able to better manage their reactions to stressful situations and circumstances. In addition, resilient individuals tend to make more effective team members and leaders (Shirey, 2012).

Problem-Solving and Decision-Making Processes

Decision making is typically viewed as but one component of problem solving. Decision making can occur without taking the time to complete a comprehensive analysis, a step that is usually required in problem solving. Also, a decision can be made without identifying the real problem. Factors that play a role in an individual's process or method of decision making include the individual's values, life experiences, preferences, and inherent ways of thinking.

Early attempts to arrive at a scientific or rational method of decision making were described in the Rational Decision-Making Model. More recently, research conducted by Vroom and Yetton (1973) and Vroom and Jago (1988) related to decision making has resulted in quantitative decision technology. This method can help managers select a decision-making style based on input and mathematical computation of effects of leader and situational variables.

The Rational Decision-Making Model

The primary assumption of the Rational Decision-Making Model, which has ties to the classic theories of economic behavior, is that of economic rationality. Economic rationality contends that people always attempt to maximize their individual economic outcomes when weighing decisions. Individuals or managers evaluate potential outcomes of their decisions based on current or prospective monetary worth. In a business decision-making situation, a manager weighs the alternative outcomes of a decision based in terms of profit-and-loss potential. The alternative selected as part of the decision-making process is the alternative that reaps the highest expected worth. *Expected worth* equals the sum of the expected values of the associated costs and benefits of the outcomes resulting from that alternative (Wagner & Hollenbeck, 2010).

Other assumptions of the model include the following:

- The problem is easy to discern and is without ambiguity.
- There is one well-defined goal to be achieved.
- All possible alternatives and consequences to action are known to the decision maker.
- There are no time or cost constraints.
- The final choice that is made will have the maximum economic payoff.

However, the assumptions of rationality often do not hold true. For example, in today's health care environment. how often does the manager have the luxury of no time or cost constraints?

Simon (1965), an economist and psychologist, concluded that most managers did not make decisions based on objective rationality. Simon proposed that there are bounds or limits to the ability of humans to make rational decisions at all times. *Bounded rationality*, a term devised by Simon, means that humans are unable to make entirely rational decisions because of the limits of human mental abilities and because of the influence of external factors on decision making. As a result, most people who make decisions do not have the time or capability to wait for the best possible solution to every problem. Decisions are made using incomplete knowledge and without attempting to determine all possible consequences. The final decision is good enough or "satisficing." Most people stop the search for alternatives when they find a satisficing alternative.

There are several influences on the decision-making process, which contribute to bounded rationality. These include intuition, personality and cognitive intelligence, EI, quality and accessibility of information, political considerations, degree of certainty, crisis and conflict, the values of the decision maker, procrastination, and decision-making styles (DuBrin, 2009).

Group Decision Making

In organizations, groups or teams of people typically make decisions rather than individuals. Group decision making is often used when the decision is complex, such as when a new process or product is being developed. Advantages of group decision making include the following: The decision made may be of higher quality because of the collective wisdom of the group members, major errors may be avoided because of the ability of the group members to evaluate each member's thinking, and commitment or "buy-in" of the group may be increased because of members' role in the outcome of the decision (DuBrin, 2009).

There are several disadvantages to group decision making. It often takes a group longer to reach a decision. In addition, decision making in groups may lead to compromises that really do not solve the problem. Because of the increased time involved for group decision making, group decision making should be reserved for problems that are multifaceted, complex, and important enough to warrant the efforts of the group (DuBrin, 2009).

An example of a group decision-making process is the nominal group technique (NGT). Use of this technique allows a manager to explore potential alternatives to a problem and the reaction to implementation of specific alternatives. NGT follows a very structured format that begins by identifying the problem and ends with developing an action plan to implement a chosen solution. Once the plan is implemented, the group reconvenes to discuss progress and to evaluate outcomes (DuBrin, 2009).

Organizational Quantitative Decision-Making Techniques

Many organizations today, particularly health care organizations, rely on data-based decision making. That is, leaders and managers in those organizations rely on results of facts and quantitative measures to make decisions although intuition and judgment still influence the decision-making process.

Examples of quantitative approaches used in decision making include the utilization of the following: Pareto diagrams for problem identification, Gantt charts and milestone charts to monitor the progress of scheduled projects, break-even analyses (a method to determine profitability of new ventures or programs), decision trees, graphic illustrations of all possible alternatives to solve a particular problem, and sophisticated inventory-control techniques (DuBrin, 2009).

Conflict Management

Conflict can be positive or negative and functional or dysfunctional, although most people tend to shy away from situations in which there may be conflict. Negative conflict can be detrimental if allowed to continue for long periods without intervention from management. In general, a conflict situation has the following characteristics:

- At least two parties are involved.
- Strong emotions and behavior, directed toward defeating or suppressing the opponent, are apparent.
- Mutually exclusive needs or values exist or are perceived to exist.
- Opposing parties attempt to gain power over each other (Katz & Lawyer, 1985).

Conflict Mode Model

When a conflict occurs, Thomas (1976) recommended that the first course of action is to discern the other party's intent in causing the conflict before determining how to respond. Response is guided by two behaviors or dimensions: cooperativeness and assertiveness. Cooperativeness is used if one is more focused on satisfying the other person's concerns. Assertiveness is used if one is more focused on satisfying one's own concerns (Thomas, 1976).

Thomas and Kilmann (1974) defined five conflict-handling modes or strategies: competing, accommodating, avoiding, collaborating, and compromising. *Competing* or *forcing* is used when the issue is important, needs speedy resolution, and "buy-in" from individuals other than the manager is unnecessary. When the issue in conflict is of relative unimportance to the manager or when the manager "gives in" to the other party involved in the conflict, *accommodation* is used. *Avoidance* should be used when emotions are still high and when the conflict is trivial; confrontation should be postponed until a more opportune time arrives. *Collaboration* is the opposite of avoidance and is used when the issue is too important to each side to be compromised; all parties want a win–win solution. *Compromise* is used for complex issues when conflicting parties are similar in power. Compromise can also be used to craft a temporary solution (Daft & Marcic, 2009).

Integrating the five conflict-handling modes with the two dimensions of cooperativeness and assertiveness results in the following conflict resolution options for managers: competing (assertive but uncooperative), collaborating (assertive and cooperative), avoiding (unassertive and uncooperative), accommodating (unassertive but cooperative), and compromising (midrange on both assertiveness and cooperation). Each option has its inherent strengths and weaknesses, and no one option is ideal for every situation.

Quality Improvement

"In God we trust. All others bring data." —W. Edwards Deming

One of the integral values of American society that has evolved in the last several decades is access to health care at reasonable cost in terms of resources. With increasing demands on health service organizations for improved quality and lower costs, the entire health care system has been forced to evaluate modes of operation. As a result, many health care organizations have incorporated concepts of QI.

QI is the commitment and approach used to scrupulously examine and continuously improve every process in every part of an organization. The ultimate intent of this methodology is meeting and exceeding customer expectations. QI empowers individuals and teams within systems to look at the way service is delivered to customers, to identify root causes of problems in the system, and then to creatively adopt solutions to the problems. Many health care organizations can accurately claim substantial improvements in both service effectiveness and efficiency as a result of this commitment and approach to quality.

In the field of QI, there exists a complex, ever-changing vocabulary. Even the term QI is not consistently used as the primary label for quality-related concepts. Other labels (and their abbreviations) frequently noted in the literature include continuous quality improvement (CQI), total quality management (TQM), total quality systems (TQS), quality systems improvement (QSI), and total quality (TQ), among others. Other related terms include performance improvement and process improvement.

The Case for Quality Improvement in Health Care

Early pioneers of QI in health care included the 19th century physician, Semmelweis, who introduced the importance of hand-washing, and Florence Nightingale, whose work led to decreasing mortality rates among English soldiers in Army hospitals by imposing strict sanitary conditions in the hospitals. Other momentous steps in QI, especially in the United States, was the formation of the Hospital Standardization Program by the American College of Surgeons, which eventually transformed into today's Joint Commission, the organization that accredits health care organizations.

In 1966, 1 year after the implementation of Medicare, Donebedian first proposed that quality could be measured by examining the structures, processes, and outcomes of care, which became the first conceptual approach widely used to measure the quality of health care (Chassin & Loeb, 2011). In 1996, the Joint Commission implemented its Agenda for Change, a quality-focused methodology to improve the systems, processes, and outcomes of care (Andel, Davidow, Hollander, & Moreno, 2012) (Table 16-3).

Despite the focus on QI and on cost reduction in the health care system, the industry in the United States remains plagued with inefficiencies and with all too common instances of poor quality. This results in alarming and unsustainable increase in costs and negatively impacts the ability of U.S. companies to remain competitive in a global economy. Aside from the staggering economic costs of an inefficient health care system, poor quality often leads to well-publicized errors, mistakes, premature deaths, and diminished quality of life for health care consumers.

Table 16-3 Health Care Quality Timeline

Date	Quality Innovation
19th century	Ignaz Semmelweis, an obstetrician, introduces hand-washing to the care of patients.
	Florence Nightingale, an English nurse, recognizes the impact of unsanitary living conditions in English Army hospitals on the morbidity and mortality of patients.
1918	The American College of Surgeons forms the Hospital Standardization Program, the predecessor of the Joint Commission, and begins on-site hospital inspections using the Minimum Standards for Hospitals, a one-page document.
1948	The modern randomized clinical trial is instituted and used in a report from the United Kingdom Research Council on the treatment of pulmonary tuberculosis.
1951	The Joint Commission on Accreditation of Hospitals (JCAH) is created.
1953	JCAH publishes Standards for Hospital Accreditation.
1965	Legislation creating Medicare is enacted. Mandatory utilization review committees are established by the law that created Medicare.
1966	Donebedian proposes the first conceptual framework for measuring health care quality.
1970	The Joint Commission modifies its traditional accreditation process, which is based on standards, to comply with Donebedian's framework.
1971	Congress creates experimental review organizations to review inpatient and ambulatory services for quality and appropriateness of care.
1972	Medicare's Professional Standards Review Organizations established by the Social Security Administration Amendment.
1983	Professional Standards Review Organizations is replaced by Medicare Utilization and Quality Control Peer Review Organizations program; later became the Quality Improvement Organization Program.
1983	Forces of Magnetism are identified as a result of the work environment study conducted by the American Academy of Nursing Task Force on Nursing Practice in Hospitals. Hospitals that were able to recruit and retain nurses at higher levels were described as "magnet" hospitals.
1989	Agency for Healthcare Policy and Research is created to replace the National Center for Health Services Research; later renamed the Agency for Healthcare Research and Quality (AHRQ). Initially, this agency was charged by Congress with developing practice guidelines and conducting health care research.
1994	University of Washington Medical Center, Seattle, becomes the first ANCC Magnet-designated organization.
1999	National Quality Forum is created; mission is to improve health care delivery by promoting the use of standardized quality measures and public reporting of resulting data and outcomes.
1999	Institute of Medicine releases the report, *To Err is Human: Building a Safer Health System.*
2000	AHRQ receives a modified mandate from Congress; no longer directly responsible for developing new clinical practice guidelines.
2001	Institute of Medicine releases the report, *Crossing the Quality Chasm: A New Health System for the 21st Century.*
2012	"Health care quality and safety are best characterized as showing pockets of excellence in specific measures or in particular services at individual health care facilities. Excellence across the board is emerging on some important quality measures. What has eluded us so far, however, is maintaining consistently high levels of safety and quality over time across all health care services and settings" (Chassin & Loeb, 2011, p. 562).

Sources: American Nurses Credentialing Center, 2013; Chassin & Loeb, 2011; Joint Commission, 2013; Institute of Medicine, 2013.

With the successful passage of national health care reform legislation, the Patient Protection and Affordable Care Act (PPACA), it is projected that approximately 32 to 45 million Americans who are currently uninsured or underinsured will be entering the health care system. PPACA makes heavy use of accountable care orgnizations and value-based purchasing. Another provision of the PPACA is that the Centers for Medicare and Medicaid Services (CMS) will no longer reimburse health care agencies for preventable readmissions and for health care facility-acquired conditions (Andel et al., 2012). Health care organizations not currently functioning at optimal levels in terms of efficiency and with the highest levels of quality outcomes are not likely to survive in today's pay for performance environment.

Quality Improvement Frameworks

For more than four decades, two Americans, W. Edwards Deming and J. M. Juran, were the primary champions of the quality movement throughout the world (Port, 1991). Deming was the developer of statistical quality control, whereas Juran was the innovator of total quality control. Both are credited with playing major roles as statistical and managerial consultants to Japanese industry in Japan's successful revitalization after the devastation of World War II. (Port, 1991).

Since the 1970s, the literature on QI has grown and many experts have contributed their ideas on QI. In the United States, the quality theories of Deming, Juran, and Crosby predominate. Deming's (1989) major thesis is that the cause of inefficiency and low quality can generally be traced back to system inadequacies rather than individual worker inadequacy. It is management's responsibility to improve the system with the involvement of all employees. This management theory focuses on improving quality, productivity, and competitive position in the marketplace and is referred to in the literature as Deming's 14 points (Box 16-4).

Deming's goal was to gear an organization's workforce to pursue specific organization-wide goals that were aimed at satisfying customer requirements for quality, price, and service. Juran (1988) defined quality as "fitness for use." To satisfy customers, a product or service must have two components—features that a customer wants and as free from deficiencies as possible. According to Juran, one or the other of these

Box 16-4 Deming's 14 Points

1. Create constancy of purpose for improvement.
2. Adopt the new philosophy.
3. Cease dependence on mass inspections.
4. End the practice of awarding business on the basis of price tags alone.
5. Institute on-the-job training and research.
6. Adopt and institute leadership.
7. Drive out fear among the organization's employees.
8. Improve constantly and forever every process for planning, production, and service.
9. Dismantle barriers between departments.
10. Eliminate slogans, exhortations, and production targets for employees.
11. Eliminate numerical quotas for employees and numerical goals for managers.
12. Remove barriers to pride of workmanship.
13. Institute a vigorous program of education and self-improvement.
14. Put everyone in the organization to work to accomplish the transformation.

Sources: Aguayo (1990); Deming (1989); Gillem (1988); Masters and Masters (1993).

Table 16-4 Juran's Trilogy: Processes Used to Maintain and Improve Quality

Process	Activities
Quality planning	Building quality into the processes and the product
Quality control	Evaluating actual performance, comparing that performance to predetermined goals, and taking action on the differences
Quality improvement (breakthrough)	Encouraging attainment of previously unprecedented levels of performance by the organization

two components alone does not constitute high quality. Juran offered three processes whereby managers can maintain and improve quality. These are commonly referred to as Juran's trilogy (Table 16-4; Juran, 1988).

Crosby (1979) emphasized the importance of systems knowledge and improvement, the disadvantages of reliance on inspections, and the need for statistical quality control. Crosby termed his major concepts the "four absolutes":

1. The definition of quality is conformance requirements.
2. The system of quality is prevention and on not relying solely on "after-the-fact" methods to improve quality.
3. The performance standard is zero defects.
4. The measurement of quality is the price of nonconformance, which involves all costs in doing things wrong. In service companies, the cost of nonconformance is 35% of operating costs, whereas the cost of conformance is a far lower figure (Crosby, 1979).

Although experts on QI differ somewhat on their approaches, their theories share several characteristics (Daft & Marcic, 2009). These include the following:

- QI is driven by the leaders of the organization.
- Customer-mindedness permeates the organization.
- A transition is made from inspection-based management to process improvement.
- Formal process-improvement methods and statistical tools are used.
- All employees are involved in the exploration and refinement of work processes.

Organizational Leadership Role and Quality Improvement

Organizational leadership has a profound impact on the successful implementation of QI. All of the experts agree that the organization's leaders must be committed to QI if an organization-wide program is to succeed. They also agree that the move to QI is not a move that can be accomplished in a short time. QI is not a "quick fix," but requires 2 to 5 years at a minimum for complete implementation (Varkey, Reller, & Resar, 2007).

The QI organization calls for changes that include a shift from individual responsibility to group or collective responsibility, a shift from administrative authority for problem solving to participative problem solving, a replacement of rigid procedures with flexibility and spontaneity, and a problem focus yielding to emphasis on continuous improvement and entrepreneurial thinking (Williams, 2009).

Quality Improvement Processes and Tools

Contemporary approaches to the measurement of quality in health care organizations today rely heavily on statistical process control, which emphasizes the use of data analytics. QI tools used in data analytics include pareto charts, cause-and-effect diagrams, run charts, and control charts, in addition to other similar methods.

Determining and measuring variation in a product or service is a key component of QI. Statistical process control is used to determine sources of variation in a process or outcome that impact service quality. For example, large variation in the quality of a product or service is indicative of an aspect that is out of control. To use a health care–related example, a health system may monitor the readmission rates of patients with sternal wound infection after open-heart surgery. Extracting data from the electronic health record (EHR), representatives of the health system will calculate the average readmission rate for all cardiac surgery patients and compare the rates to preestablished national benchmarks for open-heart surgery. Data related to readmission rates postsurgery will then be calculated by cardiac surgery practice, usually composed of a team or group of physicians, and then may be calculated relative to each specific surgeon in the practice. A cardiac surgery practice and/or a cardiac surgeon whose patients are readmitted with sternal wound infections at statistically higher rates than the average rate when compared to local and national benchmarks would most likely be asked by the health system to address the problem as more frequent infections and readmission rates would indicate a quality variance.

Approaches to QI, which started in other industries and which have been adapted for use in health care, include lean process management and Six Sigma. Lean Thinking, also referred to as Lean, originated in the 1920s in the Ford Motor Company (Ford & Crowther, 1926), while Six Sigma was introducted by the Motorola company. Six Sigma is an extension of Juran's triology as well as other QI approaches. Today, both approaches are used extensively in administration and service areas although their roots are in manufacturing (Snee & Hoerl, 2004).

Lean represented a fundamental shift from traditional Western manufacturing approaches and beliefs, which included:

1. Separation of thinking from doing for workers is essential.
2. Deficiencies in products or services can not be eliminated or avoided.
3. Organizations are most efficient when structured in a chain of command that is based on a hierarchy.
4. Inventories are essential to meet fluctuating production demands (de Koning, Verver, van den Heuvel, Bisgaard, & Does, 2006).

Japanese companies, such as Toyota, revolutionized automobile manufacturing implementing Lean Thinking processes as an alternative to the Western model of manufacturing. Lean focuses on producing what the customer wants and expects from a product—everything else is considered to be nonvalue-added activity. Another focus of Lean is reduction of waste and variability in production and in outcomes during the manufacturing process by synchronizing the flow of work. The strengths of Lean Thinking are the focus on the needs and wants of the customer and on its set of standardarized solutions to frequently occurring problems in the process (de Koning et al., 2006).

Six Sigma was introduced as a company-wide QI initiative by Motorola in the late 1980s and then adapted and developed more extensively by General Electric (GE) in the following decade. Hallmarks of the Six Sigma approach are focus on customer satisfaction with the product or service, decision making that is driven by quantitative data-analysis, and an emphasis on reducting costs. Six Sigma is a project-based QI strategy. Projects are selected and prioritized based on the importance of the project to the organizations's mission and strategic goals. Project leaders are called Black Belts (BBs) and Green Belts (GBs), a reference to skill acqusition in the martial arts. Members of upper management to whom the BB and GB report are viewed as project owners and are referred to as "champions" (de Koning et al., 2006).

The steps used in Six Sigma are somewhat analogous to the scientific method, the nursing process and similar problem-solving methods and includes five steps or phases—define, measure, analyze, improve, and control—also referred to by the acronym DMAIC. The steps of DMAIC can be used to investigate any problem in an organization regardless of the scope or scale of the problem. A cost-benefit analysis is conducted in the define stage; if the analysis is favorable to the organization, the project is accepted and then proceeds to all stages or phases of DMAIC. Once the project is accepted, it is assigned to a project team headed by a GB or BB. Strengths associated with Six Sigma include its structured, analytic and logical progression to problem-solving. Organizational buy-in at all levels to the processes used by Six Sigma is also viewed as a strength. Weaknesses of the Six Sigma approach include its complexity when used to solve smaller scale or simpler problems (de Koning et al., 2006).

Some institutions use principles from different QI methodologies on the same QI project. An example is the use of the "lean-sigma" approach, which is a combination of the lean and six-sigma approaches (Varkey et al., 2007). Link to Practice 16-2 shows how one QI project was used.

Evidence-Based Practice

In recent years, terms, such as evidence-based medicine (EBM), evidence-based practice (EBP), evidence-based nursing, evidence-based health care, and best practices guidelines (BPGs) have emerged and assumed a significant position in health care literature. These terms are probably best understood as decision-making frameworks that assist health care providers with making complex decisions utilizing research and other forms of evidence on a routine basis when formulating those decisions (Melnyk & Fineout-Overholt, 2005). Evidence-based decision frameworks are used to describe methods adopted by practitioners and others in an effort to increase the quality of health care, to decrease variability of care, and to decrease the costs related to providing health care.

Utilization of EBP and BPGs increases the quality of care by attempting to bridge the gap between the discovery of knowledge in health care and the time that knowledge is applied in practice. The Institute of Medicine (IOM) suggests that time lag may be as long as 20 years (IOM, 2001). The use of EBP and BPGs should decrease inappropriate variability in practice patterns, which often leads to increased costs. For example, a woman diagnosed with stage II breast cancer in Provo, Utah, should receive the same level of care as a woman who is diagnosed with the same stage of breast cancer in Tampa, Florida, if health care practitioners subscribe to and utilize the latest evidence-based or practice guidelines for the treatment and management of stage II breast cancer.

Link to Practice 16-2

Increasingly, QI tools and processes, such as Six Sigma, are being utilized in health care organizations. For example, staff affiliated with a 714-bed hospital in New York designed and implemented a QI project using Six Sigma methodology to correct issues associated with delayed transfer of patients to the intensive care units (ICUs) in the facility. An interdisciplinary team of clinicians and nonclinicians, led by a hospital administrator project Black Belt, analyzed components associated with inpatient transfers into the ICUs and identified eight steps which significantly impacted the transfer process.

Initially, it was determined by the team that the average time associated with a transfer from a floor bed to an ICU bed was 214 minutes; however, the time could extend to as long as 420 minutes. After conducting an initial capability analysis, the master Black Belt recommended a goal of an average of 90 minutes for average transfer time. During the improvement phase of the process, critical elements which impeded the transfer process were identified and a solution plan integrating new processes was developed. For example, the process for writing transfer orders to move patients out of the ICU was changed to ensure that transfer orders were completed by residents immediately following completion of morning rounds so that ICU beds could become available in a shorter time frame.

Following implementation of the new processes associated with transfer, data were collected and analyzed over a 1-year period (462 consecutive transfers to the ICU). The target performance goal was attained by the fourth month. The mean time for patient transfer from a floor bed to the ICU improved to 84 minutes.

Silich, S. J., Wetz, R. V., Riebling, N., Coleman, C., Khoueiry, G., Rafeh, N. A., et al. (2012). Using six sigma methodology to reduce patient transfer times from floor to critical-care beds. *Journal for Healthcare Quality, 34*(1), 44–54.

Evidence-based medicine utilizes a defined method in four major steps:

1. Eliciting, describing, defining, and refining a structured question about a target population, outcome, and, typically, an intervention
2. Systematic and comprehensive review of the literature in an attempt to answer the question
3. Evaluation of the data and data sources retrieved for methodologic rigor (i.e., data obtained as a result of randomized clinical trials as compared to data from anecdotal reports)
4. Analysis of the data uncovered to answer the question (Donald, 2002).

The limitations of EBP include the absence of organizational support and structure to properly utilize this decision-making framework; insufficient skills to frame the question, retrieve the data, or analyze the data; and gaps in the literature that make it impossible to sufficiently answer the question. In addition, some clinicians argue that EBP decreases or threatens clinical autonomy in decision making.

In 2005, Pravikoff and others surveyed over 1,000 RNs in the United States to determine nurses' readiness to implement EBP. At that time, researchers reported that nurses who responded to the survey were not ready to implement EBP for many of the reasons described above (Pravikoff, Pierce, & Tanner, 2005). Six years later, Melnyk and colleagues surveyed members of the American Nurses Association to determine the state of EBP as reported by the nurses (n = 1,015) (Melnyk, Fineout-Overholt, Gallagher-Ford, & Kaplan, 2012). In contrast to the responses of nurses in the earlier Pravikoff study, respondents in the Melnyk study reported that they are ready to implement EBP and they value EBP. In both studies, nurses reported the primary barriers to implementing EBP as lack of knowledge of the process, lack of time, and lack of EBP-knowlegable mentors. Some respondents also cited lack of an organizational culture that supports EBP as a barrier. However, nurses working in Magnet-designated facilities reported that Magnet facilities do facilitate a culture where EBP is valued and integrated.

The role of the advanced practice nurse (APN) in EBP is continuing to expand. APNs, such as Richard in the opening scenario, are often relied upon to be the clinical leaders of EBP. This leadership role includes continually researching and acquiring the most updated versions of BPGs or clinical guidelines; interpreting the guidelines for other staff and for patients and families; successfully implementing the recommendations of the guidelines; and conducting research to determine the effectiveness of the guidelines from clinical, quality, and cost perspectives after implementation. Chapter 12 contains additional information on EBP.

Summary

This chapter provides a basis for the advanced practice nurse to achieve understanding and appreciation for the utility of leadership and management theories in contemporary nursing practice. By virtue of their roles, APNs, such as Richard, are viewed as leaders and, as such, often have quite visible positions in organizations and the community.

Richard, is in a position in which he needs to define his role. To be an effective leader, he must develop a leadership style that considers his personal strengths and weaknesses and fits the needs and personality of the unit. He will also need to use a number of management concepts and principles, particularly related to motivation and change, and must also be prepared to implement QI strategies that will affect the unit to improve client care.

Assimilation of strategies to improve leadership, motivation, change, decision making, and other concepts discussed in this chapter into the practice repertoire of the advanced practitioner in nursing is crucial to the viability and sustainability of the role.

Key Points

- Leadership and management, although closely related concepts, are different.
- Characteristics of both transformational leadership and transactional leadership are crucial to effective leadership.
- Fayol's principles of Classic Management Theory are still employed in organizations today.
- Higher levels of work environment empowerment and leader-member exchange (LMX) result in greater personal transfer of knowledge in the practice setting by nurses.
- Individuals with high levels of personal resilience are valued by organizations, especially during times of turbulence and rapid change.
- QI empowers individuals and teams within systems to systematically examine processes in service delivery, to identify root causes of problems in the system, and to creatively propose and adopt solutions to the problems.
- Nurses value EBP and are ready to implement EBP.

Learning Activities

1. Analyze the leadership style of your current supervisor. Does the supervisor's leadership behavior vary from situation to situation? Would the supervisor be classified as a transformational, transactional, authentic, charismatic, visionary, or other leader? Why?
2. Assess the organization in which you work today. Are Fayol's and Taylor's principles of management evident in this organization? Give examples.
3. Think back to the last time a major change occurred in your work environment. Was the change a planned change? What were the driving forces and restraining forces? Who was the change agent? Did the change occur as planned?
4. What QI initiatives are evident in your organization? How would you find out more about Lean/Six Sigma practices? Have any nurses in your organization served in the capacity as BBs or GBs? If so, what QI projects have they led or in which projects have they been involved?

REFERENCES

Adams, J. S. (1965). Inequity in social exchanges. In L. Berkowitz (Ed.), *Advances in experimental psychology* (pp. 267–300). New York: Academic Press.

Aguayo, R. (1990). *Dr. Deming: The American who taught the Japanese about quality.* New York: Fireside.

American Nurses Credentialing Center. (2013). *History of the Magnet program.* Retrieved from http://www.nursecredentialing.org/MagnetHistory.aspx

Andel, C., Davidow, S. L., Hollander, M., & Moreno, D. A. (2012). The economics of health care quality and medical errors. *Journal of Health Care Finance, 39,* 39–50.

Avolio, B. J., & Gardner, W. L. (2005). Authentic leadership development: Getting to the root of positive forms of leadership. *The Leadership Quarterly, 16,* 315–338.

Avolio, B. J., Zhu, W., Koh, W., & Puja, B. (2004). Transformational leadership and organizational commitment: Mediating role of psychological empowerment and moderating role of structural distance. *Journal of Organizational Behavior, 25,* 951–968.

Bass, B. M., Avolio, B. J., Jung, D. I., & Berson, Y. (2003). Predicting unit performance by assessing transformational and transactional leadership. *Journal of Applied Psychology, 88*(2), 207–218.

Bennis, W. (1984). The four competencies of leadership. *Training and Development Journal, 38*(8), 15–19.

Bolino, M. C. (2007). *What about us? Relative deprivation among out-group members in LMX relationships.* Paper presented at the National Academy of Management Meeting, Philadelphia.

Bono, J. E., & Judge, T. A. (2003). Self concordance at work: Toward understanding the motivational effects of transformational leaders. *Academy of Management Journal, 46*(5), 554–571.

Burns, J. M. (1978). *Leadership.* New York: Harper & Row.

Caplan, E. (1971). *Management accounting and behavioral science.* Reading, MA: Addison-Wesley.

Carson, P. P., Carson, K. D., & Roe, C. W. (1993). Social power bases: A meta-analytic examination of interrelationships and outcomes. *Journal of Applied Psychology, 23,* 1150–1169.

Chassin, M., & Loeb, J. M. (2011). The ongoing quality improvement journey: Next stop, high reliability. *Health Affairs, 30,* 559–568.

Chemers, M., Harp, R., Rhodewalt, F., & Wysocki, J. (1985). A person–environment analysis of job stress: A contingency model explanation. *Journal of Personality and Social Psychology, 49*(3), 628–635.

Conger, J. A., & Kanungo, R. N. (1988). Behavioral dimensions of leadership. In J. A. Conger & R. N. Kanungo (Eds.), *Charismatic leadership.* San Francisco: Jossey-Bass.

Crosby, P. B. (1979). *Quality is free.* New York: McGraw-Hill.

Daft, R. L., & Marcic, D. (2009). *Understanding management* (6th ed.). Mason, OH: South-Western Cengage Learning.

de Koning, H., Verver, J. P. S., van den Heuvel, J., Bisgaard, S., & Does, R. J. M. M. (2006). Lean six sigma in healthcare. *Journal for Healthcare Quality, 28,* 4–11.

Deming, W. F. (1989). *Out of the crisis.* Cambridge, MA: Massachusetts Institute of Technology Press.

Donald, A. (2002). How to practice evidence-based medicine. *Medscape General Medicine, 5*(1). Retrieved from http://www.medscape.com/viewpublication/122_index

Drafke, M. (2009). *The human side of organizations* (10th ed.). Upper Saddle River, NJ: Pearson Prentice-Hall.

DuBrin, A. J. (2007). *Fundamentals of organizational behavior* (4th ed.). Mason, OH: Thomson South-Western.

DuBrin, A. J. (2009). *Essentials of management* (8th ed.). Mason, OH: South-Western Cengage Learning.

Fayol, H. (1949). *General and industrial management.* London, United Kingdom: Pitman & Sons.

Fiedler, F. (1967). *A theory of leadership effectiveness.* New York: McGraw-Hill.

Fiedler, F. (1969). Style or circumstances: The leadership enigma. *Psychology Today, 2*(10), 38–43.

Fiedler, F., Chemers, M., & Mahar, L. (1976). *Improving leadership effectiveness: The leader match concept.* New York: Wiley.

Ford, H., & Crowther, S. (1926). *Today and tomorrow.* Cambridge, MA: Productivity Press.

French, J., & Raven, B. (1959). The bases of social power. In D. Cartwright (Ed.), *Studies in social power.* Ann Arbor, MI: University of Michigan.

Georgopoulos, B., Mahoney, G., & Jones, N. (1957). A path-goal approach to productivity. *Journal of Applied Psychology, 53,* 345–353.

Gillem, T. (1988). Deming's 14 points and hospital quality: Responding to the consumer's demand for the best value health care. *Journal of Nursing Quality Assurance, 2*(3), 70–78.

Goleman, D., Boyatzis, R., & McKee, A. (2001). Primal leadership: The hidden driver of great performance. *Harvard Business Review, 79*(11), 42–51.

Graen, G., & Cashman, J. F. (1975). A role-making model of leadership in formal organizations: A developmental approach. In J. G. Hunt & L. L. Larson (Eds.), *Leadership frontiers* (pp. 143–165). Kent, OH: Kent State University Press.

Graen, G., & Uhl-Bien, M. (1995). Relationship-based approach to leadership: Development of the leader-member exchange (LMX) theory of leadership over 25 years: Applying a multi-level, multi-domain perspective. *Leadership Quarterly, 6,* 219–247.

Gray, E. R. (1978). The non-linear systems experiment: A requiem. *Business Horizons, 21,* 31–36.

Green, J. P. (1981). People management: New directions for the 1980s. *Administrative Management, 42,* 22–26.

Harms, P. D., & Crede, M. (2010). Emotional intelligence and transformational and transactional leadership: A meta-analysis. *Journal of Leadership and Organizational Studies, 17*(1), 5–17.

Heineken, J., & McCloskey, J. (1985). Teaching power concepts. *Journal of Nursing Education, 24*(1), 40–42.

Hellriegel, D., Jackson, S. E., & Slocum, J. W. (2008). *Management: A competency-based approach* (11th ed.). Mason, OH: Thomson South-Western.

Hersey, P., & Blanchard, K. (1977). *Management of organizational behavior: Utilizing human resources.* Englewood Cliffs, NJ: Prentice-Hall.

Herzberg, F. (1966). *Work and the nature of man.* Cleveland: World.

Hitt, M. A., Black, J. S., & Porter, L. W. (2009). *Management* (2nd ed.). Upper Saddle River, NJ: Pearson Prentice-Hall.

House, R. (1971). A path-goal theory of leader effectiveness. *Administrative Science Quarterly, 16,* 321–338.

House, R. J. (1977). A 1976 theory of charismatic leadership. In J. G. Hunt & L. L. Larson (Eds.), *Leadership: The cutting edge.* Carbondale, IL: Southern Illinois University Press.

House, R. J. (1996). Path-goal theory of leadership: Lessons, legacy, and a reformulated theory. *Leadership Quarterly, 7*(3), 323–352.

Institute of Medicine. (2001). *Crossing the quality chasm: A new health care system for the 21st century.* Washington, DC: National Academy Press.

Institute of Medicine. (2013). *Reports.* Retrieved from http://www.iom.edu/Reports.aspx

Jens, R., & Heinitz, K. (2007). Transformational and charismatic leadership: Assessing the convergent, divergent, and criterion validity of the Multifactor Leadership Questionnaire and the Conger and Kanungo Scales. *Leadership Quarterly, 18,* 121–133.

Joint Commission. (2013). *Our history.* Retrieved from http://www.jointcommission.org/assets/1/6 Joint_Commission_History.pdf

Judge, T. A., & Piccolo, R. F. (2004). Transformational and transactional leadership: A meta-analytic test of their relative validity. *Journal of Applied Psychology, 89*(5), 755–768.

Jung, D. D., & Sosik, J. J. (2006). Who are the spellbinders? Identifying personal attributes of charismatic leaders. *Journal of Leadership and Organizational Studies, 12*(4), 12–26.

Juran, J. M. (1988). *Quality control handbook.* New York: McGraw-Hill.

Kanter, R. (1977). *Men and women of the corporation.* New York: Basic Books.

Kanter, R. (1993). *Men and women of the corporation* (2nd ed.). New York: Basic Books.

Katz, N. H., & Lawyer, J. W. (1985). *Communication and conflict resolution skills.* Dubuque, IA: Kendall/Hunt.

Kay, A. (1973). Where being nice to workers didn't work. *Business Week, 1,* 98–100.

Kipnis, D. (1976). *The powerholders.* Chicago: The University of Chicago Press.

Kopelman, R. E., Prottas, D. J., & Davis, A. L. (2008). Douglas McGregor's Theory X and Y: Toward a construct-valid measure. *Journal of Management Issues, 20*(2), 255–271.

Kotter, J. P. (1995). Leading changes: Why transformation efforts fail. *Harvard Business Review,* pp. 59–67.

Lewin, K. (1951). *Field theory in social science.* New York: Harper & Row.

Lewin, K., & Lippitt, R. (1938). An experimental approach to the study of autocracy and democracy: A preliminary note. *Sociometry, 1,* 292–300.

Lindebaum, D., & Cartwright, S. (2010). A critical examination of the relationship between emotional intelligence and transformational leadership. *Journal of Management Studies, 47,* 1317–1342.

Luthans, F., & Avolio, B. J. (2003). Authentic leadership: A postivie developmental approach. In K. S. Cameron, J. E. Dutton, & R. E. Quinn (Eds.), *Positive organizational scholarship* (pp. 241–257). San Francisco: Barrett-Koehler.

Malone, E. (1975). The non-linear systems experiment in participative management. *Journal of Business, 48,* 52–64.

Maslow, A. (1968). *Toward a psychology of being.* New York: Van Nostrand Reinhold.

Maslow, A. (1971). *The farther reaches of human nature.* New York: Viking.

Masters, M. L., & Masters, R. J. (1993). Building TQM into nursing management. *Nursing Economics, 11*(5), 274–291.

May, D. R., Chan, A. Y., Hodges, T. D., & Avolio, B. J. (2003). Developing the moral component of authentic leadership. *Organizational Dynamics, 32,* 247–260.

McClelland, D. C. (1975). *Power: The inner experience.* New York: Wiley.

Melnyk, B. M., Fineout-Overholt, E., Gallagher-Ford, L., & Kaplan, L. (2012). The state of evidence-based practice in U.S. nurses. *Journal of Nursing Administration, 42*(9), 410–417.

Melnyk, B. M., & Fineout-Overholt, E. (2005). *Evidence-based practice in nursing and healthcare.* Philadelphia: Lippincott Williams & Wilkins.

Minor, J. (1980). *Theories of organizational behavior.* Hinsdale, IL: Dryden.

Morse, J., & Lorsch, J. (1970). Beyond theory Y. *Harvard Business Review, 48*(3), 61–68.

O'Boyle, E. H., Humphrey, R. H., Pollack, J. M., Hawver, T. H., & Story, P. A. (2011). The relation between emotional intelligence and job performance: A meta-analysis. *Journal of Organizational Behavior, 32,* 788–818.

Peters, T. (1987). *Thriving on chaos.* New York: Alfred A. Knopf.

Podsakoff, P. M., Bommer, W. H., Podsakoff, N. P., & Mackenzie, S. B. (2005). Relationships between leader reward and punishment behaviour and subordinate attitudes, perceptions, and behaviours: A meta-analytic review of existing and new research. *Organizational Behavior and Human Decision Processes, 99,* 113–142.

Port, O. (1991). Dueling pioneers. *Business Week,* October 25, p. 17.

Pravikoff, D. S., Pierce, S. T., & Tanner, A. (2005). Evidence-based practice readiness study supported by academy nursing informatics panel. *Nursing Outlook, 53*(1), 49–50.

Raven, B. H. (2008). The bases of power and the power/interaction model of interpersonal influence. *Analyses of Social Issues and Public Policy, 8*(1), 1–22.

Robbins, S. P., & Coulter, M. (2005). *Management* (8th ed.). Upper Saddle River, NJ: Prentice-Hall.

Robbins, S. P., & Judge, T. A. (2009). *Organizational behavior* (13th ed.). Upper Saddle River, NJ: Pearson Prentice-Hall.

Rue, L. W., & Byars, L. (1977). *Management—Theory and application.* Homewood, IL: Richard D. Irwin.

Schaubroeck, J., Lam, S. K., & Cha, S. E. (2007). Embracing transformational leadership: Team values and the impact of the leader behavior on team performance. *Journal of Applied Psychology, 92*(4), 1020–1030.

Schriesheim, C. A., Castro, S. L., Zhou, X. T., & DeChurch, L. A. (2006). An investigation of path-goal and transformational leadership theory predictions at the individual level of analysis. *Leadership Quarterly, 17,* 21–38.

Shamir, B., & Eilam, G. (2005). "What's your story?": A life-stories approach to authentic leadership development. *The Leadership Quarterly, 16,* 395–417.

Shirey, M. (2012). How resilient are your team members? *Journal of Nursing Administration, 42*(12), 551–553.

Simon, H. A. (1965). *The shape of automation for man and management.* New York: Harper Textbooks.

Snee, R. D., & Hoerl, R. W. (2004). *Six sigma beyond the factory floor.* Upper Saddle River, NJ: Pearson Education.

Tannenbaum, R., & Schmidt, W. H. (1973). How to choose a leadership pattern. *Harvard Business Review, 5,* 162–180.

Taylor, F. W. (1911). *The principles of scientific management.* New York: Harper.

Thomas, K. W. (1976). *Handbook of industrial and organizational psychology.* Chicago: Rand-McNally.

Thomas, K. W., & Kilmann, R. H. (1974). *The Thomas-Kilmann conflict mode instrument.* Tuxedo Park, NY: Xicom.

Tomey, A. M. (2009). *Guide to nursing management and leadership* (8th ed.). St. Louis: Mosby Elsevier.

Varkey, P., Reller, M. K., & Resar, R. K. (2007). Basics of quality improvement in health care. *Mayo Clinic Proceedings, 82*(6), 735–739.

Vecchio, R. P., Justin, J. E., & Pearce, C. L. (2008). The utility of transactional and transformational leadership for predicting performance and satisfaction within a path-goal theory framework. *Journal of Occupational and Organizational Psychology, 81*, 71–82.

Vroom, V. H. (1960). *Some personality determinants of the effects of participation.* Englewood Cliffs, NJ: Prentice-Hall.

Vroom, V. H. (1964). *Work and motivation.* New York: Wiley.

Vroom, V. H., & Jago, A. G. (1988). *The new leadership: Managing participation in organizations.* Englewood Cliffs, NJ: Prentice-Hall.

Vroom, V. H., & Jago, A. G. (2007). The role of situations in leadership. *The American Psychologist,* 17–24.

Vroom, V. H., & Yetton, P. W. (1973). *Leadership and decision-making.* Pittsburgh, PA: University of Pittsburgh Press.

Wagner, J. A., & Hollenbeck, J. R. (2010). *Organizational behavior: Securing competitive advantage.* New York, NY: Routledge.

Walumbwa, F. O., Avolio, B. J., & Zhu, W. (2008). How transformational leadership weaves its influence on individual job performance: The role of identification and efficacy beliefs. *Personnel Psychology, 61*, 793–825.

Wang, H., Law, K. S., Hackett, R. D., Wang, D., & Chen, Z. X. (2005). Leader–member exchange as a mediator of the relationship between transformational leadership and followers' performance and organizational citizenship behavior. *Academy of Management Journal, 48*(3), 430–432.

Washington, R. R. (2007). Empirical relationships between theories of servant, transformational, and transactional leadership. *Academy of Management Proceedings,* 1–6.

Weber, M. (1970). Bureaucracy. In W. Sexton (Ed.), *Organization theories* (pp. 39–43). Columbus, OH: Charles E. Merrill.

Williams, C. R. (2009). *Management* (5th ed.). Mason, OH: South-Western Cengage Learning.

Winter, D. G. (1973). *The power motive.* New York: Free Press.

CHAPTER 17

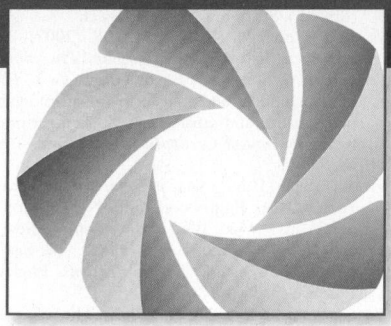

Learning Theories

Evelyn M. Wills and Melanie McEwen

Barbara Davis is a family nurse practitioner working in a community clinic. Recently, she cared for Frank Young, a 65-year-old African American who came to the clinic at his wife's insistence because of recurring, severe headaches. Mr. Young reported that his headaches started about 6 months ago; he attributed them to stress caused by his recent retirement.

Mr. Young's physical findings indicated that he was about 50 lbs overweight and that his blood pressure while sitting was 204/110 mmHg. His lower legs and feet were slightly edematous, and laboratory tests revealed a total cholesterol reading of 290 mg/dl. All other laboratory blood and urine results were normal.

Barbara explained to Mr. Young that he has high blood pressure and asked to discuss the problem with both him and his wife. She led the Youngs to a room in which they sat in comfortable chairs around a small table. Barbara began the discussion by asking if the couple had any experience with hypertension (HTN). She explained the relationship among HTN, race, age, gender, and weight and described its prevalence among various groups. She showed the Youngs a short video that used nonmedical terms to describe HTN, visually illustrated the physiologic changes that cause HTN, and then explained some of the possible complications.

After the video, Barbara questioned the Youngs to evaluate their level of understanding. A 15-minute discussion followed in which Barbara described management strategies. She gave Mr. Young two prescriptions and explained what they were for and how to take them. Following the explanation, she had him repeat the information to her. They also discussed the importance of limiting sodium intake, and Barbara gave the Youngs a booklet with pictures to show the exact types, varieties, and amounts of foods available in their region and whether the sodium content was safe, high, or too high to consume. It included condiments, with the allowed amounts, on a full-color poster that could be placed on the side of the refrigerator or attached to the door of a cabinet. There were recipes for variations on favorite foods with lowered sodium content, and the booklet also had removable shopping lists to assist Mrs. Young when she had to make quick decisions in grocery stores. Learning that both Mrs. and Mr. Young enjoyed working and gaming on the computer, Barbara included websites with helpful hints on limiting sodium and fats, and the URLs for "say NAYtoNA," a local Facebook support group page and Twitter site for social support.

At the end of the appointment, they reviewed the ways to lower Mr. Young's blood pressure and they set up an appointment with the clinic's dietitian to go over ways the Youngs could reduce the amount of fat and salt in their diet. Finally, Barbara made a follow-up appointment for the next week and encouraged Mrs. Young to accompany her husband to that meeting.

One of the most important roles of professional registered nurses (RNs) and advanced practice nurses (APNs) is teaching. Teaching performed by nurses at all levels is usually more informal than formal. That is, the nurse teaches clients and their families, or students and colleagues, more often on a one-to-one basis as the need arises than in a formal, planned teaching session in a classroom setting. But teaching includes more than just providing clients with information. Because someone has been told something does not mean that learning has occurred. Many factors are involved for learning to be successful, and providing information is only one of them.

Health information is usually foreign and difficult to understand for patients and families; the idea of health literacy as a component of health teaching is important in teaching patients/clients. Health literacy is defined as "the degree to which an individual has the capacity to obtain, communicate, process and understand basic health information and services to make appropriate health decisions" (Bastable, Myers, & Poitevent, 2014, p. 261). Although health literacy is not an educational theory, health teaching depends on the abilities of nurses to bring information and education to individuals and groups regardless of their educational level and ability to learn. Because many patients depend on someone else to help or to care for them, the caregivers must also be taught to provide assistance so that the patient may heal or live with chronic diseases or the effects of illness and trauma.

This chapter provides professional nurses with tools to facilitate learning for patients, families, and staff. Basic theories of learning can serve as a framework for the nurse in all teaching endeavors. Theories provide a way to organize thinking for what will be communicated to other people. They may offer a mechanism whereby the instructor can look at a situation in a different way when current methods are not working, or they may provide a map for charting unfamiliar territory. In any event, facilitating learning is an essential objective of the professional nurse, and application of theories helps ensure that learning is optimized.

What Is Learning?

Learning has been defined as "a relatively permanent change in behavior or in behavioral potentiality that results from experience and cannot be attributed to temporary body states such as those induced by illness, fatigue, or drugs" (Olson & Hergenhahn, 2012, p. 6). Learning occurs as individuals interact with their environment, incorporating new information into what they already know (Braungart, Braungart, & Gramet, 2014; Candela, 2012). Further, if learning is to be permanent, it must be treated as a process that occurs over time rather than an isolated event. Often, time and repeated contacts are required for an individual to acquire new knowledge that is meaningful and significant (Forrest, 2004).

Learning can be grouped into three categories: psychomotor learning (the acquisition and performance of skills), affective learning (a change in feelings, values, or beliefs), and cognitive learning (acquiring information). Examples of psychomotor learning would include a nursing student mastering certain patient care procedures (e.g., inserting an IV line or changing a sterile dressing) and a patient learning to self-inject insulin. Illustrations of affective learning include an alcoholic acquiring strategies to overcome addiction and a nurse developing cultural sensitivity when caring for immigrants. Cognitive learning generally involves the addition of new information, as when a new mother learns how to care for her infant or a novice nurse learns to recognize the signs and symptoms of heart failure. Although not always recognized, psychomotor learning tends to be more easily accomplished and measured than affective and cognitive learning (Rankin & Stallings, 2005). Nurses must understand all three types of learning and know how to facilitate each in patients and their families as well as among other nurses and ancillary staff.

The process of assimilating new knowledge into our daily lives makes all humans constant learners, because learning is necessary for survival. Although all animals can learn, humans are capable of using their knowledge to be creative, predict the future, explain the past, or deal with the present. Indeed, learning is such an important human experience that it has created the desire or curiosity to discover how people learn. This search to understand how people learn has led to the development and formalization of learning theories.

What Is Teaching?

It must be recognized that although teaching and learning are interrelated, learning occurs as a separate and individual process apart from teaching. Teaching refers to the intentional act of communicating information and is often defined as the facilitation of learning (Bastable & Alt, 2008). To accomplish this, teachers must be aware of the learning styles and learning needs of the individual and how capable that individual is of responding to the demands of instruction.

It is a common assumption that teaching is helping one to gain knowledge. While that is certainly an important component of teaching, knowledge is seldom enough to elicit a change in behavior or thinking. Knowing what should be done and acting on that knowledge are two different things. For example, a patient with chronic renal failure may *know* that salt and potassium are to be avoided in the diet, but learning has not occurred until that knowledge has been incorporated as a change in behavior.

Anyone who teaches, including a mother or father teaching a child how to put away toys, or a woman teaching a friend to crochet, has some belief regarding how learning occurs. Unfortunately, sometimes the knowledge the teacher possesses about learning is simplistic: "I told you; therefore, you should know." An individual's beliefs about learning can influence that person's behavior regarding what should happen to make learning occur. By understanding basic theories of learning, the professional nurse will be better prepared to help the learner make the transition from acquiring knowledge to learning. This chapter presents some of the many theories of learning and describes how they are used to solve problems encountered in the teaching–learning process. These theories may be used by nurses in practice or education, as well as for designing, implementing, and evaluating research projects that involved education.

Categorization of Learning Theories

Some nurses might question why it is important to understand the process of learning and to know about some of the theories of learning. Learning theories describe the processes used to bring about changes in the ways individuals understand information and changes in the ways they perform a task or skill. Further, learning theories can help provide a focus for creating an environment and conditions in which teaching can occur more effectively (Candela, 2012). Kurt Lewin is credited with the adage: "There is nothing so practical as a good theory." A good theory enables you to make choices confidently and consistently and to explain or defend why you made the choice you did. Thus, although nursing theory provides the framework for professional assessment of the client's condition or needs and the specific language the nurse uses when making a diagnosis or charting, learning theories explain *how* this information is assimilated and suggest effective ways to present it to the client as an intervention. Learning theory, then, combined with nursing theory, guides nurses as they interact with clients.

There are many different types of learning theories and only a few of the most commonly used in nursing are described in the following sections. The main categories as presented by Bigge and Shermis (1999) are the behavioral learning theories and the cognitive learning theories. Behavioral learning theories include the works of Pavlov, Skinner, and others. Cognitive learning theories include cognitive-field theories, information-processing theories, interaction theories, and developmental theories (social cognitive/social learning theory), psychodynamic theory (humanistic learning theory), and adult learning theory. Some of the major theories for each group will be discussed briefly, with examples of application from the nursing literature.

Behavioral Learning Theories

Behavioral theories were among the first to be widely recognized and used in education. Indeed, they were so pervasive in the American educational system in the 1950s and 1960s that many people still associate the term "learning theories" with behavioral theories. Behavioral learning theories served the growing American educational system well during the 20th century. They provided the rapidly expanding system with an organized, systematic approach.

Behaviorism focuses on what is directly observable in learners. It is largely based on the works of Ivan Pavlov and Edward Thorndike, who researched how both humans and animals learned, and their work became the basis for behavioral psychology (Olson & Hergenhahn, 2012; Candela, 2012). In behavioral theories, behavior (response) is viewed as the result of stimulus conditions. The behavioral learning theories that evolved from this perspective are sometimes referred to as the stimulus–response (S–R) model of learning. Some of the major behaviorist theorists include Thorndike (connectionism), Pavlov (classical conditioning), Skinner (operant conditioning), Watson (behaviorism), and Hull (reinforcement). Table 17-1 summarizes the assertions of each of these theorists.

Table 17-1 Comparison of Behavioral Learning Theories

Theorist	Theory Distinctions
Thorndike	Original stimulus–response framework; learners respond randomly to stimuli; learning is trial and error
Pavlov	Classical conditioning; responses are involuntary and based on experience
Skinner	Operant conditioning; learning produces a desirable behavior because it is reinforced or strengthened
Hull	Stimulus–response framework (based on Thorndike); includes reinforcement as a characteristic of learning
Watson	Behaviorism (based on Pavlov); classical conditioning and extinguishing behaviors

Edward L. Thorndike (1874–1949) was one of the first theorists to attempt scientific studies to understand the learning process. He perceived that learners are empty organisms who respond to stimuli in a random manner. He provided the original S–R framework for behavioral psychology. For Thorndike, learning was the result of associations formed between stimuli and responses, and the S–R connections were formed through trial and error. Such associations or habits become strengthened or weakened by the nature and frequency of the S–R pairings. The hallmark of connectionism was that learning could be adequately explained without referring to any observable internal states (Thorndike, 1932).

In a well-known study, Pavlov (1849–1936) taught his dog to salivate when a tuning fork was rung by rewarding him with meat powder placed into his mouth. Soon, the dog would salivate when the tuning fork rang even though no meat powder was provided. This involuntary reaction is known as *conditioning*. Pavlov's work is labeled as *classical conditioning* to differentiate it from other types of S–R associations that deal with voluntary behavior (Braungart et al., 2014). Classical conditioning is what one sees in a child's response to the sight of a needle. The conditioned stimulus (the sight of the needle) is able to evoke the response (crying) formerly reserved for the unconditional stimulus (actual pain from an injection). Response to the sight of a needle is learned behavior based on experience.

To B. F. Skinner (1904–1990), the purpose of psychology is to predict and control the behavior of individuals. He defined learning as a change in probability of response and coined the term *operant conditioning*. An *operant* is a set of behaviors that constitutes an individual doing something. Operant conditioning is the learning process whereby a desirable behavior is made more likely to occur in the future or to occur more frequently because it is reinforced or strengthened (Olson & Hergenhahn, 2012; Ormrod, 2012). When the desired response occurs, whether accidental or planned, a reward that is meaningful to the learner is provided, so recurrence of the desired response is increased. In the previously discussed classical conditioning, the person in question receives reinforcement no matter what he or she does, whereas in an operant conditioning situation, the individual's behavior causes the reward to happen.

John B. Watson (1878–1958) was the first American psychologist to incorporate Pavlov's work into his own. While Watson's research methods would be called into question under today's standards, he did demonstrate classical conditioning in an experiment where he subjected a young boy named Albert to a white rat. At first, the boy was not afraid of the rat. However, Watson created a loud noise whenever the boy touched the rat. Eventually, the boy associated touching the rat with the noxious stimulus and became afraid of the rat and other small animals. Watson then demonstrated the idea of "extinguishing" the conditioned behavior by offering the rat to the boy without the loud noise (Lefrancois, 2000; Ormrod, 2012). Watson's work has been used to explain and treat fears, phobias, and prejudices that people develop in response to situations and events. Watson is generally credited with originating the term *behaviorism* (Olson & Hergenhahn, 2012).

Clark L. Hull (1884–1952) based his studies on Thorndike's work but included *reinforcement* as a major characteristic of learning. Reinforcement is a complex concept that is widely used in education today. Reinforcement is a consequence of an action that makes that action more likely to be repeated. Reinforcement may be internal/external, positive/negative, self-administered, social, or impersonal (Roberts, 1975). Reinforcement can be seen in many ways, from a simple smile (or frown) to aversion therapy (e.g., the "quit smoking" clinics that have individuals smoke one cigarette after another until they become sick). Problems can arise because the behavior the teacher intends to reinforce may not be the actual behavior that is reinforced.

Box 17-1 Characteristics of Behavioral Learning Theories

- Focuses on behavior modification, reflexes, reaction, and reinforcement
- Emphasizes observable and measurable aspects of human behavior
- Posits that behavior can be controlled through rewarding desirable behavior and ignoring or punishing undesirable behavior

Behaviorists are concerned with the observable and measurable aspects of human behavior. Basically, behaviorists believe that behavior can be controlled (thus demonstrating that learning has occurred) through rewarding desirable behavior and ignoring or punishing behavior that is undesirable. Reinforcing or strengthening the behavior increases the chance of its recurrence in the future. These theorists are concerned with behavior modification and make much use of the concepts of reflexes, reactions, objective measurement, quantitative data, sequence of behavior, and reinforcement schedules (Ormrod, 2012; Ozmon, 2011). Box 17-1 summarizes characteristics of behavioral learning theories.

Teachers who subscribe to this viewpoint are considered designers and controllers of students' behavior. The teacher is responsible for what students should learn and for evaluating how, when, and if they have learned. Teachers are expected to be content experts, transmit prescribed content, control the way learners receive and use the content, and then test to determine if they have received it (Knowles, 1981). Learning objectives (also called *behavioral objectives*, *instructional objectives*, or *performance criteria*) are broken down into a large number of very small tasks and reinforced one by one. The tasks are organized so that understanding develops progressively. This premise has led to the development of programmed texts and computer-assisted instruction. Tests are used in a classroom situation to measure the amount of knowledge a student has gained.

Use of behavioral theory encourages the development of clear behavioral outcomes and methods for evaluating those desired behaviors. It works well for many of the psychomotor skills that must be accomplished for both nurses and patients. Behavioral theory, however, is not without detractors. Because the learner assumes a relatively passive role, there is a possibility that old behaviors will be resumed once the learner is removed from the highly structured and controlled environments created by behaviorally based teaching methods. In other words, without the affective and cognitive components of learning, there is no change in feelings or thinking for the learner. Once they are returned to the original environment that fostered and rewarded the undesirable behavior, chances are high that the original behavior will return. Many question whether behavioral techniques alone are capable of producing permanent changes in behavior.

Application to Nursing

Behaviorist principles are widely used by nurses, nursing educators, and staff developers. For example, learning contracts with clients are an outgrowth of this perspective. Likewise, nurses often use reinforcement when they comment on how well clients are following their treatment regimens and when they correctly repeat instructions. Also, much of nursing education is directed toward having students meet behavioral objectives, which is a hallmark of behavioral theories (see Chapter 21).

Cognitive Learning Theories

In contrast to behavioral theories, which generally ignore the thoughts, feelings, and cognitive processes of the learner, cognitive learning theories emphasize the mental processes and activities that go on within the learner (Candela, 2012). Cognitive theorists do not view reward as a condition for learning, although they do not negate the role of reinforcement. The learner's own goals, thoughts, expectations, motivations, and abilities in the processing of information are seen as the foundations for learning.

Cognitive learning theory began to gain popular momentum in the 1960s when the recognition of the limitations of behavioral theories led to the development of more complete theories to frame and explain how people learn and how permanent changes in behavior are accomplished. One of the most important theorists in cognitive science, Jean Piaget, however, developed major components of his theory in the 1920s.

Cognitive theories focus on the operations of the mind and on how thoughts influence an individual's actions in relation to the environment (Candela, 2012). Several major subcategories of cognitive learning theories have evolved over time. Those described in the following sections include gestalt (cognitive-field) theories, information-processing theories, cognitive development theories, social learning theories, psychodynamic theories, and adult learning theories. Representative examples useful for nurses are presented in the following sections.

Cognitive-Field (Gestalt) Theories

A break with behaviorism occurred when the concept of "insight" learning was introduced into the gestalt theories. "Gestalt" is a German word that refers to the configuration or patterned organization of cognitive elements (Braungart et al., 2014). The gestalt view of learning focuses on organization of a person's perceptual field to sort out and make sense of multiple parts. The scientific view underlying gestalt principles is field theory. Field theory espouses that a "field" is a dynamic, interrelated system in which any part can affect all other parts and that the whole is more than the sum of the parts (Olson & Hergenhahn, 2012). Gestalt theory and field theory have become so closely associated that they are commonly referred to as *cognitive-field theory.*

The cognitive-field psychologists consider learning to be closely related to perception. They define learning in terms of reorganization of the learner's perceptual or psychological world—his or her field. The field includes a simultaneous and mutual interaction among all the forces or stimuli affecting the person—the internal environment as well as the external environment. Experience is the interaction of a person and his or her perceived environment, whereas behavior is the result of the interplay of these forces. Consequently, perception and experiences of reality are uniquely individual, based on a person's total life experiences. Nothing exists in and of itself but only in relationship to something else. Learning, then, is the process of discovering and understanding the relationships among people, things, and ideas in the field. Learning is viewed as an active, goal-oriented process that is accomplished when information is processed and the "aha" moment is experienced. Transfer of information from the teacher to the student does not constitute learning. In order for learning to be accomplished, students must assume responsibility for learning and discover and assign their own meaning in order to understand and truly learn content. Through the learning process, the learner gains new insights or changes old ones. The purpose of learning is to think more effectively in a wide variety of situations and thus be able to solve problems.

Because cognitive-field theorists are
of the total person, they perceive self-ac
all human behavior. Motivation involve
that cause the person to want to do sc
rists who think of motivation as a driv
development are important in motivati
As an individual matures, the forces op

Kurt Lewin (1890–1947), one o
mans have a basic need to bring orde
stimulated by the ambiguity perceive
learning process, the instructor helps
of verbal explanations, showing pictu
ties, the instructor helps the individu
learner can organize the experience into a
of problems that flow hierarchically in level of difficulty and providing appro
resources for the learner to use to solve the problems, the instructor creates a motivating environment for learning (Knowles, Holton, & Swanson, 2005).

Cognitive-field theorists believe people can learn information cognitively without changing their behavior and that motivation is the key. Motivation is an extremely difficult concept to implement. In health care, one often hears reports that an individual is noncompliant, when in actuality the person is not motivated (for whatever reason) to do what the health care professionals perceive as the correct thing to do. Indeed, it often takes months and even years to find the right combination of factors that motivate an individual.

As a child, Mr. Young, from the opening case study, would probably rebel against changing his eating habits, but he may be more likely to be motivated to do so as an adult because he understands the relationship between his diet and his headaches. Box 17-2 depicts characteristics of cognitive-field theories.

Application to Nursing

Barbara, the nurse in the case study, used cognitive-field theory when she had the Youngs move into a room more conducive to learning. By controlling the external stimuli affecting the situation, she allowed the brain to focus more on the information she was presenting. By using visual models as well as her verbal explanation, she involved more senses in the learning process and thereby more of the whole person. Mr. Young's pain served as a good motivator, increasing his desire for relief and his willingness to participate in the learning process to prevent future episodes.

In reviewing recent nursing literature, cognitive-field theory and/or gestalt theory was used several times. Kelly and Howie (2011), for example, presented an overview of gestalt theory and explained how it can be used by psychiatric nurses to promote

Box 17-2 Characteristics of Cognitive-Field Learning Theories

- Learning is related to perception.
- Perceptions of reality and experiences are uniquely individual and based on life experiences.
- Thoughts influence actions.
- Motivation is key to learning.
- Self-actualization is the main motivating force.

acceptance, self-responsibility, and personal growth. In another work, ukholm (2008) analyzed nurses' writing activities and teacher interac- earched for evidence of critical thinking in an online setting. They found critical thinking and writing competence grew over time in the online activity. (2007) studied the incorporation of high-fidelity patient simulators and nurs- students' feelings of self-efficacy and confidence in performing nursing care in n intensive care situation. She found that the feelings of confidence in the ability to think critically under stress were increased in the students. Lastly, Hanson and Stenvig (2008) used cognitive field theory/gestalt theory as a framework for a study of attributes of clinical nursing educators.

Information-Processing Models

Information-processing theories emerged in the 1970s. They arose from the field of artificial intelligence as researchers attempted to create computer systems to simulate human cognitive skills (Byrnes, 2008; Candela, 2012). Learning theorists using these models are concerned with the process of acquiring information, remembering it, and using it for problem solving. These theories propose an elaborate set of internal processes to account for how learning and retention occur (Ormrod, 2012).

In information-processing theories, human memory is thought to be composed of three stores: sensory store, short-term store, and long-term store. Information from the environment passes sequentially through the stores. The sensory store (also known as the *sensory memory*, *iconic memory*, or *echoic memory*) holds incoming information long enough that preliminary cognitive processing can begin. Information stored in the sensory memory is stored basically in the form in which it was sensed—visual input is stored visually, auditory input in an auditory form. Although the sensory store has unlimited capacity, information is stored very briefly.

The short-term memory is the most active component of the memory systems. Thinking occurs within the short-term memory and determines which information will be attended to within the sensory memory. The short-term memory holds information while it is being processed from both the sensory memory and the long-term memory. Interpretation of newly received environment input is interpreted in the short-term memory.

The long-term memory is the most complicated of the memory systems and the one that has received the most research. Long-term memory is thought to have an unlimited capacity, but the experts disagree regarding how long the information remains in storage. Some experts believe it is there forever, but others believe the information is lost through a variety of forgetting processes. Information is rarely stored in the long-term memory in the form in which it is received. What is stored is the "gist" of what was seen or heard rather than word-for-word sentences or precise mental images. Individuals organize the information that is stored in the long-term memory so related pieces of information are associated together (Ormrod, 2012).

In information-processing models, learning consists of strategies to transfer information from short-term storage to long-term storage. Information in the short-term memory (also known as the *working memory*) is lost within 5 to 20 seconds if action is not taken to reinforce it (Byrnes, 2008). For example, repeating the individual's name when introduced to a new person increases the ability to recall it at a later time. It is important for an instructor using this theory to present information in an organized manner, to overlap the information with previously learned knowledge, and to show the learner how the material is organized and how it relates to what was previously learned (Ormrod, 2012). External stimuli are thought to support several different types of ongoing internal processes involved in learning, remembering, and performing. Techniques such as visual imagery facilitate learning and the recall of information.

Along with remembering is the question of why people forget. Three theories have been proposed to explain this phenomenon: decay and interference theories, and the loss of retrieval cues. Decay theory proposes that information weakens over time, if it is not practiced or used. This is similar to the "use it or lose it" theory of muscle strength. Interference theory postulates that something interferes between the information already in storage and the new information being learned. If the new information being learned interferes with previously stored information, it is called *retroactive interference*; if old information interferes with the learning of new information, it is called *proactive interference* (Ormrod, 2012). Loss of retrieval cues involves the weakening of associations among the retrieval cues and records (Byrnes, 2008). For example, a nurse frequently sees a colleague from another unit in the cafeteria. The nurse knows this person's name and recognizes him or her. When the nurse meets this same person in the grocery store in street clothes, however, the nurse knows she knows the person but may not recall from where or the name. Because the person is out of context, the associations are not readily available for recall.

Application to Nursing

Nurses in practice and research have used information-processing theories. In the opening case study, by asking the Youngs to repeat some actions they could take to assist in lowering Mr. Young's blood pressure, Barbara was helping the information to be stored in their long-term memory. In examples from the nursing literature, O'Neill, Dluhy, and Chin (2005) used an information-processing theory as a framework for creating a computerized clinical decision-making model to assist novice nurses in making clinical judgments. In another work, Chabeli (2010) presented a review of the literature describing how concept mapping is used as a teaching method to promote critical thinking in nursing education. She identified four steps to facilitate critical thinking through concept mapping, which would promote information retention and clinical application. Then, Li and Liu (2012) reported on their literature review of use of "errorless learning strategies," a process that promotes use of "implicit memory" and how it relates to long-term memory for patients with Alzheimer disease. They explained that the intent is to enhance memory rehabilitation in these patients.

Cognitive Development or Interaction Theories

Cognitive development theories assume that behavior, mental processes, and the environment are interrelated. Also termed *interaction theories*, they are concerned with the progressive development and changes in thinking, reasoning, and perception of individual learners. A major assumption of cognitive theories is that learning occurs as a sequential process. Learning takes place over time, as when a child explores and interacts with the environment.

The experiential learning model exemplifies the interaction theories, which postulate that individuals learn from their immediate experiences and that learning happens in all human settings (Kolb, 1984). Learning is how individuals adapt and cope with the environment (the world) in which they live. Because each person's experience is unique, individuals develop a preferred style for learning. Whereas behavioral objectives state what the student will learn, experiential learning focuses on the conditions of learning. The instructor's role is to create an environment for learning and the experiences that support student understanding of the whole rather than its

Box 17-3 Characteristics of Cognitive Development/Interaction Learning Theories

- Behavior, mental processes, and the environment are interrelated.
- Individuals learn from their experiences.
- Learning is how individuals adapt to and cope with their environment.
- Focus is on conditions that promote learning.

separate parts (Rogers & Freiberg, 1994). This is achieved through activities such as group process, problem-solving activities, and simulation exercises. Some of the theories noted for this perspective are Piaget's cognitive development theory, Gagne's conditions of learning, Perry's theory of intellectual and ethical development, and Bandura's social learning theories. Box 17-3 summarizes characteristics of cognitive development/interaction theories.

Piaget

Jean Piaget (1896–1980) is probably the best known of the cognitive development theorists. He believed that cognitive development occurs in stages and that the stages occur in a fixed order and are universal to persons everywhere. He identified the following stages: sensorimotor, preoperational, concrete operational, and formal operational.

According to Piaget, for learning to occur, an individual must be able to assimilate new information into existing cognitive structures or schemes; that is, the new experience must overlap with previous knowledge. Behavior becomes more intelligent as coordination between the reactions to objects becomes progressively more interrelated and complex. Cognitive development begins in the sensorimotor stage (which is evident from birth until about 2 years of age) with the baby's use of the senses and movement to explore its world. In the preoperational stage (from about 2 years old until about age 6 or 7 years), action patterns evolve into the symbolic but illogical thinking of the preschooler. In this stage, language ability grows rapidly (Berk, 2003). In the concrete operational stage, cognition is transformed into the more organized reasoning of the school-aged child (age 6 or 7 until about 11 or 12 years). Abstract reasoning begins with the formal operational stage of the adolescent where youth are able to construct ideals and reason realistically about the future (Berk, 2003; Ormrod, 2012).

In Piaget's work, it is the schemes, or psychological structures, that change with age. Individuals build new schemes by adapting their experiences into previous knowledge. Assimilation and accommodation processes make up the adaptive process (Berk, 2003).

Many adults, however, have not developed complete formal operational thinking and need concrete examples before being presented with abstract ideas. Thus, it is important for the teacher to present information in a manner appropriate for the stage of development. The nurse usually has no formal means of testing an individual's cognitive development stage but must rely on the individual's verbal interaction during the assessment process. In the case study, Barbara could do this by using a familiar example of a clogged sink to explain what was occurring inside the blood vessels.

Application to Nursing. A few nursing articles can be found that use Piaget's theory either as a conceptual framework for a research study or to interpret or describe findings or actions. For example, Dickey, Kiefner, and Beidler (2002) used Piaget's writings on development in a discussion on children's and adolescents' ability to assent, consent, or dissent to participation in medical research. Another study used Piaget's theory as the conceptual framework in a cross-cultural examination of children's fears of medical experiences (Mahat, Scoloveno, & Cannella, 2004), and a third used Piaget's work to describe the processes children use to cope with disasters (Deering, 2000). Finally, LaFleur and Raway (1999) presented a nursing study using Piaget's theory that compared the perception of pain intensity between school-aged children and adolescents. Subjects ranked the word descriptors "pain," "hurt," and "ache." Findings indicated that children and adolescents associate similar levels of intensity with each of the words but associate different experiences with each.

Gagne

Robert M. Gagne (1916–2002) believed that much of individual's learning (from sensorimotor to highly complex intellectual skills) requires different conditions for learning to be successful. He classified learning outcomes into five different categories: intellectual skills, verbal information, cognitive strategies, motor skills, and attitudes. Each category has subcategories and involves both internal and external conditions that contribute to, or interfere with, the learning process (Gagne, 1985). Gagne believed that there are eight different types of learning that proceed sequentially in a hierarchical order (Box 17-4).

For Gagne (1985), teaching means arranging the conditions that are external to the learner. When trying to get a client or patient to understand a concept (such as HTN in the case study), it is important not only to provide a definition of the concept but also to give many positive examples to illustrate the concept, while at the same time giving negative examples to illustrate what the concept is not. The nurse can test clients' understanding of a concept by asking them to think of their own examples and applications.

Application to Nursing. Gagne's principles have been used in some nursing studies. Shawler (2008) describes a strategy that uses standardized patients (actors instructed to simulate a set of symptoms) to teach graduate nursing students about complex mental disorders. In a survey of nurse anesthetists, respondents were asked to report

Box 17-4 Gagne's Types of Learning

1. *Signal learning:* An involuntary response occurs to a specific stimulus (based on Pavlov's conditioned response).
2. *Stimulus–response:* A voluntary response occurs to a specific stimulus (similar to Skinner's operant conditioning).
3. *Chaining:* Two or more stimulus-response (S–R) associations occur and a sequence of behaviors is learned.
4. *Verbal association:* A chain of verbal S–R connections is involved.
5. *Discrimination learning:* The learner responds to one stimulus but not a similar one.
6. *Concept learning:* The learner organizes different stimuli into a class and then responds to any member of that class in the same way.
7. *Principle or rule learning:* A chain of two or more concepts is constructed.
8. *Problem solving:* The combination of two or more principles or rules come together to form higher-order thinking patterns.

Source: Gagne (1985).

the frequency of their experience of one of 24 selected untoward pathophysiologic conditions in their practice. The respondents overwhelmingly believed that experiential learning was required to prepare anesthetists to manage untoward events (Fallacaro & Crosby, 2000).

Perry

William G. Perry is a cognitive theorist who did most of his work on university-age students. His work had been criticized by psychologists and educators because his initial study sample consisted mainly of young male Harvard University students from privileged backgrounds (Perry, 1999). However, since 1970, his work has been replicated numerous times and has been found to be valid and reliable. As a result, it has become influential in higher education (Candela, 2012).

Perry's theory of intellectual and ethical development is similar to Piaget's regarding how individuals learn. Like Piaget, Perry's theory posits that learners move along a developmental continuum, both logically and psychologically (Perry, 1999). Also like Piaget, Perry believes that a certain amount of disequilibrium is necessary for accommodation to occur. However, rather than first being concerned with problem solving and application of logic, Perry's model is more concerned with how learners move from a dualistic (black versus white, right versus wrong) view of the world to a more relativistic view. Accepting the relativistic view requires the learner to adopt the notion that knowledge is not absolute and that there is no absolute criteria or authority for deciding right or wrong. Also, like other learning models, Perry concludes that different learners require different learning environments (Kurfiss, 1996).

Perry's theory describes nine positions of intellectual development. The more advanced the position, the more the person is likely to utilize formal reasoning. Perry's nine positions are grouped into three periods of development. The first period, which is composed of positions 1, 2, and 3, is "dualism." The dualist considers knowledge to be absolute, and his/her belief systems are unquestioned and unanswered. Authorities are considered to have all the right answers, and to question authority is unthinkable. Position 1 is termed "basic duality" and is composed of a child's basic set of understanding of issues of truth, morality, and values.

Perry's (1999) positions 2 and 3 of the first period (dualism) are termed "multiplicity prelegitimate" and "multiplicity subordinate," respectively. In these periods, much of the knowledge base is still considered absolute, but people begin to recognize that there are some gray areas. The learner can accept multiple perspectives, but rather than evaluate and apply reason to different viewpoints, the learner will simply seek to please the teacher and "go with the flow." Ironically, as the student actively seeks "what the teacher wants," the learner begins to acquire the fundamental mechanisms of independent thought (Kurfiss, 1996).

Relativism, the second period in intellectual development (positions 4, 5, and 6), requires recognition that all knowledge is not absolute truth. In this period, students progressively develop strategies for dealing with ambiguities and begin to consider the context when making decisions about questions of knowledge. Learners view authorities and experts as fellow learners, albeit more experienced at processing and making sense of the information in a given field. As the person moves from the end of this stage to the next period, there is a realization that one is responsible for defining oneself and that the condition of one's existence is influenced by his or her own life choices.

The final period is termed "commitments" (positions 7, 8, and 9) (Perry, 1999). Here, the learner becomes skilled in rational processes and can commit to a system of values, beliefs, and opinions that is used to define the self. Decisions are made through conscious consideration of alternatives based on accumulated learning and experiences. There is willingness to accept alternate viewpoints and decisions made by others (Kurfiss, 1996).

Application to Nursing. A few citations discussing use of Perry's work in the nursing literature were identified. For example, Secomb, McKenna, and Smith (2012) cited Perry's schema of cognitive and ethical development in their study of the effectiveness of simulation on the cognitive abilities of undergraduate nursing students. In another example, Rapps, Riegel, and Glaser (2001) used Perry's theory of cognitive development as the basis for developing a predictive model to enhance critical thinking in RNs. They examined the hierarchical levels of cognitive development (dualism, relativism, and commitment) and determined that critical thinking skills were significant only in the dualistic level.

Bandura

Albert Bandura's (1977a) social learning theory was based on the concept of reciprocal determinism and concerned with the social influences that affect learning (e.g., groups, culture, and ethnicity). In this theory, environment, cognitive factors, and behavior interact with one another so each variable affects the other two. For example, people learn from the continual bombardment of environmental stimuli without being aware that they are doing so.

Bandura's theory focuses on how people learn from one another and encompasses such concepts as observational learning, imitation, and modeling (Bandura, 1977a). Many behaviors that people exhibit have been acquired through observation and modeling of others. Individuals can imitate behaviors of someone they admire. For example, teenagers often imitate the behavior of their latest movie or rock star idol, or a nursing student may imitate the behaviors of a registered nurse who exemplifies the student's concept of professionalism.

Learning by watching or listening to others (vicarious learning) can occur without imitating the behaviors observed. In this instance, people can verbally describe the behavior but may not demonstrate it until later, when there is a need to do so. The concept of vicarious learning is used frequently by schools of nursing. Because not all students can care for clients with the same condition, nursing schools have students share their clinical experiences in postconferences. Students learn from each other's experiences but may not have an opportunity to implement the learning until after they graduate.

In later years, Bandura focused more on the underpinnings of constructivism and social cognition. He stressed that the learner is actively involved with the environment through personal selection, intentionality, and self-regulation of the learning process based on his or her own "filter" of the world. People may actively select their own role models and regulate their own attitudes and actions regarding learning. An important finding of Bandura's research for health care professionals is that self-efficacy promotes learning and productive human function. This implies that nurses should promote patients' independence and confidence rather than simply accepting and endorsing dependent behaviors in order to facilitate learning and health promotion.

Application to Nursing. Numerous recent nursing articles cite using Bandura's theory. Indeed, according to a review of published research reports, Montgomery (2002) found that Bandura's social cognitive theory, the health belief model, and the health promotion model were the most significant theories for nursing research related to adolescent health promotion.

Bandura's theory has also been used by nurses to develop successful interventions. For example, Lin (2012) studied the effects of a regular community-based physical activity program on metabolic parameters in middle-aged women using social cognitive theory. The findings suggested that a regular physical activity and health education program significantly improved the risk factors for metabolic syndrome among the women. Sharpe and colleagues (2010) used social cognitive theory to study physical activity in three groups of women. In this work, one group enrolled in a 24-week behavioral intervention, a second group was exposed to a media campaign, and the third group served as a control. Finally, Rogers, Vicari, and Courneya (2010) described lessons learned in facilitating exercise adherence among breast cancer survivors in group settings using social learning theory. An important finding was that teaching and other protocols for mental health must be individualized to the individual.

In the case of the Youngs, Barbara was using Bandura's social learning theory when she gave the Youngs the URLs for Facebook and Twitter sites of other people who were living with hypertension. She understood that communicating with others living with a similar health situation forms a powerful support for learning.

Psychodynamic Learning Theory

Although not technically a group of distinct learning theories, psychodynamic theory, which was based on the work of Sigmund Freud, does have implications for learning and behavior change (Braungart et al., 2014). Some of the most important contributions to learning theory have come from the discipline of psychotherapy because psychotherapists are concerned with the reeducation of their clients. Freud contributed concepts such as the unconscious, subconscious, repression, and defense mechanism, which are used by learning theorists (Knowles et al., 2005). Freud believed emotions interfered with cognition and that human motivation comes from deep internal drives, many of which arise from the unconscious (Roberts, 1975). Individuals may or may not be conscious of their own motivations and why they think, feel, and act the way they do.

According to psychodynamic theorists, motivation for behavior can come from several sources. The most basic source of motivation comes from the primal instincts and desires we are born with. This is referred to as the *id*. According to Freud, the basic function of the *id* is to seek pleasure and avoid pain. On the other hand, motivation is also based on the function of the *superego*, which is an individual's conscience based on internalized values and societal standards. These primitive drives and highly developed conscience are mediated by the *ego*, which allows individuals to weigh decisions and make the best choices.

This psychodynamic view gives the professional nurse perspective on teaching related to a patient's ego development. Patients with healthy ego development are able to make choices about their own care and maintain sometimes difficult courses of action to achieve outcomes. On the other hand, patients with poor ego development may choose the immediately gratifying course of action. When viewed from a learning theorist perspective, knowledge may not have a profound effect on the behaviors of patients who have poor ego development. For example, simply knowing about appropriate food choices for a diabetic patient may not be enough to incorporate healthy food choices into their behavior.

While psychodynamic theory provides a framework for understanding the behavior of others, it is largely speculative and abstract in nature. Health care professionals are cautioned that while these theories may provide some insight into the behavior of a person, they should not be used to dismiss a person's behavior or as a basis for decisions about whether or not to provide teaching.

Humanistic Learning Theory

Whereas Freudian scholars saw emotions as negative influences, humanistic educators recognize that emotions can have a positive influence on the learning process. Humanistic psychologists, often referred to as "third force" psychologists, are concerned with human potential and are interested in helping individuals develop that potential. As individuals or groups achieve new abilities, the human potential improves; consequently, the individual is always "becoming." Human relations skills are one of the major human abilities that concerns humanistic educators. Humanistic educators want learners to have warm interpersonal relationships, to trust others and themselves, and to be aware of others' feelings. The teacher's role is to design experiences that help improve the learners' abilities to perceive, feel, wonder, sense, create, fantasize, imagine, and experience (Roberts, 1975).

By redefining the role of the educator and focusing on the needs and feelings of the learner, humanistic theory has given health professionals a useful tool for client-centered teaching and care. Humanistic theory is the foundation for many successful wellness programs, self-help groups, and palliative care (Braungart & Braungart, 2008).

Rogers

Carl Rogers (1902–1987), one of the leaders of the humanistic perspective, transferred his principles about "client-centered" therapy to "student-centered" teaching. For Rogers (1983), the learner is in the process of becoming, the goal of education is to develop a "fully functioning person," and the teacher's role is to facilitate the process. He believed learning is a natural process, entirely controlled internally by the learner, in which the individual's whole being interacts with the environment as the learner perceives it. The learner has both the freedom to learn and to be self directed (as opposed to teacher directed). By providing problems real and meaningful to the learner, intrinsic motivation is stimulated to solve the problem. Rogers perceived the only truly educated person to be the one who learns how to learn, knows how to adapt to changing circumstances, and is continually seeking knowledge.

Application to Nursing. Nurses often use these principles in practice. For example, Vacek (2009) used concept mapping with students to promote critical thinking in a baccalaureate nursing program. The findings were that students using concept mapping experienced enhanced learning and critical thinking. Wong and team (2008) adopted a problem-based learning approach in a clinical simulation. They found that the students learned best in a stable, safe environment and could experience the full range of learning issues without endangering themselves or their patients. Additionally, they concluded that the learning environment is also valuable to staff development.

Developmental Psychology

In addition to Piaget, other developmental psychologists have contributed to a growing understanding of learning as it is affected by characteristics such as physical capabilities, mental abilities, interests, attitudes, values, creativity, and lifestyle. Noted developmental psychologists include Abraham Maslow (1908–1970), who wrote on needs hierarchy of motivation; Erik Erikson (1902–1994), who explored personality development; and Robert Havighurst (1900–1991), who described developmental tasks or life problems that lead to readiness to learn. Other developmental psychologists have also contributed to the understanding of the impact of maturation on learning. At one time, learning was thought to cease when an individual reached the mid-20s in age. Thanks to developmental psychologists, it is now recognized that learning may occur throughout the lifespan.

Constructivism

Constructivism is one of the newer developmental learning theories and is based on Piaget's work. Constructivists believe that knowledge has no existence outside the person's mind and that learners always interpret what is presented to them using preexisting knowledge, history, and typical ways of perceiving and acting (Byrnes, 2008). The basic operating processes in learning are assimilation, accommodation, and constructivism.

Assimilation is a process whereby an individual interacts with an object or event in a way that is consistent with what is already known. *Accommodation* is a process whereby an individual modifies the existing knowledge to account for a new event. Learning occurs when the individual incorporates an experience into his or her existing knowledge base. By attempting to make sense of the new experience, the learner *constructs* new knowledge (Ormrod, 2012). Therefore, the learner constructs new knowledge rather than acquiring new knowledge. The purpose of instruction is to support this construction, rather than to communicate information (Duffy & Cunningham, 1997).

One of the significant contributions of the developmental psychologists to learning is the recognition that there is a hierarchical basis in thinking from lower forms to higher forms with age and experience. Therefore, learners need a certain amount of education, experience, or practice before being capable of highest-order thinking. If the nurse presents new information before the first information has been received and translated, the collision of the information causes the information to "jam" in the client's brain, resulting in confusion. Nurses working with older people must recognize this phenomenon and incorporate it into their practice.

It is important for nurses to realize that geriatric clients are capable of learning. It simply may take a longer period of time to do so because of the increased time it takes for information to travel through the nervous system and be interpreted. For example, a 65-year-old person who has had a stroke can relearn to use muscles just as a 45-year-old person can, but the elder client will take several weeks or months longer to do so. Even a healthy 65-year-old individual may not mentally process information as rapidly as a 45-year-old person.

Adult Learning

Malcolm Knowles (1913–1997), although not the first educator to study adult learning, is credited with popularizing the notion of andragogy in North America. *Andragogy* is concerned with a unified theory of adult learning, as opposed to *pedagogy,* which focuses on youth learning. He views pedagogy as a content model and andragogy as a process model. For Knowles (Knowles et al., 2005), the single most important thing in helping adults to learn is to create a climate of physical comfort, mutual trust and respect, openness, and acceptance of differences. By responding to the needs of the learner and providing the learning resources required for learning, teachers facilitate learning. To be effective, presenters (teachers) need to "tell it like it is" and stress "how I do it" rather than telling the learner what to do. Through self-direction, learners are responsible for their own learning. Knowles and colleagues (Knowles et al., 2005) identified six assumptions regarding andragogy (Box 17-5).

Knowles and colleagues (Knowles et al., 2005) believed that adults need to know why they need to learn something. As a result, the teacher can help learners understand

Box 17-5 Knowles' Assumptions of Adult Learners

1. *Need to know:* Adults need to know why they need to learn something.
2. *Self-concept:* As people mature, their self-concept moves from one of being dependent toward one of being self directed.
3. *Experience:* As people mature, they accumulate a large amount of experience that can serve as a rich resource for learning.
4. *Readiness to learn:* Real-life problems or situations create a readiness to learn in the adult.
5. *Orientation to learning:* As a person matures, his or her time perspective changes from one of postponed application of knowledge to immediacy of application.
6. *Motivation:* Adults are primarily motivated by a desire to solve immediate and practical problems. As a person matures, motivation to learn is stimulated by internal stimuli rather than external stimuli.

how the knowledge is important to their future or the quality of their lives. Second, Knowles recognized the importance of self-concept in the adult learner. He taught that as people mature, their self-concept moves from one of being dependent toward one of being self directed. Adult learners want others to see them as being capable of self-direction and resent having someone else's will imposed on them. A self-directing teacher avoids "talking down" to the learner, provides information that enhances the adults' ability to solve problems, and encourages independence.

A third assumption revolves around experience. Knowles and colleagues (Knowles et al., 2005) explained that as people mature, they accumulate a large amount of experience that can serve as a rich resource for learning. Adults learn better when their own experiences are incorporated into the learning process. New experiences contribute to the learner's self-identity. Ignoring or devaluing this experience is perceived as rejecting them as a person.

The fourth assumption involves readiness to learn. Real-life problems or situations create a readiness to learn in the adult. Adults are problem-oriented learners, as opposed to subject-oriented learners; they want information that will help them solve a specific problem rather than an inclusive discussion of the subject. As a person matures, readiness to learn becomes increasingly oriented to the developmental tasks of social roles. Organizing learning activities around these life experiences facilitates the learning process. Readiness to learn can be created by exposing the individual to superior models, simulation exercises, and other techniques.

Similarly, the fifth assumption centers on orientation to learning. As a person matures, his or her time perspective changes from one of postponed application of knowledge to immediacy of application. Accordingly, the orientation toward self-learning shifts from one of subject centeredness to one of problem centeredness (Knowles et al., 2005).

Finally, motivation is the cornerstone of the adult learning theories. According to Knowles and colleagues (Knowles et al., 2005), adults are primarily motivated by a desire to solve immediate and practical problems. As a person matures, motivation to learn is stimulated by internal stimuli rather than external stimuli. The learner is self directed, determines what is to be learned and how it is to be learned, and assumes the primary responsibility for learning. For example, some motivational force is exerted from external sources, such as a desire for a better paying job, but a stronger force arises from internal sources, such as job satisfaction.

Theorists subscribing to developmental approaches to learning generally agree that there is a natural progression in thinking from the lower forms to higher forms with age and experience. Therefore, people need to have a certain amount of education,

Link to Practice 17-1

Barbara Davis used Knowles' adult learning to educate another client family—the Banzas—on care of Mr. Banza's new left ventricular assist device (LVAD) at home. In her planning, Barbara considered that because the Banzas were in their 80s, they might lack literacy related to health. She quickly learned that they were both motivated to learn and had the insight and experience of their years to call upon. Before retirement, Mr. Banza had owned his own successful home maintenance business and was a licensed and skilled electrician and plumber; therefore, he would be able to understand the implanted LVAD. Mrs. Banza, however, had only finished 10th grade; therefore, she had a fairly low literacy level, and had never worked outside her home.

Barbara decided to work with the Banzas together and started by explaining the electronics and "plumbing" of the LVAD to Mr. Banza. Next, she discussed with both seniors the need for cleanliness and sterility when caring for abdominal and chest incisions. To avoid overcoming them with information, Barbara organized her teaching in steps, beginning with what they needed to know immediately. She showed both of them the daily care of the instrument and explained when and how Mrs. Banza was to summon assistance if there were problems or complications. In later sessions, Barbara gave the couple training on more complex elements of care.

Barbara saw the Banzas regularly for several months and less often for several years. They were successful in caring for Mr. Banza's device, and when Barbara saw them at their 5-year checkup, both let her know that they had organized a group of other patients with LVADs and that the support group was successful.

experience, or practice before they can perform higher order thinking (Byrnes, 2008). For example, the man with newly diagnosed diabetes, with little formal education, and little knowledge of others with diabetes will have difficulty comprehending the implications of diabetes on his lifestyle.

Application to Nursing

There are some examples of the use of Knowles' theory in the nursing literature. Hammer and Craig (2008) employed a qualitative process to study nurses returning to clinical practice after a period of inactivity. They found that the more the nurses learned that was useful directly in clinical practice, the more easily they returned to the nursing role. Last, Clapper (2010) provided a detailed explanation of the importance of using adult learning theories when developing and implementing simulations in nursing education, encouraging nursing faculty to go "beyond Knowles." The intent should be to develop self-directed, lifelong learners who understand and can use technology. See Link to Practice 17-1.

Summary of Learning Theories

As the previous discussions have illustrated, numerous learning theories have been posited over the past century. Table 17-2 summarizes the cognitive-focused theories described. Many other diverse areas of study have developed from both the behavioral and cognitive fields of learning theories. Examples include multiple intelligence

Table 17-2 Summary of Cognitive Learning Theories

Group of Theories	Key Principles	Examples of Theorists
Cognitive-field (gestalt) theories	Learning relates to perception; motivation is key; behavior is related to perception and experience.	Lewin
Information-processing theories	Memory is composed of sensory memory, short-term memory, and long-term memory; learning consists of strategies to transfer information from short-term memory to long-term memory.	Anderson Bahrick
Cognitive development (interaction) theories	Individuals learn from their experiences; learning is how individuals adapt and cope with their environment.	Gagne Piaget Bandura Perry
Psychodynamic theory; humanism	Reeducation of clients is important; focus is on human potential; emphasis is on collaboration in the learning process; recognizes that emotions can positively affect learning.	Freud Rogers
Developmental psychology	Learning is affected by many variables, including physical and mental ability, attitudes, interests, and values; learning interprets information based on previous knowledge and experiences; learning continues throughout life.	Maslow Erikson Piaget Havighurst
Andragogy (adult learning theory)	The process of learning rather than content is the focus; physical comfort, mutual trust and respect, openness, and acceptance are important concepts.	Knowles

(Gardner, 1999), whole brain learning (Maxfield, 1990), learning styles (Kolb, 1976), assimilation (Ausubel, 1978), proficiency (Knox, 1980), transformational learning (Brookfield, 1991; Mezirow, 1981), memory (Atkinson & Shiffrin, 1968), self-directed learning (Tough, 1967), self-efficacy (Bandura, 1977b), and problem solving (Newell & Simon, 1972).

Learning Styles

It is widely recognized that most individuals have a preferred style of learning. Learning style is a characteristic that allows individuals to interact with instructional circumstances in such a way that learning is produced. Learning style preference relates to the likes and dislikes a person has for certain sensory modes, learning conditions, and learning strategies. Most people have probably not thought about how they learn and if questioned would give an answer based on what they assume, rather than what is correct.

By carefully listening to verbal comments of a patient, a nurse can obtain clues about the preferred learning style. For example, if the individual says something, such as "I hear what you're saying," the preferred learning style is most likely auditory. This individual learns best by hearing a discussion, presentation, audio device, and so forth. If, however, the response is "I see what you mean," the learning style is probably visual, and the person responds better to pictures, movies, or demonstrations. Tactual and kinesthetic learners make statements such as "I feel this is very important." These learners will learn best if able to manipulate or physically maneuver material with their hands. The availability of paper and pencils for taking notes, highlighter pens for marking important information, and picture puzzles will assist these types of learners (Morse, Oberer, Dobbins, & Mitchell, 1998).

In addition to age, gender also influences one's learning style. Men tend to be more visual, tactile, and kinesthetic than women. They are also more peer oriented and nonconforming and need the freedom to move around in an informal setting (Dunn & Dunn, 1992, 1993; Dunn & Griggs, 1995). In contrast, during learning situations, women tend to be more auditory, conforming, and authority oriented than men and are more able to sit passively (Pizzo, Dunn, & Dunn, 1990).

An important factor influencing learning is whether the individual tends to learn better analytically or globally. Analytic learners learn facts step by step in a logical progression building toward a whole. Global learners, by contrast, want to understand the whole before learning about the parts. Analytic learners will listen to all the facts as long as they believe they are heading toward a goal. Global learners need to know what they need to learn and why they need to learn it.

Different environments and different teaching strategies are required for global and analytic learners. Global learners learn better with intermittent periods of concentration and relaxation in a place with soft lighting, music, or other sound while sitting informally eating snacks. Short stories, anecdotes, humor, and illustrations can be used to capture the attention of global learners (Morse et al., 1998). Conversely, the analytic learner needs a quiet, well-lit formal setting with few or no interruptions and few or no snacks (Dunn & Griggs, 1998).

Principles of Learning

A common approach for teaching either individuals or groups is the use of learning principles. Principles of learning have been derived from multiple theories and are ideas that people can agree on no matter to which learning theory they subscribe. Whereas learning theories provide explanation about the underlying mechanisms involved in the learning process, principles identify specific elements that are important for learning and describe the particular effects of these variables on learning. The following are some other learning principles that may assist nurses as they attempt to provide health information to their clients.

- Learning is facilitated if information is provided from simple to complex, concrete to abstract, and known to unknown. This generally accepted learning principle recognizes the hierarchy in learning.
- Learning is facilitated if the information is personal and individualized. Learning occurs inside individuals and is activated by learners themselves. The client is more likely to remember what is taught if actively involved in the learning process.
- Learning is facilitated if it is relevant to the learner's needs and problems. What is relevant and meaningful is decided by the learner and must be discovered by him or her. Information that is meaningful is more easily stored and retrieved than information learned by rote memorization. What the nurse perceives as important to the health of the client may not be what the client perceives as important.
- Learning is facilitated if the individual is attentive. Attention is essential for learning. Attention is the process through which information moves into the short-term memory. Any internal (e.g., fear) or external factor (e.g., noise) that distracts the client can interfere with the learning process.

- Learning is facilitated when feedback is given close to the event rather than delayed.
- Learning is sometimes painful. This is true because learning is part of the growth process. Growth involves change, and change usually involves a certain amount of anxiety. Therefore, it is more comfortable for the individual to continue his or her ordinary behavior than to deal with the accompanying emotions required to change. What seems simple to a nurse giving information to a client may be a very complex process to the client.
- Learning is an emotional process as well as an intellectual process. The nurse needs to address the emotional aspects in the learning process as well as the knowledge aspects.
- The learning process is highly unique and individual. Simply put, people learn in different ways.

Application of Learning Theories in Nursing

Professional nurses and nurses in advanced practice must remember that no theory explains everything known about learning. There is not one theory that is best used for patient education or staff education. Depending on the learner and the given situation, certain theories may be more useful than others in designing instruction. The inherent value in the discussion of the theories in this chapter is that they give the nurse an opportunity to view patients and teaching through different frameworks and perspectives. It is suggested that the nurse use a broad knowledge of different theories, rather than a specific theory alone to approach his or her teaching role. In the most pragmatic sense, the role of the nurse is to find what works best based on this broad knowledge and use it for the benefit of the client, whether that client is a patient or a colleague.

Learning theories are best contextually applied. Professional nurses must use the circumstances surrounding each different teaching situation to help decide the most useful and appropriate approach. To apply principles and adapt concepts to patient education, nurses need to ask themselves the following questions.

- How can I increase my effectiveness in teaching my clients?
- Which learning theories are most congruent with my own view of human nature and my purpose for teaching clients?
- Which techniques will be most effective for particular situations?
- What are the implications of the various learning theories for my own role and performance?
- Which learning theory should I use under what circumstances?

Many authors (Bastable & Alt, 2014; DeYoung, 2008; Fitzgerald & Keyes, 2014) have concluded that better learning outcomes are achieved when a variety of strategies, based on different learning theories, are used. By synthesizing elements from a variety of theories, the best approach for a given situation can be found.

Clients coming to nurses, however, are often in pain or frightened, factors that directly interfere with the learning process. This interference can be misinterpreted as "not paying attention" or noncompliance. During the assessment process, the nurse should be alert to any cognitive or physical problems that may interfere with learning. Potential problems include poor hearing, eyesight, or coordination, as well as impaired thinking or memory. The person's personal and cultural beliefs should also be considered when trying to teach.

Theories from psychology and sociology (e.g., motivation, change, self-efficacy, health belief) can help the nurse determine the best learning approach. Although not directly related to learning, these theories do help explain human behavior and its impact on the learning process. Creative presentations, such as making up a rap song or an acronym for essential information, are often remembered longer than dialogue alone (Bruccoliere, 2000). Presenting too much information, too fast and too soon, can lead to learner frustration and failure. Further, clients need feedback regarding what they are doing right as well as what they are doing wrong.

Nurses can also encourage clients to seek out information on their own. Many people today have access to the Internet, either at home or through their public library. By seeking answers to their own learning needs, individuals accept responsibility for their own learning; this can lead to greater self-confidence and a better self-image. The more self-confidence individuals have, the more likely they will be to take the actions necessary to correct health problems.

Summary

Professional nurses and nurses in advanced practice should study learning theories, principles, and concepts and use them to direct education efforts to best meet the needs of the learner. In the opening case study, Barbara's use of multiple techniques and interventions to work with her clients to enhance their understanding illustrates when and how learning theories can be used in nursing. The idea as discussed is learning that will result in behavior changes that will promote and maintain health.

As educational research has progressed, theorists have become interested in specific aspects of learning and have incorporated related concepts such as motivation, memory, and thinking into existing theories, or they have developed completely separate theories based on the works of others. In addition to the external environment, physical, emotional, and intellectual maturation have been recognized as affecting the learning process. The differences between child and adult learning have been explored, and new areas of learning are being investigated. As these areas are further developed, new theories regarding learning will emerge. Professional nurses must be aware of new developments in learning theory and be ready to apply new thoughts and concepts when caring for clients.

Key Points

- Learning theories provide background information as to the ways people learn.
- Critiquing learning theories allows a nurse to decide on a model to use when providing meaningful education to each group of clients.
- Many learning theories have been proposed by scholars both in psychology and in education.
- Theories of teaching emanate from learning theories and educators enact these in their teaching whether teaching children, adolescents, or adults.
- Using multiple theories can assist the nurse acting as educator to realize that different teaching methods may be needed at different times and for different health care situations.
- Knowles posited the theory of adult learning, which is a useful theory for patient/client teaching in nursing.
- Learning is personal and an individual process and nurses must be able to use many different methods to assist patients and caregivers to promote or enhance patient education.

Learning Activities

1. Consider two courses that you have participated in—one that you liked and one you did not like. Compare the teaching methodologies used in both. Determine the teachers' predominant beliefs about learning based on the classroom approach. Think about your own beliefs about learning. How did your own beliefs facilitate or hinder the learning process in each of these classes?
2. Think about the environment that you create when studying. What do you do to create an environment more conducive to your own learning? How can experience be used to create a more positive learning environment in a clinical situation?
3. Try to determine how you learn. Are you predominantly an auditory learner, visual learner, tactile learner, or some combination of these? Attempt to determine the learning style of clients in clinical situations and modify teaching interventions accordingly.
4. Think about the patients you see each time you work or are in a clinical situation. Have you noticed whether they have had effective learning experiences to help them maintain their health? Using some of the cues in this chapter, decide what form of teaching would have complemented the learning styles of a particular patient or client such that their health education would have been more effective.

REFERENCES

Atkinson, R. C., & Shiffrin, R. M. (1968). Human memory: A proposed system and its control processes. In K. W. Spence & J. T. Spence (Eds.), *The psychology of learning and motivation: Advances in research and theory* (Vol. 2, pp. 89–195). New York: Academic Press.

Ausubel, D. P. (1978). *Educational psychology: A cognitive view* (2nd ed.). New York: Holt, Rinehart & Winston.

Bandura, A. (1977a). *Social learning theory.* Englewood Cliffs, NJ: Prentice-Hall.

Bandura, A. (1977b). Self-efficacy: Toward a unifying theory of behavioral change. *Psychological Review, 84*, 191–215.

Bastable, S. B., & Alt, M. F. (2014). Overview of education in health care. In S. B. Bastable (Ed.), *Nurse as educator: Principles of teaching and learning for nursing practice* (4th ed.). Boston: Jones & Bartlett.

Bastable, S. B., Myers, G. M., & Poitevent, L. B. (2014). Literacy in the adult client population. In S. B. Bastable (Ed.), *Nurse as educator: Principles of teaching and learning for nursing practice* (4th ed., pp. 3–23, 255–311). Boston: Jones & Bartlett.

Berk, L. E. (2003). *Child development* (6th ed.). Boston: Allyn & Bacon.

Bigge, M. L., & Shermis, S. S. (1999). *Learning theories for teachers* (6th ed.). New York: Addison-Wesley.

Braungart, M. M., Braungart, R. G., & Gramet, P. R. (2014). Applying learning theories to health care practice. In S. B. Bastable (Ed.), *Nurse as educator: Principles of teaching and learning for nursing practice* (4th ed., pp. 63–123). Boston: Jones & Bartlett.

Brookfield, S. D. (1991). *Developing critical thinkers.* San Francisco: Jossey-Bass.

Bruccoliere, T. (2000). How to make patient teaching stick. *RN, 63*(2), 34–38.

Byrnes, J. P. (2008). *Cognitive development and learning in instructional contexts* (3rd ed.). Upper Saddle River, NJ: Prentice Hall/Pearson.

Candela, L. (2012). From teaching to learning: Theoretical foundations. In D. M. Billings & J. A. Halstead (Eds.), *Teaching in nursing: A guide for faculty* (4th ed., pp. 202–242). St. Louis: Elsevier/Saunders.

Carter, L. M., & Rukholm, E. (2008). A study of critical thinking, teacher–student interaction and discipline-specific writing in an online educational setting for registered nurses. *Journal of Continuing Education in Nursing, 39*(3), 133–138.

Chabeli, M. M. (2010). Concept-mapping as a teaching method to facilitate critical thinking in nursing education: A review of the literature. *Health SA Gesondheid, 15*(1), 70–77.

Clapper, T. C. (2010). Beyond Knowles: What those conducing simulation need to know about adult learning theory. *Clinical Simulations in Nursing, 6*(1), e7–e14.

Deering, C. G. (2000). A cognitive developmental approach to understanding how children cope with disasters. *Journal of Child and Adolescent Psychiatric Nursing, 13*(1), 7–16.

DeYoung, S. (2008). *Teaching strategies for nurse educators* (2nd ed.). Upper Saddle River, NJ: Prentice Hall.

Dickey, S. B., Kiefner, J., & Beidler, S. M. (2002). Consent and confidentiality issues among school-age children and adolescents. *Journal of School Nursing, 18*(3), 179–185.

Duffy, T. M., & Cunningham, D. J. (1997). Constructivism: Implications for the design and delivery of instruction. In D. H. Jonassen (Ed.), *Handbook of research for educational communications and technology* (pp. 170–198). New York: Macmillan.

Dunn, R., & Dunn, K. (1992). *Teaching elementary students through their individual learning styles: Practical approaches for grades* 3–6. Boston: Allyn & Bacon.

Dunn, R., & Dunn, K. (1993). *Teaching secondary students through their individual learning styles: Practical approaches for grades* 7–12. Boston: Allyn & Bacon.

Dunn, R., & Griggs, S. A. (1995). *Multiculturalism and learning styles: Teaching and counseling adolescents.* Westport, CT: Greenwood Press.

Dunn, R., & Griggs, S. A. (1998). Learning styles: Link between teaching and learning. In R. Dunn & S. A. Griggs (Eds.),

Learning styles and the nursing profession (pp. 11–23). New York: National League for Nursing Press.

Fallacaro, M. D., & Crosby, F. E. (2000). Untoward pathophysiological events: Simulation as an experiential learning option to prepare anesthesia providers. *Clinical Forum for Nurse Anesthetists, 11*(3), 138–143.

Fitzgerald, K., & Keyes, K. (2014). Instructional methods and settings. In S. B. Bastable (Ed.), *Nurse as educator: Principles of teaching and learning for nursing practice* (4th ed., pp. 469–515). Boston: Jones & Bartlett.

Forrest, S. (2004). Learning and teaching: The reciprocal link. *Journal of Continuing Education in Nursing, 35*(2), 74–79.

Gagne, R. M. (1985). *The conditions of learning* (4th ed.). New York: Holt, Rinehart & Winston.

Gardner, H. (1999). *Intelligence reframed: Multiple intelligences for the 21st century.* New York: Basic Books.

Hammer, V. R., & Craig, G. P. (2008). The experiences of inactive nurses returned to nursing after completing a refresher course. *The Journal of Continuing Education in Nursing, 39*(8), 358–367.

Hanson, K. J., & Stenvig, T. E. (2008). The good clinical nursing educator and the baccalaureate nursing clinical experience: Attributes and praxis. *Journal of Nursing Education, 47*(1), 38–42.

Kelly, T., & Howie, L. (2011). Exploring the influence of gestalt therapy training on psychiatric nursing practice: Stories from the field. *International Journal Mental Health Nursing, 20*(4), 296–304.

Knowles, M. (1981). *From teacher to facilitator of learning.* Follett Publishing Co., Educational Materials Catalog. Reprinted in Knowles, M., Holton, E. F., & Swanson, R. A. (2005). *The adult learner: The definitive classic in adult education and human resource development* (6th ed., pp. 251–254). Burlington, MA: Elsevier.

Knowles, M., Holton, E. F., & Swanson, R. A. (2005). *The adult learner: The definitive classic in adult education and human resource development* (6th ed.). Burlington, MA: Elsevier.

Knox, A. B. (1980). Proficiency theory of adult learning. *Contemporary Educational Psychology, 5,* 378–404.

Kolb, D. A. (1976). *The learning style inventory.* Boston: McBer.

Kolb, D. A. (1984). *Experiential learning.* Englewood Cliffs, NJ: Prentice-Hall.

Kurfiss, J. G. (1996). *Critical thinking: Theory research, practice and possibilities: ASHE-ERIC/Higher education research report.* Washington, DC: George Washington University, Graduate School of Education and Human Development.

LaFleur, C. J., & Raway, B. (1999). School-age child and adolescent perception of the pain intensity associated with three word descriptors. *Pediatric Nursing, 25,* 45–50.

Lefrancois, G. R. (2000). *Theories of human learning* (4th ed.). Belmont, CA: Wadsworth/Thomson Learning.

Leigh, G. T. (2007). High fidelity patient simulation and nursing students' self efficacy: A review of the literature. *International Journal of Nursing Education Scholarship, 5*(1), 1–17.

Li, R., & Liu, K. P. Y. (2012). The use of errorless learning strategies for patients with Alzheimer's disease: A literature review. *International Journal of Rehabilitation Research, 35*(4), 292–298.

Lin, C. (2012). Effect of a regular community-based physical activity program on metabolic parameters in middle-aged women. *TzuChi Nursing Journal, 11*(4), 84–94.

Mahat, G., Scoloveno, M. A., & Cannella, B. (2004). Comparison of children's fears of medical experiences across two cultures. *Journal of Pediatric Health Care, 18*(3), 302–307.

Maxfield, D. G. (1990). Learning with the whole mind. In R. M. Smith and associates (Eds.), *Learning to learn across the life span* (pp. 98–122). San Francisco: Jossey-Bass.

Mezirow, J. (1981). A critical theory of adult learning and education. *Adult Education, 32,* 3–27.

Montgomery, K. S. (2002). Health promotion with adolescents: Examining theoretical perspectives to guide research. *Research and Theory in Nursing Practice, 16*(2), 119–134.

Morse, J. S., Oberer, J., Dobbins, J. A., & Mitchell, D. (1998). Understanding learning styles: Implications for in-service educators. In R. Dunn & S. A. Griggs (Eds.), *Learning styles and the nursing profession* (pp. 27–40). New York: National League for Nursing Press.

Newell, A., & Simon, H. A. (1972). *Human problem solving.* Englewood Cliffs, NJ: Prentice-Hall.

Olson, M. W., & Hergenhahn, B. R. (2012). *An introduction to theories of learning* (9th ed.). Upper Saddle River, NJ: Pearson Prentice-Hall.

O'Neill, E. S., Dluhy, N. M., & Chin, E. (2005). Modeling novice clinical reasoning for computerized decision support system. *Journal of Advanced Nursing, 49*(1), 68–77.

Ormrod, J. E. (2012). *Human learning: Principles, theories and educational applications* (6th ed.). Upper Saddle River, NJ: Pearson Prentice-Hall.

Ozmon, H. (2011). *Philosophical foundations of education* (9th ed.). Upper Saddle River, NJ: Pearson.

Perry, W. G. (1999). *Forms of ethical and intellectual development in the college years: A scheme.* San Francisco: Jossey-Bass.

Pizzo, J., Dunn, R., & Dunn, K. (1990). A sound approach to reading: Responding to students' learning styles. *Journal of Reading, Writing, and Learning Disabilities International, 6,* 249–260.

Rankin, S. H., & Stallings, K. D. (2005). *Patient education in health and illness* (5th ed.). Philadelphia: Lippincott Williams & Wilkins.

Rapps, J., Riegel, B., & Glaser, D. (2001). Testing a predictive model of what makes a critical thinker. *Western Journal of Nursing Research, 23*(6), 610–626.

Roberts, T. B. (Ed.). (1975). *Four psychologies applied to education: Freudian, behavioral, humanistic, transpersonal.* New York: Schenkman.

Rogers, C. R. (1983). *Freedom to learn for the 80's.* Columbus, OH: Merrill.

Rogers, C. R., & Freiberg, H. J. (1994). *Freedom to learn* (3rd ed.). New York: Macmillan College Publishing.

Rogers, L. Q., Vicari, S., & Courneya, K. S. (2010). Lessons learned in the trenches: Facilitating exercise adherence among breast cancer survivors in a group setting. *Cancer Nursing, 33*(6), E10–E17.

Secomb, J., McKenna, L., & Smith, C. (2012). The effectiveness of simulation activities on the genitive abilities of undergraduate third-year nursing students: A randomized control trial. *Journal of Clinical Nursing, 21*(23/24), 3475–3484.

Sharpe, P. A., Burroughs, E. L., Granner, M. L., Wilcox, S., Hutto, B. E., Bryant, C. A., et al. (2010). Impact of a community-based prevention marketing intervention to promote physical activity among middle-aged women. *Health Education & Behavior, 37*(3), 403–423.

Shawler, C. (2008). Standardized patients: A creative teaching strategy for psychiatric-mental health nurse practitioner students. *Journal of Nursing Education, 47*(11), 528–531.

Thorndike, E. L. (1932). *The fundamentals of learning.* New York: Teachers College Press.

Tough, A. (1967). *Learning without a teacher.* Toronto, Canada: Ontario Institute for Studies in Education.

Vacek, J. E. (2009). Using a conceptual approach with concept mapping to promote critical thinking. *Journal of Nursing Education, 48*(1), 45–48.

Wong, F. K. Y., Cheung, S., Chung, L., Chan, K., Chan, A., To, T., et al. (2008). Framework for adopting a problem-based learning approach in a simulated clinical setting. *Journal of Nursing Education, 47*(11), 508–514.

UNIT IV

Application of Theory in Nursing

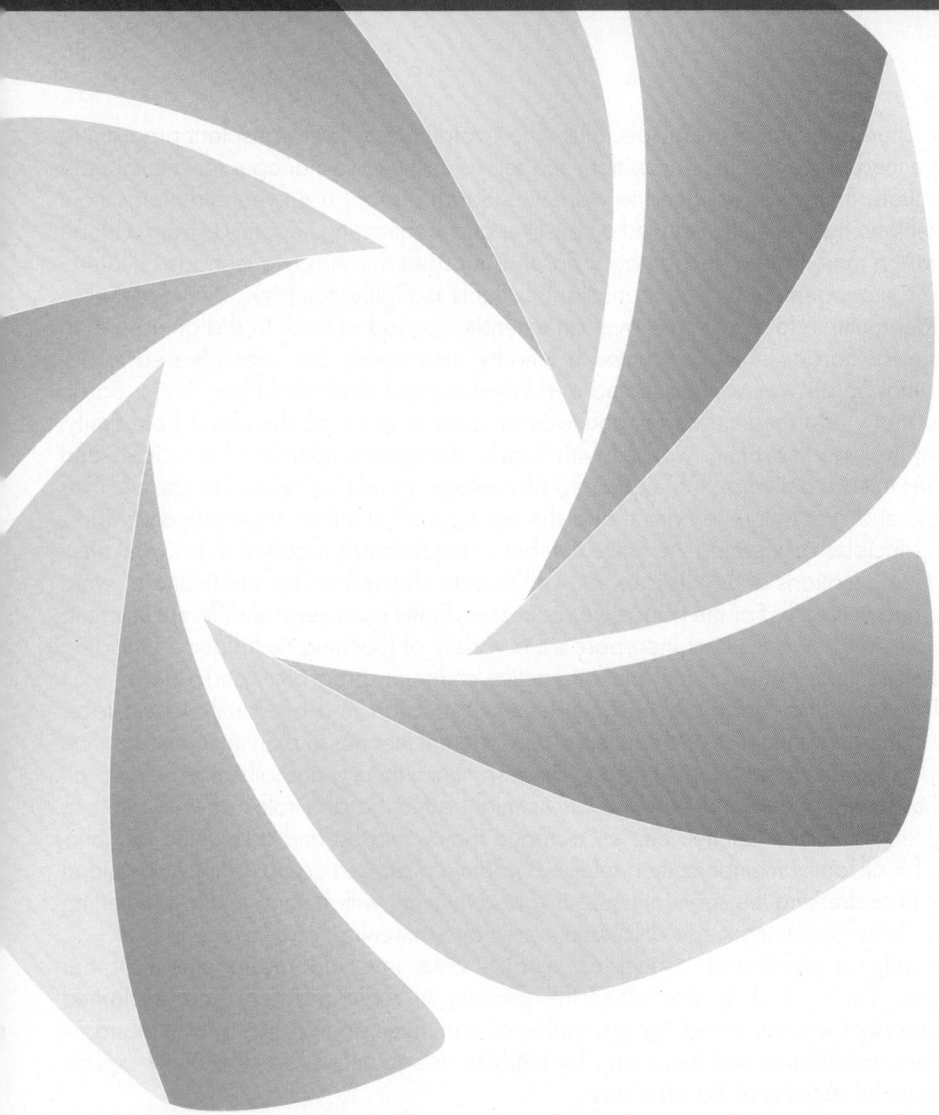

CHAPTER 18

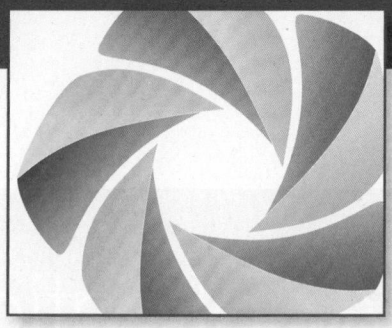

Application of Theory in Nursing Practice

Melanie McEwen

Emily Chan is a clinical nurse specialist who coordinates a liver transplant program at a large medical center. In her position, she serves as the case manager for a number of individuals. Emily was assigned to work with Sarah Bishop, a 45-year-old high school teacher who had recently received a new liver after contracting hepatitis C from a blood transfusion more than a decade ago. Sarah is married and has two teenage children.

The management of liver transplant patients is highly complex; it is essential to consider multiple facets of care over an extended period of time. In designing a plan of care for Sarah, Emily conducted a lengthy assessment. She was pleased to discover that Sarah was well educated and knew a great deal about her illness. Sarah asked many informed questions and was anxious to learn all she could from Emily. During the time that Emily worked with Sarah, she used a number of principles and theories in care delivery. She explained physiologic principles related to chronic liver disease and liver failure to Sarah, and she combined that information with pharmacologic principles concerning the large number of medications required to prevent rejection. Complications of the disease, as well as side effects from the medications, were examined at length. For the educative processes, Emily used several different learning principles and theories and incorporated a variety of teaching techniques, including one-on-one time, printed materials, interactive computer programs, and videos.

To address the many psychosocial issues that Sarah and her family would face, Emily combined principles and concepts from different theories to plan interventions. She incorporated role theory, family theory, developmental theory, and others to help Sarah and her family understand how the illness might affect Sarah's roles as wife, mother, daughter, sister, and teacher. She encouraged family support and advocated for counseling for all family members, then referred Sarah to a support group. Emily also guided Sarah in addressing the spiritual issues involved in living with a chronic, life-threatening illness. Among other concepts discussed were hope, meaning, and transcendence.

Finally, a significant aspect of Sarah's care involved management of her finances. Emily carefully described the process of reimbursement and explained what services were covered. Incorporation of principles and concepts from management and economics was necessary for Emily to adequately understand and explain the financial aspects of Sarah's care.

Theory is considered to be both a process and a product. As a process, theory has numerous activities and includes four interacting, sequential phases (analyzing concepts, constructing relationships, testing relationships, and validating relationships) that are implemented in practice. As a product, theory provides a set of concepts and relationships that may be combined to describe, explain, predict, and prescribe phenomena of interest; this information is then used to guide nursing practice (Kenney, 2013). In a practice discipline such as nursing, theory and practice are inseparable. Indeed, development and application of theory affiliated with research-based practice is considered fundamental to the development of the profession and autonomous nursing practice.

Theory provides the basis of understanding the reality of nursing; it enables the nurse to understand why an event happens. To illustrate how theory is applied in practice at a basic level, Dale (1994) used the example of a nurse who knows theories and principles of the anatomy of soft tissues and the related physiologic concept of pressure. This knowledge allows the nurse to recognize how a pressure sore can develop. Armed with this knowledge, the nurse can take steps to prevent pressure sores.

To improve the practice of nursing, nurses need to search the literature, critically appraise research findings, and synthesize empirical and contextually relevant theoretical information to be applied in practice. Further, nurses must continually question their practice and seek to find better alternatives (Litchfield & Jonsdottir, 2012). Nurses cannot afford to think of theory and research as intellectual pursuits separate from clinical performance; rather, nurses should be aware that theory and research provide the basis for practice (Marrs & Lowry, 2006; Parker & Smith, 2010; Risjord, 2010).

This chapter examines several issues related to the application of theory in nursing practice. First, the relationship between theory and practice and the concept of theory-based nursing practice are described. This is followed by a discussion of the perceived theory–practice gap that persists in nursing. Practice theories are then presented, including a discussion of how they interrelate to evidence-based practice (EBP). This chapter concludes with examples illustrating how theory is used and applied in nursing practice.

Relationship Between Theory and Practice

According to Parker and Smith (2010), the primary purpose of theory in nursing is to improve practice and thereby positively influence the health and quality of life of persons, families, and communities. In nursing, there should be a reciprocal relationship between theory and practice. Practice is the basis for nursing theory development, and nursing theory must be validated in practice. Theory is rooted in practice and refined by research, and it should be reapplied in practice. Box 18-1 shows several of the many ways in which theories influence nursing practice.

Theory provides nurses with a perspective with which to view client situations and a way to organize data in daily care. Theory allows nurses to focus on important information while setting aside less important, or irrelevant, data. Theory may assist in directing analysis and interpretation of the relationships among data and in predicting outcomes necessary to plan care. Further, a theoretical perspective allows the nurse to plan and implement care purposefully and proactively, and when nurses practice purposefully and systematically, they are more efficient, have better control over the outcome of care, and can better communicate that care with others (Masters, 2012; Parker & Smith, 2010). Thus, nurses need to use theoretical perspectives to help understand what information is important; how information, findings, and data are related; what can be predicted by relationships; and what interventions are needed to deal with special relationships.

For example, a nurse working in a postpartum maternity unit should be aware of the theoretical basis for the development of postpartum depression. That nurse

Box 18-1 Ways in Which Theory Influences Nursing Practice

- Identifies recipients/clients of nursing care
- Describes settings and situations in which practice should occur
- Defines what data to collect and how to classify the data
- Outlines actual and potential problems to be considered
- Assists in understanding, analyzing, and interpreting health situations
- Describes, explains, and sometimes predicts client's responses
- Clarifies objectives and establishes expected outcomes
- Specifies actions or interventions to be provided
- Determines standards for practice
- Differentiates nursing practice from practice of other health disciplines
- Promotes responsibility and accountability for nursing care
- Identifies areas for research

Sources: Fawcett (1992), Kenney (2013), Parker & Smith (2010).

should know risk factors for postpartum depression, its signs and symptoms, and various management strategies. Further, if the nurse suspects postpartum depression in a teenage mother, she or he must know what additional data need to be gathered to address the complex issues created by the mother's special needs and circumstances. The additional information should be analyzed and interpreted based on an understanding of the specific problems and complications posed by teen pregnancy, and an appropriate plan of care for that young woman can be developed and goals and outcomes predicted.

Similarly, a nurse working in a pediatric clinic should understand the theoretical principles of immunity and disease prevention when explaining the importance of immunization to a new mother. If the mother expresses concerns about a potential complication of the vaccine, the nurse should gather additional information from the mother to understand her specific concerns. On learning that the mother had read reports that the measles/mumps/rubella vaccine might cause autism, the nurse must be able to articulate the rationale behind immunization and to direct the mother to sources of information about vaccine safety and potential complications, including the most recent and relevant research data. This information will allow the mother to make an informed decision about the care of her infant.

Theory-Based Nursing Practice

Theory-based nursing practice is the "application of various models, theories, and principles from nursing science and the biological, behavioral, medical and sociocultural disciplines to clinical nursing practice" (Kenney, 2013, p. 333). Nursing practice is complex, and theory informs the practitioner to do what is right and just (good practice). In nursing, practice without theory becomes rote performance of activities based on tradition, common sense, and following orders (Billings & Kowalski, 2006; Marrs & Lowry, 2006; Risjord, 2010).

Theory offers the practitioner a basis for making informed decisions that are based on deliberation and practical judgment. With increasing clinical experience, nurses are able to combine theoretical and clinical knowledge with critical thinking skills to make better clinical decisions and thereby improve practice. Nursing, like all practice disciplines, uses a special combination of theory and practice in which theory guides practice and the practice grounds theory. Nurses rely heavily on theoretical understanding, and practice will be improved not just by experience but by an understanding of a wide range of theories. As Cody (2003) pointed out, "one learns to practice nursing by studying nursing theories, and one learns to practice nursing very well by studying nursing theories very intensely" (p. 226).

Dreyfus and Dreyfus (1996) believe that as nurses gain knowledge, skills, and expertise, theory and practice intertwine in a mutually supportive process; however, only if both theory and research are encouraged and appreciated can full expertise in nursing practice be realized. Theory is needed to explain the ends and means of nursing practice, and the nurse who uses theory-based practice will be able to describe, explain, predict, and control nursing events and initiate preventive actions (Kikuchi, 2004). Theory-based practice, therefore, is purposeful and controlled; it includes preventive action and can be explained by the nurse.

It is sometimes difficult to decide where, when, and how to apply theory in nursing practice. This may be particularly true for nursing students and novice nurses. The application of theory in practice requires an understanding of concepts and principles associated with the needs of a particular client, group of clients, or community, and recognition of when and how to use these concepts and principles when planning and implementing nursing care. Chinn and Kramer (2011) suggested criteria for determining when theory should be applied in practice. These are shown in Table 18-1.

Table 18-1 Guidelines for Application of Theory in Nursing Practice

Question	Process for Determining Application to Practice	Example
Are theory goals and practice goals congruent?	Examine the goal of the theory and compare it with the outcomes or goals of nursing practice (standards of practice, personal views of nursing).	A rehabilitation nurse developing a plan of care for a spinal cord injury must choose between a theory of coping and a theory of adaptation.
Is the context of the theory congruent with the practice situation?	Examine the theory to determine context for application and compare it with the context of the situation at hand.	A hospice nurse is concerned that a new agency policy on pain management is based on a theory for postsurgical pain relief.
Is there similarity between theory variables and practice variables?	Compare the theoretic variables (concepts) and the variables recognized to directly influence the practice situation to determine whether all essential concepts are addressed in the theory.	A nurse working with AIDS clients believes a learning theory might not consider the health status of the learner (the learner is assumed to be healthy) on the outcome(s) of client education.
Are explanations of the theory sufficient to be used as a basis for nursing action?	Use expert judgment about nursing actions that are implied or explicit within the theory to determine sufficiency; examine correlation between theoretical and practice variables.	A theory of therapeutic touch may be intriguing to an oncology nurse, but sufficient study should be conducted to determine when and how to apply the intervention in an oncology unit.
Does research evidence support the theory?	Conduct a review of the literature for research support of the theory; critically examine study findings for validity and applicability to practice.	Before considering implementing expensive measures that might prevent nosocomial infection, the nurse manager of a surgical ICU conducts a literature review to learn how effective the measures have been in similar settings.
How can the theory influence nursing practice and the nursing unit?	Consider ways in which an approach will affect nursing practice and a nursing unit; plan changes including observation and recording of factors relevant to the theory's application.	A theory that partially explains medication errors is being incorporated into new policies and procedures on a general medical unit, and the unit supervisor wants to be sure that the procedures include data collection for outcomes evaluation.

Source: Adapted from Chinn and Kramer (2011).

The Theory—Practice Gap

Despite the decades-long study of theory in nursing and the development and evolution of nursing theories, the notion that there is a "gap" between theory and practice is a common perception among nurses (Hatlevik, 2011; Parker & Smith, 2010; Risjord, 2010). Indeed, according to Liaschendo and Fisher (1999), nurses in clinical practice rarely use the language of nursing theory, nursing diagnosis, or the nursing process unless mandated to do so by accrediting bodies or institutional practice policies.

Risjord (2010) explains that the gap arises when the body of knowledge is not used as it should be. Several reasons for this have been suggested. Historically, for example, theory development has been regarded as the domain of nurse educators and scholars rather than the concern of practitioners. Nursing theory and practice have been viewed as two separate nursing activities, with theorists seen as those who write and teach about the ideal, separated from those who implement care in reality.

Although most scholars believe that theory and practice are, or at least should be, reciprocal, to many, the relationship between theory and practice appears to be unidirectional and hierarchical. To those nurses, theory is seen as "above" practice and is positioned to direct practice; rarely does practice appear to affect theory. This has caused confusion and apathy among practitioners who believe academic knowledge has little relevance in practice situations. Indeed, practitioners often complain that theory distorts practice, if it has any relevance to practice at all (Billings & Kowalski, 2006; Wilson, 2008).

Language also contributes to the gap in theory and practice, as many theories contain concepts and constructs that must be explained and understood before they can be applied. Further, in the ideal world of nursing theory, nursing practice is discussed as being performed as it ought to be rather than as how it is. As a result, many nurses believe that theory is irrelevant to practice because of the obscurity of academic language and focus on circumscribed, ideal situations (Doane & Varcoe, 2005).

Finally, it has been noted that practice often develops without theory, and knowing theory is not a guarantee of good practice. Furthermore, many practices resist explanation. Practice changes and develops in the light of theory, but much of the knowledge of practice is different from theory.

A different view has been taken by some. Larsen, Adamsen, Bjerregaard, and Madsen (2002) conducted a study of nursing literature and determined that there is no inherent gap between theory and practice. They concluded that although theorists and practitioners are situated in different environments, they share common and implicit understandings related to knowledge development and implementation of that knowledge in practice. Further, they contend that theoretical principles are applied daily in practice, although nurses do not always recognize their use of theory.

Closing the Theory–Practice Gap

Despite repeated calls to relate theory, practice, and research, the interaction remains fragmented or unrecognized. To promote nursing's ability to meet its obligations to society, there needs to be an ongoing, reciprocal relationship among nursing theory, nursing science, and nursing practice. This will help close the perceived gap between theory and practice.

Several factors that interfere in the reciprocal interrelationship of theory, practice, and research in nursing need to be addressed. These factors include educational issues, interaction between nursing researchers/scholars and practicing nurses, and problems or issues central to contemporary nursing practice.

Lack of exposure to theoretical principles during the basic educational program is a major impediment to closing the theory–practice gap. Because more than half of nurses in the United States have been educated in associate degree or diploma schools of nursing, they are frequently not exposed to either theory or research, as is common among baccalaureate program. This lack of focus on theory has been recognized, and in recent years, there has been momentum in nursing education to enhance emphasis on research and knowledge development (Johnson & Webber, 2010; Risjord, 2010; Walker & Avant, 2011).

It is equally important to stress theoretical concepts and principles following completion of formal education because nurses are required to continually assimilate and synthesize a sizable amount of information into their practice. The professional growth of practicing nurses is vital and, fortunately, many practicing nurses read scholarly journals, research-based literature, and practice-based journals. It is imperative that all nurses in clinical practice also be encouraged to expand their knowledge through ongoing exposure to new theoretical concepts and nursing research in continuing educational offerings or formal educational programs. These critically viewed notions of enhanced education and training, as well as lifelong learning for all nurses, were key recommendations of the Institute of Medicine (IOM) in their widely acclaimed report on *The Future of Nursing* (IOM, 2011).

A second issue relates to the disparity between the world of nursing theorists and scholars and the world of practicing nurses. Unfortunately, many nurse theorists and nurse researchers have limited clinical involvement, and time constraints restrict their ability to develop relationships with clinically based nurses. Conversely, the majority of nurses in practice have little or no direct contact with nurse theorists or nurse researchers. To address this problem, those who propose theory and conduct research have recognized the need to be directly involved in clinical practice. Further, many understand the importance of studying problems encountered in practice and using language and terminology that can be easily understood by clinical nurses who are working to implement these changes.

The final issue in closing the theory–practice gap relates to changes in health care delivery and the need to address current issues and practices from a theoretical perspective. Nurses face many challenges posed by changes in the health care delivery system. For example, the decrease in length of stay has dramatically reduced the time available for preoperative and postoperative teaching and discharge planning. Likewise, reimbursement mechanisms have dramatically influenced the availability of home health care and largely determined when and how nurses care for clients and what services are provided. These developments and anticipated changes designed to curb the inflation of health care costs may adversely affect care delivery and nursing care.

The demands of the changing health care system and attention to EBP, along with other anticipated problems must be addressed from a practice, theory, and research perspective. These problems include chronic illnesses (e.g., heart disease, cancer), aging of the population, and the increase in the number of persons from a variety of racial and cultural backgrounds. These factors contribute to the growing need to integrate multiple concepts, principles, and theories into designing, planning, and implementing effective nursing care. Thus, as nursing continues to evolve to meet the challenges described, clinical practice will need to be more heavily based on theory and research and less reliant on routine, common sense, and tradition.

Situation-Specific/Practice Theories in Nursing

Earlier chapters described different types and levels of theory used in nursing. In addition to borrowed or shared theories, this book has described grand nursing theories and middle range nursing theories. This section provides information about the theories often termed *situation-specific* or *practice theories,* which are narrow, circumscribed theories proposed for a specific type of practice. It is important to stress that they are not the only theories applied in nursing practice.

Definition and Characteristics of Situation-Specific/Practice Theories

Practice theories are nursing theories used in the actual delivery of nursing care to clients. Several characteristics are common to practice theories. First, they are used to carry out nursing interventions and often include or lead to the performance of psychomotor procedures (e.g., dressing changes, venipuncture, medication administration) or are related to communication (e.g., education, counseling). Second, practice theories may be derived from grand or middle range theories, from clinical practice, and/or from research, including literature reviews, and may describe, explain, or prescribe specific nursing practices. Third, practice theories combine a set of principles or directives for practice and often have a role in testing theories. Finally, practice theories may benefit nursing practice and the development of nursing knowledge by allowing for an in-depth analysis of a particular nursing intervention or practice.

The term *situation-specific theory* is sometimes used to describe practice theory (Chinn & Kramer, 2011; Im, 2005; Im & Chang, 2012; Meleis, 2012). Practice theories are clinically specific and reflect a particular context that may include directions or blueprints for action. Further, in comparison to grand or middle range theories, practice theories have a lower level of abstraction, are context specific, and are easily applied in nursing research and practice.

Practice theories often emerge from grounded theory research or from synthesizing and integrating research findings and applying this knowledge to a specific situation or population. Typically, the intent is to develop a framework or blueprint to understand that particular situation or group of clients. Many nursing scholars support developing theories that reflect nursing practice thus ensuring that nursing practice is a source for theory development (Im & Chang, 2012). Table 18-2 lists some areas that have been proposed for the development of practice theories for nursing.

Table 18-2 Types of Practice Theories Needed in the Discipline of Nursing

Type of Practice Theory	Examples
Theories providing explanations about client problems	Theories of healing, airway patency, fatigue, and speech
Theories describing therapeutics for client problems	Theories of suctioning, wound care, rest, and learning
Theories providing the nurse with ideas about how to approach clients	Theories of caring, empowerment, and communication
Theories providing explanations or ideas about how the nurse makes or should make decisions	Theories of clinical inference and clinical decision making
Theories providing explanations about what happens in the actual delivery of nursing care	Theories describing outcomes of client care

Source: Kim (1994).

Examples of Practice Theories From Nursing Literature

The nursing literature contains a growing number of examples of practice or situation-specific theories. In searching for illustrations, most theories that could be termed "practice theories" are those that were developed through grounded theory research or those developed through application of a grand theory or a borrowed theory to a specific aggregate or in a very defined set of circumstances. A few were identified that were reported to have resulted from quantitative research studies and literary synthesis. Also, as mentioned in Chapter 10, some of the theories that are termed by the author or others as "middle range" may be more appropriately labeled practice theories.

Examples of practice-level theories developed from qualitative, grounded theory studies include a work by Doering and Durfor (2011), who developed a theory of "persevering toward normalcy after childbirth." They identified the strategies and characteristics necessary to help manage fatigue and sleep deprivation that are key in the early weeks following childbirth. Suh (2008) examined breast cancer screening practices among immigrant Korean women in the United States. A situation-specific theory focusing on that subcultural group was proposed explaining the sociocultural context of adherence to health promotion practices. Also using grounded theory, Law (2009) developed a situation-specific theory titled "Bridging Worlds," which is intended to provide a mechanism to help hospice nurses ensure that both the physical and emotional needs of dying patients are met.

An example of a practice theory based on a grand theory is a work presented by Hannon-Engel (2008) that applied concepts and linkages from Roy's Adaptation Model to develop a theoretical framework to help practitioners manage patients with bulimia nervosa. Similarly, Mefford (2004) developed a practice theory of health promotion for preterm infants based on Levine's Conservation Model. In this theory, nursing interventions are directed toward adaptation of both the family and the infant through conservation of energy, structural integrity, personal integrity, and social integrity. Wholeness (health) of the infant and family is reflected by physiologic stability and growth, minimal structural injury, neurodevelopmental competence, and stability of the family system. Additional examples of practice or situation-specific theories and information about each are presented in Table 18-3.

Situation-Specific Theory and Evidence-Based Practice

EBP and its relationship with nursing theory was discussed in Chapter 12. As mentioned, EBP has become widely accepted in nursing as an approach to problem solving in clinical practice because it consciously and intentionally applies the currently agreed upon "best" evidence to direct care for patients (LoBiondo-Wood & Haber, 2010). A typical process used to develop EPB guidelines includes identifying a clinical problem, conducting a comprehensive literature search for relevant information about the problem, evaluating the researched evidence critically, and determining appropriate interventions.

In many ways, this process and the desired outcome mirrors the process and intent of development and implementation of situation-specific theories. Both are research based and focused on a relatively small set or subset of patients in fairly narrowly defined situations. Similarly, the desired outcome of both is to develop nursing interventions that can be applied in clinical practice to improve the health of patients.

Table 18-4 presents selected definitions of situation-specific nursing theory (micro or practice theory) and evidence-based nursing practice guidelines taken from

Table 18-3 Examples of Situation-Specific/Practice Theories and Models

Practice Theory or Model	Target Population	Development Process	Goal and Activities or Actions Prescribed
Symptom-focused diabetes care (Skelly, Leeman, Carlson, Soward, & Burns, 2008)	African American women	Review of the literature and intervention protocols	Guides community-based, culturally sensitive diabetes interventions
Midlife Women's Attitudes Toward Physical Activity (MAPA) (Im, Stuifbergen, & Walker, 2010)	Midlife women	Review of the literature; other models (e.g., Attitude, Social Influence, and Self-Efficacy Model) and a study on women's attitudes toward physical activity	Directs nursing interventions and research related to increasing participation in physical activity
Health-related behaviors of Korean Americans (Lee, Fawcett, Yang, & Hann, 2012)	Korean Americans who have or are at risk for chronic hepatitis B virus (HBV) infection	Literature review of related research and the Network Episode Model	Explanation of correlates of health-related HBV behaviors of the population; used to develop and test nursing interventions to promote positive health behaviors
Asian Immigrant Women's Menopausal Symptom Experience (Im, 2010)	Menopausal Asian immigrant women	Integrative approach to theory development (Im, 2005)	Describes Asian immigrant women's menopausal symptom experience; can be used to develop interventions and research directed to the population
Theory of Crisis Emergencies (Brennaman, 2012)	Invidious with severe, persistent mental illness	Integrative literature review, application of a middle range theory in the defined population	Theory for use by nurses in emergency department to distinguish between need for mental health crisis intervention or mental health emergency intervention
Well-being in refugee women experiencing cultural transition (Baird, 2012)	Refugee women from South Sudan immigrating to the United States	Research studies and application of transitions theory	Promotes culturally relevant interventions for nurses working with immigrant and refugee populations to foster well-being
Migration transition model (Clingerman, 2007)	Mexican and Mexican American female migrant farm workers	Qualitative research study of female farm workers	Presents the transition processes experienced by this cohort and describes their patterns of response; presents potential nursing actions or therapeutics
Situation-specific theory of self-care in diabetes mellitus (DM) (Song, 2010)	Individuals with DM	Adaption of another situation-specific theory and literature review	Describes use of health outcomes and patients' decision-making responses to signs and symptoms of DM; promote DM self-care to improve health outcomes
Maintaining hope in transition (Davidson, Dracup, Phillips, Padilla, & Daly, 2007)	People with heart failure	Application of Transition Theory to patients with heart failure	Use hope to focus on positive future orientation and emphasize the individual's ability to cope with and adjust to heart failure

Table 18-4 Definitions of Evidence-Based Nursing Practice Guidelines and Situation-Specific Nursing Theories

Evidence-Based Nursing Practice Guidelines	Situation-Specific Nursing Theories
Practice guidelines are "systematically developed statements that assist practitioners and patients [to] make decisions on appropriate care for specific client circumstances . . . created by groups of experienced experts and key affected groups who read, critique, and prioritize the pertinent evidence" (Schmidt & Brown, 2012, p. 280).	" . . . theories that focus on specific nursing phenomena, that reflect clinical practice, and that are limited to specific populations or particular fields of practice" (Im, 2005, p. 298).
Evidence-based practice clinical guidelines " . . . systematically developed practice statements designed to assist clinicians [to] make health care decisions for specific conditions or situations" (LoBiondo-Wood & Haber, 2010, p. 11).	"Theory that is developed with the sensitive consideration of context; assumes that theory . . . [takes] into account important differences across populations; draws attention to the variables that significantly affect the successful use of theory" (Chinn & Kramer, 2011, p. 256).
Evidence–based practice " . . . tracking down and applying the best available knowledge related to any specific clinical process, which specifically meets patient needs and answers critical questions related to best practices" (Malloch & Porter-O'Grady, 2010, p. 4).	[Microrange theories] " . . . focus on specific nursing phenomena . . . and offer a blueprint that is more readily operational and/or has more accessible utility in clinical situations" (Smith & Liehr, 2013, pp. 21–22).
"Evidence-based clinical practice guidelines are specific practice recommendations . . . that have been derived from a methodologically rigorous review of the best evidence on a specific topic" (Melnyk & Fineout-Overholt, 2011, p. 13).	"Situation-specific theories are coherent representations and descriptions of a set of concepts, and explanation of the relationships between those concepts and prediction of outcomes related to these relationships . . . grounded in clinical, teaching, policy or administrative situations . . . focused on a specific set of phenomena, more subscribed situations, and has a limited set of conditions" (Meleis, 2012, pp. 420–421).

the recent nursing literature. Critical review of the definitions suggests several similarities. For example, both are developed to address specific situations or phenomena and to be applied in clinical situations. For EBP, the intent is to assist clinicians make decisions in specified conditions or situations; the same is true for situation-specific theories. Additionally, although the situation-specific theory definitions do not directly or explicitly explain the source or methods used in their development, a review of the information presented previously indicates that many of them—particularly the more recently published theories—were developed through comprehensive review of the relevant health care literature as well as through research studies, which is typically the basis or starting point for the development of EBP guidelines.

Thus, it appears that situation-specific theories and EPB guidelines, standards, and protocols have much in common. As nursing researchers and nurse theorists move forward in theory development, increasing attention needs to be given to the development of situation-specific theories, with consideration of how they might be more explicitly connected to EPB guidelines.

Application of Theory in Nursing Practice

A lack of understanding of theory leads to a failure to recognize the use of theory on a day-to-day, even minute-to-minute, basis in the practice of nursing. For example, the practice of washing hands prior to client contact is based directly on the principles of germ theory and the epidemiologic concepts of disease transmission and disease prevention. Barnum (1998) used the term *implied theory* to refer to those theories used by practicing nurses during routine client care. Examples of application of theory can be taken from several sources within practice-based nursing literature. With few exceptions, as in real practice, the theoretical principles are implicit rather than explicit.

This section illustrates the application of a variety of theories, principles, and concepts in nursing journals and the nursing intervention classification system. The intent of this exercise is to show where and how nurses use theoretical principles in practice. For the most part, these theories are implied and extrapolated rather than explicitly stated in the works in question. Some readers may argue whether the theories/principles/concepts are addressed at all in the examples. Furthermore, the theories/principles/concepts discussed will most likely not be the only ones suggested in the work; indeed, there are probably countless others.

Theory in Nursing Taxonomy: Examples From the Nursing Intervention Classification System

To illustrate the use of theory in nursing taxonomies, two interventions from the Nursing Intervention Classification (NIC) system are discussed. The NIC is a comprehensive list of 554 nursing interventions grouped into 30 classes and 7 domains. Nurses in all specialties and in all types of settings perform these interventions. The NIC includes physiologic, behavioral, safety, family, and community interventions, and there are interventions for illness treatment, illness prevention, and health promotion (Bulechek, Butcher, Dochterman, & Wagner, 2013).

The intervention of intermittent urinary catheterization is used to highlight the incorporation of theories and principles from biology, physiology, and medicine into nursing. In a second discussion, theories related to behavioral interventions (i.e., learning theories and psychosocial theories and principles) are examined in the intervention of patient contracting.

Urinary Catheterization: Intermittent

Intermittent urinary catheterization refers to the "regular periodic use of a catheter to empty the bladder" (Bulechek et al., 2013, p. 406). The procedure may be performed by the nurse, another caregiver, or the client, and may be done in the home or in an institutional setting. The purposes are to eliminate residual urine in the bladder, reduce urinary infections, prevent incontinent episodes, regain bladder tone, achieve dilation of the urethra, increase client control of urinary elimination, and facilitate self-care.

The authors presented references to support the need and rationale for the intervention. The data presented in the references compared rates and are an example of the use of epidemiologic principles. Discussion of complications and side effects, including urinary tract infection and fistulas resulting from indwelling catheters, related to principles of anatomy and physiology as well as disease processes. Description of costs of alternative strategies implied the use of economic principles. Mention of reluctance to report incontinence suggested incorporation of psychosocial theories,

Table 18-5 Intermittent Urinary Catheterization: Theoretical Basis for Activities

Activity	Possible Theory Base
Perform comprehensive urinary assessment, focusing on causes of incontinence.	Physiology, certain disease processes
Teach patient/family purpose, supplies, methods, and rationale of intermittent catheterization.	Teaching/learning principles and theories
Teach patient/family clean intermittent catheterization technique.	Germ theory (principles of asepsis)
Use clean or sterile technique for catheterization.	Germ theory (principles of asepsis)
Maintain client on prophylactic antibacterial therapy for 2–3 weeks at initiation as appropriate.	Pharmacology, health promotion/prevention strategies
Establish a catheterization schedule based on individual needs.	Developmental theory, role theory, needs theory
Teach patient/family signs and symptoms of urinary tract infection.	Principles of disease processes

Source: Bulechek et al. (2013).

and encouraging self-care related to several nursing theories, such as those of Orem and Erickson, Tomlin, and Swain.

The activities that comprise the intervention of intermittent urinary catheterization largely focus on prevention and identification of infection and teaching needs related to the psychomotor skills used by nurses and others providing care. Table 18-5 lists a few of the activities for the intervention and suggests a broad theoretical basis for each.

Patient Contracting

One of the many behaviorally focused NIC interventions is patient contracting. Patient contracting is defined as "negotiating an agreement with an individual which reinforces a specific behavior change" (Bulechek et al., 2013, p. 289). Patient contracting involves analyzing patient behaviors, setting goals, determining responsibilities of interested parties and determination of consequences and reinforcement mechanisms. A written, signed contract with terms and dates may be developed.

The major theoretical basis of the intervention is principles from behavior modification and operant conditioning. The intervention also uses concepts and principles from other theories. These concepts include motivation, compliance/noncompliance, and risk factor management. In addition, patient contracting is based on the premise that all individuals have the right to self-determination to make their own choices and to be active in their own health care, and that health care providers must offer treatments that empower patients to identify their own priorities, strengths, weaknesses, and goals. These are ethical principles, which are fundamental to professional nursing practice.

Bulechek and colleagues (2013) developed a long list of activities that might be used in patient contracting. Table 18-6 lists a few of these activities and identifies a possible theoretical basis for each.

Table 18-6 Patient Contracting: Theoretical Basis for Selected Activities

Activity	Possible Theory Base
Encourage the individual to identify own strengths and abilities.	Role theory, developmental theory, needs theory
Assist the individual in identifying the health practice he or she wishes to change.	Self-determinism
Assist the client in identifying present circumstances that may interfere with achievement of goals.	Role theory, developmental theory, health beliefs, motivation theory
Encourage the individual to choose a reinforcement/reward that is significant enough to sustain the behavior.	Motivation theory

Source: Bulechek et al. (2013).

Examples of Theory From Nursing Literature

The general nursing literature is replete with examples of how theories are applied in routine nursing practice. This section presents several examples of practice—application of borrowed or "implied" theories as described earlier, as well as application of middle range and grand theories.

Application of "Borrowed" and "Implied" Theories in Nursing Practice

Examples of applying borrowed theories in practice are easily identified in the literature. For example, Blevins and Troutman (2011) looked at how several theories are applied in caring for patients with chronic renal disease. Within a general framework of "successful aging," they discussed multiple theories and concepts that should be applied when working with this population. Among them were physiologic and psychological changes in aging, developmental theory, spiritual concerns, and theories of aging. Other key concepts discussed within the "theory of successful aging" included coping, adaptation, health promotion, and decision making. The authors concluded that the theory of successful aging is useful for assisting nurses in providing comprehensive care and understanding the complexities of caring for older patients with chronic renal disease.

In another work, Cleveland, Minter, Cobb, Scott, and German (2008) explained the bases for recommendations for screening and strategies for managing lead exposure in pregnant women and children. This discussion included epidemiologic information describing risk factors and demographic data accounting for the disparities of distribution of high lead levels. Additionally, environmental concepts and theories of lead contamination and related prevention strategies were examined. Finally, the pathophysiology of lead absorption was explained, and this discussion included an overview of potential treatment for high lead levels (chelation therapy) and the related biomedical and pharmacological aspects of the therapy.

Another example of application of non-nursing theories in nursing practice comes from Morton (2008), who reported on the development and implementation of a health education program for school children. She used the Health Belief Model (HBM) as a guide to develop a series of weekly broadcasts over the participating schools' public announcement systems. Topics included head lice awareness, sleep, seat belt safety, and dental care. The intent of the education

Link to Practice 18-1

Application of "Shared" Theory in Nursing Practice

Phillips (2013) described an intervention that can be used by community health nurses who are working with older adults who smoke. She explained that because smoking is the most preventable cause of death, smoking cessation is a key public health goal. Her research-based guidelines can reduce smoking-related illness and promote health among elders. Using Bandura's self-efficacy construct as well as the HBM as a framework, the author presented five different caring options for nurses working with elders who smoke. The options discussed were (1) brief intervention sessions in which the health provider presented advice, encouragement, and assessment; (2) weekly individual behavioral counseling; (3) group behavior therapy; (4) use of pharmacotherapies; and (5) provision of self-help materials.

program was to provide health information that would enhance children's understanding of their individual risk for health threats and the perceived benefits of health promoting behaviors. In addition to HBM constructs, this program also illustrated application of other theories, models, and concepts, including learning theories, biomedical concepts (principles of infection), and epidemiology (prevention). Link to Practice 18-1 shows another example of applying non-nursing theories in nursing practice.

Application of Grand and Middle Range Theories in Nursing Practice

Articles showing how grand and middle range nursing theories have been applied in nursing practice can readily be found in the nursing literature (see Link to Practice 18-2). Bailey (2012) used Orem's self-care deficit theory to develop a plan of care for adolescent girls. Using Orem's theory as a framework, she proposed several community/public health nursing interventions to reduce vulnerability of adolescent girls. Key interventions included promoting access to reproductive health care, vocational training, and education. She also advocated health and life-skills education and participation in youth clubs to promote self-esteem. Last, she suggested multiple venues for screening and education, including school-based counseling programs.

In another work, Reedy and Blum (2010) used Meleis' Transitions Theory to develop a plan of care for bariatric surgery patients. They explained how nurses could use transitions theory to help patients enhance positive outcomes while overcoming potential negative outcomes following bariatric surgery. The different patterns of transition that bariatric patients typically undergo were explained. The transitions occur in the patients as they change the way they see the world and themselves. The authors go on to explain how relationships with family and other social and professional groups are impacted because weight loss often disrupts the family status quo.

The middle range theory of chronic sorrow was discussed by Gordon (2009). She explained how the theory can be used by nurses who care for parents of chronically ill children. She suggested that nurses must recognize how chronic sorrow is a normal grief response associated with loss, know how to assess chronic sorrow in parents of chronically ill children, and understand how to support parents

Link to Practice 18-2

Application of Nursing Theory in Practice

Nursing care for mothers-to-be who experience nausea and vomiting was addressed by Isbir and Mete (2010). The authors explained how to develop a very comprehensive and theory-based plan of care for this population based on the Roy Adaptation Model (RAM). With the primary goal of promoting adaptation, the authors first suggested evaluation of the adaptive system. It was thought that women with mild to moderate symptoms may have effective cognator and regulator systems and can cope with the symptoms and therefore would need minimal intervention, as they have adaptation at the compensatory level.

For women with severe and lasting symptoms however, their compensatory processes are not adequate and the insufficient adaption levels need to be addressed. Nurses can help coordinate regulator and cognator processes and increase adaptation to compensatory levels. The authors continued to apply the RAM to other aspects of care for pregnant women experiencing nausea and vomiting. They examined relationships among the different modes (interdependence, role function, physiologic, and self-concept modes) and focal, contextual, and residual stimuli. They concluded by describing how nursing activities and interventions (e.g., counseling about nutrition, promoting social support, identifying stressors, and reducing stress levels) can positively influence the adaptive/coping systems.

experiencing chronic sorrow by applying evidence-based strategies to promote effective coping.

Examples of how the Synergy Model has been used in guiding nursing practice can readily be found in the literature. For example, Hardin (2012) described how the Synergy Model could be used to plan and provide care to older adults with hearing loss, allowing them to participate in decision making while in a critical care unit. Then, in another work, Arashin (2010) explained how the Synergy Model could be used to develop guide rapid response teams. Table 18-7 presents additional examples of how nurses can apply a variety of theories in their practice.

Summary

Many nursing scholars believe that theory-guided practice, often in the form of EBP or situation-specific theory, is the future of nursing. As nursing progresses into the 21st century, nurses must place theory-guided practice at the core of nursing, and they must integrate relevant outcome-driven practice with the art and science of caring and healing.

As pointed out in the opening case study, advanced practice nurses like Emily routinely use concepts, principles, and theories from many disciplines, including nursing, to meet the health needs of their clients. To provide comprehensive, holistic, and effective interventions, nurses should rely on sound theoretical principles to develop and implement the plan of care.

Beginning in their basic nursing education program, all nurses should be encouraged to recognize the theoretical basis for practice and seek ways to enhance the knowledge base that supports practice. In addition, there should be an increased

Table 18-7 Application of Theory in Nursing Practice: Examples From the Literature

Reference	Situation and/or Population	Theories/Concepts Applied
Hallas, D., Fernandez, J., Lim, L., & Carobene, M. (2011). Nursing strategies to reduce the incidence of early childhood caries in culturally diverse populations. *Journal of Pediatric Nursing, 26,* 248–256.	Unmet health needs (dental care) of minority children in the United States	Leininger's culture care theory; health disparities; epidemiology; oral pathology; health promotion; health education
Senn, J. F. (2013). Peplau's theory of interpersonal relations: Application in emergency and rural nursing. *Nursing Science Quarterly, 26*(1), 31–35.	Application of concepts from Peplau's theory in communication situations between nurses and patients in the emergency department and in rural settings	Peplau's theory of interpersonal relations
Koren, M. E., & Papamiditriou, C. (2013). Spirituality of staff nurses: Application of modeling and role modeling theory. *Holistic Nursing Practice, 27*(1), 37–44.	Stresses the importance of self-care for both nurses and patients, considering that spirituality is foundational to nursing care	Modeling and role modeling theory; Erikson's developmental theory
Hardin, S. R. (2012). Engaging families to participate in care of older critical care patients. *Critical Care Nurse, 32*(3), 35–40.	Promoting optional care for older adults in critical care units by encouraging family members to participate in their care	Synergy model
Mitchell, G. (2013). Selecting the best theory to implement planned change. *Nursing Management, 23*(1), 32–37.	How nursing managers can use theory to implement changes in their work settings	Lewin's change theory, leadership theories, Herzberg's motivation theory, Lippett's change theory
Willis, D. G., & Grace, P. J. (2011). The applied philosopher-scientist: Intersections among phenomenological research, nursing science and theory as a basis for practice aimed at facilitating boys' healing from being bullied. *Advances in Nursing Science, 34*(1), 19–28.	Middle school boys who experience being bullied, largely in school situations	Roger's science of unitary human beings, Reed's theory of self-transcendence, Barrett's theory of power

emphasis on enhancing the reciprocal interaction among theory, research, and practice with a concerted effort to bridge the theory–practice gap. Through these efforts, nursing can continue to develop and use a unique knowledge base and further contribute to autonomous and professional practice.

Key Points

- Theory is both a process and a product. In the discipline of nursing, theory and practice are inseparable.
- To improve practice, nurses need to search the literature continually, critically appraise research findings, and synthesize empirical and contextually relevant theoretical information to be applied in practice.
- Theory-based nursing is the application of various models, theories, and principles from nursing science and the biologic, behavioral, medical, and sociocultural disciplines to clinical nursing practice.

- Despite the recognition of the importance of theory in nursing, there is a perceived gap between theory and practice.
- Theories may be developed by and for nurses (grand, middle range, or situation-specific nursing theories), they may be shared with other disciplines, or they may be implied (routinely used without being conscious processes).
- Nurses should promote and embrace theory-guided practice as the core of nursing. Nurses should recognize the theoretical basis for practice and seek ways to enhance the knowledge base that supports practice and bridges the theory–practice gap.

Learning Activities

1. Obtain a copy of the NIC (Bulechek et al., 2013). Select several interventions and try to identify the possible theoretical bases of each.
2. Debate the pros and cons of EBP with several classmates. Why would a focus on EBP be good for nursing? What are some drawbacks?
3. Obtain copies of recent mainstream nursing journals (e.g., *American Journal of Nursing, Nursing, RN*). Examine practice-focused articles and try to identify theories that affect the suggested nursing interventions and nursing implications.
4. Review theories and concepts described in previous chapters. Identify how they have been or could be applied in nursing practice.

REFERENCES

Arashin, K. A. (2010). Using the Synergy Model to guide the practice of rapid response teams. *Dimensions of Critical Care Nursing, 29*(3), 120–124.

Bailey, L. D. (2012). Adolescent girls: A vulnerable population, *Advances in Neonatal Care, 12*(2), 102–106.

Baird, M. B. (2012). Well-being in refugee women experiencing cultural transition. *Advances in Nursing Science, 35*(3), 249–263.

Barnum, B. S. (1998). *Nursing theory: Analysis, application, evaluation* (5th ed.). Philadelphia: Lippincott Williams & Wilkins.

Billings, D. M., & Kowalski, K. (2006). Bridging the theory-practice gap with evidence-based practice. *Journal of Continuing Education in Nursing, 37*(6), 248–249.

Blevins, C., & Troutman, M. F. (2011). Successful aging theory and the patient with chronic renal disease: Application in the clinical setting. *Nephrology Nursing Journal, 38*(3), 255–260.

Brennaman, L. (2012). Crisis emergencies for individuals with severe, persistent mental illnesses: A situation-specific theory. *Archives of Psychiatric Nursing, 26*(4), 251–260.

Bulechek, G. M., Butcher, H. K., Dochterman, J. M., & Wagner, C. M. (2013). *Nursing interventions classification (NIC)* (6th ed.). St. Louis: Elsevier.

Chinn, P. L., & Kramer, M. K. (2011). *Theory and nursing: Integrated knowledge development* (8th ed.). St. Louis: Mosby.

Cleveland, L. M., Minter, M. L., Cobb, K. A., Scott, A. A., & German, V. F. (2008). Lead hazards for pregnant women and children: Part 2. *The American Journal of Nursing, 108*(11), 40–48.

Clingerman, E. (2007). A situation-specific theory of migration transition for migrant farmworker women. *Research and Theory for Nursing Practice, 21*(4), 220–235.

Cody, W. K. (2003). Nursing theory as a guide to practice. *Nursing Science Quarterly, 16*(3), 225–231.

Dale, A. E. (1994). The theory–practice gap: The challenge for nurse teachers. *Journal of Advanced Nursing, 20*, 521–524.

Davidson, P. M., Dracup, K., Phillips, J., Padilla, G., & Daly, J. (2007). Maintaining hope in transition: A theoretical framework to guide interventions for people with heart failure. *Journal of Cardiovascular Nursing, 22*(1), 58–64.

Doane, G. H., & Varcoe, C. (2005). Toward compassionate action: Pragmatism and the inseparability of theory/practice. *Advances in Nursing Science, 28*(1), 81–90.

Doering, J., & Durfor, S. L. (2011). The process of "persevering toward normalcy" after childbirth. *MCN, 36*(4), 258–266.

Dreyfus, H. L., & Dreyfus, S. E. (1996). The relationship of theory and practice in the acquisition of skill. In P. Benner, C. A. Tanner, & C. A. Chesla (Eds.), *Expertise in nursing practice: Caring, clinical judgment and ethics* (pp. 29–47). New York: Springer.

Fawcett, J. (1992). Conceptual models and nursing practice: The reciprocal relationship. *Journal of Advanced Nursing, 17*, 224–228.

Gordon, J. (2009). An evidence-based approach for supporting parents experiencing chronic sorrow. *Pediatric Nursing, 35*(2), 115–119.

Hannon-Engel, S. L. (2008). Knowledge development: The Roy adaptation model and bulimia nervosa. *Nursing Science Quarterly, 21*(2), 126–132.

Hardin, S. R. (2012). Hearing loss in older critical care patients: Participation in decision making. *Critical Care Nurse, 32*(6), 43–50.

Hatlevik, I. K. R. (2011). The theory-practice relationship: Reflective skills and theoretical knowledge as key factors in bridging the gap between theory and practice in initial nursing education. *Journal of Advanced Nursing, 68*(4), 868–877.

Im, E. O. (2010). A situation-specific theory of Asian immigrant women's menopausal symptom experience in the United States. *Advances in Nursing Science, 33*(2), 143–157.

Im, E. O. (2005). Development of situation-specific theories: An integrative approach. *Advances in Nursing Science, 28*(2), 137–151.

Im, E. O., & Chang, S. J. (2012). Current trends in nursing thoeries. *Journal of Nursing Scholarship, 44*(2), 156–164.

Im, E. O., Stuifbergen, A. K., & Walker, L. (2010). A situation-specific theory of midlife women's attitudes toward physical activity (MAPA). *Nursing Outlook, 38*(1), 52–58.

Institute of Medicine. (2011). *The future of nursing: Leading change, advancing health.* Washington, DC: National Academies Press.

Isbir, G. G., & Mete, S. (2010). Nursing care of nausea and vomiting in pregnancy: Roy adaptation model. *Nursing Science Quarterly, 23*(2), 148–155.

Johnson, B. M., & Webber, P. B. (2010). *An introduction to theory and reasoning in nursing* (3rd ed.). Philadelphia: Lippincott Williams & Wilkins.

Kenney, J. W. (2013). Theory-based advanced nursing practice. In W. K Cody (Ed.), *Philosophical and theoretical perspectives for advanced nursing practice* (5th ed., pp. 333–351). Sudbury, MA: Jones & Bartlett.

Kikuchi, J. F. (2004). Towards a philosophic theory of nursing. *Nursing Philosophy, 5*(1), 79–83.

Kim, H. S. (1994). Practice theories in nursing and a science of nursing practice. *Scholarly Inquiry for Nursing Practice, 8*(2), 145–158.

Larsen, K., Adamsen, L., Bjerregaard, L., & Madsen, J. K. (2002). There is no gap "per se" between theory and practice: Research knowledge and clinical knowledge are developed in different contexts and follow their own logic. *Nursing Outlook, 50*(5), 204–212.

Law, R. (2009). "Bridging worlds": Meeting the emotional needs of dying patients. *Journal of Advanced Nursing, 65*(12), 2630–2641.

Lee, H., Fawcett, J., Yang, J. H., & Hann, H. W. (2012). Correlates of hepatitis B virus health-related behaviors of Korean Americans: A situation-specific nursing theory. *Journal of Nursing Scholarship, 44*(4), 315–322.

Litchfield, M. C., & Jonsdottir, H. (2012). A practice discipline that's here and now. In P. G. Reed and N. B. C. Shearer (Eds.), *Perspectives on nursing theory* (6th ed., 437–447), Philadelphia: Lippincott Williams & Wilkins.

Liaschendo, J., & Fisher, A. (1999). Theorizing the knowledge that nurses use in the conduct of their work. *Scholarly Inquiry for Nursing Practice, 13*(1), 29–41.

LoBiondo-Wood, G., & Haber, J. (2010). Integrating the processes of research and evidence-based practice. In G. LoBiondo-Wood & J. Haber (Eds.), *Nursing research: Methods and critical appraisal for evidence-based practice* (7th ed., pp. 5–26). St. Louis: Mosby.

Malloch, K., & Porter-O'Grady, T. (2010). *Introduction to evidence-based practice in nursing and health care* (2nd ed.). Sudbury, MA: Jones & Bartlett.

Marrs, J. A., & Lowry, L. W. (2006). Nursing theory and practice: Connecting the dots. *Nursing Science Quarterly, 19*(1), 44–50.

Masters, K. (2012). *Nursing theories: A framework for professional practice.* Sudbury, MA: Jones & Bartlett Learning.

Mefford, L. C. (2004). A theory of health promotion for preterm infants based on Levine's conservation model of nursing. *Nursing Science Quarterly, 17*(3), 260–266.

Meleis, A. I. (2012). *Theoretical nursing: Development and progress* (5th ed.). Philadelphia: Lippincott Williams & Wilkins.

Melnyk, B. M., & Fineout-Overholt, E. (2011). Making the case for evidence-based practice and cultivating a spirit of inquiry. In B. M. Melnyk & E. Fineout-Overhold (Eds.), *Evidence-based practice in nursing and healthcare: A guide to best practice* (2nd ed., pp. 3–24). Philadelphia: Lippincott Williams & Wilkins.

Mitchell, G. (2013). Selecting the best theory to implement planned change. *Nursing Management, 20*(1), 32–40.

Morton, J. L. (2008). "I Feel Good!" A weekly wellness radio broadcast for elementary school children. *The Journal of School Nursing, 24*(2), 83–87.

Parker, M. E., & Smith, M. C. (2010). Nursing theory and the discipline of nursing. In M. E. Parker & M. C. Smith (Eds.), *Nursing theories and nursing practice* (3rd ed., pp. 3–12). Philadelphia: F.A. Davis.

Phillips, A. (2013). Smoking cessation: Promoting the health of older people who smoke. *British Journal of Community Nursing, 17*(12), 606–611.

Reedy, S., & Blum, K. (2010). Applying middle-range nursing theory to bariatric surgery patients: Experiencing transitions. *Bariatric Nursing and Surgical Patient Care, 5*(1), 35–42.

Risjord, M. (2010). *Nursing knowledge: Science, practice and philosophy.* Oxford, United Kingdom: Wiley-Blackwell.

Schmidt, N. A., & Brown, J. M. (2012). *Evidence-based practice for nurses* (2nd ed.). Sudbury, MA: Jones & Bartlett.

Skelly, A. H., Leeman, J., Carlson, J., Soward, A. C. M., & Burns, D. (2008). Conceptual model of symptom-focused diabetes care for African Americans. *Journal of Nursing Scholarship, 40*(3), 261–267.

Smith, M. J., & Liehr, P. R. (2013). *Middle range theory for nursing* (3rd ed.). New York, NY: Springer.

Song, M. K. (2010). Diabetes mellitus and the importance of self-care. *Journal of Cardiovascular Nursing, 25*(2), 93–98.

Suh, E. E. (2008). The sociocultural context of breast cancer screening among Korean immigrant women. *Cancer Nursing, 31*(4), E1–E10.

Walker, L. O., & Avant, K. C. (2011). *Strategies for theory construction in nursing* (5th ed.). Upper Saddle River, NJ: Prentice Hall.

Wilson, J. (2008). Bridging the theory practice gap. *Australian Nursing Journal, 16*(4), 25.

CHAPTER 19

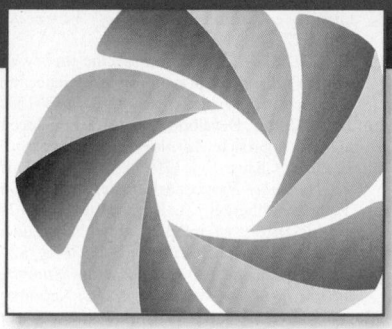

Application of Theory in Nursing Research

Melanie McEwen

Peter Jacobson is in his second semester of a master's program in nursing. He is currently a supervisor on a general medical floor of a large teaching hospital and wants to advance in nursing administration after his graduation.

Peter's program requires that all students complete either a thesis or a formal research application project, and he wants to get an early start on developing this project. During a theory course in his first semester, Peter read about Pat Benner's work (2001) detailing the process of moving from novice to expert practice in nursing, and this work intrigued him. After talking about possible research topics with one of his professors, he decides that he wants to use concepts from her theory to develop and test an orientation schedule for new graduates using selected "expert" nurses as mentors.

To better conceptualize the research study, he obtains a copy of Benner's most recent work. He also collects articles from nursing journals describing application of the novice to expert framework in different situations, including nursing practice, nursing education, and nursing research. From this information, he is able to develop an outline for his research project that uses the model as the conceptual framework.

In any discipline, science is the result of the relationship between the process of inquiry (research) and the product of knowledge (theory). The purpose of research is to build knowledge in a discipline through the generation and/or testing of theory. To effectively build knowledge, the research process should be developed within some theoretical structure that facilitates analysis and interpretation of findings. This will ultimately result in development of scientific theory. When a study is placed within a theoretical context, the theory guides the research process; forms the research questions; and aids in design, analysis, and interpretation. Thus, a theory, conceptual model, or framework provides parameters for a research study and enables the scientist to weave the facts together.

For the past several decades, nursing leaders have called for research to develop and confirm nursing knowledge and for theory to organize it. They have recognized the need to link nursing research and theory because it has been observed that research without theory results in discrete information or data, which does not add to the accumulated knowledge of the discipline (Hardin & Bishop, 2010; Chinn & Kramer, 2011).

However, it has been pointed out that the relationship between research and theory in nursing is not well understood. This may result from several factors, including the relative youth of the discipline and debates over philosophical worldviews (i.e., empiricism, constructivism, phenomenology) as described in Chapter 1.

There are also concerns regarding whether nursing should form a discrete body of knowledge without using theories from other disciplines. Nursing science is a blend of knowledge that is unique to nursing and knowledge that is imported from other disciplines (e.g., psychology, sociology, education, biology), but considerable debate continues about whether the use of borrowed theory has hindered the development of the discipline. This has contributed to problems connecting research and theory in nursing.

This chapter examines a number of issues related to the interface of research and theory in the discipline of nursing. Topics covered include the relationship between research and theory, types of theory and corresponding research, how theory is used in the research process, and the issue of borrowed versus unique theory for nursing. The chapter concludes with discussions of how theory should be addressed in a research report and the discipline's research agenda.

Historical Overview of Research and Theory in Nursing

In the discipline of nursing, research and theory were first integrated in the works of Florence Nightingale. In *Notes on Nursing,* she identified the need to organize nursing knowledge through observation, recording, and statistical inferences. Nightingale also supported her theoretical propositions through research, as statistical data, and prepared graphs were used to depict the impact of nursing care on the health of British soldiers (Kalisch & Kalisch, 2004).

After Nightingale's time, for almost a century, reports of nursing research were rare. For the most part, research and theory developed separately in nursing. Blegen and Tripp-Reimer (1994) explained that between 1928 and 1959, only 2 of 152 studies published in nursing journals reported a theoretical basis for the research design.

The amount and quality of nursing research grew dramatically, however, beginning with the initial publication of *Nursing Research* in 1952. During the last half of the 20th century, the number of nursing journals focusing on research grew to include *Research in Nursing and Health, Western Journal of Nursing Research,* and *Advances in Nursing Science.* Many other nursing journals, both general (e.g., *Journal of Nursing Scholarship, Journal of Advanced Nursing*) and specialty based (e.g., *MCN: American Journal of Maternal Child Nursing, Heart and Lung: The Journal of Critical Care, AORN Journal*), also devote significant portions of each issue to nursing research.

In the early years, research in nursing focused on education and characteristics of nurses rather than on aspects of nursing practice and nursing interventions. However, by the 1990s, clinical studies comprised over 75% of articles in research journals (Blegen & Tripp-Reimer, 1994).

Beginning in the 1970s, nurse scholars encouraged researchers to provide a theoretical or conceptual framework for research studies. At about the same time, a growing number of nurse theorists were seeking researchers to explore ways to test their models in research and clinical application. As a result, there was a push to combine research and nursing models. This emphasis on using nursing models as the framework for research was proposed to provide research into the unique perspective of nursing (Chinn & Kramer, 2011).

Despite this encouragement, however, the vast majority of research studies in nursing do not test aspects of grand nursing theories or use them as a research framework. Rather, they examine concepts, principles, and theories from a number of theoretical perspectives and disciplines. This trend persisted throughout the 1990s and into the 21st century as the focus of research and theory has moved more toward middle range, situation-specific/practice theories, and evidence-based practice (see Chapters 10, 11, 12, and 18).

Relationship Between Research and Theory

Knowledge development is cumulative, and knowledge generated from separate research studies should be integrated into a more comprehensive understanding of the subject or phenomenon being studied. The value of any research study is derived as much from how it fits with, and expands on, previous work as from the study itself. Thus, research gains its significance from the context within which it is placed—specifically from its theoretical context. The theoretical context, therefore, is the structure and system of important concepts, theoretical propositions, and theories that comprise the existing knowledge of the discipline (Chinn & Kramer, 2011; Fawcett & DeSanto-Madeya, 2013).

Moody (1990) explained that knowledge development in nursing science has lagged due to three major factors: (1) a limited theoretical base to guide practice, (2) an abundance of isolated studies that have not been tied to an integrating theoretical framework or placed in a theoretical context, and (3) inadequate efforts to link theory, measurement, and data interpretation during the research process. To further develop nursing science and strengthen the discipline, it is essential that nurse researchers and nurse scholars address these issues. This requires recognizing the relationship between research and theory and developing an understanding of how theory is used in, and developed through, research. The following sections describe this relationship.

Nursing Research

Research is the "systematic inquiry that uses disciplined methods to answer questions or solve problems" (Polit & Beck, 2012, p. 3). Research is conducted to describe, explain, or predict variables, and in a practice discipline such as nursing, research is assumed to contribute to the improvement of care. The research process consists of several essential steps that are followed in planning, implementing, and analyzing a research study (Box 19-1).

Nursing research has been defined as a "scientific process that validates and refines existing knowledge and generates new knowledge that directly and indirectly influences nursing practice" (Burns, Grove, & Gray, 2013, p. 2). It is concerned with the study of individuals in interaction with their environments and with discovering interventions that promote optimal functioning and wellness across the lifespan. In nursing, researchers have studied principles and laws governing life processes, the well-being and optimum functioning of human beings, patterns of behavior as individuals interact with their environment during critical life situations (e.g., birth, loss, illness, death), and processes that bring about positive changes in a person's health status. Furthermore, nursing research measures the impact of nursing interventions on client outcomes to provide a rational basis for practice.

Box 19-1 Steps of the Research Process

- Identify the problem to be investigated and clarify the purpose of the study.
- Review the literature.
- Define the conceptual/theoretical framework and develop conceptual definitions.
- Formulate research questions or hypotheses.
- Select a research design.
- Determine methods of measurement (instruments/tools).
- Define the population sample to be studied.
- Address legal/ethical issues related to human/animal rights.
- Develop a plan for data collection and analysis.
- Collect the data.
- Analyze the data.
- Interpret findings.
- Identify conclusions and recommendations.
- Disseminate findings.

Sources: Burns, Grove, & Gray (2013); LoBiondo-Wood & Haber (2010); Polit & Beck (2012).

Purpose of Theory in Research

Theory is integral to the research process. It is important to use theory as a framework to provide perspective and guidance to a research study. Indeed, theoretical frameworks provide direction regarding selection of the research design, identify approaches to measurement and methods of data analysis, and specify criteria for acceptability of findings as valid (Fitzpatrick, 1998).

Fitzpatrick (1998) summarized how theory can be used to guide the research process. In generating and testing phenomena of interest to nursing, theory can (1) identify meaningful and relevant areas for study, (2) propose plausible approaches to health problems to examine, (3) develop or reformulate middle range theory linked to research, (4) define concepts and propose relationships among concepts, (5) interpret research findings, (6) develop clinical practice protocols, and (7) generate nursing diagnoses based on research findings.

The Research Framework

As shown in Box 19-1, an essential step of the research process is selection of a theoretical or conceptual model that serves as a research framework. The investigator uses the conceptual model to view situations and events through a particular frame of reference, the researcher's perspective about how the concepts and variables of interest in the study fit together. The research framework describes the phenomena and problems to be studied, as well as the purposes to be fulfilled by the research. It identifies the source of the data (e.g., individuals, groups, animals, documents) and the settings in which data are to be gathered. It contributes to selection of the research design and instruments, determines procedures to be used, and identifies the methods to be used for data analysis. Finally, the framework determines the contributions of the research to the advancement of knowledge by placing the findings within the context of previous knowledge.

LoBiondo-Wood and Haber (2010) believe that using a formal and explicit framework facilitates generalizing a study's findings. This can contribute to nursing science development and promote evidence-based practice. They explain that using a framework can simplify and provide direction to the research process. Unfortunately, in many published nursing research studies, especially studies involving clinical practice problems, a study's framework is implicit rather than explicit. It may be hidden or implied in the literature review, and the reader must "tease it out."

Types of Theory and Corresponding Research

As described in Chapter 2, theory is generally classified as descriptive, explanatory, or predictive. The research designs that generate and test these theories are descriptive, correlational, and experimental, respectively (Fawcett, 1999). Prescriptive theories are also mentioned by a number of authors (Dickoff & James, 1968; Meleis, 2013) and are sometimes related to practice theories (Whall, 2005). Table 19-1 shows the three primary types of theory described in nursing literature (descriptive, explanatory, and predictive) and summarizes the examples from the following discussion.

Descriptive Theory and Descriptive Research

A descriptive theory is an integrated set of concepts that focuses on dimensions, characteristics, situations, and commonalities of a phenomenon of interest (Meleis, 2013; Norwood, 2010). A descriptive theory looks at a phenomenon and identifies its major elements or events. It may also note some relationships among the elements, but it generally only speculates about why the phenomenon occurs, how the elements relate to each other, or how changes in the elements affect each other (Barnum, 2005; Meleis, 2013).

Descriptive research involves observation of a phenomenon in its natural setting. Data are gathered by participant or nonparticipant observation and by open-ended or structured interview schedules or questionnaires. Data may be qualitative or quantitative or both. Descriptive research uses many different methods, including concept

Table 19-1 Types of Theory and Corresponding Research

Type of Theory	Type of Research	Examples From Nursing Literature
Descriptive	Descriptive or exploratory	Development of a model to examine perceptions of "feeling safe" in an intensive care unit (Lasiter, 2011)
		Development of the theory of strengthening capacity to limit intrusion (Ford-Gilboe, Merritt-Gray, Varcoe, & Wuest, 2011)
Explanatory	Correlational	Explaining the phenomenon of "maternal–fetal attachment" based on Ruben's theory of maternal role attainment and Mercer's becoming a mother (Alhusen, Gross, Hayat, Woods, & Sharps, 2012)
Predictive	Experimental	Comparing motivational-interviewing coaching with standard treatment in managing cancer pain, based on the Transtherotical Model (Thomas et al., 2012)
		Testing of multiple relationships examining women's perceptions of Caesarean birth—elements of the Roy Adaptation Model (Fawcett et al., 2011)

analysis, psychometric analyses, case studies, surveys, phenomenology, ethnography, grounded theory, and historical inquiry (McKenna & Slevin, 2008).

Descriptive research (exploratory research) answers questions such as: What are the characteristics of the phenomenon? What is the prevalence of the phenomenon? What is the process by which the phenomenon is experienced? Through systematic study of these or similar questions with a defined population or in a defined setting, a descriptive theory may result.

Nursing Studies

The nursing literature holds many excellent examples of descriptive theory and explanatory and descriptive research. For example, Cranley and colleagues (2012) used grounded theory methods to develop the "Theory of Nurses' Recognizing and Responding to Uncertainty" based on interviews with 14 experienced nurses. The theory seeks to explain how nurses respond to uncertainty in practice and how they seek information when uncertain. They outline nine major interrelated categories forming the theory. Three conditions, or uncertain patient care situations (feeling caught off-guard, encountering unfamiliar or unique orders, navigating the ethical gray areas of practice), were identified as *antecedent conditions*; three categories (figuring it out myself, collaborating with nursing colleagues and team, seeking evidence) described strategies to manage uncertainty; and three categories (resolving uncertainty, lingering doubt, learning opportunity) were consequences of managing uncertainty. Implications for nursing practice and related interventions were provided, which can be instructive for nurses seeking to address uncertainty to improve patient outcomes.

In a second example, Haggstrom, Asplund, and Kristiansen (2012) also used grounded theory methods to interview 19 nurses to develop a theory of "nursing care for patients in the ICU transitional care." The goal was to establish a "coordinated, strengthening, person-centered care for patients in transitions." Through the research process, the researchers identified a core nursing strategy, "being perceptive and adjustable," that was used throughout the process. Facilitating the transition were categories, including prepare for a change, promote recovery, and "balancing between patient's needs and caregiver resources." Subcategories of interventions and strategies used by the nurses identified in the study included elicit trust, make the unknown known, create an alliance, reinforce the patient's will, orienting and integrating, and attempting to implement the patient's own strengths.

Last, Kanacki, Roth, Georges, and Herring (2012) conducted a grounded theory study of 25 widows to explore perceptions of their husbands' end-of-life care. They identified three major themes: (1) awareness of impending death, (2) care and comfort connections, and (3) bereaved responses, which were connected by a "core phenomenon" of "being together." The result was a theoretical model identified as "Shared Presence: Caring for a Dying Spouse."

Explanatory Theory and Correlational Research

Explanatory theories specify relationships between dimensions or characteristics of individuals, groups, situations, or events. They explain why, and the extent to which, one phenomenon is related to another. Explanatory theories are composed of concepts and propositions (Norwood, 2010).

Explanatory theories are typically generated and tested by correlational research. Correlational research requires measurement of the dimensions or characteristics of phenomena in their natural states. Data are usually gathered by nonparticipant observation or a self-report instrument. Instruments can include fixed-choice, open-ended questionnaires, or interview schedules. Correlational research yields qualitative or quantitative data or both. Statistical analysis uses various nonparametric or parametric measures of association (LoBiondo-Wood & Haber, 2010).

Nursing Studies

Using a correlational study design, Esposito and Fitzpatrick (2011) examined the relationships between nurses' beliefs regarding the benefits of exercise, their exercise behaviors, and their recommendation of exercise. Guided by Pender's Health Promotion Model, this study surveyed 112 nurses using two research tools: the Exercise Benefits/Barriers Scales (EBBS) and the Health-Promoting Lifestyles Profiles II (HPLP-II). The researchers identified positive correlations between exercise benefits, physical activity, and recommendation of exercise to patients. Further, nurses who believe in health promotion and engage in healthy behaviors are more likely to be positive role models and teach health behaviors to their patients.

Another study (Weiss & Lokken, 2009) used a correlational design to examine predictors and outcomes of postpartum mother's perception of readiness for discharge after childbirth using Meleis' Transitions Theory as the conceptual framework. In total, 119 patients completed all phases of data collection, which included three surveys and a postdischarge telephone interview. The team determined that Transitions Theory was useful in conceptualizing the transition home after childbirth, which focused attention on relevant variables including the quality of discharge teaching, coping difficulty, readiness for discharge, and utilization of family support and health care services.

Finally, Othman, Kiviniemi, Wu, and Lally (2012) reported on a correlational study undertaken to determine the influence of demographic characteristics, breast cancer knowledge, fatalistic beliefs, health beliefs, and subjective norms on Jordanian women's intention to undergo mammography. The researchers used constructs from both the Health Belief Model and the Theory of Reasoned Action and determined that Jordanian women lacked knowledge about breast cancer. Further, social norms and self-efficacy influenced their intention to have a mammogram. It was concluded that interventions need to focus on providing knowledge and skills to empower women to seek screening.

Predictive Theory and Experimental Research

Predictive theories move beyond explanation to the prediction of relationships between characteristics or phenomena among different groups. Predictive theories are generated and tested by experimental research.

Experimental research involves the manipulation of some phenomenon to determine how it affects or changes some dimension or characteristic of another phenomenon. Experimentation encompasses many different designs, including pretest–posttest–noncontrol group design, quasi-experiments, time series analyses, and true experiments. Experimental research requires quantifiable data. Statistical analyses, involving various nonparametric and parametric tests, are used to measure differences. Qualitative data can be collected but generally must be coded to be tested statistically (LoBiondo-Wood & Haber, 2010).

Nursing Studies

Experimental research studies, and corresponding predictive theories, are relatively uncommon in nursing literature. Examples from recent nursing literature include a study by Dougherty, Thompson, and Kudenchuk (2012), which used a randomized experimental clinical trial comparing two interventions designed to improve outcomes for partners following receipt of an implantable cardioverter defibrillator (ICD). In a work guided by Bandura's Social Cognitive Theory, the researchers identified concerns and issues common to partners of patients who receive an ICD. Based on the ability to anticipate or predict common concerns, they designed and are currently testing nursing interventions to address them.

A second example using an experimental design is a study by Rogers, Keller, Larkey, and Ainsworth (2012). The team used Roy's Adaptation Model as a framework to study the efficacy of 12-week intervention employing "sign chi do" (SCD) exercises (meditative movements similar to tai chi) to promote physical activity among sedentary, community-dwelling elders. Using a randomized experimental design with repeated measures, they examined the effect of SCD (intervention) on physiologic function adaptation and self-concept adaptation. Among the findings were that self-concept adaptation measures were not significantly different between the groups but that physiologic adaptation (balance and physical function) improved for the SCD group. This suggests that SCD is useful for improving physiologic functioning among sedentary elders. Then, a quasi-experimental design was used to test application of Pender's health promotion model (Shin, Kang, Park, Cho, & Heitkemper, 2008). Using structural equation modeling of a large sample ($n = 389$) of elderly Korean women, the researchers sought to predict health-promoting behaviors. They determined that health-promoting behaviors were explained by multiple factors: commitment to a plan of action, behavior-specific cognitions and affect, environmental influences, prior health-related behaviors, biologic factors, psychologic factors, and sociocultural factors. It was concluded that to precipitate health-promoting behaviors that will improve quality of life, nursing interventions should involve those factors.

How Theory Is Used in Research

Theory brings organization to the variables of interest and the concepts reflected in a study. It provides a guide for developing a study and allows the findings to be placed in, or linked to, a larger body of knowledge. Therefore, a theoretical perspective increases the scientific value of a study's findings.

Both nursing and non-nursing theories have relevance for problems studied by nursing researchers, and theories tend to show up in the research process in one of three ways. A theory can be generated as the outcome of a study. In other cases, a research project is undertaken for the specific purpose of testing a theory. Most frequently, a theory is used in a research framework as the context for a study (McEwen, 2013). Each of these three ways that theory is used in research is described in the following sections.

Theory-Generating Research

Research that generates theory (i.e., descriptive research) is designed to develop and describe relationships between and among phenomena without imposing preconceived notations of what these phenomena mean (Chinn & Kramer, 2011). It is inductive and includes grounded theory, field observations, and phenomenology. During the theory-generating process, the researcher moves by logical thought from fact to theory by means of a proposition stated as an empirical generalization.

Norwood (2010) explained several steps in the process of theory generation. First, the researcher identifies observations with shared characteristics or common themes in an identified group or in a particular setting. Second, the researcher translates these observations into more abstract concepts by determining what general phenomenon these observations represent. The third step involves identifying patterns of relationships between observations and concepts. Next, the researcher translates observations of relationships into propositional statements and finally weaves the concepts and propositions together into a framework or tentative theory. In some

NURSING EXEMPLAR 1: THEORY-GENERATING RESEARCH

The following study is a good example of theory generation using grounded theory research techniques. The study is analyzed using the steps described by Norwood (2010).

Dyess, S. M., & Chase, S. K. (2012). Sustaining health in faith community nursing practice: Emerging processes that support the development of a middle-range theory. *Holistic Nursing Practice, 26*(4), 221–227.

Identify common themes in an identified group: The researchers provided background information explaining how most people older than 65 years live with chronic illnesses (e.g., heart disease, hypertension, hearing and vision impairment, cognitive loss, arthritis, cancer, diabetes). Further, they suggest that these individuals and their families need holistic approaches in symptom management and coping strategies.

Translate observations into abstract concepts: Faith community nurses were asked to submit "stories" of nursing situations from their practice. These were reviewed and four "core processes" of nursing practice within communities of faith were identified. These were (1) entering the private world of other (the faith community nurse seeks to know and understand the individual in the context of his or her life), (2) connecting to faith (actions that link to traditions and mores of the faith [e.g., praying, attending luncheons, Bible study]), (3) mutually transforming experience (the nurse and patient perceive a "profound transformation" or sense of awe in being changed by the encounters), and (4) sustaining health (nurse identifies and addresses gaps in health care).

Patterns of relationships identified: "Many community-dwelling older adults living with chronic illness desire comprehensive whole-person support" (Dyess & Chase, 2012, p. 221). Faith communities are well positioned to provide cost-effective, holistic care for adults living with chronic illness. Nurses can facilitate positive relationship between patient and health care providers by understanding and utilizing the four "core processes" as they plan and implement care.

Weave concepts and propositions together into a framework or rudimentary theory: The four core processes can become the foundation of a middle range theory of faith community nursing. The theory explains and supports the intimacy of the nursing relationship that enhances the holistic approach that includes beliefs and meaning and that can contribute to future research and be used to organize education and support nurses entering the specialty.

cases, the researcher may identify an existing theory that these concepts and relationships represent. Nursing Exemplar 1 analyzes a grounded theory study to further illustrate the steps involved in theory-generating research.

Nursing Studies

Theory-generating research studies can readily be found in nursing literature. As mentioned, a number of nursing theories have been developed using grounded theory research techniques. For example, Rempel, Ravindran, Rogers, and Magill-Evans (2012) used grounded theory methods to develop a theoretical explanation of the process they termed "Parenting Under Pressure" to describe how parents of young children with life-threatening congenital heart disease learn to manage the responsibilities of monitoring and caring for their children at home.

Often, new theories are developed from existing theories. For example, Kelly (2008) reportedly developed the middle range "commitment to health theory" from the Transtheoretical Model of Behavior Change, and Dobratz (2011) developed the middle range theory "Psychological Adaptation in Death and Dying" based on aspects of the Roy Adaptation Model. In another example, the middle range theory of Self-Care of Chronic Illness (Riegel, Jaarsma, & Stromberg, 2012) contained concepts and elements consistent with Orem's grand theory of self-care. Finally, Reimer and Moore's (2010) middle range theory of "flight nursing expertise" includes elements identified by Benner (2001).

Theory-Testing Research

Sometimes a study is conducted for the purpose of testing a theory or assessing its explanatory value in a specific situation. In theory-testing research, theoretical statements are translated into questions and hypotheses. Theory testing requires a deductive reasoning process that also follows several steps.

First, the researcher chooses a theory of interest and selects a specific propositional statement from the theory (rather than the entire theory) to be tested. Next, the researcher develops a hypothesis or hypotheses that must have specific measurable variables that reflect the propositional statement. The researcher conducts the study and interprets findings. The interpretation determines if the study supports or contradicts the propositional statement and, thus, the theory. Finally, the researcher determines if there are any implications for further use of the theory in nursing practice (LoBiondo-Wood & Haber, 2010; Norwood, 2010).

Examples of theory testing are fairly rare in nursing literature. One reason for this is the lack of clarity about what constitutes theory testing. Silva (1986) pointed out that serious misconception exists among some researchers and theorists that if a conceptual model has been used as a theoretical framework for research, then this constitutes theory testing. It does not, however, because theory testing requires detailed examination of theoretical relationships and necessitates that the study be designed to accept or refute these relationships.

Another reason there has been little theory-testing research relates to interpretation and evaluation of the research. Acton, Irvin, and Hopkins (1991) developed criteria for evaluating theory-testing research (Box 19-2, p. 441) that will help those who are interested in conducting this type of study as well as those using the criteria. In addition, Nursing Exemplar 2 gives an example of the evaluation of a theory-testing study using these criteria.

NURSING EXEMPLAR 2: THEORY-TESTING RESEARCH

The following is a review of an excellent example of theory-testing research. This study tested the Theory of Health Promotion for Preterm Infants based on Levine's Conservation Model of Nursing. Here, the research is evaluated using the criteria suggested in Box 19-2.

Mefford, L. C., & Alligood, M. R. (2011). Testing a theory of health promotion of preterm infants based on Levine's Conservation Model of Nursing. ***The Journal of Theory Construction & Testing, 15*****(2), 41–47.**

Purpose: "The purpose of this study was to perform an exploratory test of the middle range Theory of Health Promotion for Preterm Infants based on Levine's Conservation Model of nursing" (Mefford & Alligood, 2011, p. 41).

Explicit summary of theory: The theoretical framework, including goals of nursing care and subjects of nursing care (preterm infants and family), are discussed.

Definitions: Seven theoretical concepts (termed "latent variables") (physiologic immaturity at birth, structural immaturity at birth, neurologic immaturity at birth, family system characteristics at birth, etc.) are defined.

Previous studies: The theoretical framework section described the process involved in development of the middle range theory and provided detail on both Levine's model and related information, as well as a description of application and previous testing.

Hypotheses: Hypotheses were not specified. However, a path diagram model was provided that explained anticipated relationships among the latent variables in the theory to be used for statistical testing.

Operational definitions: Operational definitions are clearly described as "measurement variables" for each of the theoretical concepts (latent variables).

Study design: The design was a descriptive correlational *ex post facto* study using data collected from existing databases of a level III neonatal intensive care unit (NICU) and an associated intermediate care nursery.

Instruments: A number of measures were used for the study. Data were collected on such variables as "surfactant therapy," birth weight, Apgar scores, maternal age, prenatal care, and consistency of nursing caregivers. They also created a measure of "heath status" that assessed such indictors as postconceptual age at discharge, weight at discharge, and "morbidity score" (bronchopulmonary dysplasia, intraventricular hemorrhage, nosocomial infect, etc.).

Sample: The convenience sample included 235 infants with a gestational age at birth of less than 37 weeks who were treated in the study NICU.

Statistics: Measures of univariate and multivariate normality were submitted to LISREL program for structural equation modeling.

Data analysis: The structural equation modeling carried out indicated that the "overall good fit of the model to the data . . . [had] a Goodness of Fit Index of 0.905." (Mefford & Alligood, 2011, p. 46). Each of the relationships originally posited were discussed and most of the relationships presented in the original model were supported.

Research report: The findings indicated that the middle range theory was supported as "the model fit and path directions and strengths were congruent with relational propositions of the theory" (Mefford & Alligood, 2011, pp. 46–47).

Significance of theory for nursing: The authors concluded that the findings validate the theoretical assertion that nursing care supports adaptive efforts of the infant and family and facilitates attainment of health. Further, the researchers noted that consistency of nursing caregivers is very important to promoting health for preterm infants.

Recommendations: The study provided evidence that the Theory of Health Promotion for Preterm Infants holds promise as a theoretical framework to guide neonatal nursing practice and improve health outcomes of these tiny patients.

Nursing Studies

Some studies testing theories were found in recent nursing literature. Not surprisingly, most of those studies identified tested grand or middle range nursing theories or theories derived from grand nursing theories.

Research testing grand nursing theories included a study conducted by Gigliotti (2004). In this work, elements of Neuman's systems model were tested by examining maternal–student role stress. This study was designed to examine the moderating capabilities of the psychological and sociocultural variables in the flexible line of defense. In the study, 135 women were given questionnaires to measure role stress, maternal and student role involvement, and social support. It was concluded that the effect of student role involvement on maternal–student role stress is contingent upon low network support. Also, the effect of maternal role involvement on maternal–student role stress is significantly enhanced for women age 37 years and older.

Research that tested theories or models derived from grand or middle range nursing theories included a work by Hodgins, Wuest, and Malcolm (2011), which tested the middle range caregiving theory (Wuest, 2001) in women who were caregivers of family members with dementia. Another example (Fawcett et al., 2011) tested multiple relationships within the Roy Adaptation Model examining women's perception of Caesarean birth.

Box 19-2 Criteria for Evaluating Theory-Testing Research

- The purpose of the study is to examine the empirical validity of the constructs, concepts, assumptions, or relationship from the identified theory.
- The theory is explicitly described and summarized.
- The constructs and concepts to be examined are theoretically defined.
- An overview of the previous studies that are based on the theoretic framework, or that clearly show the derivation of the concepts being tested, must be included in the review of the literature.
- The research questions or hypotheses are logically derived from the definitions, assumptions, and propositions of the theory.
- The research questions or hypotheses are specific enough to put the theory at risk for falsification.
- The operational definitions are clearly derived from the theory.
- The design is congruent with the level of theory described.
- The instruments are theoretically valid and reliable.
- The theory guides the sample selection.
- The statistics used are the most robust possible.
- Data analysis provides evidence for supporting, refuting, or modifying the theory.
- The research report includes an interpretative analysis of the finding in relation to the theory being tested.
- The significance of the theory for nursing is discussed in the report.
- The researcher makes recommendations for further research on the basis of the findings.
- Researchers should identify theory-testing studies in their abstracts, publication titles, and library retrieval key words.

Box 19-3 Use of a Theory as a Conceptual Framework in a Nursing Study

- The framework's concepts are used as variables in the study.
- The conceptual definitions are drawn from the framework.
- The data collection instrument is congruent with the framework.
- Findings are interpreted in light of explanations provided by the framework.
- The researcher identifies whether the study's findings support or challenge the framework.
- Implications for nursing practice are based on the explanatory power of the framework.
- Recommendations for further research address the concepts and relationships in the framework.

Source: Norwood (2010)

Theory as the Conceptual Framework or Context of a Study

The most common way of incorporating a theory into the research process is by using the theory to drive the entire study (McEwen, 2014). In these cases, the problem being investigated is fitted into an existing theoretical framework, which guides the study and enriches the value of its findings.

The process of using a theory as a conceptual framework also involves several steps. Typically, during the process of conducting the literature review, the researcher identifies an existing framework that can be meaningfully applied to the study or develops a conceptual framework that is unique to the study (Norwood, 2010). When a framework is used as the context, it is integrated into the study in a number of ways (Box 19-3). Nursing Exemplar 3 presents an evaluation of a published research study illustrating how a nursing theory is used as a conceptual framework.

NURSING EXEMPLAR 3: THEORY AS A CONCEPTUAL FRAMEWORK

The following is a good example of using a nursing theory (the Roy Adaptation Model) as the conceptual framework for a research study. The criteria suggested in Box 19-3 were used to evaluate this work.

DeSanto-Madeya, S. (2009). Adaptation to spinal cord injury for families post-injury. *Nursing Science Quarterly, 22*(1), 57–66.

Research problems consistent with the framework: The purpose of this study was to "identify individuals' and family members' perspectives of the physical, emotional, functional, and social components of adaptation and their adjustment to spinal cord injury" (DeSanto-Madeya, 2009, p. 58).

Conceptual definitions derived from the framework: Concepts studied were derived from the Roy Adaptation Model. Concepts described were adaptive systems (families) in constant interaction with changing focal stimuli (time since injury) and contextual stimuli (level of injury and factors that help or hinder their adaptation).

Instruments congruent with the framework: The research instruments were described in detail. They included the Adaptation to Spinal Cord Injury Interview Schedule (developed by the researcher for a previous study) and a detailed background data sheet.

Findings interpreted based on the framework: The findings were interpreted based on explanations of the Roy Adaptation Model.

Relationship of findings to framework: The researchers described the findings in relation to the Roy Adaptation Model by explaining how family members' responses fell within Roy's Modes of Adaptation. An "adaptation score" was calculated for spinal cord–injured individuals and their family members, and adjustment to spinal cord injury was evaluated at year 1 and year 3. Factors that help or hinder adaptation were also assessed.

Implications for nursing: It was concluded that family relationships and refocusing of values positively influenced adaptation to spinal cord injury. Additionally, it was noted that depression is common for both the injured person and the family members, an observation that is very important for nurses providing care.

Recommendations for future research: The researchers noted that further inquiry should be conducted with a larger sample to determine the utility and adequacy of applying aspects of Roy's model to caring for individuals with spinal cord injury.

If the conceptual framework used by the researcher is an existing framework, the process can be termed *theory fitting*. In theory fitting, the researcher formulates a research purpose or research question and then proceeds to the literature to search for a theory to guide the study. The theory that best fits the research study is then selected. There are potential problems with this practice, however. The concepts or relationships from the original theory may be incorrectly applied, the work may appear forced, or the study may fail to lead to meaningful conclusions. To be effective, theory fitting requires an extensive search of the literature and an understanding of theoretical progress in nursing and other fields (Moody, 1990).

Nursing Studies

A number of current studies using both nursing and non-nursing theories as the research framework were identified. For example, a recent research review focused on symptom investigation and management in patients with brain tumor based on the Theory of Unpleasant Symptoms (Cahill, LoBiondo-Wood, Bergstrom, & Armstrong, 2012). In other examples, the AACN's Synergy Model (AACN, 2013) was the framework to develop a study identifying "tele-intensive care competencies" in ICU nurses (Goran, 2011). Lastly, a correlational study examining the relationships between spirituality and health-promoting behaviors among homeless women was conducted by Hurlbut, Robbins, and Hoke (2011) based on Pender's Health Promotion Model.

Non-nursing theories are frequently used as conceptual frameworks, and numerous examples are found throughout the nursing literature. For example, Zhou, Stoltzfus, Houldin, Parks, and Swan (2010) used the Theory of Reasoned Action (Theory of Planned Behavior) as their conceptual framework studying the knowledge, attitudes, and behaviors of oncology advanced practice nurses (APNs) regarding advanced care planning for cancer patients. Also, as discussed previously, Dougherty and colleagues (2012) used Bandura's Social Cognitive Theory as the framework for their experimental study on assisting partners of patients with ICD to adjust to relationships and health care utilization, and Othman and colleagues (2012) used the Health Belief Model and the Theory of Reasoned Action to examine self-efficacy and barriers to mammography screening among Jordanian women.

Nursing and Non-Nursing Theories in Nursing Research

As explained in previous chapters, there has been significant debate in the discipline of nursing regarding the source of the theories used in nursing research. Some scholars have emphasized the importance of using only nursing theories for research to ensure that what results is, indeed, nursing research. But it has also been shown that nurses depend on and use knowledge drawn from various sources in developing nursing research and that this practice does not negate the importance of the findings to nurses.

Rationale for Using Nursing Theories in Nursing Research

Some nursing theorists and nursing researchers believe that it is essential to use only nursing theories and models in nursing research. They assert that only nursing models truly deal with the scope and direction of nursing interventions; therefore, they provide a sound conceptual framework for nursing research. Additionally, their use as frameworks for research is one way of ensuring that the study will be relevant to the discipline (Fawcett & DeSanto-Madeya, 2013).

Proponents argue that conceptual models of nursing and nursing theories can be used to guide all forms of nursing research. They believe that nursing theories help nurse researchers identify the phenomena of central interest to the discipline and assist in designing studies that reflect nursing's distinctive perspective of people and their environment in matters of health. Fawcett (2000), in particular, questioned whether using a theory from another discipline resulted in nursing research, even if a nurse conducted the research. To address her concerns about using theories and concepts from other disciplines, she challenged researchers to base studies in the context of conceptual models of nursing and nursing theories.

One common criticism regarding the use of nursing models to direct research is a practice used by the editors of many nursing journals. It has been reported that if a nursing theory is used as a conceptual framework, the authors are often asked (by the journal's editors) to rewrite an article to delete the notation of the nursing theory component. Roberts (1999) concluded that it appears that "editors and reviewers of clinical specialty journals are anxious to protect the reader from nursing theory . . . to make the article more readable" (p. 300).

Concerns Over Reliance on Nursing Models to Direct Nursing Research

In response to repeated calls to focus research only on nursing theories and models, Brink (2000) wrote that many manuscripts that include a nursing theory or conceptual model treat the model or theory as an appendage. She pointed out that, in many cases, reporting of the conceptual framework consists of a single-paragraph description of the model, which often has nothing to do with the rest of the manuscript. She explained that the theory does not direct the literature review, the models, or the problem under study and never relates to the conclusions, and the author is asked to delete the paragraph. Brink argued that borrowed theories or practice theories can readily be used to describe and explain phenomena that affect nursing and concluded that to limit nurses to using only nursing theories in nursing research is shortsighted.

Tripp-Reimer (1984) described the difference between theories *of* nursing and theories *for* nursing. She believed that grand theories are theories *of* nursing and describe the nature and scope of the discipline to assist nurses in their general approach to care. On the other hand, theories *for* nursing identify what nurses should do to achieve the best client care. She noted that too often, superimposing a grand theory as a conceptual framework is confusing, and theories or concepts that are being studied do not underlie the nursing models, even though they may be congruent with them. Although the theories are congruent with the nursing models, they do not underlie the models; thus, the relationship appears forced.

Tripp-Reimer (1984) wrote that research should develop and test theories *for* nursing practice. Research should focus on testing which interventions work best with certain types of clients in specific clinical situations. This is being accomplished with the increasing interest in the development and testing of middle range nursing theories (see Chapters 10 and 11) and practice/situation specific theories (see Chapter 12).

Other Issues in Nursing Theory and Nursing Research

To enhance understanding of the use of theory in nursing research, other issues should be addressed. Two significant issues are:

1. Recognizing the importance of adequately describing the theory in the research report
2. Examining how theory fits into the discipline's research agenda

The Research Report

To clearly illustrate the impact of the theoretical framework in developing the research study and to show the context within which the findings should be interpreted, discussion of the theoretical framework should be incorporated into several sections of the research report (Norwood, 2000). First, the framework should be introduced and briefly described in the problem statement.

Second, the framework is usually described in detail under its own heading at the end of the literature review. In this section, the description of the theory or concepts should be drawn from primary sources. The concepts should be clearly defined, and proposed relationships need to be described. A model or diagram that depicts both the framework and how it is being translated or applied to the present study may be added. Additionally, if the study is using an existing framework, the section should describe previous research application of the framework.

Third, how the framework is operationalized should be delineated in the methodology section. This will explain how the framework influences or is reflected in the study's design, data collection strategies, and data analysis methods. If an instrument has been developed for the study, the specific items that are used as indicators of the concepts in the framework need to be identified (Norwood, 2000).

Fourth, the framework needs to be referred to in the Discussion section of the research report. The findings should be discussed in terms of how they illustrate, support, challenge, or contradict the framework.

Finally, suggestions for changing nursing practice or conducting further research that are consistent with the framework's concepts and propositions should be offered in the report's conclusion (Norwood, 2000). Box 19-4 presents an outline for inclusion of the theoretical framework in the research report.

Box 19-4 Guidelines for Writing About a Research Study's Theoretical Framework

In the Study's Problem Statement
- Introduce the framework.
- Briefly explain why it is a good fit for the research problem area.

At the End of the Literature Review
- Thoroughly describe the framework and explain its application to the present study.
- Describe how the framework has been used in studies about similar problems.

In the Study's Methodology Section
- Explain how the framework is being operationalized in the study's design.
- Explain how data collection methods (such as questionnaire items) reflect the concepts in the framework.

In the Study's Discussion Section
- Describe how study findings are consistent (or inconsistent) with the framework.
- Offer suggestions for practice and further research that are congruent with the framework's concepts and propositions.

Source: Norwood (2000)

Nursing's Research Agenda

There is a need for nurses to increase research that addresses significant clinical problems and adds to the knowledge base of the discipline. To accomplish this, research themes must be significant to the discipline's theory and practice, and research must build on previous knowledge to lead to knowledge accumulation. Recommendations for future nursing research are to move beyond descriptive studies to explanatory and predictive studies, to promote study replication, and to conduct meta-analyses in areas where experimental studies have been conducted. Finally, it is important that nurses explicate the theoretical perspective of the research design in the research report to demonstrate how the study fits into the current body of knowledge.

The National Institute for Nursing Research (NINR) began as a center within the National Institutes of Health in 1986 and became an institute in 1993. The NINR supports clinical and basic research to establish a scientific basis of the care of individuals across the life span. This includes caring for individuals during illness and recovery, reduction of risks for disease and disability, promotion of healthy lifestyles, promotion of quality of life in those with chronic illness, and care for individuals at the end of life. Research priorities of the NINR (2011) are:

- Enhance health promotion and disease prevention
- Improve quality of life by managing symptoms of acute and chronic illness
- Improve palliative and end-of-life care
- Enhance innovation in science and practice
- Develop the next generation of nurse scientists.

(See Link to Practice 19-1 for more information).

To build the body of nursing knowledge, nurses must consider these issues from a theoretical perspective and must avoid looking at them in isolation.

In a well-supported essay, Hinshaw (2000) identified "areas of evolving nursing science" (p. 119) that should be targeted for directed nursing research (Box 19-5).

Link to Practice 19-1

The NINR (see www.ninr.nih.gov) provides significant funding for nursing research. Graduate students and potential nurse researchers should review the research priorities set by the NINR to understand its major areas for funding priorities. The NINR has indicated that it will invest in basic clinical and translation research to:

1) Enhance health promotion and disease prevention.
   - Develop innovative behavior interventions to promote health and prevent illness in diverse populations.
   - Study the behavior of systems that promote the development of personalized interventions.
   - Translate scientific advances to effect positive health behavioral change.
2) Improve quality of life by managing symptoms of acute and chronic illness.
   - Improve knowledge of biologic and genomic mechanisms associated with symptoms and symptom clusters.
   - Study the multiple factors that influence management of symptoms.
   - Develop strategies to assist individuals and their caregivers in managing chronic illness.
3) Improve palliative and end-of-life care.
   - Study complex issues and choices in palliative and end-of-life care.
   - Develop and test biobehavioral interventions that provide palliative care.
   - Determine the impact of providers trained in palliative and end-of-life care on health care outcomes.
4) Enhance innovation in science and practice.
   - Develop new technologies and informatics-based solutions to promote health.
   - Use genetic and genomic technologies to advance knowledge.
5) Develop the next generation of nurse scientists.
   - Support ongoing development of investigators at all stages of their research careers.
   - Facilitate more rapid advancement from student to scientist.
   - Expand research knowledge through established infrastructure (NINR, 2011).

Box 19-5 Areas of Evolving Nursing Science

- Critical health needs of communities and vulnerable populations
- Practice strategies and outcomes
- Family health and transitions
- Health promotion/risk reduction
- Biobehavioral manifestations of health and illness
- Women's health
- Health and illness of older adults
- Environments for optimizing client outcomes
- Genetics research
- End-of-life research

These areas should receive priority attention in nursing theory and nursing research in the 21st century. Additionally, according to Hinshaw, research programs should focus on intervention research to provide a stronger, more predictable base for nursing practice.

Hinshaw (2000) also called for interdisciplinary collaboration and multidisciplinary research partners. She wrote that this will more effectively address complex problems and provide a global perspective for care. However, it is important to recognize that interdisciplinary and multidisciplinary research will necessitate familiarity with theories, concepts, and principles of other disciplines.

In addition to the research priorities listed in Box 19-5 on page 447, nursing knowledge must be developed that will direct nursing practice, nursing administration and management, and nursing education. Table 19-2 gives suggestions for further research in these three areas that will be beneficial for the development of the discipline.

Table 19-2 Examples of Research Priorities in Nursing Practice, Nursing Administration/Management, and Nursing Education

Nursing Practice	Nursing Administration and Management	Nursing Education
Client needs related to health and illness (e.g., health promotion/illness prevention, symptom management, enhancing quality of life)	Development and evaluation of new patient care delivery models	Use of instructional technology (e.g., new approaches to laboratory and simulated learning)
Providing and testing nursing care interventions and measuring outcomes of care	Provision and maintenance of healthful work/practice environments	Development, implementation, and evaluation of new pedagogies
Evidence-based nursing practice (multiple areas)	Development of provider and patient safety guidelines	Development, implementation, and evaluation of flexible curriculum designs
Identification, prevention, and management of common health problems/threats in specific community-based settings (e.g., worksites, homes, schools)	Implementation and evaluation of use of technology to complement patient care	Development of new models for teacher preparation and faculty development
Reducing health disparities (e.g., delivery of culturally competent care, enhancing access to and utilization of health care)	Evaluation of outcomes of care related to cost effectiveness and quality	Methods for teaching evidence-based practices
Enhancing nursing care provision related to specific health problems or issues (by specialty area, setting, or other category) (e.g., pain management, reducing incidence of low-birth-weight infants, improving immunization compliance, prevention of nosocomial infection, reduction of HIV infection, prevention of lower back strain)	Program planning, implementation, and evaluation	Evaluation of processes for grading, testing, and evaluation of students, faculty, and curricula
Examination of appropriate application of genetics information and knowledge in nursing practice	Strategies to improve nurse retention and satisfaction	Strategies to enhance community-based learning and service strategies

Sources: Websites of American Association of Colleges of Nursing; American Organization of Nurse Executives; International Council of Nurses; National League for Nursing; American Association of Operating Room Nurses

Summary

The relationship between research and theory is undeniable, and it is important to recognize the impact of this relationship on the development of nursing knowledge. This chapter has provided details on the interface of theory and research and given examples of when, where, and how theory and research interface.

In the discipline of nursing, research may be theory generating or theory testing. Or, as in the opening case scenario, a theory may be used as the conceptual framework that drives the study. The source of the theory for a research study may be unique to nursing (such as using Benner's Novice to Expert model by the student in the case scenario) or borrowed from another discipline, but the theoretical base should be explicit and appropriate.

As an evolving science, nurses should avoid research in isolation. It is imperative that nursing research respond to important questions and issues from nursing practice, administration and management, and education. This will provide a sound base of knowledge, which will further strengthen the discipline.

Key Points

- The purpose of research is to build knowledge through generation and/or testing of theory.
- Nursing research is the "scientific process that validates and refines existing knowledge and generates new knowledge that directly and indirectly influences nursing practice" (Burns et al., 2013).
- One of the essential steps of the research process is the selection of a theoretical or conceptual model that serves as a research framework.
- Several types of theory and corresponding research are commonly found in nursing. Among them are (1) descriptive theory and descriptive research, (2) explanatory theory and correlational research, and (3) predictive theory and experimental research.
- Theory is typically used in nursing research in one of three ways: (1) as an outcome or product of research (the research generates theory), (2) the research is undertaken to test a theory, (3) theory is used as a framework or context for the research.
- Both nursing and non-nursing theories are useful in directing nursing research.
- Research priorities for nursing should include theoretical bases or foundations.

Learning Activities

1. Find a research article from a recent journal that purports to test a theory. Use the guidelines from Box 19-2 on page 441 to evaluate the research study (see the example in Nursing Exemplar 2, p. 440).
2. Find a research article from a recent nursing journal that uses a grand or middle range theory as a conceptual framework. Use the guidelines from Box 19-3 on page 442 to evaluate how well the conceptual framework is used to guide the research project (see the example in Nursing Exemplar 3, p. 442).

REFERENCES

American Association of Critical-Care Nurses. (2013). The AACN synergy model for patient care. Retrieved from http://www.aacn.org/wd/certifications/content/synmodel.pcms?menu=certification

Acton, G. J., Irvin, B. L., & Hopkins, B. A. (1991). Theory-testing research: Building the science. *Advances in Nursing Science, 14*(1), 52–61.

Alhusen, J. L., Gross, D., Hayat, M. J., Woods, A. B., & Sharps, P. W. (2012). The influence of maternal-fetal attachment and health practices on neonatal outcomes in low-income, urban women. *Research in Nursing & Health, 35*(2), 112–120.

Barnum, B. S. (2005). *Nursing theory: Analysis, application, evaluation* (5th ed.). Philadelphia: Lippincott Williams & Wilkins.

Benner, P. (2001). *From novice to expert: Excellence and power in clinical nursing practice* (commemorative edition). Englewood Cliffs, NJ: Prentice-Hall.

Blegen, M. A., & Tripp-Reimer, T. (1994). The nursing theory–nursing research connection. In J. C. McCloskey & H. K. Grace (Eds.), *Current issues in nursing* (4th ed., pp. 87–91). St. Louis: Mosby.

Brink, P. J. (2000). A response to Fawcett. *Western Journal of Nursing Research, 22*(6), 653–655.

Burns, N., Grove, S. K., & Gray, J. R. (2013). *The practice of nursing research: Appraisal, synthesis and generation of evidence* (7th ed.). St. Louis: Elsevier.

Cahill, J., LoBiondo-Wood, G., Bergstrom, N., & Armstrong, T. (2012). Brain tumor symptoms as antecedents to uncertainty: An integrative review. *Journal of Nursing Scholarship, 44*(2), 145–155.

Chinn, P. L., & Kramer, M. K. (2011). *Theory and nursing: Integrated knowledge development* (8th ed.). St. Louis: Mosby.

Cranley, L. A., Doran, D. M., Tourangeau, A. E., Kushniruk, A., & Nagle, L. (2012). Recognizing and responding to uncertainly: A grounded theory of nurses' uncertainty. *Worldviews on Evidence-Based Nursing, 9*(3), 149–158.

DeSanto-Madeya, S. (2009). Adaptation to spinal cord injury for families post-injury. *Nursing Science Quarterly, 22*(1), 57–66.

Dickoff, J., & James, P. (1968). A theory of theories: A position paper. *Nursing Research, 17*(3), 197–203.

Dobratz, M. C. (2011). Toward development of a middle-range theory of psychological adaptation in death and dying. *Nursing Science Quarterly, 24*(4), 370–376.

Dougherty, C. M., Thomson, E. A., & Kudenchuk, P. J. (2012). Development and testing of an intervention to improve outcomes for partners following receipt of an implantable cardioverter defibrillator in the patient. *Advances in Nursing Science, 35*(4), 359–377.

Dyess, S. M., & Chase, S. K. (2012). Sustaining health in faith community nursing practice: Emerging processes that support the development of a middle-range theory. *Holistic Nursing Practice, 26*(4), 221–227.

Esposito, E. M., & Fitzpatrick, J. J. (2011). Registered nurses' beliefs of the benefits of exercise, their exercise behavior and their patient teaching regarding exercise. *International Journal of Nursing Practice, 17*, 351–356.

Fawcett, J. (1999). *The relationship of theory and research* (3rd ed.). Philadelphia: F. A. Davis.

Fawcett, J. (2000). But is it nursing research? *Western Journal of Nursing Research, 22*(5), 524–525.

Fawcett, J., Abner, C., Haussler, S., Weiss, M., Meyers, S. T., Hall, J. L., et al. (2011). Women's perceptions of caesarean birth: A Roy international study. *Nursing Science Quarterly, 24*(40), 352–362.

Fawcett, J., & DeSanto-Madeya, S. (2013). *Contemporary nursing knowledge: Analysis and evaluation of nursing models and theories* (3rd ed.). Philadelphia: F. A. Davis.

Fitzpatrick, J. J. (1998). *Encyclopedia of nursing research.* New York: Springer.

Ford-Gilboe, M., Merritt-Gray, M., Varcoe, C., & Wuest, J. (2011). A theory-based primary health care intervention of women who have left abusive partners. *Advances in Nursing Science, 34*(3), 198–214.

Gigliotti, E. (2004). Etiology of maternal–student role stress. *Nursing Science Quarterly, 17*(2), 156–164.

Goran, S. F. (2011). A new view: Tele-intensive care unit competencies. *Critical Care Nurse, 31*(5), 17–29.

Haggstrom, M., Asplund, K., & Kristiansen, L. (2012). How can nurses facilitate patient's transitions from intensive care? A grounded theory of nursing. *Intensive and Critical Care Nursing, 28*, 224–233.

Hardin, S. R., & Bishop, S. M. (2010). History and philosophy of science. In A. M. Tomey & M. R. Alligood (Eds.), *Nursing theorists and their work* (7th ed., pp. 16–25). St. Louis: Mosby.

Hinshaw, A. S. (2000). Nursing knowledge for the 21st century: Opportunities and challenges. *Image: Journal of Nursing Scholarship, 32*(2), 117–123.

Hodgins, M. J., Wuest, J., & Malcolm, J. (2011). Modeling the effects of past relationship and obligation on changes in the health and health promotion of women caregivers of family member with dementia. *Research in Nursing & Health, 34*, 440–456.

Hurlbut, J. M., Robbins, L. K., & Hoke, M. M. (2011). Correlations between spirituality and health-promoting behaviors among sheltered homeless women. *Journal of Community Health Nursing, 28*(1), 81–91.

Kalisch, P. A., & Kalisch, B. J. (2004). *The advance of American nursing* (4th ed.). Philadelphia: Lippincott Williams & Wilkins.

Kanacki, L. S., Roth, P., Georges, J. M., & Herring, P. (2012). Shared presence: Caring for a dying spouse. *Journal of Hospice and Palliative Nursing, 14*(6), 414–425.

Kelly, C. W. (2008). Commitment to health theory. *Research and Theory for Nursing Practice: An International Journal, 22*(2), 148–160.

Lasiter, S. (2011). Older adults' perceptions of feeling safe in an intensive care unit. *Journal of Advanced Nursing, 67*(12), 2649–2657.

LoBiondo-Wood, G., & Haber, J. (2010). Integrating evidence-based practice. In G. LoBiondo-Wood & J. Haber (Eds.), *Nursing research: Methods, critical appraisal, and utilization* (7th ed., pp. 5–26). St. Louis: Mosby.

McEwen, M. (2014). Theoretical frameworks for research. In LoBiondo-Wood & Haber (Eds.), *Nursing research: Methods, critical appraisal, and utilization* (8th ed.). St. Louis: Mosby.

McKenna, H. P., & Slevin, O. D. (2008). *Nursing models, theories and practice.* Oxford, United Kingdom: Blackwell Publishing.

Mefford, L. C., & Alligood, M. R. (2011). Testing a theory of health promotion for preterm infants based on Levine's conservation Model of Nursing. *The Journal of Theory Construction & Testing, 15*(2), 41–47.

Meleis, A. I. (2013). *Theoretical nursing: Development and progress* (5th ed.). Philadelphia: Lippincott Williams & Wilkins.

Moody, L. E. (1990). Developing a theoretical design for research. In L. E. Moody (Ed.), *Advancing nursing science through research* (pp. 211–248). Newbury Park, CA: Sage.

National Institute for Nursing Research. (2011). Bringing science to life: NINR strategic plan. Retrieved from https://www.ninr.nih.gov/sites/www.ninr.nih.gov/files/ninr-strategic-plan-2011.pdf

Norwood, S. L. (2000). *Research strategies for advanced practice nurses.* Upper Saddle River, NJ: Prentice-Hall Health.

Norwood, S. L. (2010). *Research essentials: Foundations for evidence-based practice.* Upper Saddle River, NJ: Prentice Hall.

Othman, A. K., Kiviniemi, M. T., Wu, Y. W., & Lally, R. M. (2012). Influence of demographic factors, knowledge and beliefs on Jordanian women's intention to undergo mammography screening. *Journal of Nursing Scholarship, 44*(1), 19–26.

Polit, D. F., & Beck, C. T. (2012). *Nursing research: Generating and assessing evidence for nursing practice* (9th ed.). Philadelphia: Lippincott Williams & Wilkins.

Rempel, G. R., Ravindran, V., Rogers, L. G., & Magill-Evans, J. (2012). Parenting under pressure: A grounded theory of parenting young children with life-threatening congenital heart disease. *Journal of Advanced Nursing, 69*(3), 619–630.

Riegel, B., Jaarsma, T., & Stromberg, A. (2012). A middle-range theory of self-care of chronic illness. *Advances in Nursing Science, 35*(3), 194–204.

Reimer, A. P., & Moore, S. M. (2010). Flight nursing expertise: Towards a middle-range theory. *Journal of Advanced Nursing, 66*(5), 1183–1192.

Roberts, K. L. (1999). Through a looking glass: Nursing theory and clinical nursing research. *Clinical Nursing Research, 8*(4), 299–301.

Rogers, C. E., Keller, C., Larkey, L. K., & Ainsworth, B. E. (2012). A randomized controlled trial to determine the efficacy of Sign Chi Do exercise on adaptation to aging. *Research in Gerontological Nursing, 5*(2), 101–113.

Shin, K. R., Kang, Y., Park, H. J., Cho, M. O., & Heitkemper, M. (2008). Testing and developing the Health Promotion Model in low-income, Korean elderly women. *Nursing Science Quarterly, 21*(2), 173–178.

Silva, M. C. (1986). Research testing nursing theory: State of the art. *Advances in Nursing Science, 9*(1), 1–11.

Thomas, M. L., Elliott, J. E., Rao, S. M., Fahey, K. F., Paul, S. M., & Miaskowski, C. (2012). A randomized, clinical trial of education or motivational-interviewing-based coaching compared to usual care to improve cancer pain management. *Oncology Nursing Forum, 39*(1), 39–49.

Tripp-Reimer, T. (1984). Commentaries. *Western Journal of Nursing Research, 6*(2), 195–197.

Weiss, J. A., & Lokken, L. (2009). Predictors and outcomes of postpartum mothers' perceptions of readiness for discharge after birth. *Journal of Obstetric, Gynecologic, and Neonatal Nursing, 38,* 406–417.

Whall, A. L. (2005). The structure of nursing knowledge: Analysis and evaluation of practice, middle range and grand theory. In J. J. Fitzpatrick & A. L. Whall (Eds.), *Conceptual models of nursing: Analysis and application* (3rd ed., pp. 13–26). Norwalk, CT: Appleton & Lange.

Wuest, J. (2001). Precarious ordering: Toward a formal theory of women's caring. *Health Care for Women International, 22,* 167–193.

Zhou, G., Stoltzfus, J. C., Houldin, A. D., Parks, S. M., & Swan, B. A. (2010). Knowledge, attitudes and practice behaviors of oncology advance practice nurses regarding advanced care planning for patients with cancer. *Oncology Nursing Forum, 37*(6), E400–E410.

CHAPTER 20

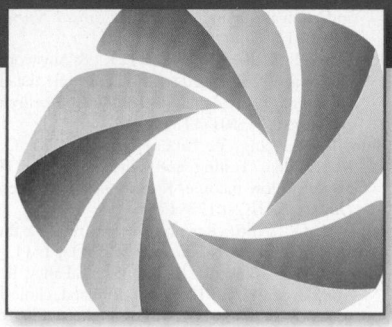

Application of Theory in Nursing Administration and Management

Melinda Granger Oberleitner

Greta Martin is a family nurse practitioner who has been employed for several years as part of a multiphysician practice. Most of her practice has been focused on managing the care of adults with chronic illnesses, such as congestive heart failure and diabetes.

Although she enjoys her work very much, Greta has always been interested in exploring one of the entrepreneurial opportunities that a career in nursing has to offer. Recently, she has focused on combining her interests in computers and the Internet with her expertise as an advanced practice nurse (APN). Along with several investors, she is in the process of creating an Internet-based disease management company. As envisioned, the company will focus on the needs of older adults and will hire APNs and other registered nurses (RNs) to provide clinical services and to serve as case managers for plan members diagnosed with chronic illnesses.

As she began the planning process for the project, Greta found that she had much to learn in regard to applying management and administration principles. In particular, she needed to learn more about organizational design. As the company is established, she must examine issues such as chain of command, control, authority, and responsibility. The group must determine how the company will be structured and who will be responsible for day-to-day operations.

The group is also looking at case management models to select or modify one that is appropriate for use with its anticipated clientele and the method of delivery. Finally, Greta realized that she should learn about her leadership style and develop her leadership abilities to direct the new company. Recognizing her deficiencies in administration and management, Greta sought information from a number of sources to learn about administration theories and how to apply them in her new enterprise.

Nursing practice, including advanced nursing practice, occurs within a larger context and framework that is shaped by traditional and prevailing theories, models, and frameworks of administration and management. Even if only one nurse is employed by an organization, that nurse's practice is shaped and influenced by models and principles of leadership, management, and administration used by the leaders of the organization. To be most effective in the advanced practice role, an APN should be able to recognize and adapt to the specific organizational characteristics that define the organization in which she or he practices.

This chapter expands on concepts and principles presented in Chapter 16. It explores specific applications of administration and management theories, models, and frameworks in nursing and health care. These concepts include organizational design; shared governance; transformational leadership; patient care delivery models; case management; disease/chronic illness management; quality management (QM)/performance improvement processes, tools, and techniques; and evidence-based practice (EBP).

Organizational Design

The structure of an organization provides a formal framework in which management processes occur. This formal framework historically serves many purposes, including provision of a chain of administrative command or authority that should be evident to all employees, a formal system of communication between management and staff, and a method to accomplish the work of the organization effectively and efficiently. The right structure enables the organization to reach its organizational goals.

Six elements of structure that were formulated by management theorists in the 1900s still provide a guide to the design of organizations in the 21st century. These six elements are listed in Box 20-1, and each is discussed briefly in the following sections (Robbins & Judge, 2009).

Work Specialization

Work specialization is having each step of the work process performed by a different individual rather than the whole process being done by one person. Proponents of work specialization argue that it makes the most efficient use of worker skills, attributes, and characteristics. Medication administration can be used to illustrate the concept of work specialization. Physicians determine the need for a medication order and determine the composition of that order; hospital pharmacists then review the order and fill the prescription as directed by the physician. The nurse on the unit administers the medication ordered by the physician and prepared by the pharmacist.

Box 20-1 Elements of Organizational Structure

1. Work specialization
2. Chain of command
3. Span of control
4. Authority and responsibility
5. Centralization versus decentralization
6. Departmentalization

In the traditional hospital structure, pharmacists work in an isolated group to prepare all medications to be delivered by nurses to patients in the facility.

In recent years, recognition that work specialization can lead to boredom, low productivity, and poor quality has led to a reexamination of the concept. In many cases, this has resulted in assigning employees a variety of activities to accomplish and encouraging employees to work in teams. In some hospitals, a clinical pharmacist is part of a team of health care workers assigned to accomplish the work of the unit and resides, along with the traditional nursing staff, on the clinical unit. Some unit-based clinical pharmacists engage in tasks, such as medication administration, which was once considered the exclusive domain of nursing.

The usual configuration of clinical nurse specialists (CNSs) is perhaps the most vivid representation of work specialization. For example, a neuroscience CNS would not be considered interchangeable with a cardiovascular CNS because of the extreme degree of work specialization in the role of the CNS. The CNS is educationally prepared as an expert in a specific specialty area and is not considered a generalist.

Chain of Command

Fayol (1949), Weber (1970), and Taylor (1911) (see Chapter 16) advocated that an employee should be administratively responsible to, or report to, only one supervisor. This arrangement is termed the chain of command. Chain of command refers to formal lines of communication and authority and can usually be determined by looking at an organizational chart. However, as organizations have become increasingly complex, individuals in organizations may find themselves administratively responsible to more than one individual.

Although the nurse working on the 7 PM to 7 AM shift in the intensive care unit (ICU) is ultimately administratively responsible to the ICU director, there is usually a different chain of command on the night shift; this may include the night charge nurse and the night house supervisor.

APNs in today's health care organizations may be administratively responsible to a variety of individuals, some of whom may not be nurses, such as product or service line managers. Some APNs may also assume managerial roles, as in the case of a nurse anesthetist who is administratively in charge of a group of nurse anesthetists.

Span of Control

The third element of management, span of control, can also be determined from the organizational chart. Span of control refers to the number of employees directed by a manager. The classical management theorists recommended narrow spans of control for workers performing complex jobs. There is no consensus regarding the optimal number of employees one manager should have in his or her span of control—suggested ranges are from 3 to 50 employees. Several contingencies play a role in the variability of the range of numbers of employees in span of control. These contingencies include the quality and experience of the manager, the abilities and maturity of the employees, the complexity of the task, and, in some cases, the geographic location of the work setting. The most recent research results indicate a significant level of improvement in nurse engagement when the manager is responsible for 50 or fewer direct reports (Cathcart, 2004).

In recent years, because of cost-cutting initiatives in health care and other organizations, management layers have been decreased and span of control for managers has increased. Communication patterns between manager and employees and between employee and employee change when span of control changes. Graicunas (1937) developed a mathematical model to illustrate the changes in numbers of communication patterns when span of control is changed. This mathematical model demonstrated that as the number of employees reporting to a manager increases, the number of interactions increases geometrically. As a result of this geometric increase, Graicunas recommended that a span of six or seven employees was the maximum that a manager could handle effectively. In his mathematical computations, Graicunas did not consider contingency factors or variables, such as the manager's experience, the maturity of the employees, or the stability or predictability of the work being performed, which may also influence the effectiveness of a manager with a given span of control.

Several factors should be considered when contemplating altering managerial span of control on inpatient nursing units. These factors include skill mix and expertise of the unit staff, duties of first-level managers (i.e., charge nurses) when the middle-level manager is not present, and the potential savings in salary expenses.

Authority and Responsibility

Line authority and *staff authority* are two distinctions that describe formal relationships in an organization. When looking at an organizational chart, line authority refers to chain of command, superior–subordinate, and leader–follower relationships. For example, the chief nursing officer delegates authority to the unit manager, who then delegates to a subordinate, the charge nurse. The command relationship is a direct "line" between supervisor and subordinate.

In larger organizations, managers can be designated as top-level, middle-level, or first-level managers. Top-level managers include the organization's chief executive officer (CEO) and the highest nursing administrator. Middle-level managers, as the name implies, coordinate management activities between the top management level and first-level managers. Middle-level managers are usually involved in long-range planning and in policy decisions that affect one unit or multiple units. This manager is usually responsible for day-to-day activities of the units. Titles in nursing that represent middle-level managers include unit managers, unit directors, unit supervisors, and head nurses. First-level managers are assigned to one unit and are concerned with that specific unit's work. First-level managers, such as charge nurses, team leaders, and primary care nurses, are crucial to the success of the unit's work. APNs are most often administratively responsible to either top-level or middle-level managers. APNs who assume administrative responsibilities in the organization may be top-level or middle-level managers.

In some organizations, APNs are in *staff* positions as opposed to *line* positions. Staff authority supports the work of the line manager without having any line authority or responsibility. Employees in staff positions support, assist, and advise those in line authority positions. In a staff position, the APN is not responsible for the hiring, firing, directing, or disciplining of other employees. This lack of authority could be a disadvantage to the APN in accomplishing the tasks of the role because the APN often must work through others to accomplish goals. Even when the APN is in a staff position, the APN is responsible to a line manager, who is either a top-level or middle-level manager.

Centralization Versus Decentralization

Centralization and *decentralization* are degrees of how decision making is dispersed or diffused throughout the organization. In organizations with centralized decision making, decisions are made by one individual or a small group of individuals at the top of the organizational structure. Decentralization refers to decision making that occurs at the lowest levels feasible. Most of today's organizations are really neither totally centralized nor decentralized but are a combination of the two. With the advent of performance improvement initiatives over the past 30 to 40 years, the trend in American organizations has been toward decentralization in an effort to involve employees directly responsible for the work product in the decision-making process. In nursing, organizational designs, such as shared governance, have gained popularity as a method to empower and engage staff in the decision-making process.

Departmentalization

The primary purpose of *departmentalization* is to subdivide the work of the organization so that specialization of the work can be accomplished. Departmentalization emphasizes specialization of skills. Hospitals have historically implemented departmentalization with traditional departments, such as central supply, pastoral care, and patient care departments, among others. A typical manufacturing plant, although different from a hospital, is probably organized in much the same way as the hospital. For example, both probably have marketing, accounting, and human resources departments. Grouping activities in this manner is known as functional departmentalization.

Other types of departmentalization include product, customer, geographic, and process departmentalization. Today, hospitals and other organizations use cross-disciplinary teams to accomplish the organization's performance initiatives that transcend traditional departmental boundaries to better focus on customer needs (Robbins & Judge, 2009).

Shared Governance

Shared governance is "a structural model through which nurses can express and manage their own practice with a higher level of professional autonomy" (Porter-O'Grady, 2003, p. 251). Nursing shared governance, an organizational structure and process, was introduced in the late 1970s as an alternative to traditional or industrial bureaucratic organizational design (Christman, 1976; Cleland, 1978; Laschinger & Finegan, 2005). In this design, professional nurses use self-directed work teams at the unit level to make professional practice decisions and to accomplish the work of the unit.

Porter-O'Grady, Hawkins, and Parker (1997) described the major components of shared governance as the creation of partnerships, equity, accountability, and ownership. Much of the effort directed at restructuring the nursing organization to implement shared governance was done to empower nurses to join with each other and with other health care decision makers to better confront issues affecting the practice of professional nursing (Porter-O'Grady, 1994). In the shared governance model, staffs, not managers, are empowered to make patient care decisions at the staff level (Kramer et al., 2008).

Implementation of shared governance is usually accompanied by the simultaneous implementation of participation and decentralization. Participation and decentralization are not substitutes for shared governance and should not be used synonymously with the term *shared governance*. Participative models call for employees to be involved in the decisions that involve them. However, management still determines the breadth and depth of employee participation. Decentralization allows employees at lower levels of the hierarchical structure to have greater involvement in decision making and to have some authority to implement the decisions. However, management usually retains the real authority and power in terms of which decisions are to be implemented. In short, both participation and decentralization rely on management discretion to determine the amount of employee involvement in decision making, whereas shared governance does not.

Nursing shared governance models have always focused on nurses controlling their professional practice. A comparative analysis by Kramer and Schmalenberg (2003), who interviewed 279 nurses at 14 magnet hospitals, found that the highest staff nurse ownership of practice issues and outcomes occurred when there were visible, viable, and recognized structures devoted to nursing control over practice. To be able to control practice, nurses must have control over resources that impact professional practice and they must also have influence over themselves as a professional group (Lake, 2007).

Porter-O'Grady (2012) advances the idea that in order for true interprofessional team-based models of accountability to thrive in health services organizations, five principles govern the practice and relationships of the teams and are needed to sustain shared governance:

- Professions are driven by practice and practitioners—the locus of control for decision making in terms of what constitutes professional practice, quality, competence, and knowledge generation must be retained by the practitioner. The farther away the decision making is from the knowledge worker (the professional), the lower the decision quality and the higher the cost of the decision.
- Structure is key—there must be direct alignment between organizational structure and intended behaviors and outcomes. Organizational structures that are ineffective in producing the most effective outcomes for knowledge workers such as RNs include traditional bureaucratic structures such as vertical, hierarchical structures in which management has ultimate control of decision and policy making.
- Accountability is central to professional practice—true accountability by professionals can only thrive in environments in which the organizational structure is such that accountability is within the control of the practitioner at the point of practice.
- Control of accountability must be purposefully designed into the shared governance structure—shared governance facilitates distributive decision making. In a true shared governance model, practitioners retain control over professional practice—not management.
- Leadership by management is crucial to the effectiveness of shared governance—the competencies of managers and leaders in shared organization are different than in traditional organizations. These competencies include distributive decision-making, effective servant leadership, and assisting practice peers to create work environments in which knowledge workers can practice to the fullest extent (Porter-O'Grady, 2012).

Three general models of shared governance are:

1. Councilor model—the most common model; utilizes a coordinating council to integrate decisions made by staff and managers in subcommittees that report to the coordinating council
2. Administrative model—the organizational chart is split to resemble two tracks—a management track and a clinical track; membership in both tracks includes managers and staff
3. Congressional model—uses a democratic process to empower nurses to vote on issues

Structure of the models is not important; what is important is control over practice that leads to improved patient, nurse, and organizational outcomes (Anthony, 2004; Hess, 2004; Kramer et al., 2008; Weston, 2008).

Research-based studies have attempted to evaluate the outcomes of shared governance from the perspectives of the organization, the nurse, and the patient. From an organizational perspective, in general, research supports the finding of an improved financial posture for the organization after implementation of shared governance. The improved finances stem from either cost savings or cost reductions. Reported examples of cost savings and reductions range from a decrease in overall meeting time for staff to multimillion dollar reductions in the use of temporary or agency nurses once shared governance has been fully implemented. Research studies indicate implementation of shared governance has resulted in improving the work environment of nurses, which could lead to increased nurse satisfaction and ultimately to improved nurse retention.

Detractors of the shared governance model point to the expense of introducing and maintaining the model, the longer time it takes to arrive at decisions using the model, and the fact that not all nurses want to have a role in decision making or want accountability for decisions.

Transformational Leadership in Nursing and in Health Care

Historically, nursing and health care organizations were built on old paradigm beliefs of hierarchical structures with an emphasis on rationality and logical decision making. The old paradigm is evolving to a new paradigm that values mutuality, affiliation, cooperation, networking, and an emphasis on human relations. In nursing, the shift has led to decentralization, participative management and decision making, and shared governance.

In transformational leadership, the leader and the follower have the same purpose. Barker (1994) proposed that it is easier to study the *results* of transformational leadership than the *process*. Transformational leadership is moral and philosophical leadership rather than technical leadership. Bennis and Nanus (1985) conceptualized four strategies for transformational leadership: (1) creating a vision, (2) building a social architecture that provides the framework for generating commitment to the vision and for establishing an organizational identity, (3) developing and sustaining organizational trust, and (4) attending to the self-esteem of others in the organization. Cottingham (1988) proposed six strategies for a transformational leader (Box 20-2).

Porter-O'Grady (1992) suggested that transformational nursing leaders should focus on relationships and develop personal skills such as paradigm assessment, process ambiguity, staff decision making, and shared governance. Transformational leadership is not leading and controlling; rather, it is coordinating, integrating, and facilitating. Transformational leaders should strive to build coalitions and networks among disciplines and departments by bringing diverse groups together toward a shared vision or goal while at the same time managing the complexity of the organization.

One essential element of the Magnet recognition model is evidence of transformational leadership in the organization. Clavelle, Drenkard, Tullai-McGuinness, & Fitzpatrick (2012) explored leadership practices of 225 chief nursing officers (CNOs) in Magnet facilities. The results of this study revealed increased education and experience of the CNO was positively correlated with transformational leadership characteristics. CNOs 60 years old and older and those with doctoral degrees scored significantly higher in the transformational leadership practices of inspiring

Box 20-2 Strategies for a Transformational Leader

Know the people you work with: Find out about their interests outside of the work environment; be visible and accessible.

Help people to learn and develop: Expose them to new ideas and methods; encourage attendance at seminars to help team members learn as much as possible about their roles.

Provide frequent feedback about performance: Give feedback quickly rather than waiting for a formal evaluation meeting. Feedback should be specific enough to enable the person to correct deficiencies; criticism should be positive rather than negative.

Award responsibility and status to coworkers: Give them the opportunity to participate in work projects that will allow for growth and increased responsibility. Recognize the potential in others and give them the opportunity to realize that potential.

Reward coworkers for a job well done: Monetary rewards should be as high as possible within the framework of the organization.

Make information available to all involved: Involve coworkers in decision making and problem solving and support their efforts.

a shared vision and challenging the process (Kouzes & Posner, 2008). The top two transformational leadership practices of the CNOs in this study, as measured by the Leadership Practices Inventory: Self Instrument, were enabling others to act and modeling the way for others.

McGuire and Kennerly (2006) also explored the transformational and transactional leadership characteristics of nurse managers ($n = 63$) and the relationship to commitment to the organization by RNs ($n = 500$) working on those managers' units. The study findings revealed that nurse managers who were viewed as transformational leaders were more likely to inspire a higher sense of commitment to the organization in staff nurses working on their units than those nurse managers who were viewed by staff nurses as more transactional leaders. This study also indicated that transformational nurse managers who were viewed by staff nurses as charismatic with high integrity, ethical, and moral character and who exhibited risk-taking behaviors brought a competitive advantage to the organization and played a large role in cultivating a healthier professional work environment on their units.

Patient Care Delivery Models

Nursing care in the acute care setting is delivered most often utilizing a group practice model. The group practice model provides the structure and context for the delivery of care (Brennan & Anthony, 2000). Practice models range from those that are based on patient assignments (such as team nursing), accountability systems (primary nursing), and managed care (case management) to models that are designed to incorporate professional practice concepts of autonomy, decision making, participation, and professional values (shared governance model) (Anthony, 2004).

Assignment systems for nursing staff or patient care delivery models change in response to changing needs. For example, in the 1920s, the *case method* and *private duty nursing* models of total patient care were the systems most often implemented. By the 1950s, *functional nursing* was introduced as a response to a shortage of nurses. *Team* or *modular nursing* was also introduced in the 1950s to capitalize on the expertise of professional nurses and to use nonprofessional team members in the provision of nursing care. *Primary nursing*, a shift back to care of individual patients by professional nurses, was commonly used in the 1960s and 1970s. The method that has most recently appeared in the literature is *patient-focused care* (PFC).

Each of the delivery methods has inherent advantages and disadvantages. These patient care delivery methods are used primarily in hospitals, but they can be adapted for use in other settings. Factors to consider prior to implementation of a particular method or system include type and acuity of patients, complexity of the tasks to be performed, availability or supply of RNs, skill and expertise of the staff, and the economic resources of the organization.

Total Patient Care (Functional Nursing)

Total patient care, the oldest delivery method, was accomplished by nurses in the home and hospital settings. Most of the patients were assigned to nurses as cases; one nurse attended to all of the patient's needs during the course of the nurse's shift. The major disadvantage of this method is cost, particularly in times of nursing shortages.

Evolving as a result of the nursing shortage that occurred during World War II, the functional method of providing patient care was derived from the principles of scientific management; that is, emphasis on efficiency, division of labor, and rigid controls (Marriner-Tomey, 2009). In this method, the patient's physical needs are attended to primarily by unlicensed workers (i.e., nursing aides), with RNs responsible primarily for managerial functions. The focus of this method was on the completion of certain tasks, such as administering medication or performing treatments, rather than on meeting all of the needs of the patient by one nurse, as was accomplished in total patient care methods.

Although patient care appears to be delivered efficiently and there would appear to be little confusion regarding responsibilities for tasks and assignments with this method, functional nursing has several disadvantages. These disadvantages include the need for greater coordination of care, fragmentation of care, the majority of care being provided by nonprofessional and unlicensed workers, de-emphasis on the psychological needs of the patient, and the repetitive nature of the work. In times of nursing shortages, health care administrators often return to a hybrid of functional nursing, including the use of unlicensed health care workers or unlicensed assistive personnel (UAP).

Team Nursing

Team nursing was developed after World War II in an effort to alleviate the fragmented care associated with functional care. In the team nursing approach, a professional or technical nurse is the team leader of a group of other health care workers that may include other professional and technical nurses and unlicensed personnel such as nursing assistants. The team is responsible for the provision of care to a group of patients on a nursing unit.

The team leader is the coordinator of the group and is responsible for assigning team members to specific patient assignments. The team leader may or may not have a patient assignment. The team leader is responsible for knowing about the conditions and needs of all of the patients assigned to the team and for communicating with physicians. Duties that cannot be performed by other team members because of lack of skill, expertise, or licensure are performed by the team leader. Team members report to the team leader, who in turn reports to the unit manager.

Advantages of team nursing are the democratic nature of the method, the focus on the entire patient rather than on specific tasks to be accomplished, the autonomy provided to the team to accomplish the work, and increased satisfaction with the method by workers and patients. Disadvantages of team nursing include the high degree of coordination and planning required and the dependence on the unique skills of the team leader to make the concept work efficiently and effectively. Team nursing has rarely been implemented in its purest form. Instead, a combination of team and functional nursing has most frequently been implemented.

Primary Nursing

Primary nursing was initiated in the late 1960s and early 1970s in response to professional nurses who decried the lack of personal contact with patients and who were unhappy with the provision of fragmented care. Primary nursing uses some of the concepts on which total patient care was based (i.e., during work hours, the primary nurse, an RN, would be responsible for planning care and providing total patient care to a group of patients). When the primary nurse was not on duty, an associate nurse (another RN) would provide care to the patients based on a care plan developed by the primary nurse. However, the primary nurse retained responsibility for the assigned patient load 24 hours a day while the patient was hospitalized.

Job satisfaction is high in primary nursing because of the high degree of autonomy and responsibility afforded to the primary nurse. Continuity of care is greatly facilitated by the primary nursing model. Disadvantages to primary nursing include the numbers of RNs required to implement primary nursing and the high degree of coordination and professional nursing expertise required for the role. Primary nurses who are inadequately trained or incompetent to implement the role may be incapable of fulfilling the primary nurse role.

Patient-Focused Care/Patient-Centered Care

The PFC model was developed in an effort to decrease the cost of providing health care while improving the quality of the service (Myers, 1998). The principles of PFC are derived from total quality management/continuous quality improvement in that PFC brings patient care needs as close as possible to the bedside. A goal of PFC is to decrease the number of health care workers needed while simultaneously increasing the time nurses would have to spend with patients. Theoretically, the cost of care should decrease while quality of care increases.

Mang (1995) described principles of implementation of PFC. These principles are summarized in Box 20-3 and are discussed briefly in the following text. *Patient redeployment* involves placing patients with similar needs and diagnoses in the same geographic location. The optimal number of patients with similar needs and diagnoses

Box 20-3 Principles of Patient-Focused Care

- Patient redeployment
- Support services decentralization
- Worker cross-training
- Creation of multidisciplinary teams
- Patient involvement
- Task simplification

on a unit should be between 50 and 100 to create an economy of scale and to ensure predictable census and workload. *Decentralization of support services* refers to relocation of ancillary services (i.e., pharmacy, radiology, admissions, and laboratory) closer to the patient to allow for more efficient use of personnel.

Creation of *multiskilled workers*, or cross-trained workers, is accomplished by combining appropriate types of tasks. For example, the multiskilled worker would be responsible for housekeeping, food service, and other unskilled tasks for a group of patients. However, Mang (1995) does not advocate training unskilled workers to perform tasks that traditionally would require a worker to be licensed. The goal of creating the multiskilled worker is to decrease the number of workers the typical patient comes in contact with by up to 75% (Clouten & Weber, 1994).

Over time, patient-focused care evolved into a model in which patients and families are active participants in decision making about care. Four concepts are associated with contemporary patient- and family-centered care models: dignity and respect; information sharing; participation; and collaboration (Johnson et al., 2008). Indeed, in this model, patients must be well informed and included in all decision making related to the plan of care. In addition, *task simplification* would be applied to every aspect of the patient's care to allow for greater efficiency and time savings, which results in earlier discharge for the patient.

The goals of PFC are to (1) transform the health care organization into a customer-focused organization; (2) improve continuity of care for patients; (3) improve professional relationships among doctors, nurses, and other caregivers; (4) minimize the movement of patients throughout hospitals; (5) increase the proportion of direct care activities as compared to other activities in the organization; (6) reconfigure the clinical environment to truly meet the needs of the patients; and (7) empower direct caregivers to plan and implement work in ways that are most responsive to the needs of patients (Zarubi, Reiley, & McCarter, 2008). Two industry leaders in integrating patient- and family-centered care are Planetree, Inc., and the Institute for Patient- and Family-Centered Care (Warren, 2012).

The results of some studies evaluating the PFC model indicate that patient and staff satisfaction improve after implementation of PFC, as does physician satisfaction in relationship with nursing staff. In terms of savings, some institutions reported a decrease in time of the admission process, a decrease in inventory, and an improvement in costs. Quality indicators, such as direct patient care time, patient satisfaction, continuity of care, and nosocomial infection rates, revealed positive trends after implementation of PFC. Zarubi and colleagues (2008) describe adoption of patient and family-centered care (PFCC) as the model for patient care delivery in a health system in Arizona. One goal of the health system was to provide greater opportunities for patients and families to be involved in decision making at all organizational levels. As a result, the health system adopted a philosophy that integrates key concepts and principles of PFCC as identified by the Institute for Family-Centered Care (2009). An example of a change that reflected a focus on PFCC was the elimination of the standard, preset 10 AM to 8 PM hospital visiting policy so that visiting hours could be determined by patients and family according to their wishes and needs. Since implementation in 2006, the authors state, "At this point, we realize that there is no turning back. Now that we have empowered our patients and families to question our policies and practices and offer their opinions, we find we can no longer use the excuse 'that's the rule' when a patient or family member voices a concern about the way something is done." (Zarubi et al., 2008, p. 280).

Some health care organizations have extended the patient and family-centered care model by engaging former patients and family members in an advisory capacity to assist the organization with patient satisfaction, quality, and safety concerns (Warren, 2012). These advisors relate their experiences from past care encounters in the organization or facility with the goal of improving the care experiences of other patients and families in the future. Patient and family advisors have assisted health care facilities with making changes to policies (Kelly, 2007), the physical environment, and aspects of clinical care delivery (Foley, 2001; Muething, 2007), as well as with staff education and development (Dokken, Moretz, Black, & Ahmann, 2007).

There is considerable new and renewed interest in patient- and family-centered care models as a result of provisions of the newly enacted Patient Protection and Affordable Care Act, which focus on patient satisfaction and which have the potential to significantly impact reimbursement for care provided in health care organizations. For example, The Hospital Consumer Assessment of Healthcare Providers and Systems (HCAHPS) initiative provides a mechanism for health care facilities to benchmark patient satisfaction trends in their facilities with expected national outcomes; outcomes are tied to financial incentives for health care institutions (Cropley, 2012). Implementation of patient- and family-centered care models may lead to improved patient/family experiences, which results in increased satisfaction scores and financial incentives for the institution providing the care.

Use of Patient Care Delivery Models Today

Rarely do pure forms of any of the patient care delivery methods described earlier exist in practice today. Typically, components of several of the methods, or a combination of the methods, are used to accomplish patient care. Delivery methods usually differ between inpatient and outpatient areas and from unit to unit, depending on the nature of the patient care unit and the skill mix of the staff assigned to the unit.

Kangas, Kee, and McKee-Waddle (1999) explored the differences and relationships among job satisfaction of RNs, patient satisfaction with nursing care, nursing care delivery models, organizational structure, and organizational culture. In this study, there were no differences in nurse job satisfaction or patient satisfaction with nursing care in different organizational structures (i.e., shared governance) or where different nursing care delivery methods (i.e., primary, team, functional) were used. A "supportive" environment was most crucial to the job satisfaction of the RNs. More recently, a growing body of research related to organizational attributes of health care organizations that support clinical practice has been conducted. Organizational attributes that support professional clinical practice include elements such as decentralization of authority, support from management, interdisciplinary collaboration, effective communication, access to adequate resources for the provision of patient care, and control over professional practice (Flynn, 2007). Support of clinical practice translates to improved patient care and quality clinical outcomes.

The Nursing Work Index-Revised (Aiken & Patrician, 2000) has been used to measure attributes of the work environment of professional nurses that support professional clinical practice. These attributes include organizational support for nursing practice, specifically, adequacy of resources to support the practice of professional nursing, including adequate RN staffing, autonomy for nurses, nurse control of nursing practice, and collegial nurse–physician relationships. When these attributes are present to a sufficient degree, nurse job satisfaction is higher and burnout rates and physical disability rates are lower. Improved patient-related outcomes such as decreased adverse events, lower mortality, and higher levels of patient satisfaction with care are noted (Flynn, 2007).

Aiken, Clarke, Sloane, Sochalski, and Silber (2002) attempted to explicate the evidence linking nurse staffing to patient outcomes. In a study that was based on an analysis of outcomes of 232,342 patients in 168 Pennsylvania hospitals over a 20-month period, risk of death following common surgical procedures increased by 7% for each patient added to the nurse's workload over a nurse-to-patient ratio of 1:4. The difference in mortality for surgical patients in hospitals in which nurses cared for an average of eight patients was 30% higher than in hospitals in which nurses cared for four patients or fewer. Failure-to-rescue rates for patients with complications were 30% higher in the hospitals in which nurses cared for an average of eight patients as compared to the hospitals in which the nurses cared for four or fewer patients (Clarke & Aiken, 2003). The result is that nurses employed by hospitals that enforce large patient loads are significantly less likely to save the life of a patient who develops a serious complication. In addition, increased needlestick injuries for nurses (Clarke, Sloane, & Aiken, 2002), increased patient and family complaints, falls with injuries, medication errors, and hospital-acquired infections are more likely to occur when the nurse-to-patient ratio is higher (Aiken, Clarke, & Sloane, 2002; Cho, Ketefian, Barkauskas, & Smith, 2003.

Higher patient-to-nurse ratios are also associated with increased nurse burnout and job dissatisfaction rates. Each patient over a 4:1 ratio increased nurse burnout by 235 and job dissatisfaction by 15% (Aiken et al., 2002). More recently, Cimiotti, Aiken, Sloane, and Wu (2012) documented a significant association between patient-to-nurse ratio and incidence of urinary tract and surgical site infections. When using a statistical model that controlled for patient severity and nurse and hospital characteristics, only RN burnout was significantly associated with urinary tract and surgical site infections. In hospitals that reduced burnout by at least 30%, more than 6,000 fewer infections were noted, for an annual cost savings of up to $68 million. These findings become even more significant when examined in light of new provisions associated with the Patient Protection and Accountable Care Act, which include loss of reimbursement to health care organizations for facility-acquired conditions such as urinary tract and surgical site infections (Andel, Davidow, Hollander, & Moreno, 2012).

In 1999, California became the first state in the United States to pass legislation to enforce minimum nurse staffing levels in hospitals. Implementation of the legislation began in 2004. The stated goal of the legislation was to improve the quality of care for patients in California hospitals. Spetz (2008) conducted research to examine whether nurses who work in hospitals in California were more satisfied with staffing levels and other job attributes since minimum staffing levels were enacted. The results of this research indicate that nurse satisfaction did increase from 2004 to 2006. Nurse satisfaction with the adequacy of RN staffing, time for patient education, benefits, and amount of clerical support was increased.

After implementation of the California Safe Staffing Law, some studies failed to substantiate a relationship between increased nurse staffing levels and improved patient outcomes (Donaldson et al., 2005; Burnes-Bolton et al., 2007; Hickey, Gauvreau, Jenkins, Fawcett, & Hayman, 2011). However, a study conducted by Aiken and colleagues (2010) concluded that mandatory staffing levels in California were associated with lower patient mortality and with improved nurse retention. Tellez and Seago (2013) explored the effect of California's minimum staffing legislation on changes to the California RN workforce, particularly the direct care nurse in the acute care setting. The most meaningful finding of this research is the increase in nurse satisfaction after the minimum staffing law was enacted. Aiken, Clarke, Sloane, Lake, and Cheney (2008) empirically examined whether better hospital nurse care environments resulted in lower patient mortality and better nurse outcomes independent of nurse staffing levels and the educational level of the RN workforce in the hospital. Results of this study indicate that attributes of the care environment must be optimized, in addition to nurse staffing and nurse educational levels, to achieve the highest level of quality care. Specifically, the researchers state, "It seems reasonable to assume that the actual number of patient deaths that could be averted annually by improved care environments, nurse staffing, and nurse education is somewhere in the range of 40,000 per year" when extrapolating study results across the United States. The results of this study imply that if all hospitals had better care environments, a 4:1 patient-to-nurse ratio, and if 60% of staff nurses were BSN prepared, the overall mortality rate would be significantly decreased, as would the failure-to-rescue rate.

Using data extracted from 665 adult acute care general hospitals in four of the nation's largest states and from surveys of nurses working in the study hospitals, Aiken and colleagues (2011) attempted to determine the conditions under which the impact of three variables—nurse-patient staffing ratios, nurse educational level, and work environment—are associated with patient outcomes, such as inpatient mortality rate and failure-to-rescue rates. The general hospitals were located in California (n = 271), Pennsylvania (n = 153), Florida (n = 168), and New Jersey (n = 73) and represented 86% of general acute care hospitals in those states. These four states account for more than 20% of annual hospitalizations in the United States.

The results of this study reveal that lowering the patient-to-nurse ratio by one patient per nurse in hospitals with good work environments, as measured by the Practice Environment Scale of the Nursing Work Index revised (PES-NWI), significantly improved patient outcomes, slightly improved outcomes in hospitals with average practice environments, and had no effect in hospitals with poor environments. Increasing the numbers of nurses with the bachelor of science in nursing degree by 10% decreased the odds of patients dying by 4%, which confirms previous findings by Aiken and colleagues (2003). This positive influence was observed independently of staffing and quality of the work environment and was consistent across all hospitals (Aiken et al., 2011).

American Nurses Credentialing Center Magnet Recognition Program

The Magnet Recognition Program originated as a result of a 1983 landmark policy study (McClure, Poulin, Sovie, & Wandelt, 1983) conducted by the American Academy of Nursing to identify characteristics common to hospitals with environments of nurse recruitment and retention. At that time, during a national nursing shortage, 41 hospitals became the focus of intensive research efforts. The characteristics identified were referred to as the "Forces of Magnetism" (Wolf, Triolo, & Ponte, 2008).

The Magnet Recognition Program was developed by the American Nurses Credentialing Center (ANCC) in the early 1990s to recognize health care organizations that provide exemplary nursing care and that uphold the traditions within nursing of professional nursing practice. The program also serves as a method or means to disseminate successful best practices and strategies in nursing among institutions. Magnet hospitals have incorporated proven solutions to address nurse recruitment and retention and to foster nursing leadership (Kirkley, Johnson, & Anderson, 2004).

In 2005, the Commission on Magnet (COM) approved 26 recommendations for change to the Magnet program. The recommendations were primarily focused on changes to the appraisal process. Once these changes were ratified, the Commission began work on a new conceptual model of the forces of magnetism in an effort to clarify the role of the forces in pursuit of excellence in nursing practice. Research related to the 14 forces revealed there was redundancy among the forces, which have

Box 20-4 Components of the Magnet Model

- Transformational leadership
- Structural empowerment
- Exemplary professional nursing practice
- New knowledge, innovations, and improvements
- Empirical quality results

been reconfigured into seven domains or clusters of evidence: leadership, resource utilization and development, nursing model, safe and ethical practice, autonomous practice, research, and quality processes. In addition, an eighth domain, focusing on outcomes or results, was added in recognition of the importance of outcomes of care when referring to a culture of excellence and innovation, such as Magnet recognition (Triolo, Scherer, & Floyd, 2006; Wolf et al., 2008).

The 2005 model for Magnet that was adopted by the COM comprises five components that lead to empirical quality outcomes. Overarching the five components is the concept of global issues in nursing and health care. The five components are presented in Box 20-4.

The Magnet Recognition Program is based on quality indicators and standards of nursing practice as defined in the American Nurses Association's *Scope and Standards for Nursing Administrators* (2004). The Magnet designation process includes the appraisal of both qualitative and quantitative factors in nursing. As of early 2013, a total of 390 health care organizations in the United States, as well as three organizations in Australia, one in Lebanon, and one in Singapore, have achieved Magnet designation. Magnet hospitals have low nurse turnover (Janzen, 2003; McClure & Hinshaw, 2002); are safer workplaces (Aiken, Sloane, Lake, Sochalski, & Weber, 1999); and have better patient outcomes (Aiken, Havens, & Sloane, 2000), shorter lengths of stay (Aiken et al., 1999), higher patient satisfaction, and lower Medicare patient mortality rates (Aiken, Smith, & Lake, 1994) than non-Magnet designated hospitals. Lastly, Houston and colleagues (2012) reported that involvement in decision making in a study of staff nurses (n = 5,000) is higher in Magnet-designated facilities than in non-Magnet facilities. Empowered decision making is an integral component of creating a patient-centered work environment in which continual quality improvement and improved patient outcomes are paramount.

Case Management

The Case Management Society of America (CMSA) defines case management as "a collaborative process that assesses, plans, implements, coordinates, monitors, and evaluates options and services to meet an individual's health needs through communication and available resources to promote quality cost-effective outcomes" (Yamamoto & Lucey, 2005). Case management is a role developed in the late 1980s and early 1990s in response to the prospective payment system and diagnosis-related groups (DRGs). An expansion of the total patient care system, case management originated in outpatient settings. For example, community and public health nurses carry a caseload of patients for which they plan, coordinate, and evaluate care. Rarely do these nurses implement the care personally; however, they retain responsibility for patient outcomes.

As a result of the proliferation of managed care in hospitals, case management was also adopted in inpatient facilities, which is sometimes referred to as "within the walls" case management (Yamamoto & Lucey, 2005). Most inpatient case management systems are based on one of two models: the New England Medical Center Model, which focuses primarily on managing patient care to control resources; or the St. Mary's (or Carondelet) Model, in which the role of the case manager is to control or lower costs associated with patient stays, while simultaneously reducing the length of stay and producing optimal patient outcomes.

The minimal recommended educational requirement for nurse case manager roles is the baccalaureate degree in nursing. However, although not all case managers may need to perform case management duties at the advanced level, many organizations prefer advanced educational preparation and specialization for nurses in the role of case manager. Advantages of the APN as opposed to the BSN in the case management role include recognition of the APN as expert practitioner, change agent, researcher, manager, teacher, and consultant—roles for which the BSN nurse has not been educated in a comprehensive fashion (Blass & Reed, 2003; Stanton, Swanson, Sherrod, & Packa, 2005).

Although case management implementation varies from institution to institution, one variation is to assign a case manager to a group of high-risk patients within a specific population. For example, one hospital may have case managers in pediatrics, neuroscience, oncology, cardiovascular, orthopedics, and other specialty areas. The case manager does not coordinate the care of all the patients in a specialty. Instead, coordination of care by a case manager occurs only for those patients who have been designated as "high risk" because of age, comorbidities, and other factors that would place that patient at risk for greater consumption of resources or prolonged length of stay.

Ideally, the case manager coordinates the care of the patient from preadmission to the time of discharge and perhaps beyond discharge. This coordination of care requires interdisciplinary collaboration and cooperation. The case manager's role in this model transcends geographic or unit boundaries. The neuroscience case manager, for example, may first meet the patient in the neurosurgery clinic or at the neurosurgeon's office and would play a role in coordinating preadmission testing. Following surgery, the case manager would track the progress of the patient from the ICU, to an intermediate care unit, to the neurology floor, then to a rehabilitation unit if required. The case manager would then be involved in establishing postdischarge home care if necessary.

The literature is replete with reports of improved patient outcomes, coupled with reduced costs, as a result of the implementation of case management processes. Organizations use aggregated data derived from case management activities for benchmarking purposes as part of overall performance improvement initiatives. As the caseloads of individuals with chronic illnesses increase in conjunction with the increase in the aging population, case management holds even greater promise for patients as well as for health care providers.

Case managers are employed not only by hospitals but also by health maintenance organizations (HMOs), other managed care organizations, insurance companies, and disease management companies. Case managers serve as the liaison between patients and families, health plans, care providers, and purchasers to determine the extent of coverage and probable costs and to coordinate treatment at a lower cost and outside of inpatient care if possible.

As an example of the integral role that case managers play in coordinating care outside of inpatient facilities, a joint venture between Banner Health and Blue Cross

Blue Shield of Arizona Advantage provides at least one home visit by a case manager for members who qualify for case management services. Patients who qualify for the visits are typically no longer eligible for home health and are recovering at home from major conditions or chronic illnesses such as stroke, heart attack, heart failure, and/or chronic obstructive pulmonary disease. The program also targets individuals who were admitted following fractures and related health problems resulting from a fall. The home visit is focused on conducting a home assessment to decrease the client's risk for subsequent falls. The primary goal of the home visit initiative is to reduce readmission rates into acute care facilities. Since the program was established, readmission rates for all age groups have dropped by 13% (Case Management Advisor, 2013).

Although RNs constitute the largest professional group in case management, the role is becoming increasingly multidisciplinary, with social workers, respiratory therapists, physical therapists, and other health care professionals joining organizations as case managers. However, many recognize the unique capabilities of the RN in optimizing the role of case manager.

Disease/Chronic Illness Management

The onset and eventual progression of many chronic illnesses is considered by many to be preventable. *Disease management* has been defined in the literature as a patient care approach that emphasizes comprehensive, coordinated care along a disease continuum and across health care delivery systems (Ellrodt et al., 1997). Disease management is the redirection of patient care services from inpatient to outpatient settings and is viewed as a proactive rather than a reactive approach to providing health care services (Rossiter et al., 2000). In essence, disease management programs use medical, prescription drug, and other health-related data to identify individuals with chronic illnesses who are at high risk of experiencing serious health problems and to provide early intervention to avoid or minimize those problems (Marlowe, 2000).

People diagnosed with chronic illnesses (e.g., asthma, diabetes mellitus, congestive heart failure [CHF], AIDS, lower back pain, and certain forms of cancer) are potential candidates for disease management interventions. Kongstvedt (1997) offered a set of criteria by which to evaluate what types of chronic illnesses are appropriate for disease management (Box 20-5).

Box 20-5 Criteria for Evaluating Need for Disease Management Services

- A high percentage of complications associated with the disease are preventable.
- The effect of a disease management program would be evident within 1–3 years after implementation.
- The conditions that are manifested can be managed in a nonsurgical, outpatient setting.
- There is a high rate of noncompliance with treatment protocols; however, the noncompliance is amenable to change.
- Practice guidelines are available (or there is potential to develop such guidelines) that outline optimal treatments of the disease.

The potential of disease management to reduce health care costs associated with common chronic illnesses seems significant. With the aging of the large "baby boomer" cohort of the population, a precipitous rise in the incidence of chronic illnesses, such as diabetes and CHF, seems to be a foregone conclusion. At current rates, the economic burden related to the treatment of just three chronic illnesses (heart disease, diabetes mellitus, and asthma) in the United States is staggering, with an estimated 80% of all health care dollars in the United States spent on managing a relatively small number of chronic illnesses (Wojcik & Bradford, 2000).

Disease Management Models

Historically, disease management programs were developed by pharmacy benefits management (PBM) organizations, which were mainly owned by pharmaceutical companies that had a financial stake in management of diseases. The theory was that if disease management programs were successful, the drug manufacturing company sponsoring the program would sell more drugs to the individual. As interest in disease management has grown, PBMs, as disease management program sponsors, represent only a small segment of the business. Other more recent sponsors and advocates of disease management programs include managed care companies, individual state Medicaid agencies, provider organizations, and independent vendors. Independent disease management vendors are the most rapidly growing segment in the disease management arena because of the potential for profitability. Many of the independent vendors are web-based providers of disease management services.

Managed care and managed care organizations (MCOs) evolved in an attempt to control costs associated with traditional fee-for-service insurance reimbursement practices. MCOs are held clinically and financially responsible for health outcomes of their enrolled members on a capitated fee basis. Many MCOs have implemented disease management and wellness programs that utilize a case management approach to improve clinical outcomes (Sackett, Pope, & Erdley, 2004). The method of disease management implementation in Medicaid and other state programs varies by state and is becoming more widely used, with states reporting disease management programs to cover asthma, diabetes, CHF, and other chronic illnesses.

Clinical outcomes have been tracked using disease management indicators since the inception of the program. Examples of disease management indicators related to patients with CHF, for example, include tracking the percent of patients with appropriate use of drugs, such as ACE inhibitors and beta-blockers, inappropriate use of calcium channel blockers and NSAIDs, hospital admission rates, use of emergency departments, and regular primary care or cardiology visits as well as other indicators.

Among the most notable outcomes of this disease management program are increases in the percentages of patients with improved HbA1c levels, improved LDL levels, and the increased use of aspirin in the diabetic population. Clinical improvements were also observed in the CHF population, in patients with asthma and in patients with HIV. Cancer-related screening practices also improved including increased use of mammography, PAP, and PSA testing (Horswell et al., 2008).

Sackett and colleagues (2004) write of the need to demonstrate return on investment (ROI) for disease management programs. Disease management programs that are appropriately designed and implemented can reduce health care costs by controlling utilization of services.

Accountable Care Organizations and Medical Home Models of Care

Newer initiatives in health care include the formation of accountable care organizations or ACOs and patient-centered medical homes (PCMHs) models of care coordination. According to the U.S. Government's Centers for Medicare and Medicaid Services, "ACOs are groups of doctors, hospitals, and other health care providers, who come together voluntarily to give coordinated high-quality care to the Medicare patients they serve" (Centers for Medicare and Medicaid Services [CMS], 2013). The goal of ACOs is well-coordinated care that is accomplished across care settings. Some challenges associated with achieving this goal include enhancing the collaboration, communication, and teamwork skills of physicians and other providers associated with ACOs. While many medical, nursing, and other health sciences curricula now include content, such as the situation, background, assessment, recommendation (SBAR) communication technique, older physicians and nurses may not have been exposed to these techniques and skills while in school and will require professional development education in these areas (Press, Michelow, & MacPhail, 2012).

The goals of PCMHs include improving health care quality by improving care coordination while reducing costs associated with care. PCMHs emphasize preventive care and primary care and were first introduced in the care of pediatric patients in the 1960s. The PCMH approach is focused on increased coordination of care, which results in enhanced patient outcomes, as opposed to the more common volume-based models of care in which providers are reimbursed based on the numbers of patients seen and the numbers of procedures for which they are able to bill. PCMHs seem to hold great promise in providing effective chronic disease management at lower costs (DeVries et al., 2012).

The growing need to manage chronic illnesses is creating an unprecedented opportunity for nurses, particularly APNs, who by virtue of their educational credentials and clinical expertise, are uniquely positioned to become leaders in disease management. Roles for APNs include coordination of care for persons with chronic illnesses in for-profit and not-for-profit health care organizations in which APNs provide an array of direct services to plan members. APNs use published practice guidelines to manage and coordinate care of individuals with chronic illnesses across health care settings. Nurses are the best prepared for the scope of this care coordinator role, particularly those prepared as nurse practitioners (NPs) and CNSs, who have specialized in caring for patients with one or more chronic illnesses.

Quality Management

In 2001, the Institute of Medicine (IOM) released the publication, *To Err Is Human.* The release of this document, which asserted that medical errors were responsible for between 44,000 and 98,000 deaths annually in the United States, spurred demands for greater accountability and quality in the U.S. health care system (Kohn, Corrigan, & Donaldson, 2000). Since that time, many quality improvement or quality management (QM) initiatives have been undertaken in health care systems and organizations that directly impact the discipline of nursing.

Although there is some variation in the emphasis placed on specific aspects of QM between organizations, seven key principles or elements are viewed as integral components of all QM programs. These elements include focus on the customer, process improvement, variance analysis, leadership, employee involvement, scientific method, and benchmarking (Baker & Gelmon, 1996).

In the QM environment, quality is defined in terms of what is acceptable to the customer; that is, the customer determines expectations of quality. Comprehensive knowledge of the customer's needs and expectations is integral to providing the best in quality customer service. There are two types of customers: customers who are external to the organization and customers who are internal. In health care, for example, external customers are patients, families, physicians not employed by the organization, payers, and communities. Internal customers are staff members employed by the organization to provide a service to external customers. For example, the staff on a nursing unit is a customer of pharmacy services. The nursing staff relies on the pharmacy staff to provide accurate medications in a timely fashion to the nursing unit to enable the external customer, the patient, to receive medications appropriately and on time.

Process improvement involves scrupulously examining work processes involved in achieving a work product. For example, in a hospital setting, the process of transferring a patient from an orthopedic unit to a rehabilitation unit may have 20 or more steps and may involve five or six different departments. The more steps (and people) involved, the greater the likelihood that the transfer will be delayed or that an error will be made during the transfer, which leads to increased costs. Process improvement dictates that every aspect of patient transfer must be examined to determine whether each step in the process is really needed to accomplish the transfer. Members of each department or unit involved in the transfer are included on a process improvement team to examine the process for redundancies and lapses in service and to streamline the process.

Monitoring and analysis of variation in processes is crucial, particularly in health care organizations. There are two types of variation, common cause variation, which occurs no matter how well a system operates, and special cause variation. Special cause variation is variation that occurs outside of what is to be expected and can be caused by employee error and equipment or systems failure. The scientific method used to distinguish between common cause and special cause variation is statistical control (Varkey, Reller, & Resar, 2007).

Leadership in a QM environment has two components: comprehensive knowledge and an understanding of concepts and techniques of quality improvement and personal involvement. Leaders must be familiar with the terminology, the concepts, and the statistical techniques used in QM. Essential roles and responsibilities of leaders in QM include being personally committed to the philosophy, providing resources that include training others in the philosophy, reviewing progress on a regular basis, giving recognition, and managing resistance while empowering others.

To initiate and sustain a successful, meaningful quality improvement program, all members of the organization should have education and training related to QM. Employees should come away from the training with a clear understanding of their individual roles and responsibilities related to quality improvement. A broad range of employees should be encouraged to participate on quality improvement teams to design and improve work processes. Organizations that have been successful in implementing QM have empowered employees at all levels to search for better ways to redesign work processes to achieve customer satisfaction.

True quality improvement activities are based on scientific and statistical methods rather than on trial-and-error approaches to problem identification and problem-solving. The scientific method is a precise, systematic, orderly, planned, and organized method of problem solving that can be replicated and understood by employees of the organization. Several problem-solving methods can be used by health care organizations, including the most commonly used approach for rapid improvement in health care, the plan-do-stay-act (PDSA) cycle (Varkey et al., 2007). Other quality improvement methods utilized in contemporary health care organizations are Six Sigma and lean strategies. Problem analysis tools (also called statistical process control tools) used in the problem-solving process include flow charts, cause-and-effect diagrams, and run charts.

Benchmarking, a process originally implemented by the Xerox Corporation in 1979 (Camp & Tweet, 1994), is the identification, adaptation, and dissemination of best practices among competitors and noncompetitors that lead to their superior performance. In other words, quality can be improved in an organization by analyzing and then copying the methods of leaders in a field such as health care. Effective benchmarking involves identifying specific key indicators of a process (i.e., length of endotracheal intubation in postoperative patients), comparing this process with other organizations, determining the best process, and then using knowledge of the best process internally to design new processes or improve existing ones (Baker & Gelmon, 1996).

Many governmental, public, and private groups are working to make health care rankings and information available to consumers. For example, using the websites Healthcare.gov and Medicare.gov, Medicare enrollees and other consumers can search for and compare the quality of physicians, hospitals, nursing homes, home health agencies and dialysis facilities. For example, comparisons of hospitals include patient satisfaction survey results, timely and effective care results, readmission, complications and death rates, and number of Medicare patients by diagnosis type treated in the facility. From these sites, a prospective patient can determine areas of the hospital's performance that need improvement and can compare the hospital's performance in some categories with state and national results (benchmarking data).

Quality Improvement Initiatives in Nursing

Examples of quality improvement initiatives in nursing and health care abound in the literature and range from simple one-team solutions to complex multisite collaborations. Pappas (2008) describes a quality improvement study whose objective was to establish a methodology for nursing leaders to determine the cost of nurse sensitive adverse events (e.g., medication errors, patient falls, urinary tract infection, pneumonia, and pressure ulcers) from hospital cost accounting systems. A further objective of the study was to determine whether relationships existed between the occurrence of nurse-sensitive adverse events in selected medical and surgical patients, the level of nurse staffing, and the actual cost of patient care for an inpatient hospital admission. The results of this study revealed that in both medical and surgical patients, the occurrence of an adverse event (although only a small number of adverse events occurred in the study time period) was the best predictor of cost per case. In other words, when an adverse event occurred, the costs for the inpatient visit increased by an average of $659 for medical patients and by an average of $903 for surgery patients.

In this study, the occurrence of pneumonia in the surgery patient study group was the only significant relationship found between quantity of nurse staffing and the occurrence of a nurse-sensitive adverse event. Other implications related to quality improvement included the finding that age and severity were the best predictors of adverse events. The author recommends that this information be used to influence staffing decisions at the individual unit level to reduce the risk of future occurrence of adverse events. The results of this research also contribute to the growing body of evidence related to the role of adequate nurse staffing in preventing patient complications, which may lead to increased morbidity and mortality and ultimately to poorer quality outcomes and increased health care costs.

Experts predict that financial pressures for hospitals and health systems will be more intensive in the future than in the past. The only way for these organizations to control costs will be through operational and clinical improvements. Health care institutions that can provide documented successes in quality improvement that result in improved clinical and cost outcomes will be the institutions most heavily courted by MCOs, by private and government insurers, and by consumers.

Also, as a result of new Internet-based rating mechanisms, health care consumers are becoming increasingly savvy about checking quality "report cards" of health care facilities and providers. Health care–related sites are among those most sought after among Internet users. At the same time, Americans age 50 years and older, the segment of the population that uses the most health care services, are using the Internet in ever-increasing numbers. Institutions that are implementing best practices and continually striving to improve performance while decreasing costs will be the biggest winners in the competitive health care environment of the future (Health Care Strategic Management, 2000). Link to Practice 20-1 presents how one health care facility used a quality improvement team to ensure greater safety.

Link to Practice 20-1

Quality Improvement to Promote Safety

Occurrence of a major adverse event in a patient care setting often serves as the impetus for change in terms of quality improvement. After a patient safety issue was identified at a children's hospital related to the use of "smart pumps" in the administration of intravenous medications, a performance improvement team was assembled to increase use of medication safety software by nurses. The quality improvement team utilized the Deming Cycle performance improvement method to increase adherence and compliance with intravenous medication delivery software. Strategies implemented by the team to improve compliance included improved communication with nurses who were direct caregivers, staff education related to safety software specifics, acquisition of additional technology, and implementation of the medication safety champion role. Adherence monitoring was also incorporated. Following implementation of the performance improvement strategies, nurse adherence improved dramatically from 28% at baseline to greater than 85%, an adherence rate that exceeded nationally accepted benchmark adherence rates.

Gavriloff, C. (2012). A performance improvement plan to increase nurse adherence to use of medication safety software. *Journal of Pediatric Nursing, 27*(4), 375–382.

Evidence-Based Practice

Health care consumers expect quality care, and most health care practitioners want to provide quality care. Pressure for cost containment compels providers to demonstrate that interventions produce cost-effective outcomes that do not sacrifice the quality of health care. Further, selected interventions must be not only effective but also justified and congruent with acceptable standards.

EBP is a problem-solving approach that enables clinicians to provide the highest quality of care to patients and their families by integrating the following approaches:

- Critical appraisal and critique of the most recent and relevant research (evidence)
- Considering the clinician's own clinical expertise
- Considering preferences and values of the patient (Melnyk & Fineout-Overholt, 2005).

For EBP to take root and flourish in an organization, there must be institutional support and commitment from administrators. This support stems from the mission, goals, and culture of the organization. Without this support, necessary resources and infrastructure components, such as access to databases, dedicated personnel, and computer support, which are integral to a successful EBP program, may not be allocated or made fully available and accessible (Melnyk & Fineout-Overholt, 2005).

APNs must make clinical decisions on the best evidence available. They must also select interventions that are linked to cost-effective outcomes. This integrated approach allows the APN to use critical thinking skills to determine whether scientific evidence and clinical practice guidelines are relevant and consistent with the applicable health care situation and with the patient's values, preferences, and life context (Glanville, Schirm, & Wineman, 2000).

In one example, Drenning (2006), an APN, describes a collaborative approach that was utilized to implement an EBP change to address the knowledge and comfort level of RNs in discussing advanced directives with patients. Members of the team included staff nurses, nursing managers, directors, an APN with clinical expertise in palliative care, and a doctorally prepared nurse educator and researcher. The team identified the need for a practice change, clarified the practice problem, and identified desired patient and clinical outcomes. The team also researched relevant and evidence-based interventions related to the identified problem and proposed solutions for implementation.

An inpatient asthma education quality improvement program at Children's Hospital in Boston utilizes evidence-based guidelines and a team approach of an inpatient asthma nurse practitioner (IANP), other APNs, and unit-based RNs to provide patient and family education using individualized asthma action plans. The education is based on 2007 National Heart, Lung, and Blood Institute/National Asthma Education and Prevention Program guidelines, which recommend that care providers teach and reinforce asthma self-management techniques during every care encounter. Acute care encounters are especially valuable as parents and other caregivers are likely to want to participate in activities that prevent further emergency room visits and inpatient stays. (McCarty & Rogers, 2012).

Chapter 12 contains additional information about EBP. See also Link to Practice 20-2 for a novel approach to encouraging EBP.

Link to Practice 20-2

Promoting Evidence-Based Practice

Nursing administrators in a hospital district in Houston hosted a Sacred Cow Contest as a strategy to promote a culture that values clinical inquiry and to stimulate nurse interest in EBP. As part of the contest, nurses were encouraged to challenge the routines inherent in clinical practice, such as changing bed linens daily, performing "routine" vital signs, and the necessity for all nurses to listen to shift report on all patients on a given unit. Nurses were asked to consciously think of activities and procedures they performed daily and to question why the activity or procedure was necessary. When a practice was questionable, the nurses were asked to consider if it may be a sacred cow and were asked to submit entries challenging the practice. Sample entry categories for the contest were cash cow, mad cow, holy cow, and put the cow out to pasture, among others. More than 100 Sacred Cow Contest entries were received from inpatient and outpatient settings and from individual nurses as well as teams of nurses. After winning entries were named, a message communicating contest follow-up actions was sent to the nursing staff. Nurses were asked to adopt a sacred cow and were offered support and resources to establish EBP workgroups on the nursing units to address the sacred cow issue identified.

Mick, J. (2011). Promoting clinical inquiry and evidence-based practice. *Journal of Nursing Administration, 41*(6), 280–284.

Summary

This chapter has provided examples of the application of specific theories, models, and frameworks in nursing administration and management. The models, which were described along with related historical and contemporary applications, should provide the APN with a foundation for navigating the complex, ever-changing environment of health care organizations today and in the future.

Health care organizations of the future hold great promise for APNs, such as Greta from the opening case study, who are willing to assume entrepreneurial and intrapreneurial roles in providing cost-effective quality health care. A more detailed understanding of some of these models will be necessary in certain circumstances (e.g., as in the case study), but it is hoped that this chapter has provided a basis for further investigation for those who need more detailed information.

Key Points

- Organizational structure and design are key elements in determining efficiency and effectiveness of work processes and quality of outcomes in health care organizations.
- Shared governance is imperative to nurses controlling professional practice.
- Transformational leaders bring a competitive advantage to an organization and play an important role in cultivating healthy professional work environments.

- Nursing care in the acute care setting is most often delivered using a group practice model. Attributes of the work environment such as nurse staffing ratios and nurse educational level have significant and direct impact on patient outcomes such as infection, failure-to-rescue, and mortality rates.
- Implementation of concepts associated with patient- and family-centered care models, including dignity and respect, information-sharing, participation, and collaboration, lead to improved patient and staff satisfaction.
- Case management and disease management play crucial roles in acute care facilities and in other models of coordinated health care such as HMOs, MCOs, ACOs, and PCMHs.
- Quality improvement and evidence-based practice are concepts that are inextricably linked in today's highest performing health care organizations.

Learning Activities

1. Interview a middle-level manager in a hospital to determine recent changes in span of control. Has the span of control for the manager decreased or increased in the past 2 to 3 years? What impact has the manager noticed related to decreased or increased span of control? What is the manager's preference in terms of numbers of employees in his or her span of administrative control?
2. What are the roles of APNs employed by health care organizations in quality improvement activities in your community? Are APNs the leaders of quality improvement teams? What significant contributions have occurred as a result of APN involvement on QI teams?
3. Talk with APNs who are employed in hospitals in your area. Determine the following:
   a. Are the APNs unit based? If so, what is the method of patient care delivery on the unit, that is, primary nursing, team nursing, PFC? What are the advantages and disadvantages to the APN role related to each of the different delivery methods?
   b. Do the APNs have staff or line authority? What are the advantages and disadvantages to the role of each type of authority?
   c. Administratively, do the APNs report to a senior or middle-level manager?
   d. Do any of the APNs work in a shared governance environment?
4. What roles do nurses, especially APNs, play in HMOs, MCOs, ACOs, and PCMHs in your area? Are these nurses in case management roles? Do they work independently or are they part of an interdisciplinary team of case managers?
5. What EBP activities have APNs in your area spearheaded? Have health care consumers benefited?

REFERENCES

Aiken, L. H., Cimiotti, J. P., Sloane, D. M., Smith, H. L., Flynn, L., & Neff, D. M. (2011). Effects of nurse staffing and nurse education on patient deaths in hospitals with different nurse work environments. *Medical Care, 49*(12), 1047–1053.

Aiken, L. H., Clarke, S. P., Cheung, R. B., Sloane, D. M., & Silber, J. H. (2003). Educational levels of hospital nurses and surgical patient mortality. *Journal of the American Medical Association, 290,* 1617–1623.

Aiken, L. H., Clarke, S. P., & Sloane, D. M. (2002). Hospital staffing, organization, and quality of care: Cross-national findings. *International Journal of Quality Health Care, 14*(1), 5–13.

Aiken, L. H., Clarke, S. P., Sloane, D. M., Lake, E. T., & Cheney, T. (2008). Effects of hospital care environments on patient mortality and nurse outcomes. *Journal of Nursing Administration, 38*(5), 223–229.

Aiken, L. H., Clarke, S. P., Sloane, D. M., Sochalski, J., & Silber, J. H. (2002). Hospital nurse staffing and patient mortality, nurse burnout and job dissatisfaction. *The Journal of the American Medical Association, 288*(16), 1987–1993.

Aiken, L. H., Havens, D. S., & Sloane, D. M. (2000). The magnet nursing services recognition program: A comparison of two groups of magnet hospitals. *American Journal of Nursing, 100*(3), 26–36.

Aiken, L. H., & Patrician, P. (2000). Measuring organizational attributes of hospitals: The revised Nursing Work Index. *Nursing Research, 49*(3), 146–153.

Aiken, L. H., Sloane, D., Cimiotti, J. P., Clarke, S. P., Flynn, L., Seago, J. A., et al. (2010). Implications of the California nurse staffing mandate for other states. *Health Services Research, 45*(2), 1–18.

Aiken, L. H., Sloane, D. M., Lake, E. T., Sochalski, J., & Weber, A. L. (1999). Organization and outcomes of inpatient AIDS care. *Medical Care, 37*(8), 760–772.

Aiken, L. H., Smith, H. L., & Lake, E. T. (1994). Lower Medicare mortality among a set of hospitals known for good nursing care. *Medical Care, 32*(8), 771–787.

American Nurses Association. (2004). *Scope and standards for nurse administrators* (2nd ed.). Silver Springs, MD: Author.

Andel, C., Davidow, S. L., Hollander, M., & Moreno, D. A. (2012). The economics of health care quality and medical errors. *Journal of Health Care Finance, 39*(1), 39–50.

Anthony, M. K. (2004). Shared governance models: The theory, practice, and evidence. *Online Journal of Issues in Nursing, 9*(1). Retrieved from http://www.nursingworld.org/MainMenuCategories/ANAMarketplace/ANAPeriodicals/OJIN/TableofContents/Volume92004/No1Jan04/SharedGovernanceModels

Baker, G. R., & Gelmon, S. B. (1996). Total quality management in health care. In J. A. Schmele (Ed.), *Quality management in nursing and health care* (pp. 66–87). Boston: Delmar.

Barker, A. M. (1994). An emerging leadership paradigm: Transformational leadership. In E. C. Hein & J. M. Nicholson (Eds.), *Contemporary leadership behavior: Selected readings* (4th ed., pp. 81–86). Philadelphia: J. B. Lippincott.

Bennis, W., & Nanus, B. (1985). *Leaders: Strategies for taking charge*. New York: Harper & Row.

Blass, T. C., & Reed, T. L. (2003). Case management serves as an alternative career for advanced practice nurses. *Nursing Management, 34*(10), 81–83.

Brennan, P. F., & Anthony, M. K. (2000). Measuring nursing practice models using multi-attribute utility theory. *Research in Nursing and Health, 23*(5), 372–382.

Burnes-Bolton, L., Aydin, C. E., Donaldson, N., Brown, D. S., Sandhu, M., Fridman, M., et al. (2007). Mandated nurse staffing ratios in California: A comparison of staffing and nursing-sensitive outcomes pre-and post-regulation. *Policy Politics and Nursing Practice, 8*(4), 238–250.

Camp, R. C., & Tweet, A. G. (1994). Benchmarking applied to health care. *Journal of Quality Improvement, 20*(5), 229–238.

Case Management Advisor. (2013). Home visit help to reduce Medicare readmissions. *Case Management Advisor, 24*(2), 15–16.

Cathcart, D. (2004). Span of control matters. *Journal of Nursing Administration, 34*(9), 395–399.

Centers for Medicare and Medicaid Services. (2013). *Accountable care organizations (ACOs): General information*. Retrieved from http://innovation.cms.gov/initiatives/ACO/

Cho, S. H., Ketefian, S., Barkauskas, V. H., & Smith, D. G. (2003). The effects of nurse staffing on adverse events, morbidity, mortality, and medical costs. *Nursing Research, 52*(2), 71–79.

Christman, L. (1976). The autonomous nursing staff in the hospital. *Nursing Administration Quarterly, 1*(1), 37–44.

Cimiotti, J. P., Aiken, L. H., Sloane, D. M., & Wu, E. S. (2012). Nurse staffing, burnout, and health care associated infection. *American Journal of Infection Control, 40*, 486–490.

Clarke, S. P., & Aiken, L. H. (2003). Failure to rescue: Measuring nurses' contributions to hospital performance. *American Journal of Nursing, 103*, 42–47.

Clarke, S. P., Sloane, D. M., & Aiken, L. (2002). Effects of hospital staffing and organizational climate on needlestick injuries to nurses. *American Journal of Public Health, 92*(7), 1115–1119.

Clavelle, J. T., Drenkard, K., Tullai-McGuinness, S., & Fitzpatrick, J. J. (2012). Transformational leadership practices of chief nursing officers in Magnet organizations. *Journal of Nursing Administration, 42*(4), 195–201.

Cleland, V. S. (1978). Shared governance in a professional model of collective bargaining. *Journal of Nursing Administration, 8*(5), 39–43.

Clouten, K., & Weber, R. (1994). Patient-focused care . . . playing to win. *Nursing Management, 25*(2), 34–36.

Cottingham, C. (1988). Transformational leadership: A strategy for nursing. *Today's OR Nurse, 10*(6), 24–27.

Cropley, S. (2012). The relationship-based care model: Evaluation of the impact on patient satisfaction, length of stay and readmission rates. *Journal of Nursing Administration, 42*(6), 333–339.

DeVries, A., Li, C.-H., Sridhar, G., Hummel, J. R., Breidbart, S., & Barron, J. J. (2012). Impact of medical homes on quality, healthcare utilization, and costs. *The American Journal of Managed Care, 18*(9), 534–544.

Dokken, D., Moretz, J., Black, J., & Ahmann, E. (2007). The many roles of families in "family centered care" part 5. *Pediatric Nursing, 33*(4), 356–358.

Donaldson, N., Burnes-Bolton, L., Aydin, C., Brown, D., Elashoff, J., & Sandhu, M. (2005). Impact of California's licensed nurse-patient ratios on unit-level nurse staffing and patient outcomes. *Policy Politics and Nursing Practice, 6*, 198–210.

Drenning, C. (2006). Collaboration among nurses, advanced practice nurses, and nurse researchers to achieve evidence-based practice change. *Journal of Nursing Care Quality, 21*(4), 298–301.

Ellrodt, G., Cook, D. J., Lee, J., Cho, M., Hunt, D., & Weigarten, S. (1997). Evidence-based disease management. *Journal of the American Medical Association, 278*(20), 1687–1692.

Fayol, H. (1949). *General and industrial management*. London, United Kingdom: Pitman & Sons.

Flynn, L. (2007). Extending work environment research into home health settings. *Western Journal of Nursing Research, 29*(2), 200–212.

Foley, G. V. (2001). Forming partnerships, moving pain management forward. *Cancer Practice, 9*(4), 163.

Gavriloff, C. (2012). A performance improvement plan to increase nurse adherence to use of medication safety software. *Journal of Pediatric Nursing, 27*(4), 375–382.

Glanville, I., Schirm, V., & Wineman, N. M. (2000). Using evidence-based practice for managing clinical outcomes in advanced practice nursing. *Journal of Nursing Care Quality, 15*(1), 1–11.

Graicunas, A. (1937). Relationships in organizations. In L. Gullick & L. Urwick (Eds.), *Papers on the science of administration* (pp. 181–188). New York: Institute on Public Administration.

Healthcare.gov. http://www.healthcare.gov/prevention/index.html

Health Care Strategic Management. (2000). While quality, best outcomes have been "nice to do," they will become essential for survival in coming years. *Health Care Strategic Management, 1*(Suppl.), 11–13.

Hess, R. G. (2004). From bedside to boardroom—nursing shared governance. *Online Journal of Issues in Nursing, 9*(1), 2.

Hickey, P. A., Gauvreau, K., Jenkins, K., Fawcett, J., & Hayman, L. (2011). Statewide and national impact of California's staffing law on pediatric cardiac surgery outcomes. *Journal of Nursing Administration, 41*(5), 218–225.

Horswell, R., Butler, M. K., Kaiser, M., Moody-Thomas, S., McNabb, S., Besse, J., et al. (2008). Disease management programs for the underserved. *Disease Management, 11*(3), 145–152.

Houston, S., Leveille, M., Luquire, R., Fike, A., Ogola, G. O., & Chando, S. (2012). Decisional involvement in Magnet, Magnet-aspiring, and non-Magnet hospitals. *Journal of Nursing Administration, 42*(12), 586–591.

Institute for Family-Centered Care. (2009). http://www.familycenteredcare.org/faq.html

Janzen, S. K. (2003). Testimony before the House of Representatives Committee on Veteran Affairs, Subcommittee on Oversight and Investigation.

Johnson, B., Abraham, M., Conway, J., Simmons, L., Levitan, S. E., Sodomka, P., et al. (2008). *Partnering with patients and families to design a patient-and-family-centered health care system. Recommendations and promising practices.* Bethesda, MD: Institute for Family-Centered Care in Collaboration with the Institute for Healthcare Improvement. Retrieved from http://www.familycenteredcare.org/tools/downloads.html

Kangas, S., Kee, S., & McKee-Waddle, R. (1999). Organizational factors, nurses' job satisfaction, and patient satisfaction with nursing care. *Journal of Nursing Administration, 29*(1), 32–42.

Kelly, M. (2007). Achieving family-centered care: Working on or working with stakeholders? *Neonatal, Paediatric and Child Health Nursing, 10*(3), 4–11.

Kirkley, D., Johnson, A. P., & Anderson, M. A. (2004). Technology support of nursing excellence: The magnet connection. *Nursing Economics, 22*(2), 94–98.

Kohn, L. T., Corrigan, J. M., & Donaldson, M. S. (Eds.). (2000). *To err is human: Building a safer health system.* Washington, DC: National Academy Press.

Kongstvedt, P. R. (1997). *Essentials of managed health care* (2nd ed.). Gaithersberg, MD: Aspen.

Kouzes, J., & Posner, B. (2008). *The leadership challenge.* San Francisco, CA: Jossey-Bass Publications.

Kramer, M., & Schmalenberg, C. E. (2003). Magnet hospital nurses describe control over nursing practice. *Western Journal of Nursing Research, 25*(4), 424–452.

Kramer, M., Schmalenberg, C. E., Maguire, P., Brewer, B. B., Burke, R., Chmielewski, L., et al. (2008). Structures and practices enabling staff nurses to control their practice. *Western Journal of Nursing Research, 30*(5), 539–559.

Lake, E. T. (2007). The nursing practice environment: Measurement and evidence. *Medical Care Research and Review, 64,* 1045–1225.

Laschinger, H. K., & Finegan, J. (2005). Empowering nurses for work engagement and health in hospital settings. *Journal of Nursing Administration, 35*(10), 439–448.

Mang, A. L. (1995). Implementation strategies of patient-focused care. *Hospital and Health Services Administration, 40*(3), 426–435.

Marlowe, J. F. (2000). Disease management: Managed care's new thing. *Journal of Compensation and Benefits, 16*(3), 48–55.

Marriner-Tomey, A. (2009). *Guide to nursing management and leadership* (8th ed.). St. Louis: Mosby Elsevier.

McCarty, K., & Rogers, J. (2012). Inpatient asthma education program. *Pediatric Nursing, 38*(5), 257–263.

McClure, M. L., & Hinshaw, A. S. (2002). *Magnet hospitals revisited: Attraction and retention of professional nurses.* Washington, DC: American Nurses Publishing.

McClure, M. L., Poulin, M. A., Sovie, M. D., & Wandelt, M. A. (1983). *Magnet hospitals: Attraction and retention of professional nurses.* Washington, DC: American Nurses Publishing.

McGuire, E., & Kennerly, S. M. (2006). Nurse managers as transformational and transactional leaders. *Nursing Economics, 24*(4), 179–185.

Melnyk, B. M., & Fineout-Overholt, E. (2005). *Evidence-based practice in nursing and health care.* Philadelphia: Lippincott Williams & Wilkins.

Mick, J. (2011). Promoting clinical inquiry and evidence-based practice. *Journal of Nursing Administration, 41*(6), 280–284.

Muething, S. (2007). Family-centered care evolves as more and more collaboration occurs. *Family Education Management, 14*(1), 1–3.

Myers, S. (1998). Patient-focused care: What managers should know. *Nursing Economics, 16*(4), 180–188.

Pappas, S. H. (2008). The cost of nurse-sensitive adverse events. *Journal of Nursing Administration, 38*(5), 230–236.

Porter-O'Grady, T. (1992). Transformational leadership in an age of chaos. *Nursing Administration Quarterly, 17*(1), 17–24.

Porter-O'Grady, T. (1994). Whole systems shared governance: Creating the seamless organization. *Nursing Economics, 12*(4), 187–195.

Porter-O'Grady, T. (2003). Researching shared governance: A futility of focus. *Journal of Nursing Administration, 33*(4), 251–252.

Porter-O'Grady, T. (2012). Reframing knowledge work: Shared governance in the postdigital age. *Creative Nursing, 18*(4), 152–159.

Porter-O'Grady, T., Hawkins, M., & Parker, M. (1997). *Whole systems shared governance: Architecture for integration.* Gaithersburg, MD: Aspen.

Press, M. J., Michelow, M. D., & MacPhail, L. H. (2012). Care coordination in accountable care organizations: Moving beyond structure and incentives. *The American Journal of Managed Care, 18*(2), 778–780.

Robbins, S. P., & Judge, T. A. (2009). *Organizational behavior* (13th ed.). Upper Saddle River, NJ: Prentice-Hall.

Rossiter, L. F., Whitehurst Cook, M. Y., Small, R. E., Shasky, C., Bovbejerg, B. E., Penberthy, L., et al. (2000). The impact of disease management on outcomes and cost of care: A study of low income asthma patients. *Inquiry—Blue Cross and Blue Shield Association, 37*(2), 188–202.

Sackett, K., Pope, R. K., & Erdley, W. S. (2004). Demonstrating a positive return on investment for a prenatal program at a managed care organization: An economic analysis. *Journal of Perinatal and Neonatal Nursing, 18*(2), 117–127.

Spetz, J. (2008). Nurse satisfaction and the implementation of minimum nurse staffing requirements. *Policy, Politics, and Nursing Practice, 9*(1), 15–21.

Stanton, M. P., Swanson, M., Sherrod, R. A., & Packa, D. R. (2005). Case management evolution: From basic to advanced practice role. *Lippincott's Case Management, 10*(6), 274–286.

Taylor, F. W. (1911). *The principles of scientific management.* New York: Harper.

Tellez, M., & Seago, J. A. (2013). California nurse staffing law and RN workforce changes. *Nursing Economic$, 31*(1), 18–26.

Triolo, P. K., Scherer, E. M., & Floyd, J. M. (2006). Evaluation of the magnet recognition program. *Journal of Nursing Administration, 36*(1), 42–48.

Varkey, P., Reller, M. K., & Resar, R. K. (2007). Basics of quality improvement in health care. *Mayo Clinic Proceedings, 82*(6), 735–739.

Warren, N. (2012). Involving patient and family advisors in the patient and family-centered care model. *MEDSURG Nursing, 21*(4), 233–239.

Weber, M. (1970). Bureaucracy. In W. Sexton (Ed.), *Organization theories* (pp. 39–43). Columbus, OH: Charles E. Merrill.

Weston, M. J. (2008). Defining control over nursing practice and autonomy. *Journal of Nursing Administration, 38*(9), 404–408.

Wojcik, J., & Bradford, M. (2000). Online disease management. *Business Insurance, 34*(45), 23.

Wolf, G., Triolo, P., & Ponte, P. R. (2008). Magnet recognition program: The next generation. *Journal of Nursing Administration, 38*(4), 200–204.

Yamamoto, L., & Lucey, C. (2005). Case management "within the walls." *Critical Care Nursing Quarterly, 28*(2), 162–178.

Zarubi, K. L., Reiley, P., & McCarter, B. (2008). Putting patients and families at the center of care. *Journal of Nursing Administration, 38*(6), 275–281.

CHAPTER 21

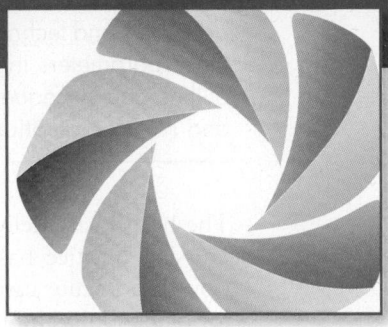

Application of Theory in Nursing Education

Evelyn M. Wills and Melanie McEwen

Linda Washington is a supervisor on a surgical floor of a large teaching hospital. Her responsibilities require her to work closely with the faculty from two area nursing schools and help place students with preceptors. Because of her enjoyment in working with students and faculty, Linda decided that she would like to become a nursing educator and enrolled in a master's degree program. This semester, she is taking a course on nursing education, and she is learning a great deal about how nursing programs are structured and the underlying rationale. The course requires a project in which a small group of students designs a nursing curriculum that will meet the changing needs of the health care system and the changing profile of nursing students in the 21st century. Initially, this project seemed daunting for Linda and her colleagues, and they were unsure where to begin.

During one class period, Linda's professor explained how a curriculum is derived from the faculty's philosophy of nursing and nursing education. She explained that a conceptual framework is then developed from the philosophy, and it is from this framework that the curriculum is built. The students also learned that in most nursing programs, the conceptual framework is an eclectic blend of concepts and processes, although some programs use grand nursing theories as their basis.

In a brainstorming session, Linda and her group agreed on a philosophy of nursing education, describing what they saw as the interplay of the metaparadigm concepts and concepts of teaching and learning. But there was considerable discussion and significant differences among group members about what other concepts or theories should be used as the basis for the curriculum framework. In addition, there was disagreement on what would be the best teaching strategy to meet the needs of older nursing students and students from diverse backgrounds. Some members of the group favored a structured, traditional type of program, in which the faculty member was responsible for directing learning experiences, whereas other group members preferred to focus on less rigid instructional techniques and incorporate more web-based options and simulation.

The discussions were enlightening, and finally Linda's group compromised. They would use "caring" as a central concept and draw heavily from Jean Watson's

(1996) work to structure the curriculum. They would also incorporate adult learning principles and technologically based instructional strategies into their program. With these parameters in place, the group began to describe courses, write objectives, outline course sequencing, discern outcome measures, identify teaching strategies, and set up evaluation methods.

The health care delivery system has changed dramatically during the past 15 years. Nursing practice has also changed, requiring it to adapt to a move from institution-based acute care to community-based care with an enhanced focus on caring for older adults and individuals with chronic conditions, as well as understanding the importance of cultural differences. Nursing education has been slow to respond to changes and anticipated trends in health care, and "in general nurses are late adopters of technology" (Schmitt, Sims-Giddens, & Booth, 2012, p. 2). This is contrary to assertions by nursing leaders and nursing organizations who believe that "it is the responsibility of nursing education, in collaboration with practice settings, to shape practice, not merely respond to changes in the practice environment" (American Association of Colleges of Nursing [AACN], 1999, p. 60).

The literature is awash with buzzwords for nursing education. Problem-based learning, caring, lifelong learning, informatics, evidence-based education, quality/performance improvement, culturally relevant care, interpersonal communication, and excellence are only a few. Furthermore, new trends for curricula reflect increased emphasis on evidence-based practice, population diversity, patient outcomes, health promotion, and informatics (Speziale & Jacobson, 2005). Other evolving emphases in nursing education include a greater focus on economics of health care, increasing use of simulation, along with more attention to interprofessional educational collaborations and distance education (Institute of Medicine [IOM], 2011; Keating, 2011a). Terms and trends commonly found in nursing education discussions include computer simulation, accelerated programs, concept-based curricula (Giddens, Wright, & Gray, 2012; Hardin & Richardson, 2012), virtual communities (Carlson-Sabelli, Giddens, Fogg, & Fielder, 2011), and distance learning/education (Jeffries, 2012).

A well-developed and articulated theoretical or organizational framework gives a nursing program the perspective that shapes the content and the methods that guide students' learning; eventually these methods have an impact on nursing practice (Iwasiw, Goldenberg, & Andrusyszyn, 2009; Keating, 2011a. A theoretical basis provides a foundation that helps nursing students define their professional philosophies and values. It identifies and describes essential concepts and significant problems and suggests approaches to structure and methods that the student may use in continuing to develop her or his knowledge. Additionally, the theoretical framework or model for the nursing program can influence the means by which material is presented and the methods by which learning is evaluated.

Barnum (1998) wrote that theoretical principles drawn from a number of sources directly affect a curriculum whether faculty members recognize it or not. Indeed, a nursing curriculum conveys a theory (or theories) of nursing by virtue of the content selected. In general, a program's curricular framework may be focused on a single or specific nursing theory adopted (or adapted) by the faculty, or the faculty may employ an eclectic approach in which the organizational framework is designed using concepts and threads taken from multiple theories, frameworks, and resources (Boland, 2012). Likewise, the means of presenting the content, the structure of courses, and evaluation methods are heavily based on theory.

In general terms, theoretical principles, concepts, and models are used in two major ways in nursing education. First, they are used to determine the content and organization and structure of a program's curriculum. Second, they are used to determine the instructional processes and strategies used by faculty to teach students. Both of these contributions of theory to nursing education are discussed in this chapter.

Theoretical Issues in Nursing Curricula

Curriculum refers to the content and processes by which learners gain knowledge and understanding, develop skills, and alter attitudes, appreciation, and values under the auspices of a given school or program. The curriculum of a school of nursing typically includes philosophy and mission statements; an organizational or conceptual framework; lists of outcomes, competencies, and objectives for the program; individual courses, course outlines and syllabi; educational activities; and evaluation methods (Dillard & Siktberg, 2012). Furthermore, most curricula specify essential nursing content and means of application in clinical practice (Keating, 2011b). Specific components of the curriculum of a given program of study are summarized in Box 21-1.

Several issues that relate to the incorporation of theoretical principles and frameworks into nursing curricula are reviewed in this section. These include basic curriculum design, the impact of regulating organizations on nursing curricula, components of curricular conceptual/organizational frameworks, and the processes involved in designing and organizing nursing curricula. The section concludes with a short discussion of current issues in nursing curriculum development.

Curriculum Design in Nursing Education

A *curriculum* is a "formal plan of study that provides the philosophical underpinnings, goals, and guidelines for the delivery of a specific educational program" (Keating, 2011a, p. 1). The curriculum provides faculty with a means of conceptualizing and organizing the knowledge, skills, values, and beliefs critical to the delivery of a coherent program of study that facilitates the achievement of the desired outcomes (Boland, 2012; Ruchala, 2011).

The curricula of most nursing programs are based on the Tyler Curriculum Development Model, which was published in 1949. Bevis (1989a, 1989b) stated that the incorporation of the Tyler model within nursing curricula began in the 1950s and continued throughout the 1960s and 1970s. According to Bevis (1989b), introduction of Tyler's concepts in the 1950s, along with her first book on curriculum development (Bevis, 1973) and Mager's (1962) publication of *Preparing*

Box 21-1 Components of a Curriculum

- A defined philosophy or mission statement
- An organizing framework
- Anticipated outcomes, competencies, and/or objectives to be achieved
- Selected content with specific sequencing of the content
- Educational activities and experiences to facilitate learning
- Means of evaluation

Source: Dillard and Siktberg (2012).

Instructional Objectives, led to the development of Tyler-type curricula throughout nursing education. Eventually, the Tyler model became the primary model used in developing nursing curricula for all levels of nursing education—diploma, associate degree, and baccalaureate.

The Tyler model begins with identification of the educational purposes or objectives for the program. It then differentiates what learning experiences should be selected to attain the objectives. The third issue addressed by the Tyler model is how to organize learning experiences for effective instruction. Finally, the model focuses on evaluation of behaviors to determine if objectives have been met (Bevis, 1989b). The Tyler model values effectiveness, efficiency, and predictability, and it emphasizes individualism and competition. It assumes that knowledge consists of facts, generalizations, principles, and theories and that events or phenomena can be explained by cause-and-effect relationships that can be deductively examined (Diekelmann, 1987).

Nursing Curricula and Regulating Bodies

The impact of the Tyler model on nursing curricula and nursing education cannot be overstated; it has directly influenced not only state boards of nursing but also the accreditation process. State boards of nursing set rules and requirements regarding nursing educational programs and curricula; these boards eventually based criteria for licensure of nursing programs on the Tyler model (Bevis, 1987; Rentschler & Spegman, 1996).

According to Bevis (1989b), the Tyler-based curriculum development process has been translated into essential curricular components, and without evidence of these components, state boards will not grant program approval. The rules and regulations set by state boards of nursing typically specify content areas that must be covered, minimum hours that must be spent by all students in clinical settings, and competencies or skills that all students must possess at the completion of the nursing program (Boland & Finke, 2012). A stated or defined conceptual framework is required for program approval by many state boards of nursing (National Council of State Boards of Nursing [NCSBN], 2009, 2011).

Similar to the impact on state board criteria, the Tyler model has heavily influenced the framework for accreditation by the National League for Nursing (NLN). Through the accreditation process, the NLN has had a great impact on the development, implementation, and evaluation of undergraduate nursing curricula (Boland & Finke, 2012). The first NLN accreditation visits were in 1939, and soon NLN accreditation requirements became the standard for nursing education (Bevis, 1989a; Flood, 2011). Beginning in 1972, the NLN criteria for bachelor's (BSN) programs included a criterion requiring that the curriculum be based on a conceptual framework that was consistent with the stated philosophy, purposes, and objectives of the program (Kelley, 1975; NLN, 1972; Wu, 1979). Likewise, in the 1970s, accreditation requirements for associate degree in nursing (ADN) programs required that the "conceptual framework of the program of learning is clearly stated and implemented" (NLN, 1977, p. 14).

Meleis (2012) observed that the recognition of the potential of nursing theories to be used as guidelines for the conceptual frameworks of nursing curricula and programs in the 1960s and 1970s coincided with the development of most of the nursing theories. Indeed, nursing education promoted theory development in the search for a coherent presentation of nursing to guide and structure curricula.

Over the ensuing years, accreditation criteria changed somewhat. During this time, "the requirements for a conceptual framework were a major source of confusion and concern among nurse educators" (Tanner, 1989, p. 8). Because of this confusion, guidelines were changed, and since the mid-1980s, they have been more flexible. Most recently, the National League for Nursing Accrediting Committee (NLNAC)'s accreditation standards, for example, state that the curriculum must "incorporate established professional standards, guidelines and competencies . . . clearly articulate student learning outcomes and program outcomes" (NLNAC, 2013, p. 82). In addition, the "professional standards/guidelines" can be from "nationally recognized nursing organization for use in the development and evaluation of a nursing curriculum" (NLNAC, 2013, p. 5). Thus, while not explicitly requiring a defined conceptual framework, some type of specific organizational strategy must be used to structure the program.

Since the mid-1990s, the AACN Commission on Collegiate Nursing Education (CCNE) has also been accrediting baccalaureate and master's nursing programs. In its accreditation standards, like the NLNAC, the CCNE does not specify an organizing framework, per se. Rather, the need for a curricular framework is implied as Standard III states that the "curriculum is . . . logically structured to achieve expected individual and aggregate student outcomes" (CCNE, 2009, Standard III-C). See Link to Practice 21-1.

Conceptual/Organizational Frameworks for Nursing Curricula

As mentioned previously, the conceptual or organizational framework of a nursing program should be an outgrowth of the philosophy of the faculty, which typically reflects the faculty's philosophical beliefs about the metaparadigm concepts (Boland, 2012; Keating, 2011b). Scales (1985) explained that the interrelationship of these concepts is the basic organizational framework of the curriculum, and as the concepts are further defined within the framework, the curriculum becomes established. Additional concepts and theories selected to comprise the conceptual framework are likewise taken from the philosophy (Boland, 2012).

According to Bevis (1989a), a curriculum conceptual framework is an "interrelated system of premises that provides guidelines or ground rules for making all curricular decisions—objectives, content, implementation, and evaluation" (p. 26). The conceptual framework may be referred to as the curriculum framework, the framework for curriculum development, the conceptual system, the curriculum theory,

Link to Practice 21-1

Application of Theoretical Information for Nursing Educators

Linda, the nurse from the opening case study, was surprised at the organizational structure of nursing education as she studied the elements of teaching and of curriculum. She perused the Baccalaureate Essentials of the CCNE (AACN, 2008) to learn more about requirements for BSN education. As the nursing program she was attending was preparing for accreditation, she asked to be allowed to attend faculty meetings to gain more insight into the process. The chair of the committee welcomed Linda to the accreditation preparation meetings, and her attendance formed an informative learning experience regarding curriculum design and instructional strategies.

Access the CCNE Web site at: http://www.aacn.nche.edu/education-resources/essential-series to learn more.

a theory of education, or the theoretical framework, but regardless of the name, it is the conceptualization and articulation of concepts, facts, propositions, postulates, theories, and variables relevant to the specific nursing program.

Purposes of the Conceptual Framework

The conceptual or organizational framework for a curriculum serves several purposes. First, it allows faculty to determine what knowledge is important to nursing (i.e., the concepts, principles, skills, and theories to be covered) and how that knowledge should be defined, categorized, and linked with other knowledge. It also helps explain how these ideas or concepts apply to nursing practice. Second, the conceptual framework facilitates the sequencing and prioritizing of knowledge in a way that is logical and internally consistent (Boland, 2012). Finally, "an organizing framework provides faculty with a means of delivering a cohesive curriculum to give students learning experiences necessary to achieve the desired educational outcomes" (Dillard & Siktberg, 2012, p. 84).

McEwen and Brown (2002) completed a large-scale, nationwide study that examined the curricular frameworks of BSN, ADN, and diploma nursing programs. The findings illustrated trends at that time in structuring the conceptual frameworks of nursing curricula. In general, the nursing process was the most commonly used component of conceptual frameworks for nursing curricula, being used by 55% of all programs. Simple-to-complex organization (37% of all programs), a biopsychosocial model (36% of all programs), and nursing theorists (33% of all programs) were the other most frequently reported components. Of those identifying a nursing theory as part of the conceptual framework, the most commonly reported nursing theorists were Orem, Roy, Watson, Neuman, and Benner. The most commonly used non-nursing theories reported were systems theory, Maslow's and Erickson's theories, and adaptation.

Designing a Curriculum Conceptual Framework

Boland (2012) stated that there are two approaches to determining or developing an organizational framework for a nursing curriculum. Faculty members may choose a single, specific nursing theory or model on which to build the framework, or they may choose a more eclectic approach, selecting concepts from multiple theories or models. She explained that use of a single theory to develop the conceptual framework helps by providing a single image with a defined vocabulary that is shared by both the learner and the teacher. In some cases, however, it was observed that the language of the theory and the definitions of the central concepts may be too abstract to be helpful. If a single theory is used as the framework, the faculty will adopt the theory and use its definitions and relationships to structure and organize content.

Several articles in recent nursing literature describe the use of nursing theories as the basis for the curriculum framework of nursing programs. In one example, Berbiglia (2011) provided a detailed explanation of how Orem's Self-Care Deficit Theory (SCDT) can be used as the conceptual framework in BSN programs. Also focusing on Orem's SCDT, Secrest (2008) described the process of tool development in an Orem-based curriculum and the role of faculty in bringing a curriculum revision to fruition. Beckman, Boxley-Harges, and Kaskel (2012) discussed the processes used by faculty at their nursing program as their program transitioned from an associated degree program to a BSN program using the Neuman Systems Model as the curricular framework.

To avoid being constrained by a single nursing theory or model, most faculty choose an eclectic approach that combines many theories and concepts in framework development (Boland, 2012; Keating, 2011b). Often, two or three organizing themes are used to build a curriculum grid. These themes can be variables, such as life phases, body systems, and the nursing process.

A criticism of the eclectic approach to constructing conceptual frameworks is that it impedes the development of a body of knowledge that is uniquely nursing. If the eclectic approach is taken, a combination of many theories, concepts, or processes is used, and borrowed concepts must be specifically defined for the program. Relationships between and among the concepts must also be explained. On the other hand, an advantage to an eclectic approach is the ability to incorporate concepts and definitions that best fit the faculty's beliefs and values (Boland, 2012).

Components of the Curricular Conceptual Framework

The two major areas to be addressed during development of a curriculum framework are as follows: (1) What concepts will be covered? (2) What will be the structure, ordering, or sequencing for introducing the concepts and delineating the relationships between and among them?

Curriculum Concepts. Once a conceptual framework for a nursing program is agreed on, the task is to identify the major elements or concepts that will appear and reappear as "threads" at each level of the curriculum, and thus provide a basis for the organization and sequencing of content. Most undergraduate nursing conceptual frameworks minimally describe the concepts of health, person, environment, and nursing. Other concepts, such as caring, self-care, growth and development, nursing process, and adaptation, may be added to expand or clarify the framework. Each of the central concepts should be defined, and the linkages between and among the concepts should be explained to unify or interrelate the details.

The conceptual framework may then use additional constructs or devices to help structure or organize the material. It may use developmental stage, acute/chronic concepts, health/illness continuum, settings, or the nursing process as the chief organizer. In addition, "process threads" or themes are usually present throughout the curriculum. These might include the nursing process, problem solving, interpersonal relationships, communication, research, change, and teaching. Each of these constructs or devices should also be defined and explained.

Curriculum Structure or Sequencing. The curriculum is designed to provide a sequence of learning experiences that will enable students to achieve desired educational outcomes. Content may be structured or organized based on such variables as location (e.g., hospital, clinics, community), developmental stage (e.g., infant, child, adolescent, adult, elder), or physiologic systems (e.g., musculoskeletal, gastrointestinal, cardiovascular, reproductive). Factors to be considered in sequencing the curriculum include consideration of the relationships among the concepts and the sequences in which the content should be ordered so that the organization supports the selected relationships. The conceptual properties (attributes) of the concepts to be learned, and the sequence in which the content is ordered, should be logically consistent. Table 21-1 gives examples of how sequencing can be used to organize courses based on several parameters (i.e., metaparadigm concepts, attributes of the person, subconcepts, activities, and complexity).

In most programs, sequencing moves from concepts that are relatively simple to concepts that are more complex, or from wellness to progressively serious illnesses (Keating, 2011b). It has been noted that both of these organizational strategies can be problematic because the self-evident needs of the ill client(s) may be easier for the

Table 21-1 Methods for Sequencing Used in Nursing Curricula

Basis of Sequencing	Beginning Level	Intermediate Levels	Final Level
Sequencing based on metaparadigm concepts	Introduction to the concepts and discussion that there are interrelationships	Focus on relationship between person(s) and nursing; move toward focus on interrelationships of person(s), nursing, and health	Focus on interrelationship of all concepts (persons, nursing, health, environment)
Sequencing based on the attributes of person(s)	Concept of personhood established (individual, family, community)	Focus on individual; move to focus on family and groups	Focus on community
Sequencing based on relationships of concepts	Person (individual, family, community) identified; nursing focused on restoration, maintenance, or promotion; health on a continuum; environment is controlled	Focus on relationship of individual and the nursing goal of health restoration; environment is controlled. Move to focus on nursing of family and/or groups and the goal of health maintenance; environment is less controlled	Focus on relationship of community and the nursing goal of health promotion; environment is open and less confined
Sequencing based on activities	Student is an observer	Student is an observer-participant	Student is a participant-practitioner
Sequencing based on complexity	Examines health care environments with few variables	Examines health care environments with many variables	Examines health care environments with complex variables

Source: Scales (1985).

novice nurse to recognize and understand than the more subtle health needs of the well client(s) (Scales, 1985).

Patterns of Curricular Conceptual Frameworks

There are two common patterns of curriculum organization in nursing programs. Probably the more common one is that of *blocking* course content. When courses are blocked, content is generally structured around a particular clinical specialty area, client population, or body systems. In this organizational scheme, content can be organized according to specific practice settings (e.g., medical-surgical nursing, mental health nursing, critical care nursing), developmental stages (birth, infancy, childhood, adulthood, older adult), or body systems (e.g., respiratory system, circulatory system, digestive system). This approach produces a curriculum that is highly structured (Boland & Finke, 2012).

Boland and Finke (2012) explained that blocking has some advantages because it facilitates course assignments and complements faculty expertise. Also, in a blocked course design, it is easy to trace placement of content within the curriculum. However, there are some concerns. Blocking of content often causes the content to become isolated from previous or following courses. This may impede the student's ability to integrate knowledge and to transfer concepts, information, and expertise across courses. Another concern is that each area is self-contained and based on a different set of premises because every major block of study is derived from a different theoretical base. For example, Barnum (1998) explained that fundamentals nursing focuses on skills, medical-surgical nursing focuses on body systems, obstetrics is a life event–based specialty, psychiatric nursing is based on client behavior, and public health nursing is based on principles of epidemiology.

The second curriculum pattern is that of integrating or *threading* course content. Integrating course content is a more conceptual approach to curriculum design. In the integrated curriculum, faculty members identify concepts considered core to nursing practice and then integrate or thread these concepts throughout the curriculum. A nursing theory, for example, may be used to define core concepts across the program. Concepts that are frequently integrated include lifespan development, nutrition, and pharmacology (Boland & Finke, 2012).

Current Issues in Curriculum Development

There have been several recent shifts in nursing curricula. First, increasingly, community-based and population-focused components are being added to basic curricula. This has been encouraged by changes in the health care delivery system that has moved much of patient care out of the acute care hospital. With that shift, there has been a growing tension between curricula that focus on technology and pathophysiology and those that focus on a more humanistic, holistic concept of nursing. Other recent changes in nursing education involve less focus being given to skills and tasks, with a corresponding increased focus on the integration of content and problem-solving strategies and concept-based curricula (Cannon & Boswell, 2012; Hardin & Richardson, 2012; Secrest, 2008).

Nursing educators recognize that the content, concepts, principles, and theories taught in nursing programs should be regularly updated. For example, there has been a focus related to strengthening nursing curricula, particularly in the areas of spiritual care (Burkhart & Schmidt, 2012), safety and quality (Barnsteiner et al., 2013; Bednash, Cronenwett, & Dolansky, 2013; Chenot & Daniel, 2010), genetics (Daack-Hirsch, Dieter, & Quinn-Griffin, 2011; Giarelli & Reiff, 2012; Williams et al., 2011), gerontology (Azzaline, 2012; Skiba, 2012), and end-of-life care/palliative care (Lewis, 2012; Moreland, Lemieux, & Myers, 2012; Stapleton, 2009). A number of areas in which enhanced content in nursing programs should be addressed to meet current and future health care needs have been identified in the nursing literature (Heller, Oros, & Durney-Crowley, 2000; Lewis, 2012; Stokowski, 2011). These are listed in Box 21-2.

Box 21-2 Content Areas in Nursing Education to be Enhanced

- The aging population
- Evidence-based practice
- Cultural diversity and health disparities
- Spiritual care
- Technology (informatics, electronic medical records, telehealth)
- The globalization of health problems (threat of spread of diseases)
- Alternative or complementary therapies
- Genetics and genomics
- Palliative care/end-of-life care
- Population health
- Health care reform and reimbursement
- Health policy and regulation issues
  - Safety/quality
  - Leadership

Source: Heller et al., 2000; Lewis, 2012; Stokowski, 2011.

Theoretical Issues in Nursing Instruction

To accommodate changing student profiles and address the needs of students from different generations (e.g., baby boomers, generation X, millennial), students from a variety of cultural backgrounds, students with family responsibilities, and students from remote or rural areas, nursing educators have observed that changes or modifications in methods of instruction are warranted. To this end, new teaching strategies, based on sound educational theories and research, should be developed and promoted.

What is taught in nursing programs can be divided into three categories: (1) cognitive content, (2) psychomotor tasks, and (3) application of content and skills in nursing practice. Cognitive content refers to all the information the nurse learns as background for functioning (e.g., anatomy, physiology, pathology, psychology, medical procedures, nursing techniques). Psychomotor tasks are the acts or skills nurses perform according to a given rationale by applying accepted techniques (e.g., administering medications, changing dressings, inserting intravenous lines). Application of cognitive knowledge and skills involves recognizing and interpreting phenomena in the clinical setting and adapting care based on the interpretation.

Teaching strategies are different for each of the three areas. Cognitive content is easily transmitted through a variety of means: lectures, discussions, programmed learning, or reading assignments. Acquisition of cognitive content can be achieved in the absence of skilled teaching if another source of information (i.e., a textbook) is available. Psychomotor skills require demonstration, return demonstration with corrective feedback, and skill development through practice. Learning to apply cognitive knowledge and psychomotor skills in practice is the most complex learning task and takes time as learning accumulates from multiple clinical experiences in varied settings. Increasingly, simulation is being utilized to develop and refine psychomotor skills.

The following sections examine two major issues in nursing instruction. These are incorporation of multiple theory-based strategies in teaching and the use of technology in nursing education. Use of multiple teaching strategies is important to enable nursing students to attain cognitive content and psychomotor skills and, most importantly, enable them to apply these in clinical settings. Technologic instruction is included because it is becoming increasingly important in nursing education, and the use of distance education methods is anticipated to become even more common.

Theory-Based Teaching Strategies

To best meet the learning needs of students at the beginning of the 21st century, nursing educators are encouraged to move beyond reliance on traditional techniques of lecture and reading assignments to incorporate other teaching strategies that are based on sound theoretical principles. Some theories suggested by Barnum (1998) are dialectic learning, problem-based learning, operational instruction, and logistic teaching. Each of these strategies is presented in this section, along with examples from the nursing literature showing how they have been applied in education.

Dialectic Learning

Traditional dialectic teaching leads students to develop and expand their own thoughts on a given subject, primarily through the use of well-constructed questions. Questioning can lead to demonstration of inconsistencies in, or contradictions to, the student's position. In dialogue, the student moves from a narrow conception of the subject matter to a broader and more comprehensive understanding that encompasses more events and more complexities. Dialogue often results in self-revelation because the student is required to think through issues while considering answers to complex questions (Barnum, 1998).

Application to Nursing. Dialectic teaching is used frequently in nursing education. For example, it is commonly used in clinical situations and postclinical conferences. Dialectic teaching has shown to be effective in updated examples of clinical post-conferences as described by Schams and Kuennen (2012) and Yehle and Royal (2010). Heise and Himes (2010) presented an example of a course council that used open dialogue, questioning, and reflection to promote problem solving, critical thinking, and professional responsibility among students.

Online discussions provide an environment for dialectic learning. In one example, Kuhn, Hasbargen, and Miziniak (2010) presented an analysis of the effectiveness of an online discussion format using structured questioning to improve thinking skills. In a similar work, Anderson and Tredway (2009) designed an online critical thinking course using problem-based learning methods. The students were cast as stakeholders in the project. In a third example, Guhde (2010) combined online discussions, personal reflection, and faculty and peer input with simulation to improve student's clinical decision making. Finally, Dreifuerst (2012) provided a detailed account of a study of "debriefing for meaningful learning," a process for debriefing students following simulation experiences in which they reflected on their experiences to improve their clinical reasoning skills.

Problem-Based Learning Strategies

Problem-based learning (PBL) involves the use of predefined clinical situations and case studies to enhance or stimulate students to acquire specific skills, knowledge, and abilities (Rowles, 2012). Simulated clients may be used, or the student might be given a real problem in an actual clinical case; the objective of PBL is to determine how to manage the person's care.

Problem-based learning allows the instructor to manipulate multiple variables to add increasingly complex issues or circumstances that must be considered in problem resolution. For beginner students, the teacher may identify the problems but let the students seek solutions. Or the teacher may use the case as a problem-seeking exercise, teaching students how to find the important facts among the array of available data (Barnum, 1998).

In addition, PBL encourages self-direction, interpersonal communication, and use of information technology. Typically, small groups of students work together in self-directed teams; the case studies challenge them to improve their critical thinking capabilities, learn self-evaluation strategies, and promote communication among peers (Bently, 2004; Rowles, 2012). Although it is an effective learning strategy, PBL can be time intensive to implement because it requires faculty to develop realistic scenarios that usually focus on problems encountered by a single individual and/or family in a changeable clinical situation (Bently, 2004; Kane, 2004).

Application to Nursing. Problem-based learning techniques are commonly used in nursing education. For example, Wong and colleagues (2008) devised and tested a PBL framework in a simulated clinical setting. They noted that PBL is difficult in the real clinical setting because the needs of the patient take precedence; however, they found a simulated PBL situation successful. Cooper and Carver (2012) presented their findings of their use of problem-based learning in teaching mental health nursing, noting that the format helped students gain confidence in their practice.

In another example, Chan (2012) described how PBL and role playing were used in a classroom setting to promote teamwork, problem-solving skills, and critical thinking.

Operational Teaching Strategies

Operational teaching strategies focus on presenting various perspectives regarding an agent or issue. A symposium that uses speakers with different perspectives on the same subject matter or a debate is an example. Other operational strategies focus on providing different or atypical activities for the learner. Using educational games or viewing nonmedical videos for illustration are considered to be operational teaching activities (Barnum, 1998).

Application to Nursing. Many nursing faculty use operational teaching techniques to make learning more interesting and enjoyable and to provide a different perspective on a particular topic (Herrman, 2011; Robb, 2012). Use of games to enhance students' decision making, critical thinking, and teamwork was described by Stanley and Latimer (2011). In other examples, Hogan, Kapralos, Cristancho, Finney, and Dubrowski (2011) reported on an effort that employed an interactive, virtual learning environment or "serious game" used to acquire community health nursing skills, and Anderson (2008) used simulation game playing with a multidisciplinary theme in which the students act as physician, social worker, and chaplain as well as the nurse to assess and intervene with an obstetric patient. Use of movies, films, and television as a method to engage nursing students was described by several nursing educators (Briggs, 2011; DiBartolo & Seldomridge, 2009, 2010; Edmonds, 2011).

Logistic Teaching Strategies

Logistic teaching strategies are based on the concept of mastery of sequential learning. Logistic teaching techniques generally divide the material to be learned into learning sequences, where acquisition of one section of the material is a necessary prerequisite to acquisition of another component. Logistic strategies teach the student clearly defined components and provide for reinforcement and testing of each component as the program progresses. As sections of the material are added and related to each other, knowledge accumulates (Barnum, 1998).

Formative testing is a logistic teaching strategy because a course is conceived as consisting of separate and definite units and tests are constructed to measure attainment of each unit. Other strategies include use of self-instructional modules and portfolios; these are typically logistic in nature because they follow a pattern of assembling information that is built on previously explained material (Rowles, 2012).

Application to Nursing. Logistic or sequential teaching is common in nursing curricula and has been effective because courses are sequenced and must be passed, and objectives or outcomes met, before students can progress to the next course or level. Examples from recent nursing literature include a work by Wassef, Riza, Maciag, Worden, and Delaney (2012), which described a mechanism in which graduate students were required to maintain and periodically submit electronic portfolios to document academic progress. Also describing how portfolios can be used effectively as summative assessment for nursing students progression were Hill (2012) and Timmins and Dunne (2009). Use of modules to promote learning was described in several situations. Examples include using a modular format to teach ethics to undergraduate BSN students (Hsu & Hsieh, 2011), graduate students about complementary and alternative therapies (Swanson et al., 2012), and disaster management for public health nurses (Chiu, Polivka, & Stanley, 2011)

Use of Technology in Nursing Education

The use of technology-based distance learning methods, such as the Internet and interactive video conferencing, has become widespread in nursing programs. In addition, computer-assisted instruction, which has been available since the early 1990s, is becoming more sophisticated and more widely used (Zwirn & Muehlenkord, 2012).

Three main types of technology-based educational methods are available to nursing educators. Interactive distance learning includes the use of two-way video and audio broadcasts carried over telephone lines, Internet courses, and video classrooms in widely dispersed geographic locations. This technology, called *synchronous delivery*, requires that teacher and student be available to each other simultaneously. Another interactive distance learning technique uses virtual classrooms that are available to students who have Internet carriers. These interactive virtual classrooms are available at all hours via a server. Finally, computer-based virtual reality simulations allow students under the guidance of the nursing educator to rehearse psychomotor interventions in realistic nursing situations prior to placing the patient into the learning situation as what happens in a practicum (Cannon & Boswell, 2012).

Familiarity with both synchronous (immediate or real-time access) and asynchronous (delayed access) technology makes it possible to use multiple teaching strategies. Virtual classrooms may combine both synchronous and asynchronous technology. Synchronous technology (e.g., video conferencing, chat rooms, and real-time online classrooms) allows students to have personal contact with the instructor with immediate feedback, similar to face-to-face instruction, although the depth of the discussion may suffer. Asynchronous methods (e.g., LISTSERV email lists, discussion boards, and bulletin boards) permit students to fit learning into their busy lifestyles. Asynchronous methods allow students to answer in greater depth because they have time to consider an answer.

Synchronous methods, such as video conferencing, offer slightly more traditional pedagogy than strict reliance on Internet delivery, as the instructor is seen and heard and, through multiple media, can present a broad and diverse lecture format. Depending on the depth and difficulty of the materials, students may respond less frequently in the video classroom than on a chat facility in the virtual classroom.

Use of both synchronous and asynchronous methods supports adult learning more effectively than any single method alone. It is recognized that a combination of methods is preferable to many students, who express greater satisfaction with both methods than with either method alone (Peterson, Hennig, Dow, & Sole, 2001).

Virtual reality simulation is an innovation in clinical skills education and often employs use of high-fidelity human patient simulators. Some of these computerized mannequins produce motion and sounds that allow realistic situations as students practice assessing, planning, and carrying out interventions. The faculty preprogram the simulator with clinical situations to allow students to practice skills in a patient-safe environment (Cannon & Boswell, 2012; Jeffries & Clochesy, 2012).

The high-fidelity patient simulator is the closest thing to virtual reality currently in existence for nursing education. It consists of a mannequin and the apparatus within, which is programmed and accessed using a laptop, desktop, or handheld computer. Several current models simulate patients of all ages providing students with opportunities to assess heart, lung, and bowel sounds and initiate interventions to deal with multiple situations and patient responses (Jeffries & Clochesy, 2012; Jeffries, 2012).

Issues in Technology-Based Teaching

Several issues should be considered when applying technologic innovations in nursing instruction. Institutional issues include the provision of the technology, software, and facilities for its use (Hodson-Carlton, 2012; Zwirn & Muelenkord, 2012). Faculty responsibilities include design or modification of the curriculum and the course content to reflect technology-based delivery. Other faculty concerns are the type of media to be used, faculty–student interaction, technology management, student evaluation, and faculty and course evaluation (Anderson & Tredway, 2009; Jeffries, 2012; Cannon & Boswell, 2012).

Instructors who use distance education by electronic modalities should be familiar with the technology at the user level and must carefully design courses for students involved in self-paced, independent study. Further, faculty using electronic educational methods should be familiar with principles of adult learning (Knowles, 1980) when constructing the curricula and the course work for electronic delivery.

Numerous programs are available to educators that permit multiple methods of interface between the teacher and student. These programs allow students to gain access to the course materials on their own schedule and to have real-time experiences with the instructor, such as is found in a chat facility or on a real-time face-to-face video and telephone-based format such as Skype. Some also allow testing and provide security parameters to authorize only the teacher and student to have access to the student's records. E-mail, bulletin boards, and wikis permit messages between instructor and students and among students or groups of students.

To take full advantage of up-to-date electronic teaching methods, the instructor needs to become proficient in multiple methods of conveying content and should be prepared to apply learning theories. Technology-based distance education embraces adult educational principles. Indeed, the content is presented in useful form, the immediacy of the student's need for knowledge is supported, and the student's ability to rely on previous knowledge base to provide a foundation for her or his questioning are all present in the typical interactive web-based classroom. The use of multiple ways of presenting the material in a course conducted using interactive technology-based education/learning creates the stimulus for learning and expands the educator's abilities in conveying course content.

Although the rewards of teaching by electronic methods are many, there are also issues of which faculty who are teaching web-based and online courses should be made aware. Distance methods such as web-based teaching–learning require considerably more time than in-class, face-to-face strategies (Anderson & Avery, 2008; Halstead & Billings, 2012). The necessary time to spend on this activity is becoming more recognized but has still not been adequately addressed by educational administrators. The usual 6 hours of preparation to 1 hour of class time for face-to-face classroom instruction may expand to as much as 12 or more hours to each hour of web-based class time as the educator learns new electronic teaching methods. Indeed, the time that instructors invest in teaching web-based and online courses can be overwhelming to both novices and experienced educators.

The advantage of the method is that communication can be carried on all hours of the day, 7 days weekly, by web-based classroom, virtual chat, discussion boards, e-mail, fax, and telephone (Halstead & Billings, 2012). Although the educator becomes a facilitator of adult education and the strategies are organized to take advantage of the self-directed, independent nature of the learners, the educator involved in this strategy soon learns it is important to manage time so as to avoid becoming overwhelmed (Friesth, 2012; Halstead & Billings, 2012). Although electronic web-based online learning frees students from travel and necessity of reorganizing their already busy lives, it does not lighten the instructor's load and adds hours to preparation and teaching activities (Anderson & Avery, 2008). The immediacy of the needs of the students who have continuous access to educators may tempt faculty members to spend excessive time reading e-mail and in other communication efforts.

Educators who are contemplating using web-based teaching–learning strategies should consult with seasoned faculty mentors. They should be encouraged to take advantage of their experience with the methods of delivery for electronic education, peruse the literature about the issues of time and recognition, and negotiate from a position of knowledge to obtain the required time and promise of recognition.

Application to Nursing. Although technology-based instruction in nursing is still relatively new, an increasing number of examples have appeared in the literature describing how technology is being used in nursing education and discussing successes and lessons learned. Billings and Kowalski (2007) identified podcasting as a nursing educational tool. They found that implementing podcasting is a means of accessing the current generation of learners that allows educators to "take the learning to the learners" (p. 57). Fetter (2009) found that competencies in information technology could be integrated into an undergraduate curriculum.

Because simulation has become so widely used, the literature is full of examples illustrating how simulation activities can be used in nursing education. For example, Berragan (2011) gave an overview or summary look at simulation and determined that it is highly effective as a pedagogic tool for nursing education. In other examples, McCormick, de Slavy, and Fuller (2013) used an unfolding case simulation to teach nursing students about Parkinson disease, and Carlson (2012) described how it can be used in pediatric nursing education. Among many other examples, simulation has been used to teach nurses and nursing students diabetes care (Tschannen, Aebersold, Sauter, & Funnell, 2013), postoperative care in the cardiothoracic intensive care unit (Powell, 2013), wound care (Ayer, 2013), how to perform during a code (Delac, Blazier, Daniel, & Wilfong, 2013), and home health care nursing (Smith & Barry, 2013). Thus, it is very evident that use of "low fidelity," "high fidelity," and many other iterations and combinations of integrated, participatory simulated experiences will grow in nursing. As these educational experiences are developed, however, faculty must ensure that they are developed using appropriate learning theories and recognized and evidence-based teaching strategies.

Summary

This chapter has presented two major areas relevant to the use of theoretic principles and models in nursing education: curriculum design and instruction. In the opening case study, Linda and her classmates learned that it is necessary to have a sound, identified theoretical base to serve as the framework for a nursing program. They also recognized that it is important to select multiple teaching strategies to deliver the material in a manner that will best support student learning.

Likewise, it is essential that all nurse educators be aware of how theoretical principles are used in education. They should be able to articulate the conceptual framework of their program and recognize how the framework shapes the program. Nursing educators should also use multiple strategies and techniques for instruction to enable students to develop their knowledge base and to develop critical thinking abilities and problem-solving skills. Finally, nursing educators should recognize that technology will play an increasingly important role in nursing education and be prepared to incorporate distance education methods and virtual reality simulation into instruction.

Whether the focus is continuing education of practicing nurses or fundamental education of students of the discipline, modern teaching and learning methods make educational efforts more available to a wide variety of individuals with a variety of educational and learning needs. It is therefore imperative that nursing educators understand relevant principles and theories to address these needs.

Key Points

- Curricula are created by faculty to fulfill their ideals of nursing education and to provide the community with effective, safe, well-educated nurses.
- Curricula are best organized around a guiding principle, be it a nursing theory or a collection of nursing and shared theories; the outcome is to provide the students with intellectual and clinical development as professional nurses.
- Nursing programs are evaluated and accredited by several bodies, including state boards of nursing, the American Association of Colleges of Nursing's Commission on Collegiate Nursing Education, and the National League for Nursing's Accrediting Commission.
- Experiential methods are being initiated to enhance learning using computerized and electronic means including clinical simulations and virtual reality classrooms.
- Innovations such as critical thinking, problem-based learning, and simulation are part of many nursing curricula.
- Learning environments have evolved. Today they include fully face-to-face, in-class learning; hybrid models in which some content is presented via web-based methods; and totally web-based courses in which all of the content is presented online.

Learning Activities

1. Select one of the courses in a nursing program and modify it to be delivered using some type of distance learning (e.g., Internet delivery, such as podcasting, or other innovative online methods). How will presentation of the material be accomplished? How will students interact with each other and with the instructor? What activities will be added? What activities will be deleted?
2. Search recent nursing literature for research on technology-based nursing education. Do these techniques appear to be as effective as traditional class work in ensuring that students achieve the goals or competencies of the nursing program?
3. Discuss the use of patient simulators in clinical nursing staff education. Consider the cost and upkeep of the equipment for simulators and faculty training and education, and the need for technical support of the equipment.

REFERENCES

American Association of Colleges of Nursing. (1999). A vision of baccalaureate and graduate nursing education: The next decade. *Journal of Professional Nursing, 15*(1), 59–65.

American Association of Colleges of Nursing. (2008). *Essentials of baccalaureate education.* Retrieved from http://www.aacn.nche.edu/education-resources/BaccEssentials08.pdf

Anderson, C. (2008). Simulation game playing—A nursing instructional strategy. *Clinical Simulation in Nursing Education, 4,* e7–e15.

Anderson, K. M., & Avery, M. D. (2008). Faculty teaching time: A comparison of web-based and face-to-face graduate nursing courses. *International Journal of Nursing Education Scholarship, 5*(1), 1–12, article 2.

Anderson, M. S., & Tredway, C. A. (2009). Transforming the nursing curriculum to promote critical thinking online. *Journal of Nursing Education, 48*(2), 111–115.

Ayer, M. (2013). Does simulation enhance nursing student's knowledge of skin and wound care? *Journal of Wound, Ostomy & Continence Nursing, 40*(3S), S82.

Azzaline, J. B. (2012). Creative strategies for a stand-along gerontology course for the nursing curriculum. *Nursing Education Perspectives, 33*(3), 199–200.

Barnum, B. S. (1998). *Nursing theory: Analysis, application, evaluation* (5th ed.). Philadelphia: Lippincott Williams & Wilkins.

Barnsteiner, J., Disch, J., Johnson, J., McGuinn, K., Chappell, K., & Swartwout, E. (2013). Diffusing QSEN competencies across schools of nursing: The AACN/RWJF Faculty Development Institutes. *Journal of Professional Nursing, 29*(2), 68–74.

Beckman, S. J., Boxley-Harges, S. L., & Kaskel, B. L. (2012). Experience informs: Spanning three decades with the Neuman systems model. *Nursing Science Quarterly, 25*(4), 341–346.

Bednash, G. P., Cronenwett, L., & Dolansky, M. A. (2013). QSEN: Transforming education. *Journal of Professional Nursing, 29*(2), 66–67.

Bently, G. W. (2004). Problem-based learning. In A. J. Lowenstein & M. J. Bradshaw (Eds.), *Fuszard's innovative teaching strategies in nursing* (3rd ed., pp. 83–106). Sudbury, MA: Jones & Bartlett.

Berbiglia, V. A. (2011). The self-care deficit nursing theory as a curriculum conceptual framework in baccalaureate education. *Nursing Science Quarterly, 24*(2), 137–145.

Berragan, L. (2011). Simulation: An effective pedagogical approach for nursing. *Nurse Education Today, 31*(6), 660–663.

Bevis, E. O. (1973). *Curriculum building in nursing: A process.* New York: National League for Nursing Press.

Bevis, E. O. (1987). History of curriculum development. In National League for Nursing, *Curriculum revolution: Mandate for change* (publication no. 15-2224, pp. 27–40). New York: National League for Nursing Press.

Bevis, E. O. (1989a). *Curriculum building in nursing: A process* (3rd ed., publication no. 15-2277). New York: National League for Nursing Press.

Bevis, E. O. (1989b). Illuminating the issues: Probing the past, a history of nursing curriculum development—The past shapes the present. In E. O. Bevis & J. Watson (Eds.), *Toward a caring curriculum: A new pedagogy for nursing* (publication no. 15-2278, pp. 13–35). New York: National League for Nursing Press.

Billings, D. M., & Kowalski, K. (2007). Using podcasts for nursing education. *Journal of Continuing Education in Nursing, 38*(2), 56–57.

Boland, D. L. (2012). Developing curriculum: Frameworks, outcomes and competencies. In D. M. Billings & J. A. Halstead (Eds.), *Teaching in nursing: A guide for faculty* (4th ed., pp. 138–159). St. Louis: Elsevier.

Boland, D. L., & Finke, L. M. (2012). Curriculum designs. In D. M. Billings & J. A. Halstead (Eds.), *Teaching in nursing: A guide for faculty* (4th ed., pp. 119–136). St. Louis: Elsevier.

Briggs, C. L. (2011). Engaging students using feature films. *Journal of Nursing Education, 50,* 360.

Burkhart, L., & Schmidt, W. (2012). Measuring effectiveness of a spiritual care pedagogy in nursing education. *Journal of Professional Nursing, 28*(5), 315–321.

Cannon, S., & Boswell, C. (2012). *Evidence-based teaching in nursing: A foundation for educators.* Sudbury, MA: Jones & Bartlett.

Carlson, K. L. (2012). Re-envisioning pediatric nursing education. *MCN, 37*(6), 379–385.

Carlson-Sabelli, L. L., Giddens, J. F., Fogg, L., & Fielder, R. A. (2011). Challenges and benefits of using a virtual community to explore nursing concepts among baccalaureate nursing students. *International Journal of Nursing Education Scholarship, 8*(1), 1–14.

Chan, Z. C. Y. (2012). Role-playing in the problem-based learning class. *Nurse Education in Practice, 12*(1), 21–27.

Chenot, T. M., & Daniel, L. G. (2010). Frameworks for patient safety in the nursing curriculum. *Journal of Nursing Education, 49*(10), 559–564.

Chiu, M., Polivka, B. J., & Stanley, S. A. R. (2011). Evaluation of a disaster-surge training for public health nurses. *Public Health Nursing, 29*(2), 136–142

Commission on Collegiate Nursing Education. (2009). *Standards for accreditation of baccalaureate and greater nursing education programs.* Washington, DC: American Association of Colleges of Nursing. Retrieved from http://www.aacn.nche.edu/ccne-accreditation/standards09.pdf

Cooper, C., & Carver, N. (2012). Problem-based learning in mental health nursing: The students' experience. *International Journal of Mental Health Nursing, 21*(2), 175–183.

Daack-Hirsch, S., Dieter, C., & Quinn-Griffin, M. T. (2011). Integrating genomics into undergraduate nursing education. *Journal of Nursing Scholarship, 43*(3), 223–230.

Delac, K., Blazier, D., Daniel, L., & Wilfong, D. (2013). Five alive: Using mock code simulation to improve responder performance during the first 5 minutes of a code. *Critical Care Nurse, 36*(2), 244–250.

DiBartolo, M. C., & Seldomridge, L. A. (2009). Cinemeducation: Teaching end-of-life issues using feature films. *Journal of Gerontological Nursing, 35*(8), 30–36.

DiBartolo, M. C., & Seldomridge, L. A. (2010). From community outreach to reaching students: Using public access television as an educational strategy. *Nurse Educator, 35*(3), 114–117.

Diekelmann, N. (1987). Curriculum revolution: A theoretical and philosophical mandate for change. In National League for Nursing, *Curriculum revolution: Mandate for change* (publication no. 15-2224, pp. 137–157). New York: National League for Nursing Press.

Dillard, N., & Siktberg, L. (2012). Curriculum development: An overview. In D. M. Billings & J. A. Halstead (Eds.), *Teaching in nursing: A guide for faculty* (4th ed., pp. 76–91). St. Louis: Elsevier.

Dreifuerst, K. T. (2012). Using debriefing for meaningful learning to foster development of clinical reasoning in simulation. *Journal of Nursing Education, 51*(6), 326–333.

Edmonds, M. L. (2011). Use of film in teaching multiculturalism to future nurse educators. *Journal of Nursing Education, 50,* 544.

Fetter, N. S. (2009). Curriculum strategies to improve baccalaureate nursing information technology outcomes. *Journal of Nursing Education, 48*(2), 78–85.

Flood, M. E. (2011). Best laid plans: A century of nursing curricula. In S. B. Keating (Ed.), *Curriculum development and evaluation in nursing* (2nd ed., pp. 5–31). Philadelphia: Lippincott Williams & Wilkins.

Friesth, B. M. (2012). Teaching and learning at a distance. In D. M. Billings & J. A. Halstead (Eds.), *Teaching in nursing: A guide for faculty* (4th ed., pp. 380–400). St. Louis: Elsevier.

Giarelli, E., & Reiff, M. (2012). Genomic literacy and competent practice: Call for research on genetics in nursing education. *Nursing Clinics of North America, 47*(4), 529–545.

Giddens, J. F., Wright, M., & Gray, I. (2012). Selecting concepts for a concept-based curriculum: Application of a bench mark approach. *Journal of Nursing Education, 51*(9), 511–515.

Guhde, J. (2010). Clinical decision-making: Using online exercise and patient simulation to improve students' clinical decision-making. *Nursing Education Perspectives, 31*(6), 387–389.

Halstead, J. A., & Billings, D. M. (2012). Teaching and learning in online learning communities, In D. M. Billings & J. A. Halstead (Eds.), *Teaching in nursing: A guide for faculty* (4th ed., pp. 401–421). St. Louis: Elsevier.

Hardin, P. K., & Richardson, S. J. (2012). Teaching the concept curricula: Theory and method. *Journal of Nursing Education, 51*(3), 155–159.

Heller, B. R., Oros, M. T., & Durney-Crowley, J. (2000). The future of nursing education: 10 trends to watch. *Nursing and Health Care Perspectives, 21*(1), 9–13.

Herrman, J. W. (2011). Keeping their attention: Innovative strategies for nursing education. *The Journal of Continuing Education in Nursing, 42*(10), 449–456.

Hill, T. L. (2012). The portfolio as a summative assessment for the nursing students. *Teaching and Learning in Nursing, 7*(1), 140–145.

Heise, B. & Himes, D. (2010). The course council: An example of student-centered learning. *Journal of Nursing Education, 49*(6), 343–345.

Hodson-Carlton, K. E. (2012). The learning resource center. In D. M. Billings & J. A. Halstead (Eds.), *Teaching in nursing: A guide for faculty* (4th ed., pp. 335–351). St. Louis: Elsevier.

Hogan, M., Kapralos, B., Cristancho, S., Finney, K., & Dubrowski, A. (2011). Bringing community health nursing education to life with serious games. *International Journal of Nursing Education Scholarship, 8*(1), 1–14.

Hsu, L. L., & Hsieh, S. I. (2011). Effects of a blended learning module on self-reported learning performances in baccalaureate nursing students. *Journal of Advanced Nursing, 67*(11), 2435–2444.

Institute of Medicine. (2011). *The future of nursing: Leading change, advancing health.* Washington, DC: National Academies Press.

Iwasiw, C. L., Goldenberg, D., & Andrusyszyn, M. A. (2009). *Curriculum development in nursing education* (2nd ed.). Sudbury, MA: Jones and Bartlett.

Jeffries, P. E. (2012). *Simulation in nursing education: From conceptualization to evaluation.* Philadelphia: Lippincott Williams & Wilkins.

Jeffries, P. R., & Clochesy, J. M. (2012). Clinical simulations: An experiential, student-centered pedagogical approach. In D. M. Billings & J. A. Halstead (Eds.). *Teaching in nursing: A guide for faculty,* (4th ed., pp. 352–368). St. Louis: Elsevier.

Kane, V. (2004). Example: Problem-based learning: The use of the exemplar family as the basis for learning health promotion and illness/injury prevention. In A. J. Lowenstein & M. J. Bradshaw (Eds.), *Fuszard's innovative teaching strategies in nursing* (3rd ed.). Sudbury, MA: Jones & Bartlett.

Keating, S. B. (2011a). Introduction to the history of curriculum development and curriculum approval process. In S. B. Keating (Ed.), *Curriculum development and evaluation in nursing* (2nd ed., pp. 1–4). Philadelphia: Lippincott Williams & Wilkins.

Keating, S. B. (2011b). Components of the curriculum. In S. B. Keating (Ed.), *Curriculum development and evaluation in nursing* (2nd ed., pp. 149–194). Philadelphia: Lippincott Williams & Wilkins.

Kelley, J. (1975). The conceptual framework in nursing education. In National League for Nursing, *Curriculum development, part VI: Curriculum revision in baccalaureate nursing education* (publication no. 15-1576, pp. 15–20). New York: National League for Nursing Press.

Knowles, M. S. (1980). *The modern practice of education: From pedagogy to androgogy* (2nd ed.). New York: Cambridge Books.

Kuhn, J., Hasbargen, B., & Miziniak, H. (2010). Pretest online discussion groups to augment teaching and learning. *CIN: Computers, Informatics, Nursing, 28*(5), 297–304.

Lewis, D. Y. (2012). Incorporating national priorities into the curriculum. *Journal of Professional Nursing, 28*(2), 105–109.

Mager, R. F. (1962). *Preparing instructional objectives.* Belmont, CA: Fearon Publishers.

McCormick, M. J., de Slavy, J. R., & Fuller, B. (2013). Embracing technology: Using an unfolding case simulation to enhance nursing student's learning about Parkinson disease. *Journal of Neuroscience Nursing, 45*(1), 14–20.

McEwen, M., & Brown, S. C. (2002). Conceptual frameworks in undergraduate nursing curricula: Report of a national survey. *Journal of Nursing Education, 41*(1), 5–14.

Meleis, A. I. (2012). *Theoretical nursing: Development and progress* (5th ed.). Philadelphia: Lippincott Williams & Wilkins.

Moreland, S. S., Lemieux, M. L., & Myers, A. (2012). End-of-life care and the use of simulation in a baccalaureate nursing program. *International Journal of Nursing Education Scholarship, 9*(1), 1–16.

National Council of State Boards of Nursing. (2011). *Nursing regulation; Boards of nursing contact information.* Retrieved from https://www.ncsbn.org/247.htm

National League for Nursing. (1972). *Criteria for the appraisal of baccalaureate and higher degree programs in nursing.* New York: National League for Nursing Press.

National League for Nursing. (1977). *Criteria for evaluation of educational programs in nursing leading to an associate degree* (5th ed.). New York: National League for Nursing Press.

National League for Nursing Accrediting Committee. (2013). *Standards and criteria.* Retrieved from http://www.acenursing.net/manuals/SC2013.pdf

Peterson, J. Z., Hennig, L. M., Dow, K. H., & Sole, M. L. (2001). Designing and facilitating class discussions in an internet class. *Nurse Educator, 26*(1), 28–32.

Powell, F. A. (2013). Using simulation training in a cardiothoracic intensive care unit. *AORN, 97*(6), 739–745.

Rentschler, D. D., & Spegman, A. M. (1996). Curriculum revolution: Realities of change. *Journal of Nursing Education, 35*(9), 389–393.

Robb, M. K. (2012). Managing a large class environment: simple strategies for new nurse educators. *Teaching and Learning in Nursing, 7*(1), 47–50.

Rowles, C. J. (2012). Strategies to promote critical thinking and active learning. In D. M. Billings & J. A. Halstead (Eds.), *Teaching in nursing: A guide for faculty* (4th ed., pp. 258–284). St. Louis, Elsevier.

Ruchala, P. L. (2011). Curriculum development and approval processes in changing educational environments. In S. B. Keating (Ed.), *Curriculum development and evaluation in nursing* (2nd ed.). New York: Springer.

Scales, F. S. (1985). *Nursing curriculum: Development, structure, function.* Norwalk, CT: Appleton-Century-Crofts.

Schams, K. A., & Kuennen, J. K. (2012). Clinical postconference pedagogy: Exploring evidence-based practice with millennial-inspired "building blocks." *Creative Nursing, 18*(1), 13–16.

Schmitt, T. L., Sims-Giddens, S. S., & Booth, R. G. (2012). Social media use in nursing education. *Online Journal of Issues in Nursing, 17*(3), 2.

Secrest, J. (2008). The role of tool development in an Orem-based curriculum. *Self-Care, Dependent Care and Nursing, 16*(2), 25–33.

Skiba, D. J. (2012). Technology and gerontology: Is this in your nursing curriculum? *Nursing Education Perspectives, 33*(3), 207–209.

Smith, S. J., & Barry, D. G. (2013). The use of high-fidelity simulation to teach home care nursing. *Western Journal of Nursing Research, 35*(3), 297–312.

Speziale, H. J. S., & Jacobson, L. (2005). Trends in registered nurse education programs 1998–2008. *Nursing Education Perspectives, 26*(4), 230–235.

Stanley, D., & Latimer, K. (2011). "The Ward": A simulation game for nursing students. *Nurse Education in Practice, 11*(1), 20–25.

Stapleton, V. (2009). End of life care skills are essential for all students. *Nursing Standard, 24*(1), 32–33.

Stokowski, L. A. (2011). Overhauling nursing education. *Medscape Nursing.* Retrieved from http://www.medscape.com/viewarticle/736236

Swanson, B., Zeller, J. M., Keithley, J. K., Fung, S. C., Johnson, A., Suhayda, R., et al. (2012). Case-based online modules to teach graduate-level nursing students about complementary and alternative medical therapies. *Journal of Professional Nursing, 28*(2), 125–129.

Tanner, C. A. (1989). An analysis of the historical and political background of the revision of the NLN's criteria for the appraisal of baccalaureate and higher degree programs. In N. Diekelmann, D. Allen, & C. Tanner (Eds.), *The NLN criteria for appraisal of baccalaureate programs: A critical hermeneutic analysis* (publication no. 15-2253, pp. 3–10). New York: National League for Nursing Press.

Tschannen, D., Aebersold, M., Sauter, C., & Funnell, M. M. (2013). Improving nurses' perceptions of competence in diabetes self-management education through the use of simulation and problem-based learning. *The Journal of Continuing Education in Nursing, 44*(6), 257–263.

Timmins, F., & Dunne, P. J. (2009). An exploration of the current use and benefit of nursing student portfolios. *Nurse Education Today, 29*(3), 330–341.

Wassef, M. E., Riza, L., Maciag, T., Worden, C., & Delaney, A. (2012). Implementing a competency-based electronic portfolio in a graduate nursing program. *CIN: Computers, Informatics, Nursing, 30*(5), 242–248.

Watson, M. J. (1996). Watson's theory of transpersonal caring. In P. H. Walker & B. Neuman (Eds.), *Blueprint for use of nursing models: Education, research, practice and administration* (publication no. 14-2696, pp. 141–186). New York: National League for Nursing Press.

Williams, J. K., Prows, C. A., Conley, Y. P., Eggert, J., Kirk, M., & Nichols, F. (2011). Strategies to prepare faculty to integrate genomics into nursing education programs. *Journal of Nursing Scholarship, 43*(3), 231–238.

Wong, F. K. Y., Cheung, S., Chung, L., Chan, K., Chan, A., To, T., et al. (2008). Framework for adopting a problem-based learning approach in a simulated clinical setting. *Journal of Nursing Education, 47*(11), 508–514.

Wu, R. R. (1979). Designing a curriculum model. *Journal of Nursing Education, 18*(3), 13–21.

Yehle, K. S., & Royal, P. A. (2010). Changing the postclinical conference: New time, new place, new methods equal success. *Nursing Education Perspectives, 31*(4), 256–258.

Zwirn, E. E., & Muehlenkord, A. (2012). Using media, multimedia, and technology-rich learning environments. In D. M. Billings & J. A. Halstead (Eds.), *Teaching in nursing: A guide for faculty* (4th ed., pp. 369–385). St. Louis: Elsevier.

CHAPTER 22

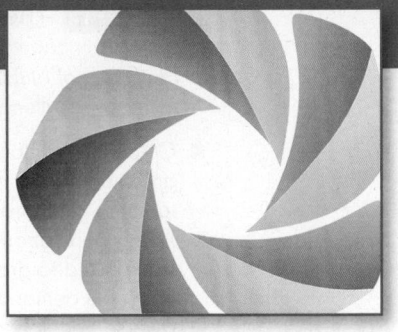

Future Issues in Nursing Theory

Melanie McEwen

Rebecca Jackson will graduate from a master's program in nursing in only a few weeks. She has learned a great deal about nursing practice, research, administration and management, and education from the various courses she has taken, and she is enthusiastic about the career opportunities she is considering. When she started the program, she was confident that she wanted to become a nurse administrator, but midway through her studies, she decided to focus on research. She ultimately wants to get a doctorate and become an educator and researcher.

Currently, Rebecca is working as a clinical supervisor at the public health department in a major metropolitan area. In the 10 years Rebecca has been with the health department, she has witnessed tremendous growth in the diversity of the population served. There are immigrant families from several Spanish-speaking countries, as well as from the Southeast Asian countries of Cambodia, Laos, Vietnam, and the Philippines. Recently, there has been an influx of refugees from Iraq, Croatia, Bosnia, and eastern Africa. Rebecca is intrigued by these groups' divergent perceptions of health and ways to promote health. Furthermore, she is concerned with communication issues and how to motivate health promotional practices. She has determined that this is particularly important in working with children and in teaching parents ways to improve their health.

In her position, Rebecca has had several opportunities to be involved in funded research. At present, she is working with a sociologist, an anthropologist, a clinical psychologist, and an epidemiologist to write a grant for a research project that will examine and compare health beliefs, health practices, and health promotional behaviors among various cultural groups in the city. The study will have multiple levels and phases and will incorporate both quantitative and qualitative data collection techniques and analysis.

Rebecca helped develop the conceptual framework for the study, which combines aspects of the Health Belief Model and Leininger's Culture Care Diversity Theory. The framework identifies cultural beliefs, practices, and values and incorporates them with knowledge of health threats and perceptions of illness severity, seriousness, and value for taking action. The researchers expect that the information provided by the study will allow the health department to develop a series of health programs that are sensitive to the needs, beliefs, and practices of the many cultural groups in the department's catchment area.

Box 22-1 The Future of Nursing—Health Care Challenges

In *The Future of Nursing*, the Institute of Medicine (IOM, 2011) identified five major "health care challenges" facing the U.S. health care system in the 21st century. These are:

- Chronic conditions (e.g., diabetes, hypertension, arthritis, cardiovascular disease, and mental health conditions): Prevalence of these conditions are expected to increase and to be exacerbated by growing rates of obesity.
- Aging population: The proportion of the U.S. population aged 65 years and older is expected to grow from 12.7% in 2008 to 19.3% in 2030. This will dramatically affect the demand for health care services.
- Diverse population: Minority groups are projected to increase from about a third of the U.S. population to 54% by 2042. Diversity involves various ethnic and racial groups, language, immigrant status, socioeconomic status, and other cultural features.
- Health disparities: Inequities in the burden of disease, injury, or death experienced by socially disadvantaged groups. Health disparities are not only partially caused by deleterious socioenvironmental conditions and behavior risk factors but may also be influenced by bias that results in unequal, inferior treatment.
- Limited English proficiency: Related to the increasingly diverse population is the problem of limited English proficiency. To be effective, health information must be accessible, understandable, and culturally relevant. Limited English proficiency and varying cultural and health practices contribute to the complex challenges that health care providers must address.

During the last two decades, a number of shifts occurred in the demographic patterns of the United States. This has been coupled with major changes in the health care delivery system and changes in the causes of illness, disability, and death. The Patient Protection and Affordable Care Act of 2010 (ACA) has contributed to the growing emphasis on health care financing, community-based care, health promotion, and access to care. Additionally, significant cost reductions, restructuring of health care services, and growth in integrated health care systems using managed care strategies are anticipated. Consequently, the increased severity of illness among persons in inpatient facilities and the increased incidence of chronic illnesses, particularly in the growing number of elderly, have taxed the health care system. Box 22-1 describes current and future health care challenges that the discipline of nursing and nursing science must recognize, understand, and address (Institute of Medicine [IOM], 2011).

In the face of system-wide changes associated with implementation of the ACA and other initiatives, major problems remain and must be addressed. For example, the health care system is not designed to provide convenient care to all who need it. The system is organized according to physicians' specialties and schedules, not according to the needs of their patients. Hospitals are used inappropriately, with access to care, supplemental insurance, and home care services still unevenly distributed.

There is also a growing need for health care providers, including nurses, who can meet the challenges of the changing system and evolving health and illness patterns. Nurses of the future must be capable of ensuring access to care and promoting high-quality outcomes. The American Association of Colleges of Nursing (AACN) (2008) has described the skills and practice capabilities currently expected for nurses (Box 22-2). In short, essential competencies include critical thinking and clinical judgment skills, ability to work in a variety of health care settings and with patients who have complex health problems, effective organizational and teamwork skills, understanding of evidence-based care, recognition of the influence of culture

Box 22-2 Competencies and Skills Needed by Generalist Nurses

Practice from a holistic, caring framework.
Practice from an evidence base.
Promote safe, quality patient care.
Use clinical/critical reasoning to address simple to complex situations.
Assume accountability for one's own and delegated nursing care.
Practice in a variety of health care settings.
Care for patients across the health–illness continuum.
Care for patients across the lifespan.
Care for diverse populations.
Engage in care of self in order to care for others.
Engage in continuous professional development.

Source: AACN (2008).

on health and ability to care for individuals from diverse backgrounds and across the lifespan; and a commitment to personal accountability and professional development.

The IOM's (2011) publication on the *Future of Nursing* has been viewed as a challenge and strategy to (1) make quality health care accessible to the diverse populations of the United States, (2) intentionally promote wellness and disease prevention, (3) improve health outcomes, and (4) provide compassionate care across the lifespan. The IOM goes on to describe a future health system in which:

- Primary care and prevention are central drivers.
- Interprofessional collaboration and coordination are the norm.
- Payment for services rewards value rather than volume.
- Quality care is affordable for individuals and society.

To plan for the future health care system, the discipline of nursing should give increasing attention to related theories, concepts, and models. Among these are primary health care (as opposed to "illness care"), health promotion, health protection, motivation, health as a resource for everyday life, health economics, patient safety, and quality of life. Frameworks for practice will embrace community-based and community-focused care, changing identification of the client (population/aggregate/group versus individual), interprofessional collaboration, noninstitutional care settings, innovation, technology transformation, and multiple levels of decision-making authority (Manojlovich, Barnsteiner, Bolton, Disch, & Saint, 2008; Porter-O'Grady & Malloch, 2011; Rutherford, 2008).

This chapter describes the current state and some of the anticipated changes that will affect the discipline of nursing during the next decade and examines how these changes will influence theory and knowledge development. Topics covered include future issues in nursing science and future issues in theory development. This is followed by an exploration of future theoretical issues related to nursing practice, research, administration and management, and education.

Future Issues in Nursing Science

Nursing science is concerned with answering questions of interest to the profession and adding to its body of knowledge. Knowledge development is accomplished through the study of concepts, relationships, and theories relevant to the discipline and generally occurs within the broad domain of one of the major worldviews of the discipline.

As discussed in Chapter 1, a paradigm is a pattern, model, or global concept accepted by most people in an intellectual community; it is a set of systematic beliefs or a worldview. Paradigms provide scientists with a general orientation to phenomena, a way of organizing perceptions, criteria for selecting problems, guidelines for investigations and methods, and limitations on possible solutions. The paradigm, or worldview, provides a guiding framework for resolving problems, conducting research, and deriving theories and laws in the discipline.

Nursing science has two predominant paradigms, broadly classified as empiricist and constructivist, which hold fundamentally opposing views of knowledge development and reality. Chapter 1 described the ongoing debate within the scientific nursing community about the appropriateness of the two philosophies and methodologies for directing and conducting research, as well as identifying questions of relevance to the discipline.

Most in the profession today find the philosophical debate inconclusive, frustrating, and not particularly germane to promoting nursing. Many scholars believe that nursing should emphasize the benefits of inquiry per se, rather than the supremacy of one paradigm over the other, because neither method is more scientific than the other, and the process of inquiry is the same despite the methods used to acquire knowledge (Chinn & Kramer, 2011; Norwood, 2010; Risjord, 2010).

In the 21st century, nursing science should work to eliminate obstacles to nursing research and promote acceptance of multiple methods of inquiry and use of research findings—or "translation"—in practice. Because the problems of nursing are so diverse, use of differing viewpoints and paradigms are needed to help answer questions and provide solutions to questions of interest. Because multiple perspectives encourage appreciation of the uniqueness of individuals, use of various perspectives will encourage identification of answers to important problems. Also, applying different viewpoints provides new insights that can help nurses formulate new ideas for study.

Combining or triangulating methods can maximize the strengths and minimize the weaknesses of each method and should be encouraged. Integration of qualitative and quantitative methods has been suggested as one way to advance nursing science because research traditions from both paradigms are complementary although the approaches are different. Qualitative methods can describe phenomena of interest in nursing and generate theories that propose relationships between identified concepts. Quantitative methods can test the relationships of qualitatively developed theories and suggest whether the theory should be accepted or revised (Bekhet & Zauszniewski, 2012; Norwood, 2010). Indeed, Chinn and Kramer (2011) observed that blending and using a variety of research processes and techniques in knowledge development indicates growing maturity in nursing scholarship. Nurses should be encouraged to be pragmatic regarding research methodology and use the right method for the task.

Future Issues in Nursing Theory

According to the AACN (2006, 2011) nurses in advanced practice should be prepared to critique, evaluate, and use theory. Nurses should be able to integrate and apply a wide range of theories from nursing and other sciences into a comprehensive and holistic approach to care. Thus, in addition to nursing theories, nurses prepared at the graduate level should be exposed to relevant theories from a wide range of fields, including natural sciences, social sciences, biologic sciences, and organizational

Box 22-3 Theoretical Knowledge and Skills for DNPs

The doctor of nursing practice (DNP) program prepares the graduate to:

1. Integrate nursing science with knowledge from ethics and the biophysical, psychosocial, analytical, and organizational sciences as the basis for the highest level of nursing practice.
2. Use science-based theories and concepts to:
   a. Determine the nature and significance of health and health care delivery.
   b. Describe actions and advanced strategies to enhance, alleviate, and ameliorate health and health care, and deliver phenomena as appropriate.
3. Evaluate outcomes. Develop and evaluate new practice approaches based on nursing theories and theories from other disciplines.

Source: AACN (2006, p. 9).

and management concepts. Basic theoretical knowledge and skills proposed by the AACN are listed in Box 22-3.

As explained in Chapter 2, the discipline of nursing is currently in the "integrated knowledge stage" of theory development. In this stage, there is an increasing emphasis on conducting research that will produce knowledge to support practice. Additionally, in this stage, there has been a shift in focus to application of "evidence" from across all health-related sciences (translational research). It is anticipated that the importance of middle range and situation-specific/practice theories will continue to be emphasized, and there will be less attention given to grand theories and conceptual frameworks. See Chapters 10, 11, 12, and 18 for detailed discussions of middle range, situation-specific theories, and evidence-based practice (EBP) guidelines.

In a study of nursing theory instructors in master's programs, McEwen (2000) identified the issues that were perceived as "essential" for graduate nursing students. These were, in order: introduction to theory, the relationship of theory and research, middle range theories, grand nursing theories, nursing's metaparadigm, theory analysis, concept analysis, and theory evaluation. This study also identified content that instructors felt was overemphasized in graduate theory courses. The most commonly cited content areas were grand nursing theories and theory development/theory construction. On the other hand, content that nursing theory instructors believed needed increased emphasis were application of theory in practice; middle range theory; and the interdependent relationship of theory, research, and practice with additional stress on the interrelationship with EBP.

Implications for Theory Development

The discipline of nursing has recognized several new trends for theory development. These include development of middle range theories, situation-specific (practice) theories, and EBP protocols/procedures as the latest steps in knowledge development.

There has been broad acceptance of the need to develop middle range theories to support nursing practice (Chinn & Kramer, 2011; Kim, 2010; Meleis, 2012; Smith & Liehr, 2014). This call for development of middle range theory is consistent with a desire to focus increased attention on substantive knowledge development. In the future, as additional middle range theories are developed, there will be a growing need to consider their analysis and evaluation (whether formal or informal). Indeed, nurses should direct considerable effort toward developing, testing, evaluating, and refining middle range theories to develop the discipline's substantive knowledge base.

In recent years, there has been enhanced attention to the application of theory in practice and the relationship of theory, practice, and research. Development of situation-specific (practice) theories and EBP models has consequently become increasingly emphasized (Chinn & Kramer, 2011; Im & Chang, 2012; Meleis, 2012). Furthermore, many nurse researchers use theories from other disciplines in their studies and, as a result, more emphasis and discussion should be given to borrowed theory, along with recognition that this practice does not negate the findings or make them less valuable to nursing.

It is important that nurses understand the interrelationship between theory, research, and practice and recognize the importance of this reciprocal relationship to the continuing development of nursing as a profession. In a practice discipline such as nursing, theory and practice are inseparable, and development and application of theory affiliated with research-based practice have been seen as fundamental to the development of professionalism and autonomous practice. Despite repeated calls to merge theory, practice, and research, there remains a confusing and fragmented mix. Progress has been made, however, because there has been increased emphasis on the interchange and interaction among research, clinical practice, and theory development. This trend should continue.

Theoretical Perspectives on Future Issues in Nursing Practice, Research, Administration and Management, and Education

With accessibility, cost containment, and provision of quality care driving health care reform, the discipline of nursing must anticipate how these forces will affect nursing within the changing health care system. With implementation of the ACA and other health system changes early in the 21st century, nurses are expected to assume a central role in helping to achieve cost-effective, quality health services. How these changes and related theoretical implications will affect nursing practice, nursing research, nursing administration and management, and nursing education are examined separately.

Future Issues and Nursing Practice

A transformation is occurring in nursing practice. This has been driven by socioeconomic factors as well as by developments in health care delivery. Many nursing leaders have identified relevant factors. Among these are changing demographics and increasing racial and ethnic diversity and related health disparities, the explosion of technology and information systems, globalization of the world's economy, more educated consumers, increasing acceptance and use of alternative therapies, explosion of genomic information, a shift to population-based care, and increasing complexity of care and concerns over end-of-life issues (IOM, 2011; Porter-O'Grady & Malloch, 2013; Risjord, 2010; Stokowski, 2011).

Increasingly, nurses are finding employment in home health and other ambulatory settings in which they provide care for well or chronically ill clients. These trends will most likely continue throughout the near future and, in response, nursing interventions will focus more on comprehensive assessment and care planning, case management, and client teaching to achieve the goals of health promotion, health maintenance, and disease prevention. Further, in the future, nurses will routinely use diagnosis and intervention databases, as well as expert systems, to assist with decision making.

Nurses, particularly advanced practice nurses (APNs), need to be prepared to function in some type of community-based health care system. They must be able to collaborate and cooperate within a multidisciplinary team and to demonstrate critical thinking and decision-making capabilities. They will be asked to resolve conflicts and effect health care at both the individual and aggregate level. Nurses must also have at least a basic knowledge of several disciplines, including public health, biostatics, and behavioral sciences. In addition, they must possess management and administrative skills. Specific nursing practice competencies needed for today's health care system were identified from a study of nurse administrators (Utley-Smith, 2004); these are shown in Table 22-1.

Theoretical Implications for Nursing Practice

Based on current and anticipated changes, a number of models, concepts, and theories need to be developed and applied in nursing practice and then studied and refined. New models should be based on community-based practice, population focus, case management, and interprofessional and interagency collaboration. Concepts and theories should be developed that focus on cultural competence, resource management, health promotion, risk reduction, motivation, management

Table 22-1 Nursing Practice Competencies for Today's Health Care System

Competency	Examples of Activities
Health promotion—Activities to enable clients to improve health, maximize health potential, and enhance well-being	Teach prevention and health promotion activities. Educate patients about lifestyle and its effect on health. Use community resources to enhance care. Advocate for policy change to promote health.
Supervision—Ability to coordinate the implementation of the plan of nursing care by ancillary or subordinate members of the health care team	Supervise ancillary nursing staff. Delegate and monitor work tasks of ancillary staff. Assume responsibility for personnel under direct supervision.
Interpersonal communication—Use relationship skills to work effectively on an interdisciplinary team	Organize daily routine in an efficient manner. Function as a participating member of the health care team. Function effectively in problem-solving situations. Apply effective communication skills. Collaborate with other members of the health care team.
Direct care—Appropriately use psychomotor and/or technical skills in delivering patient care	Administer medications. Perform activities of daily living (ADLs) for assigned patients. Perform major care tasks (e.g., catheterization, Levine tube insertion).
Computer technology—Ability to use electronic and technologic equipment to access, retrieve, and store information that assists in the delivery of effective care	Demonstrate computer literacy. Access and retrieve electronic data necessary for patient care. Use information technology to facilitate communication, manage data, and solve patient care problems.
Caseload management—Ability to coordinate care of a number of clients	Organize care for a group of 2–10 patients (depending on the nurse's experience and responsibilities, patient needs, and patient acuity)—involves direct care, time management, and resource management.

Source: Utley-Smith (2004).

of chronic diseases, normal aging, maternal–child welfare, and social epidemics, among others.

The concept of EBP has grown dramatically and will help fill the gap among research, theory, and practice (Chinn & Kramer, 2011; Jensen, 2012; Hudson, Duke, Haas, & Varnell, 2008; Walker & Avant, 2011). This focus on EBP should assist in the integration of research findings into clinical practice. As discussed in Chapter 12, EBP is relatively new in nursing because many nursing practices are based on experience, tradition, intuition, common sense, and untested theories. Although the encouragement to move to EBP is growing, implementation has been stalled somewhat. This is attributed to the delay in implementation of nursing research findings in practice. More effort will be needed to identify and define "best practices" and to communicate them to both providers and consumers of health care. As the conceptualization of EBP becomes more established within nursing, however, the relationship between EBP and theory must become more explicit. Nursing theorists and scholars should focus attention on melding middle range theory and EBP, and turn attention to recognizing the association between EBP and situation-specific or prescriptive theories.

Future Issues and Nursing Research

The new century challenges nursing research with many critical imperatives for improving health care. Health and illness challenges of the 21st century will necessitate reshaping health research as well as health care delivery. Likewise, the changes in the nation's population, its health needs and expectations, and changes in the health care financing will have a dramatic impact on the direction of nursing research. Changes in technology and hospital systems, changes in staffing patterns, and scientific emphasis in areas such as genetics must also be addressed in nursing research. Furthermore, greater emphasis must be placed on reporting nursing research activities and findings to other researchers, clinicians, the media, and the public (National Institute of Nursing Research [NINR], 2011).

During the last three decades, there has been a significant increase in the amount and quality of nursing research. In the last 10 years, research priorities focused on topics such as end-of-life/palliative care, chronic illness experiences (e.g., managing symptoms, avoiding complications of disease and disability, supporting family caregivers, and promoting health behaviors), quality of life, and quality of care. Additional areas of interest related to these themes as well as additional ones have been identified by the NINR (2011) for more focused study in the future (Table 22-2).

Theoretical Implications for Nursing Research

With the identification and promotion of these nursing research priorities, a number of concepts and theories should be studied and further developed over the next decade. These include such phenomena as transitions, quality of life, motivation, changing lifestyle habits, health promotion, symptom management, palliative care, economics of care, caregiver support, disparity, vulnerability, gender differences, informatics, telehealth, genetics, decision making and self-determination, and family interactions.

To improve health care and ultimately promote nursing science, nurses should continue developing and testing middle range and practice theories. They should test conceptual relationships and combine the study of concepts and relationships from various theories. Use of techniques such as meta-analysis and triangulation to synthesize findings will become increasingly important.

Table 22-2 Future Areas for Nursing Research Emphasis

Themes	Areas Targeted for Specific Study
Enhance health promotion and disease prevention.	Develop innovative behavior interventions to promote health and prevent illness in diverse populations and across the lifespan. Study the behavior of systems (e.g., family units, populations and/or organizations) that promote the development of personalized interventions. Improve the understanding of behavioral patterns and incentives for behavioral change. Develop and test models of lifelong preventive care. Create innovative communication strategies for individuals, families, clinicians, and communities that promote health and improve health literacy. Translate scientific advances to effect positive health behavioral change. Incorporate interdisciplinary, community, and other health care partnerships in the design or conduct of health promotion research.
Improve quality of life by managing symptoms of acute and chronic illness.	Improve knowledge of biologic and genomic mechanisms associated with symptoms and symptom clusters. Design interventions to improve the assessment and management of symptoms over disease trajectories. Study the multiple factors that influence the management of symptoms and apply this knowledge to design of personalized interventions. Develop strategies to improve self-management of chronic illness across the lifespan. Develop strategies to assist individuals and their caregivers in managing chronic illness, including analyses of caregiver burden and cost-effectiveness.
Improve palliative and end-of-life care.	Improve understanding of the complex issues and choices underlying palliative and end-of-life care. Develop and test biobehavioral interventions that provide palliative care for chronically ill individuals across the lifespan, including those from diverse populations. Develop and test strategies to minimize the physical and psychological burden on caregivers, particularly when the person for whom they are caring nears the end of life. Determine the impact of providers trained in palliative and end-of-life care on health care outcomes. Create new communication strategies among clinicians, patients, families, and communities to promote decision making regarding complex treatment and care options in the face of life-threatening illness.
Enhance innovation in science and practice.	Develop new technologies and informatics-based solutions that promote health, including comprehensive high-throughput technologies. Develop and apply new and existing knowledge to the implementation of health information technology, including electronic health records. Expand knowledge and application of health care technologies to facilitate decision support, self-management, and access to health care. Use genetic and genomic technologies to advance knowledge of the "symptom," including the biologic underpinnings of symptoms associated with chronic illness. Encourage risk taking, innovation, reinvention, and creativity including high-risk/high-return concepts.
Develop the next generation of nurse scientists.	Support ongoing development of investigators at all stages of their research careers. Facilitate more rapid advancement from student to scientist. Recruit and enlist young nurse investigators, including those from underrepresented communities. Support innovative models of trans-institutional learning and interdisciplinary training to leverage the research experience of other scientists in different fields of study. Expand research knowledge through established infrastructures including Web-based workshops, summer institutes, and virtual training methods. Mobilize technology to form global partnerships with international schools of nursing in scientific areas central to NINR's mission.

Source: NINR (2011).

Box 22-4 Issues Affecting Nursing Administration and Management in the Future

- Cost of health care
- Challenge of managed care
- Impact of health policy and regulation
- Interdisciplinary education for collaborative practice
- Nursing shortage
- Opportunities for lifelong learning and workforce development
- Significant advances in nursing science and research

Source: Roy (2000)

Future Issues and Nursing Leadership and Administration

A number of issues and developments will dramatically affect nursing leadership and administration in the future (Box 22-4). Concerns about health care costs affect nursing by determining how work is organized and treatment planned, and influencing clients' perception of, and participation in, care. Calls for significant change in health care financing will dramatically change reimbursement mechanisms. With implementation of the ACA, there will be an increase in state and federal regulations related to costs, care coordination, and managed care, and states will continue to define, measure, and assess quality and serve as contractors for corporate entities while enforcing accountability of health care providers, insurance companies, and managed care organizations.

Case management will lead to greater levels of interprofessional and collaborative practice. Addressing problems related to the anticipated nursing shortage and the essential need to promote integration of care through systems thinking and collaboration among health teams and changes in practice models to promote autonomy, empowerment, and professional development are particularly important issues facing nursing administrators (Ellis & Hartley, 2012; Huston, 2010; Porter-O'Grady & Malloch, 2013).

In nursing administration, collaboration and care coordination will be increasingly important with enhanced efforts to contain the costs associated with managing complex client needs, particularly within the context of implemention of the ACA. As a result, there should be some degree of interdisciplinary competence in all health professions. This will necessitate corresponding changes in leadership and management priorities that promote unity and collaboration. Competencies needed by future nurse managers include leadership skills, financial/budgeting knowledge, business acumen, communication skills, technology understanding, human resource and labor relations skills, as well as collaboration and team building skills.

Nursing administrators must be able to identify institutional strengths and weaknesses and to assess human resources and environmental issues. Nursing administrators should also focus on maximizing human potential and accountability and work to encourage growth and development of employees. There is a need to use proven motivational techniques to encourage both staff and clients. The challenge is to integrate services in an efficient and effective way to improve care outcomes, while managing costs and meeting satisfaction needs.

Theoretical Implications for Nursing Administration and Management

For the future, models of care delivery must be developed that will achieve desired client outcomes and contribute to staff satisfaction, retention, and productivity.

Furthermore, these models must contribute to the financial integrity of the organization for which they are developed because there is a need to make the system efficient and cost effective, while ensuring quality care. Data management and processing of information are essential in every area, and administrators must be able to quantify changes in client acuity and to provide exact information about clients.

Models of care should provide greater integration of health services, more intense management of services, an increase in outcome-oriented management, and an increase in ambulatory and community-based health care. There will also be an increased emphasis on bioinformatics and communication skills, and health care financing will continue to be of paramount importance. Concepts to be developed and examined in nursing administration and management include cost, value, competency, utilization, quality measurement, productivity, innovation, integration, safety, and outcomes (Porter-O'Grady & Malloch, 2013; Rutherford, 2008). Quinless and Elliot (2000) recommended that nursing students and administrators learn to apply basic economic theories and concepts and be aware of the costs involved in providing complex health care for the growing population. They also suggested that nurses understand how to balance care and cost and design cost-effective health care delivery. Finally, all nurses should constantly consider the ethical considerations that underlie health services.

Future Issues and Nursing Education

In the past, nursing education supported passive learning, using structured, professional instruction and supervised practice. Nursing students have been socialized using mechanistic, rigid standards, where faculty demand that they meet the minimum standards of objective-based learning. To survive in the highly complex, challenging, and rapidly changing health care system, however, it will be increasingly important for nurses to use and apply creative and critical thinking skills. Nursing leaders have recognized that significant changes are needed in nursing education to promote these skills. Further, issues such as the shortage of nursing faculty, coupled with a serious shortage of nurses educated to teach nursing, the growing acceptance of virtual education and simulation, the increase in nontraditional students, the explosion of accelerated programs, and the widespread acceptance of the doctor of nursing practice (DNP) degree have challenged previous nursing education models and traditions (Billings & Halstead, 2012; Dahnke & Dreher, 2011; IOM, 2011; Stokowski, 2011).

In recent years, nurse educators have been called to review old assumptions and methods for educating nurses. Because nurses must be able to think critically and independently, content and learning experiences must be revamped to produce graduates with the competencies needed for current and future practice. A nationwide study for nursing education programs (Speziale & Jacobson, 2005) identified several content areas that will need enhanced emphasis now and in the future. These include diversity, informatics, and EBP. Furthermore, nursing educators expect to place greater emphasis in use of distance learning and Internet course simulations, case studies, active learning strategies, concept mapping, computer-assisted instruction, and virtual reality simulations in nursing programs in the future. Other teaching strategies or modalities that will be used increasingly in the future include LISTSERV email lists, problem-based learning, simulation, e-learning, mentoring, and videoconferencing.

To support these changes, nursing educators need to teach thinking skills as well as content. They should use active learning strategies to foster student responsibility for learning. They may restructure clinical experiences and change content to place less emphasis on hospital experiences and narrow medical specialty areas to de-emphasize illness care and emphasize wellness care. In addition, nursing students must learn to evaluate the effectiveness of nursing interventions.

Suggestions for curricular changes in future nursing education include increased emphasis on the process and procedure of learning (Benner, Sutphen, Leonard, & Day, 2010; Stokowski, 2011; Tanner, 2007). Among the recommendations are these: Integrate teaching and learning in classroom and clinical settings more effectively, shift to competency-based curricula, focus on "knowledge management," and promote interprofessional education. Other suggestions to broaden understanding include encouraging the use of group work to promote communication and social skills, and increasing use of projects that require months to complete to enhance understanding of the complexity of the real world as well as providing greater diversity in clinical experiences,. The Link to Practice 22-1 presents recommendations of the IOM of changes in nursing education to meet current and future health care needs.

Theoretical Implications for Nursing Education

Rather than teach traditional specialties (e.g., maternity nursing, pediatrics, psychiatric nursing), nursing educational programs in the future should stress essential concepts, theories, and models. These should include issues such as aging and care of elders, aspects of pharmacology, human growth and development, vulnerable populations, genetics, complementary and alternative therapies, environmental health issues, health policy, palliative care, and culture. Models should incorporate high-tech care, EBP, and patient safety. Pathophysiology of chronic illnesses, health promotion, disease prevention, self-care, community health care, decision making, change processes, and management and leadership models should also be part of nursing curricula (AACN, 2008; Benner et al, 2010; IOM, 2011; Stokowski, 2011).

Curricula should shift from being primarily content driven and controlled by the faculty to being outcome driven and focused on the needs of the learner, the profession, and the public. A diversity of theoretical and practice experiences should be encouraged, and experiences should include involvement in discharge planning, caring for clients in outpatient and ambulatory care settings, assisting families in well-baby clinic visits, and assisting individuals in gaining access to community resources. Further, interprofessional learning and collaborative practice experiences are essential.

Content for nursing education in the future should include leadership development, critical thinking and problem-solving skills, EBP, clinical competency in a variety of settings, collaboration and communication, outcomes focus, cultural competence, and appreciation of research directed toward practice and educational evaluation. Other concepts to be stressed in nursing education programs are safety, teaching and learning, health promotion, illness prevention, lifelong learning, and professional development.

Experiential knowledge and active participation in learning can lead to the development of a knowledge base and a better ability to think critically and independently. Contemporary educational systems must provide opportunities for students to practice and use critical and creative processes within their basic nursing education. Programs should emphasize group and resource management, organizational and leadership skills, clinical management and coordination, technologic capabilities, and professional judgment.

Link to Practice 22-1

Recommendations From the IOM

Transforming Nursing Education

- Nursing education needs to provide understanding of, and experience in, care management, quality improvement methods, systems change management, and reconceptualized roles of nurses in a reformed health care system.
- Nursing education should serve as a platform for continued lifelong learning and include opportunities for seamless transition to higher degree programs.
- Accrediting, licensing, and certifying organizations need to mandate demonstrated mastery of core skills and competencies to complement the completion of degree programs and written board examinations.
- The nursing student body must become more diverse in response to underrepresentation of racial and ethnic minority groups and men in the nursing workforce.
- Nurses should be educated with physicians and other health professionals as students and throughout their careers.

Transforming Nursing Practice

Among the recommendations from the IOM with regard to practice are the following. Nurses can:

Improve access to primary care—APNs can be utilized to build the primary care workforce as access to coverage, service settings, and services increase under the ACA.

Improve quality of care—Nurses are crucial in preventing medication errors, reducing infection, and facilitating transition from hospital to home.

Create new opportunities for nurses in new and expanded capacities. Suggestions include:

- Accountable care organizations—a group of primary care providers, a hospital, and perhaps some specialists who share the risk and rewards of providing care at a fixed reimbursement rate.
- Medical/health homes—a specific type of primary care practice that coordinates and provides comprehensive care; promotes a relationship between patient and provider; and measures, monitors, and improves quality of care.
- Community health centers—clinics that provide high-value, quality primary and preventive care in poor and underserved areas.
- Nurse-managed health centers—clinics run by nurses and including other professionals such as physicians, social workers, health educators, and outreach workers as part of a collaborative team. Services include primary care, family planning, mental/behavior care, and health promotion.
- Information technology—Develop technology to aid providers to plan, deliver, document, and review clinical care.

IOM, 2011

Summary

Increasingly, nurses will be coordinators of teams of care, where they will manage multiskilled workers and share accountability for clinical and financial outcomes. They will need to become adept at care coordination, delegation, interprofessional collaboration, standards setting, and outcomes monitoring across the continuum of care. For the future, it is important that the discipline continue to develop the broad knowledge base of nursing and work to understand the integration of theory, research, and practice. Additionally, the discipline should recognize how this reciprocal arrangement affects nursing practice, administration and management, and education.

Rebecca, the nurse in the opening case study, recognized some of the changes described in this chapter (e.g., increasing cultural diversity, the need to focus on health promotion, communication challenges) and wanted to address them in her practice and research. She also understood that to respond to these changes, she had much to learn about issues in nursing practice, research, administration and management, and education, particularly related to theory and development of nursing science.

Nurses are committed to a holistic view of the person, and as the health profession with the largest number of providers, nursing has the potential to have the greatest impact on health and health care delivery. But to prepare for the future, nurses must more clearly identify and communicate what they do. Ongoing development, application, analysis, and evaluation of concepts, principles, theories, and models are vital to this process; nurses must be encouraged to continue these activities to develop the discipline.

Key Points

- As the health care delivery system changes and evolves in response to changes in demographics, health care needs, and health care financing, the discipline of nursing must respond.
- The Institute of Medicine's landmark report *The Future of Nursing* provides guidelines and recommendations for nursing to meet the health needs of individuals, families, groups, and populations in the future.
- In the future, nursing theory will increasingly focus on development, application and testing of middle range theories, situation-specific theories, and EBP protocols as the latest steps in knowledge development.
- Nursing practice will be dramatically influenced by changes in the health system subsequent to full implementation of the ACA as well as other system changes. Practice models will increasingly be community based and population focused. Interprofessional collaboration will be encouraged. Attention will be on concepts/needs including health promotion, resource management, informatics, and case management.
- Nursing research will focus more on "mixed-methods" or combining or triangulating research methods that will more completely and accurately address the complex issues and clients found in contemporary health care. Themes for enhanced research and related theory development include interventions for health promotion, symptom management, end-of-life issues, effective use of technology, and development of future nursing scientists.
- Nursing leadership and administration will need to address such pressing issues as quality and safety, cost management, collaboration, and the need to effectively integrate care. Cultivation of communication skills, leadership skills, technology acumen, and knowledge of human resources and economics are vital.

- Nursing education for the future will incorporate changes in modes of delivery including increasing use of simulation and better, more focused integration of clinical and classroom learning. Competency-based curricula, lifelong learning, and seamless academic progression will all be stressed.
- In the future, nurses must more clearly identify and communicate what they do through development, application, analysis, and evaluation of concepts, principles, theories, and models.

Learning Activities

1. Talk to a nurse administrator, a nurse educator, a nurse researcher, and an APN (nurse practitioner or clinical nurse specialist) about future issues in nursing and health care delivery. What changes do they anticipate in the next few years? How should currently practicing nurses prepare for future changes?
2. Select a nursing journal that deals primarily with education, research, or administration (e.g., *Journal of Nursing Education, Nursing Research, Journal of Nursing Administration*), and review issues from the past 3 years to analyze trends. What are the "hot topics"? Can any predictions be made for future issues?
3. Select a nursing journal that primarily discusses scholarly issues or topics related to nursing science (e.g., *Advances in Nursing Science, Image: Journal of Nursing Scholarship*) and review issues from the past 3 years to analyze trends. What are the "hot topics"? Can any predictions be made for future issues?
4. Select a nursing specialty journal (e.g., *MCN The American Journal of Maternal Child Nursing, Pediatric Nursing, Journal of Community Health Nursing*) that is primarily concerned with practice and review issues from the past 3 years to analyze trends. What are the "hot topics"? Can any predictions be made for future issues.
5. Join a LISTSERV related to an advanced nursing role (e.g., education, administration, advanced practice) to examine current issues and to communicate with members about future issues.

REFERENCES

American Association of Colleges of Nursing. (2006). *The essentials of doctoral education for advanced nursing practice.* Washington, DC: Author. Retrieved from http://www.aacn.nche.edu/publications/position/DNPEssentials.pdf

American Association of Colleges of Nursing. (2008). *The essentials of baccalaureate education for professional nursing practice.* Washington, DC: Author. Retrieved from http://www.aacn.nche.edu/education-resources/BaccEssentials08.pdf

American Association of Colleges of Nursing. (2011). *The essentials of master's education in nursing.* Washington, DC: Author. Retrieved from http://www.aacn.nche.edu/education-resources/MastersEssentials11.pdf

Bekhet, A., & Zauszniewski, J. (2012). Methodological triangulation: An approach to understanding data. *Nurse Researcher, 20*(2), 40–43.

Benner, P., Sutphen, M., Leonard, V., & Day, L. (2010). *Educating nurses: A call for radical transformation.* San Francisco, CA: Jossey-Bass.

Billings, D. M., & Halstead, J. A. (2012). *Teaching in nursing: A guide for faculty* (4th ed.). Philadelphia: Elsevier.

Chinn, P. L., & Kramer, M. K. (2011). *Theory and nursing: Integrated knowledge development* (8th ed.). St. Louis: Mosby.

Dahnke, M. D., & Dreher, H. M. (2011). *Philosophy of science for nursing practice: Concepts and application.* New York: Springer.

Ellis, J. R., & Hartley, L. (2012). *Nursing in today's world: Trends, issues and management.* Philadelphia: Lippincott Williams & Wilkins.

Hudson, K., Duke, G., Haas, B., & Varnell, G. (2008). Navigating the evidence-based practice maze. *Journal of Nursing Management, 16*(6), 409–416.

Huston, C. J. (2010). *Professional issues in nursing: Challenges & opportunities* (2nd ed). Philadelphia: Lippincott Williams & Wilkins.

Im, E. O., & Chang, S. J. (2012). Current trends in nursing theories. *Journal of Nursing Scholarship, 44*(2), 156–164.

Institute of Medicine. (2011). *The future of nursing: Leading change, advancing health.* Washington, DC: The National Academies Press.

Jensen, E. (2012). Linking theory, research and practice. In N. A. Schmidt & J. M. Brown (Eds.), *Evidence-based practice for nurses: Appraisal and application of research* (2nd ed., pp. 122–139). Sudbury, MA: Jones and Bartlett.

Kim, H. S. (2010). The nature of theoretical thinking in nursing (3rd ed.). New York: Springer.

Manojlovich, M., Barnsteiner, J., Bolton, L. B., Disch, J., & Saint, S. (2008). Nursing practice and work environment issues in the 21st century. *Nursing Research,* 57(1S), S11–S14.

McEwen, M. (2000). Teaching theory at the master's level: Report of a national survey of theory instructors. *Journal of Professional Nursing, 16*(6), 354–361.

Meleis, A. I. (2012). *Theoretical nursing: Development and progress* (5th ed.). Philadelphia: Lippincott Williams & Wilkins.

National Institute of Nursing Research. (2011). *NINR strategic plan: Bringing science to life.* Retrieved from https://www.ninr.nih.gov/sites/www.ninr.nih.gov/files/ninr-strategic-plan-2011.pdf

Norwood, S. L. (2010). *Research essentials: Foundations for evidence-based practice.* Upper Saddle River, NJ: Pearson Education.

Porter-O'Grady, T., & Malloch, K. (2011). *Quantum leadership: Advancing innovation, transforming health care* (3rd ed.). Sudbury, MA: Jones & Bartlett.

Porter-O'Grady, T., & Malloch, K. (2013). *Leadership in nursing practice: Changing the landscape of health care.* Sudbury, MA: Jones & Bartlett.

Quinless, F. W., & Elliot, N. L. (2000). The future in health care delivery: Lessons from history, demographics, and economics. *Nursing and Health Care Perspectives, 21*(2), 84–89.

Risjord, M. (2010). *Nursing knowledge: Science, practice and philosophy.* Oxford, United Kingdom: Wiley-Blackwell.

Roy, C. (2000). A theorist envisions the future and speaks to nursing administrators. *Nursing Administration Quarterly, 24*(2), 1–12.

Rutherford, M. M. (2008). The how, what and why of valuation and nursing. *Nursing Economics, 26*(6), 347–352.

Smith, M. C., & Liehr, P. R. (2014). Preface. In M. J. Smith & P. R. Liehr (Eds.), *Middle range theory for nursing* (3rd ed., pp. xiii–xvi). New York: Springer.

Speziale, H. J. S., & Jacobson, L. (2005). Trends in registered nurse education programs 1998–2008. *Nursing Education Perspectives, 26*(4), 230–235.

Stokowski, L. A. (2011). *Overhauling nursing education.* Medscape today news. Retrieved from http://www.medscape.com/viewarticle/736236

Tanner, C. A. (2007). The curriculum revolution revisited. *Journal of Nursing Education, 46*(2), 51–52.

Utley-Smith, Q. (2004). Five competencies needed by new baccalaureate graduates. *Nursing Education Perspectives, 25*(4), 166–170.

Walker, L. O., & Avant, K. (2011). *Strategies for theory construction in nursing* (5th ed.). Upper Saddle River, NJ: Pearson Education.

GLOSSARY

Adaptation The ability of the body to incorporate different ways of working as a result of changes in bodily makeup, chemistry, or the environment.

Agent In epidemiology, refers to those factors, such as biologic organisms, chemical agents, or physical factors, whose presence or absence can result in disease in the host.

Andragogy Description of Knowles' theory of adult learning. Knowles believed that the most important thing in helping adults to learn is to create a climate of physical comfort, mutual trust and respect, openness, and acceptance of differences.

Antecedent That which necessarily goes before; a cause that must precede an effect. For example, the presence of food on the table is antecedent to dinner.

Assumptions Beliefs about phenomena one must accept as true to accept a theory about the phenomenon as true; they cannot be empirically testable.

Beck's Postpartum Depression Theory Proposes interventions to alert nurses to the incidence and impact of postpartum depression. The model stresses the importance of identifying new mothers who might be suffering from postpartum depression and suggested interventions.

Behavioral learning theories Referred to as the stimulus–response (S–R) models of learning. Some of the major behaviorist theorists include Thorndike (connectionism), Pavlov (classical conditioning), Skinner (operant conditioning), Watson (behaviorism), and Hull (reinforcement).

Behavioral systems model Dorothy Johnson's human needs-based model.

Benner's Model of Skill Acquisition in Nursing Pat Benner's theoretical model, which outlines and explains five stages of skill acquisition in nursing: novice, advanced beginner, competent, proficient, and expert.

Cancer theory Theory that cancer begins with an event that leaves a cell premalignant; this is followed by a number of promotional steps that increase the potential for an initiated cell to become malignant.

Caring Science as Sacred Science Jean Watson's theory of nursing that incorporates spiritual dimensions of nursing with the ideals of the unitary process theories but reflects the interactive processes of nursing.

Change In a system, a state of flux which can elicit feeling of uncertainty, anxiety, and upheaval.

Chaos theory The study of unstable, aperiodic behavior in deterministic (nonrandom), nonlinear, dynamic systems. Chaos theory focuses on finding the underlying order in the apparent disorder of natural and social systems and understanding how change occurs in nonlinear dynamical systems over time.

Cognitive behavioral theory (Beck) Behavior theory based on the observation that biased cognitions are faulty; these thoughts are labeled *cognitive distortions.*

Cognitive development theories (interaction theories) Assume that behavior, mental processes, and the environment are interrelated. Cognitive development theories are concerned with the progressive development and changes in thinking, reasoning, and perception of individual learners. A major assumption of cognitive theories is that learning is experiential and occurs as a sequential process, over time. Major cognitive development theorists include Piaget, Gagne, Perry, and Bandura.

Cognitive distortions Habitual errors in thinking that are formed in the conscious mind. These distorted cognitions create a false basis for beliefs, particularly regarding the self; influence one's basic attitude about the self; and may lead to inaccurate conclusions about the self.

Cognitive-field (Gestalt) theories View that considers learning to be closely related to perception. In Gestalt theory, learning is seen in terms of reorganization of the learner's perceptual or psychological world—his or her field. The field includes a simultaneous and mutual interaction among all the forces or stimuli affecting the person. Experience is the interaction of a person and his or her perceived environment, whereas behavior is the result of the interplay of these forces. Consequently, perception and experiences of reality are uniquely individual, based on a person's total life experiences. Learning is the process of discovering and understanding the relationships among people, things, and ideas in the field.

Cognitive learning theories Group of theories that explain that learning relies on the assimilation of facts and information that can be tested by having the person repeat the facts, steps, reasons, and information back to the teacher and act on the knowledge gathered.

Cognitive restructuring The process of changing cognitive distortions.

Comfort Theory Katherine Kolcaba's theory, which explains that patients experience needs for comfort in stressful health care situations. These needs are identified by the nurse, who then seeks to implement interventions to meet them.

Concept A word or term that refers to phenomena that occur in nature or thought; formulated in words that enable people to communicate meaning about reality in the world.

Concept analysis Explores the meaning of concepts to promote understanding.

Concept development The rigorous process of bringing clarity to the definition of concepts used in science.

Conceptual framework A set of interrelated concepts that symbolically represents and conveys a mental image of a phenomenon.

Conceptual model A set of interrelated concepts that symbolically represents and conveys a mental image of a phenomenon.

Concrete terms That which can be known by human senses, measurable, visible by some means, often predictable.

Conflict theories Centered on the observation that in human societies, elements of inequality, power/authority, domination/subjugation, interests, and conflict are common. These elements result in "conflicts" that may potentially change the society.

Consequence The result or outcome of a situation or action.

Conservation Model Myra Levine's model, which focuses on the interactions of nurse and client and considers multiple factorial interactions to produce predictable results using probability as the reality.

Construct A complex concept composed of more than one concept and typically built or "constructed" to fit a purpose.

Critical social theory Uses societal awareness to expose social inequalities that keep people from reaching their full potential. Proponents of critical social theory maintain that social exchanges should stimulate the evolution to a more just society.

Cultural bias Interpreting and judging phenomena in relation to one's own culture (e.g., racism, sexism, classism, and ageism).

Culture Care Diversity and Universality Theory Madeline Leininger's theory, which recognizes and demonstrates to nurses the importance of considering the impact of culture on health and healing. Major concepts of the model are culture, culture care, and culture care differences (diversities) and similarities (universals) pertaining to transcultural human care.

Curriculum The content and processes by which learners gain knowledge and understanding; develop skills; and alter attitudes, appreciation, and values under the auspices of a given school or program.

Curriculum conceptual framework An interrelated system of premises that provides guidelines or ground rules for making all curricular decisions—objectives, content, implementation, and evaluation.

Descriptive theories Theories that describe, observe, and name concepts, properties, and dimensions but don't generally explain the interrelationships among the concepts or propositions.

Discipline Distinctions between bodies of knowledge found in academic settings; a branch of education instruction or a department of learning or knowledge.

Disease causation A force or factor that contributes to a condition that disturbs the normal functioning of an organism; failure of an organism to respond to or adapt to its environment, leading to a disease state.

Driving forces In Planned Change Theory, driving forces encourage or facilitate movement to a new direction, goal, or outcome.

Dynamical In chaos theory, it refers to the time-varying behavior of a system.

Emotional intelligence (EI) Refers to the ability to manage one's self and one's relationships effectively. EI includes understanding one's own feelings, sensitivity, and empathy for others and the regulation of emotions.

Empiricism Philosophical school of thought that values observation, perception by senses, and experience as sources of knowledge. Empiricism is founded on the belief that what is experienced is what exists; these experiences must be verified through scientific methodology.

Empowerment The transfer or delegation of responsibility and authority from managers to employees; the sharing of power, vision, mission, knowledge, expertise, decision making, and resources necessary for employees to reach organizational goals.

Environment In grand nursing theory, the external elements that affect the person; internal and external conditions that influence the organism; significant others with whom the person interacts; and an open system with boundaries that permit the exchange of matter, energy, and information with human beings.

Environment/environmental factors In the epidemiologic triangle, refers to events, physical elements or properties, biologic entities (e.g., animals, plants), or social/economic considerations that may influence whether an individual will develop a disease.

Epidemiologic triangle Classic epidemiologic model frequently used to illustrate the interrelationships among the host, agent, and environment with regard to disease causation. A change in any of the three components can result in the disease process.

Epistemology Study of knowledge or ways of knowing; how people come to have knowledge.

Evidence The facts that lead to the belief in the truth about a situation.

Evidence-based practice An approach to problem solving that conscientiously uses the current "best" evidence in the care of patients. Evidence-based practice involves identifying a clinical problem, searching the literature, critically evaluating the research evidence, and determining appropriate interventions.

Evidence-based nursing The integration of nursing theory with the best available research evidence as well as the expertise of the nurses, the available resources including professional expertise along with patient-family preferences, and quality improvement findings.

Exhaustion Final stage of the stress response in Selye's work in which the body has exhausted all its resources and a diseased state can occur.

Exchange theories Theories based on utilitarianism, which supports the notation that maximization of each individual's satisfaction automatically leads to maximum satisfaction of the wants of all. In exchange theories, individuals are motivated to maximize material benefits from exchanges with others.

Exemplar An item that is exactly what a concept or idea is about; a true example of the concept.

Explanatory theories Theories that relate concepts to one another and describe and specify associations or interrelations between and among concepts.

Feminist theories Based on the observation that gender differences and subordination have traditionally been viewed as both natural and inevitable. A core assumption in feminist theories is that women are oppressed and that gender is socially constructed and tends to justify the subordination and exploitation of women.

Fight-or-flight response First stage of stress response in Selye's work; alarm reaction that mobilizes the body's defense forces, putting the body in a state of disequilibrium.

Gate control theory (GCT) Theory that posits that a gating mechanism occurs in the spinal cord. Pain impulses are transmitted from the periphery of the body by nerve fibers, and the impulses travel to the dorsal horns of the spinal cord, specifically to the area of the cord called the *substantia gelatinosa*. The cells of the *substantia gelatinosa* can inhibit or facilitate pain impulses, and if the activity of the transmission cells is inhibited, the gate is closed and impulses are less likely to be conducted to the brain. The GCT suggests that if pain medication is administered before the onset of pain (i.e., before the gate is opened), it will help keep the gate closed longer and fewer pain impulses will be allowed to pass through.

General adaptation syndrome (GAS) Selye's work that explains the physiologic responses to stress in three stages: "fight-or-flight syndrome," resistance, and exhaustion.

General systems theory (GST) A "grand" theory that explains that systems are composed of both structural and functional components that interact within a boundary that filters the type and rate of exchange with the environment. Input, throughput, output, and feedback are common to systems. One basic tenet of GST is that systems are composed of subsystems, each with its own function systems. Also, systems contain energy and matter and may be open or closed.

Genetic theories and principles Concept that a gene is the fundamental and functional unit of heredity. A gene mutation is an alteration in DNA coding that results in a change in the protein product. Mutations in some genes cause clinical disease because of the absence of the normal protein. Gene discoveries have provided information on genetic disorders that cause symptoms in a large proportion of persons who have abnormal genotypes.

Germ theory Early theory of disease infection proposed by Louis Pasteur. Pasteur theorized that a specific organism (i.e., a germ) was capable of causing an infectious disease.

Grand theories Theories that are composed of relatively abstract concepts that are not operationally defined and attempt to explain or describe very comprehensive aspects of human experience and response; may incorporate numerous other theories.

Great man theory of leadership A trait theory that asserts that leaders possess certain characteristics (i.e., physical or personality traits and talents) that nonleaders do not.

Health In grand nursing theory, the ability to function independently; successful adaptation to life's stressors; achievement of one's full life potential; and unity of mind, body, and soul.

Health as Expanding Consciousness Margaret Newman's nursing theory, which posits that persons are identified by pattern and organization and are consciousness rather than merely having consciousness. Health is a pattern of the individual.

Health Belief Model A widely used social psychology theory that explains health behavior in terms of several constructs: perceived susceptibility of the health problem, perceived severity, perceived benefits, perceived barriers, self-efficacy, and cues to action.

Health literacy Describes how well an individual can read, interpret, and comprehend health information for maintaining an optimal level of wellness.

Health Promotion Model Nola Pender's framework for integrating nursing and behavioral science perspectives on factors that influence health behaviors. The model may be used as a guide to explore the biopsychosocial processes that motivate individuals to engage in behaviors directed toward health.

Homeodynamics The idea that health is achieved through continuous interaction of human and environmental energy systems.

Host/host factors In the epidemiologic triangle, refers to factors (e.g., age, gender, race/ethnicity, marital status, economic status, state of immunity, lifestyle factors) that may influence whether an individual develops a disease.

Humanbecoming Paradigm Rosemary Parse's theory, which states that humanbecoming is a separate paradigm of nursing in which nurses guide patients in choosing the possibilities in changing health process through intersubjective processes.

Human needs theory Maslow's description of the hierarchy of dynamic processes that are critical for human development and growth. There are six incremental stages: physiologic needs, safety needs, love and belonging needs, self-esteem needs, self-actualizing needs, and self-transcendent needs. The goal of Maslow's theory is to attain the sixth level or stage: self-transcendent needs. Motivation is the key to Maslow's theory because individuals are seen as striving for self-actualization.

Human science The study of human life by valuing the lived experience of persons and seeking to understand life in its matrix of patterns of meaning and values. Knowledge is created to provide understanding and interpretation of phenomena.

Immune system Refers to a complex, coordinated group of systems that produces physiologic responses to injury or infection. The purpose of the immune system is to neutralize, eliminate, or destroy microorganisms that invade the body. Extensive interactions affect the manufacture of products that alter the structure and function of cells.

Immunity State or process of being immune to a disease state; involves specific recognition of what is designated as an antigen, memory for particular antigens, and responsiveness on reexposure.

Implied theory Refers to those theories used by practicing nurses during routine client care without conscious consideration.

Intention Main determinant in the Theory of Reasoned Action/Theory of Planned Behavior; the cognitive representation of the individual's readiness to perform a behavior and is determined by attitude, subjective norms, and perceived behavioral control.

Interpersonal theory Sullivan's developmental theory based on the premise that an individual cannot exist apart from his or her relationships with other people. Development is dependent on interpersonal situations which continue throughout the person's life. The sequence of interpersonal events to which a person is exposed from infancy to adulthood and ways in which these situations occur contribute to the individual's development.

Intersystem Model Barbara Artinian's model explaining the interactions between patient and nurse systems. These become more complex when the interaction is between and among community systems and health care systems.

Knowledge The awareness or perception of reality acquired through insight, learning, or investigation. In a discipline, knowledge is what is collectively seen to be a reasonably accurate understanding of the world perceived by members of the discipline.

Learning A relatively permanent change in behavior that results from experience. Learning occurs as individuals interact with their environment, incorporating new information into what they already know.

Learning styles The many ways a person may learn including preferences for learning formats. Some people learn best by reading, some by being told, others by being shown; many learners need a motor component to the learning, and others prefer computer learning methods.

Maternal Role Attainment/Becoming a Mother Ramona Mercer's work on identification of the factors that influence the development and evolution of relationships between key maternal and infant variables that determine maternal role attainment.

Metatheory A theory about theory; focuses on broad issues such as the processes of generating knowledge and theory development.

Methodology The means of acquiring knowledge.

Middle range theories Theories that are substantively specific and encompass a limited number of concepts and a limited aspect of the real world.

Model A graphic or symbolic representation of phenomena or reality. Models objectify and present certain perspectives or points of view about nature or function or both.

Modeling and role-modeling (MRM) theory A deductive theory developed by Erickson, Tomlin, and Swain that focuses on the interpersonal interactions between nurse and client.

Motivation–hygiene theory (Herzberg's two-factor theory) Explains differences between factors that are true motivators for individuals (i.e., recognition for a job well done, opportunities for promotion or advancement, challenging and rewarding work), and hygiene or maintenance factors (e.g. salary, quality of supervision, interpersonal relationships with coworkers, and good working conditions).

Natural History of Disease model A model that explains the progression of a disease process in an individual over time using two stages: prepathogenesis and pathogenesis. The model also describes the three levels of prevention—primary prevention, secondary prevention, and tertiary prevention.

Neuman Systems Model Betty Neuman's systems-based approach focused on human needs and relief from stress in the nursing care of vulnerable patients.

Nursing In grand nursing theory, a science, an art, and a practice discipline that involves caring. Goals of nursing include care of the well, care of the sick, assisting with self-care activities, helping individuals attain their human potential, and discovering and using nature's laws of health. The purposes of nursing care include placing the client in the best condition for nature to restore health, promoting the adaptation of the individual, facilitating the development of an interaction between the nurse and the client in which jointly set goals are met, and promoting harmony between the individual and the environment.

Nursing metaparadigm A worldview or global perspective of the discipline. Nursing's metaparadigm is generally thought to consist of the concepts of person, environment, health, and nursing.

Nursing philosophy The belief system of the profession; provides perspective for nursing practice, scholarship, and research.

Nursing research A scientific process that validates and refines existing knowledge and generates new knowledge that directly and indirectly influences nursing practice. Nursing research is concerned with the study of individuals in interaction with their environments and with discovering interventions that promote optimal functioning and wellness across the lifespan.

Nursing science The substantive, discipline-specific knowledge that focuses on the human-universe-health process articulated in nursing frameworks and theories. The system of relationships of human responses in health and illness addressing biologic, behavioral, social, and cultural domains.

Nursing: What it is, what it is not Florence Nightingale's organized definition of professional nursing. Nightingale's work served as the basis for modern nursing by focusing on the needs of vulnerable patients for nursing care.

Ontology The study of being; what is or what exists; nature of reality.

Operant conditioning B. F. Skinner's term for the manipulation of selected reinforcers. According to Skinner, an individual performs a behavior (discharges an operant) and receives a consequence (reinforcer) as a result of performing the behavior. The consequence is either positive or negative, and the consequence will most likely determine whether the behavior will be repeated.

Operational definition The actual measurement of a concept, term, or phenomenon for a research study.

Paradigm A worldview or overall way of looking at a discipline and its science. It is an organizing framework that contains concepts, theories, assumptions, beliefs, values, and principles that form the way a discipline interprets the subject matter with which it is concerned. Paradigm shift occurs when the traditional theories no longer describe the world as newer information has been learned.

Parsimony That which is as constrained as possible so that only those elements that are needed are included.

Patient Centered Approaches to Nursing Abdellah's grand theory, based in the human needs of patients and focused on education and practice of nursing care of the ill in home or hospital.

Path–Goal Theory An expectancy theory in which situational factors (i.e., nature and scope of the task, the employee's perceptions and expectations, and the role of the leader) are examined. The leader is responsible for helping the employee determine and clarify the path the worker is to take to reach the goal and to provide motivation and reward. The leaders also must identify and remove obstacles from the path of the worker to enable him or her to successfully attain the goal.

Pathogenesis Second stage of the Natural History of Disease model. After exposure or interaction, the stage moves from early pathogenesis to the disease course to resolution—either death, disability, or recovery.

Person In grand nursing theory, a being composed of physical, intellectual, biochemical, and psychosocial needs; a human energy field; a holistic being in the world; an open system; an integrated whole; an adaptive system; and a being who is greater than the sum of his parts.

Phenomenology The study of phenomena; emphasizes the appearance of things as opposed to the things themselves. In phenomenology, understanding is the goal of science, and it recognizes the connection between one's experience, values, and perspectives.

Phenomenon That which may be sensed or not but which exists in the real world.

Philosophy A study of problems that are ultimate, abstract, and general. These problems are concerned with the nature of existence, knowledge, morality, reason, and human purpose. A statement of beliefs and values about human beings and the world.

Planned change theory Lewin's theory describing change process that occurs by design (rather than spontaneously or by chance). There are two forces involved in change, *driving forces* and *restraining forces.* Change is a move from the status quo that results in a disruption in the balance of forces or disequilibrium between opposing forces and often leads to feelings of uneasiness, uncertainty, and loss of control. In planned change, driving forces should be identified and accentuated, and restraining forces should be identified and minimized to achieve the desired outcome or change. Effective change is the return to equilibrium as a result of balancing opposing forces. Three phases must occur if planned change is to be successful: unfreezing the status quo, moving to a new state, and refreezing the change to make it permanent.

Positivism A term often equated with empiricism. Positivism supports mechanistic, reductionist principles where the complex can best be understood in terms of its basic components.

Postmodernity Generally regarded as a new social and political epoch that succeeded the "modern era" or "modernity." Postmodernity is highly sceptical of explanations that claim to be valid for all groups, cultures, traditions, or races, and instead focuses on the relative truths of each person.

Postmodern theory A philosophical reaction to the underlying assumptions and universalizing tendency of the doctrine of positivism and scientific objectivity characterized by "modernity."

Power The influence wielded by an individual or group of individuals to change behaviors and attitudes and to sway decisions; implies a dependency relationship.

Practice (or applied) science A science that uses the knowledge of basic science for a practical end. Research is largely clinical and action oriented.

Practice-based evidence Evidence from large practice databases that include findings not only from research studies but also from benchmarking data, clinical expertise, data from cost-effectiveness and quality improvement studies, infection control, medical records, and include national standards of care as well as patient and family preferences.

Predictive theories Theories that describe precise relationships between concepts; are able to describe future outcomes consistently and include statement of causal or consequential relatedness.

Prepathogenesis First stage of the Natural History of Disease model occurring prior to interaction of the disease agent and human host when the individual is susceptible.

Prescriptive theories Theories that prescribe activities necessary to reach defined goals. In nursing, prescriptive theories address nursing therapeutics and predicate the consequence of interventions.

Problem-based learning (PBL) The use of predefined clinical situations and case studies to enhance or stimulate students to acquire specific skills, knowledge, and abilities. PBL allows the instructor to manipulate multiple variables to add increasingly complex issues or circumstances that must be considered in problem resolution.

Profession A learned vocation or occupation that has a status of superiority and precedence within a division of work.

Psychic energy Term used by Freud to explain how the human as an energy system is composed of instincts, whereby instincts are the sole energy source for human behavior.

Psychoanalytic theory Theory developed by Freud in which behavior is the product of an interaction among the three major systems of the personality: the id, ego, and superego.

Psychodynamic theories Theories that attempt to explain the multidimensional nature of behavior and understand how an individual's personality and behavior interface; also provide a systematic way of identifying and understanding behavior.

Psychosocial Developmental Theory Erikson's theory, which describes eight stages of a person's life that are formed by social influences that interact with the physical/psychological, maturing organism. The first four stages occur in infancy and childhood, the fifth stage occurs in adolescence, and the last three stages occur during the adult years. Erikson believed that each stage of development builds on the next, thus contributing to the formation of the total person.

Quality improvement (QI) The commitment and approach used to scrupulously examine and continuously improve every process in every part of an organization. The ultimate intent of QI is meeting and exceeding customer expectations.

Randomized, controlled clinical trials Research studies in which an intervention is tested against another intervention. The interventions are randomly assigned to the subjects who are in the study to form at the minimum two groups: a research group and a control group. The data are collected and statistically analyzed to indicate the results of the research.

Rational Emotive Theory Ellis' theory, which describes the interconnectedness between thoughts, feelings, and actions. The underlying premise is that an individual has the cognitive ability to think, decide, analyze, and do and that the individual thinks either rationally or irrationally. The repetition of irrational thoughts reinforces dysfunctional beliefs, which, in turn, produce dysfunctional behaviors. These dysfunctional beliefs lead to self-defeating behaviors. Ellis posited that if behaviors are learned, they can be unlearned.

Research The systematic inquiry that uses disciplined methods to answer questions or solve problems. Research is conducted to describe, explain, or predict variables, and in a practice discipline such as nursing, research is assumed to contribute to the improvement of care.

Resistance The second stage of the stress response in Selye's work; the body's physiologic responses to regain homeostasis.

Restraining forces In the planned change theory, restraining forces block or impede progress toward a goal.

Role theory A theory that contends that normative expectations and requirements, such as culturally defined behavioral rules, are attached to positions (status) in social organizations (e.g., family, corporation, society). Roles can be assumed to carry rights and privileges as well as duties and obligations.

Roy Adaptation Model (RAM) Callista Roy's model, which focuses on assisting the client to adapt to and overcome the stresses of illness and environmental factors.

Science A way of explaining observed phenomena as well as a system of gathering, verifying, and systemizing information about reality (i.e., it is both a process and a product).

Science of Unitary and Irreducible Human Beings Martha Rogers' theory synthesized from theories of the sciences to incorporate the proposition that the human is an open system embedded in larger open systems; living systems are pattern and organization; and man is sentient, capable of awareness, feeling, and choosing.

Self-actualization In humanistic theories (e.g., Maslow), refers to the process of developing human potential and talents.

Self-Care Deficit Nursing Theory (SCDNT) Dorothea Orem's work, consisting of three nested theories: the theories of self-care, self-care deficit, and nursing systems. This needs-based theory seeks to provide for as many contingencies as possible in the care of the patient, ill or well.

Self-transcendence In Reed's theory, a characteristic of developmental maturity in which there is an expansion of self-boundaries and orientation toward broadened life perspectives and purposes.

Shared (or borrowed) theory Theories that arise or are derived from other disciplines but are applied in nursing situations.

Simultaneity Conceptualization in which humans and environment including the universe are in constant interaction all at the same time.

Simultaneity paradigm Parse's depiction of a group of theories based on the science of unitary and irreducible human beings and meaning that the paradoxes of living go on all at once, continuously. The human is a system embedded in the universal energy system and enters into all that is taking place, in some way, at all times.

Situation-specific theories (practice theories) Theories that are specific, narrow in scope, contain few concepts, and are easily defined. They tend to be prescriptive.

Stress, coping and adaptation theory Lazaurs and Folkman's explanation of the psychological responses that occur as a person copes with stressful situations. Successful coping results in adaptation, which is the capacity of a person to survive and flourish.

Symbolic interactionism A sociologic paradigm that synthesizes the concepts of self, mind, and society. In this viewpoint, humans adapt to and survive in their environment by sharing common symbols, both verbal and nonverbal. Within symbolic interactions, humans can imagine themselves in social roles and internalize the attitudes, values, and norms of a social group.

Synergy Model A model that describes nurses' contributions, activities, and outcomes with regard to caring for critically ill patients. The model identifies eight patient needs or characteristics and eight competencies of nurses in critical care situations. When patient characteristics and nurse competencies match and synergize, outcomes for the patient are optimal.

Teaching The intentional act of communicating information; may be defined as the facilitation of learning.

The Future of Nursing A publication from the Institute of Medicine (IOM), which has been viewed as a challenge and strategy to (1) make quality health care accessible to the diverse populations of the United States, (2) intentionally promote wellness and disease prevention, (3) improve health outcomes, and (4) provide compassionate care across the lifespan.

Theoretical framework A set of interrelated concepts that symbolically represents and conveys a mental image of a phenomenon.

Theory A systematic explanation of an event in which constructs and concepts are identified and relationships are proposed and predications made; a set of interpretive assumptions, principles, or propositions that help explain or guide action.

Theory-based nursing practice Application of various models, theories, and principles from nursing science and the biologic, behavioral, medical, and sociocultural disciplines to clinical nursing practice.

Theory evaluation (or theory analysis) The process of systematically examining a theory and ascertaining how well the theory serves its purpose; results in a decision or action about the use of the theory.

Theory of Chronic Sorrow A theory that initially described grief observed in the parents of children with mental deficiencies; expanded to include individuals who experience a variety of loss situations and to their family caregivers.

Theory of Goal Attainment and Transactional Process Imogene King's nursing framework, which focuses on the transactions between nurse and client to attain the goals of the nurse–patient relationship.

Theory of Reasoned Action/Theory of Planned Behavior A theory that explains the relationship among beliefs, attitudes, intentions, and behavior. According to the theory, the most important determinant of a person's behavior(s) is intention.

Theory of Self-Transcendence Pamela Reed's explanation of the expansion of self-boundaries and orientation toward broadened life perspectives and purpose in which the individual moves beyond the immediate or constricted view of self and the world. The theory can be used by nurses to develop interventions to attend to spiritual and psychosocial expressions of self-transcendence in clients who are confronted with end-of-life issues.

Theory of Unpleasant Symptoms A theory that seeks to improve understanding of the symptom experience in various contexts and to provide information useful for designing effective means to prevent, ameliorate, or manage unpleasant symptoms and their negative effects.

Theory–practice gap The notion that there is a "gap" between theory and practice; a common perception among nurses because nurses in clinical practice rarely use the language of nursing theory, nursing diagnosis, or the nursing process.

Totality paradigm The paradigm in which the person and the world are known by the sum of their parts and the workings thereof.

Transactional Leader A leader who is viewed as the traditional manager, one who is concerned with day-to-day operations.

Transformational Leader A leader who is a long-term visionary able to inspire and empower others with his or her vision.

Transitions Theory Afaf Meleis' theory, which describes the interactions between nurses and patients, explaining how nurses are concerned with the experiences of people as they undergo transitions, whenever health and well-being are the desired outcome. The goal of nursing is to address the potential problems that individuals encounter during transitional experiences and develop preventative and therapeutic interventions to support the patient during these occasions.

Uncertainty in Illness Theory Merle Mishel's theory describing how individuals process illness-related stimuli and structure meaning for those events. Adaptation is the desirable end-state achieved after coping with the uncertainty. Nurses may develop interventions to influence the person's cognitive process to address the uncertainty, which should produce positive coping and adaptation.

Unitary Concept in which all things are part of a universal energy system and in constant and changing interaction.

Utilitarianism Philosophical perspective that considers and supports "the greatest good for the greatest number."

Variable A phenomenon that has properties that can differ or change based on circumstances; anything that varies.

Web of causation (chain of causation) A disease model used to explain chronic diseases or disability not attributable to one or two factors or causative agents; rather, they result from the interaction of multiple factors.

Worldview The philosophical frame of reference used by a social or cultural group to describe that group's outlook on and beliefs about reality.

AUTHOR INDEX

Note: Page numbers followed by b indicate material in boxes, those followed by f indicate material in figures, and those followed by t indicate material in tables.

A

Abdellah, F.
assumptions, concepts, and relationships, 139–141
background, 139
nursing theory, 31, 34t, 119, 124t, 139–142
parsimony of theory, 141
patient-centered approach, 139–142
philosophical underpinnings of theory, 139
publications, 141t
testability of theory, 141
usefulness of theory, 141
value in extending nursing science, 142

Abner, C.
research on cesarean birth, 434t, 441

Abraham, M.
patient-focused care, 462

Abraham, P. J.
model of skill acquisition in nursing, 232

Abraham, S.
human needs theory, 317
interpersonal theory, 312
natural history of disease, 339

Achatz, M. I. W.
genomics in cancer care, 346

Acton, G. J.
theory-testing research, 439

Adam, E.
nursing theory, 35t, 119

Adams, J. S.
Equity Theory, 368

Adams, S.
Iowa Model, of evidence-based practice, 267

Adamsen, L.
theory–practice gap, 416

Ade-Oshifogun, J. B.
prescriptive theories, 77–78

Adkins, C. S.
principle-based concept analysis, 66

Aebersold, M.
technology in nursing education, 493

Agazio, J.
stress theories, 321

Aguayo, R.
Deming and quality improvement, 377t

Ahlstrom, G.
Theory of Chronic Sorrow, 109, 250

Ahmann, E.
patient-focused care, 463

Aiken, L. H.
California Safe Staffing Law, 464
Magnet Recognition Program, 466
nurse staffing and patient outcomes, 464–465
Nursing Work Index-Revised, 463

Ainsworth, B. E.
experimental study of "sign chi do" exercises, 437

Ajzen, I.
Theory of Reasoned Action/Planned Action, 222–223, 322–326, 325f, 327t

Akyuz, A.
cancer theories, 348
Postpartum Depression Theory, 251

Albrecht, S. A.
Postpartum Depression Theory, 251

Alexander
critical social theory and feminism, 293

Alexander, J. C.
cultural diversity and cultural bias, 293

Alhusen, J. L.
correlational research, 434t

Allan, H.
psychoanalytic theory, 309

Alligood, M. R.
grand theory categorization, 118–119
middle range theory, 214
Nightingale, 134
nursing theory, 24, 25, 27t–28t
theory evaluation, 97, 106, 126
Theory of Goal Attainment, 177
theory-testing research, 440–441

Alper, P.
infection prevention, 334

Altmann, T. K.
cultural care diversity and universality theory, 234

Altpeter, T.
Caring Science as Sacred Science, 186

Ames, S. W.
general adaptation syndrome, 319–320

Andel, C.
nurse staffing and patient outcomes, 464
quality improvement, 375, 377

Anderson, C.
operational teaching, 490
Theory of Goal Attainment, 176

Anderson, E. S.
Theory of Comfort, 246

Anderson, J.
stress theories, 321

Anderson, K. M.
technology in nursing education, 492

Anderson, M.
postmodern social theory, 300

Anderson, M. A.
Magnet Recognition Program, 465

Anderson, M. S.
dialectic learning, 489
technology in nursing education, 492

Anderson, R. A.
general systems theory, 283

Andrews, H. A.
metaparadigm, 43t

Andrist, L. C.
nursing theory development, 30

Andrusyszyn, M. A.
nursing education, 480

Anthony, M. K.
patient care delivery models, 459
shared governance, 458

Antonofski, A.
Artinian Intersystem Model, 165t

Arashin, K. A.
Synergy Model, 426

Arcamone, A. A.
Health Promotion Model, 236

Archbold, P. G.
role theory, 288

Ardizzone, L. L.
infection prevention, 334

Arhin, A. O.
generational differences, 287

Armola, R.
Theory of Unpleasant Symptoms, 247

Armstrong, T.
Theory of Unpleasant Symptoms, 443
Uncertainty of Illness Theory, 244

Arndt, M.
critical social theory, 293

Artinian, B.
assumptions, concepts, and relationships, 165–168, 167b, 167t
background, 164
Intersystem Model, 159, 160, 164–169
models, 82
nursing theory, 36t, 131, 164–169
parsimony of theory, 169
philosophical underpinnings of theory, 164, 165t, 166f
testability of theory, 168–169
usefulness of theory, 168
value in extending nursing science, 169

Askey-Jones, S.
cognitive behavioral therapies, 315
Asplund, K.
theory of ICU transitional care, 435
Transitions Theory, 238
Atkinson, R. C.
memory, 405
Attewell, A.
Nightingale, 132, 133, 135, 136
Attree, M.
general systems theory, 282
Audain, C.
Nightingale, 133
Ausubel, D. P.
assimilation, 405
Auvil-Novak, S. E.
prescriptive theories, 40
Avant, K.
associational statements, 80
concept derivation, 59, 59b
concept development, 58–59, 58b, 60t, 67, 68t
evidence-based practice, 261, 263, 504
grand theories, 74, 127
immune function, 343
metatheory, 37, 74
middle range theories, 74
postmodernism, 10
practice-based evidence, 262
practice theories, 74
relationship among levels of theory, 75
statement development, 87, 87b
theory analysis, 96, 97, 98t, 100, 101t, 106, 107t, 124, 126, 127
theory concepts, 79
theory development, 73
theory development process, 86
theory–practice gap, 417
theory synthesis, 88, 88b
Averill, J. B.
Theory of Comfort, 246
Avery, M. D.
technology in nursing education, 492
Avolio, B. J.
authentic leadership, 364
transformational leadership, 363
Aydin, C. E.
California Safe Staffing Law, 464
Ayer, M.
technology in nursing education, 493
Azzaline, J. B.
nursing curriculum, 487

B

Baca-Zinn, M.
conflict theories, 289, 289b, 290
feminist theory, 290
Bacon, F.
empiricism, 8
philosophy, overview, 7
Baiardi, J.
Roy Adaptation Model, 181
Bailey, C. A.
infection prevention, 334
Bailey, D. E.
Uncertainty of Illness Theory, 241, 244
Bailey, L. D.
psychosocial developmental theory, 310
Self-Care Deficit Nursing Theory, 425
Bailey, M.
infection prevention, 334
Bailey, P. H.
comparison of concept development models, 67
concept development, 51
Bairan, A.
cultural care diversity and universality theory, 233
Baird, M. B.
well-being in refugee women experiencing cultural transition, 420t
Baker, D.
Health Belief Model, 326
Baker, G. R.
quality improvement, 470
Baldwin, C. M.
Modeling and Role-Modeling, 172
Ball, E.
Artinian Intersystem Model, 168
Ballard, J.
concept analysis, 69–70
Banasik, J. L.
cancer theories, 347
genetics, 344
immune system, 343
Bandera, E. V.
cancer theories, 348
Bandura, A.
self-efficacy, 405
social learning theory, 222, 396, 399–400
Barber, D.
psychoanalytic theory, 309
Barkauskas, V. H.
nurse staffing and patient outcomes, 464
Barker, A. M.
transformational leadership, 458
Barker, P.
chaos theory, 298
tidal model, 231t
Barnoy, S.
genetic counseling, 345
Barnsteiner, J.
future issues in nursing, 499
nursing curriculum, 487
Barnum, B. S.
descriptive theories, 75–76
descriptive theory, 434
explanatory theories, 76
implied theory, 422
nursing education/curriculum, 480, 486
teaching strategies, 488–490
theory evaluation, 98t, 100, 100b, 106, 107t
Barone, C. P.
gate control theory, 349
Barone, S. H.
Roy Adaptation Model, 181
Barrett, E. A. M.
nursing science, 12
Power as Knowing Participation in Change, 196
Rogerian theory, 196
Barron, J. J.
disease management, 470
Barry, D. G.
technology in nursing education, 493
Bartlett, R.
interpersonal theory, 313
Bartoszek, G.
web of causation, 335
Bass, B. M.
transformational leadership, 363
Bastable, S. B.
definition of teaching, 388
health literacy, 387
learning theories, 407
Bauermeister, J.
stress theories, 321
Bayoumi, M.
human needs theory, 317
Bazini-Barakat, N.
Public Health Nursing Practice Model, 224, 231t
Beal, J. A.
Health as Expanding Consciousness, 201
Beanlands, H.
critical social theory, 293
Beaton, J. L.
research methodology, 17
Beck, A. T.
cognitive theory, 314, 327t
Beck, C. T.
Postpartum Depression Theory, 248, 250–251
research defined, 432
research process, 433b
Beck, D. M.
Nightingale, 132, 133, 135, 136
Becker, M. H.
Health Belief Model, 222, 323f
Beckman, S. J.
nursing curriculum, 484
Beckstrand, R. L.
Postpartum Depression Theory, 251
Bednarz, J. L.
symbolic interactionism, 286
Bednash, G. P.
nursing curriculum, 487
Beery, T.
genetics, 343, 345
Beidler, S. M.
Piaget's cognitive development theory, 396–397
Bekel, G.
Orem, 142
Bekhet, A.
methodological triangulation, 500
Beland, I. L.
patient-centered approach, 139–142

Belcher, A.
Conservation Model, 163
Bell, A. F.
principle-based concept analysis, 66
Bell, S. E.
social justice, 44
Bellar, A.
allostasis, 340
Belot, C.
Health Belief Model, 326
Benedict, L.
humanbecoming paradigm, 205
Benedict, S.
critical social theory, 293
Benham-Hutchins, M.
chaos theory, 298
Benkert, R.
social justice, 44
Benner, P.
Dreyfus model, 222
middle range theory, 214, 230
model of skill acquisition in nursing, 230–233, 430, 439
nursing curriculum, 508
nursing theory, 36t, 119, 230–233
theory to practice to theory approach, 84
Bennis, W.
charismatic leadership, 364
transformational leadership, 458
Benoit, R.
risk factors for pressure ulcers, 218
Benson, H.
relaxation response, 221
Benson, S.
Johnson model, 149
Bently, G. W.
problem-based learning, 489
Berbiglia, V. A.
nursing curriculum, 484
Bergquist, S.
parish nursing model, 231t
Bergstrom, N.
Theory of Unpleasant Symptoms, 443
Uncertainty of Illness Theory, 244
Berk, L. E.
Piaget's cognitive development theory, 396
Bernard, C.
homeostasis, 340
Berragan, L.
technology in nursing education, 493
Berry, D.
Health as Expanding Consciousness, 202
Berson, Y.
transformational leadership, 363
Besse, J.
disease management, 469
Betker, C.
practice to theory approach, 85
Bevis, E. O.
Caring Science as Sacred Science, 186
nursing curriculum, 481–482
Bezerra, S. T. F.
Theory of Goal Attainment, 177
Biasio, H. A.
nursing as discipline, 4
philosophy, overview, 6
Bienemy, C.
Health Belief Model, 326
Bigge, M. L.
learning theory, 389
Biggs, A.
Orem, 145
Bill, R.
infection prevention, 334
Billings, D. M.
future issues in nursing education, 507
technology in nursing education, 492, 493
theory-based nursing practice, 414
theory–practice gap, 416
Bisgaard, S.
quality improvement, 379–380
Bishop, S. M.
nursing theory development, 33t
theoretical statements, 79
theory and research, 431
theory components, 79
theory concepts, 79
theory structure and linkages, 81
variable *vs.* nonvariable concepts, 52
Bjerregaard, L.
theory–practice gap, 416
Bjorklund, P.
psychosocial developmental theory, 310
Black, J.
patient-focused care, 463
Black, J. M.
germ theory, 333
immune system, 342
Black, J. S.
behavioral theories of leadership, 357
Contingency Theory of Leadership, 361
Blackburn, S.
nursing theory, 27t–28t
philosophy, overview, 6
Blanchard, K.
situational leadership theory, 362
Blass, T. C.
case management, 467
Blattner, W. A.
cancer theories, 347, 348t
Blau, P.
social exchange theory, 280
Blazier, D.
technology in nursing education, 493
Blegen, M. A.
middle range theory, 214, 216
nursing theory–nursing research connection, 431
Blevins, C.
theory of successful aging, 424
Blugis, A.
human needs theory, 317
Blum, K.
Transitions Theory, 238–239, 425
Blumer, H.
symbolic interactionism, 285
Blyler, D.
Uncertainty of Illness Theory, 244
Bodley, J. H.
cultural diversity and cultural bias, 293, 294t
Bogue, R.
Theory of Goal Attainment, 176
Bokhour, B.
Transitions Theory, 239
Boland, D. L.
nursing education/curriculum, 480–487
Bolino, M. C.
Leader–Member Exchange Theory, 358
Bolton, L. B.
future issues in nursing, 499
Bommer, W. H.
Path–Goal Theory, 361
Bond, M. L.
Artinian Intersystem Model, 168
Bonhomme, N.
natural history of disease, 339
Bonin, J.
Roy Adaptation Model, 181
Bono, J. E.
transformational leadership, 363
Boore, J.
nursing care for patients at risk for suicide, 218
Boostridge, M.
Nightingale, 133, 134, 136
Booth, A.
cognitive behavioral therapies, 315
Booth, R. G.
nursing education, 480
Bositis, A.
Conservation Model, 163
Boswell, C.
nursing curriculum, 487
technology in nursing education, 491, 492
Boughton, M. A.
Uncertainty of Illness Theory, 244
Bournes, D. A.
Parse and humanbecoming paradigm, 203, 207
Bovbejerg, B. E.
disease management, 468
Bowers, B. J.
Theory of Genetic Vulnerability, 220
theory to research to theory approach, 86
Bowes, S.
Theory of Chronic Sorrow, 109, 250
Boxley-Harges, S. L.
nursing curriculum, 484
Boyatzis, R.
emotional intelligence, 356–357
Boykin, A.
caring as central construct, 45
Caring Science as Sacred Science, 186
nursing theory, 36t, 118, 119
Braden, C. J.
self-help model, 242t

Bradford, M.
disease management, 469
Bramlett, M. H.
Rogerian theory, 196
Braungart, M. M.
learning theory in health practice, 387, 390, 392, 400, 401
Braungart, R. G.
learning theory in health practice, 387, 390, 392, 400, 401
Bredown, T. S.
theory evaluation, 106
Breidbart, S.
disease management, 470
Brennaman, L.
Theory of Crisis Emergencies, 420t
Brennan, P. F.
patient care delivery models, 459
Brenner, A.
stress theories, 321
Brewer, B. B.
shared governance, 456, 457, 458
Briggs, C. L.
operational teaching, 490
Brink, P. J.
reliance on nursing models in research, 444
Brinkman, K. S.
humanbecoming paradigm, 205
Brixey, M. J.
model of skill acquisition in nursing, 232
Brockopp, D.
Caring Science as Sacred Science, 186
Brookfield, S. D.
transformational learning, 405
Brosch, L. R.
Health Belief Model, 326
Broschard, D.
Self-Transcendence Theory, 248
Brown, C. G.
Health Belief Model, 326
Brown, D. S.
California Safe Staffing Law, 464
Brown, E.
nursing theory development, 30
Brown, J. M.
evidence-based practice, 32, 259, 260, 421t
Brown, J. W.
Newman and Newman theory, 198, 201
Brown, S. C.
nursing curriculum, 484
Brown, V. B.
role theory, 288
Brownmiller, S.
radical feminism, 291
Brozaitiene, J.
Social Readjustment Rating Scale, 342
Bruccoliere, T.
learning approaches, 408
Brunssen, S.
Maternal Role Attainment/Becoming a Mother, 252
Bryant, C. A.
Bandura's social learning theory, 400
Bryant, L. G.
Theory of Comfort, 246
Buchanan, K.
Health Belief Model, 326
Budreau, G.
Iowa Model, of evidence-based practice, 264
Buet, A.
infection prevention, 334
Buettner-Schmidt, K.
concept analysis, 57
Bulechek, G. M.
Nursing Intervention Classification system, 422–423, 423t, 424t
prescriptive theories, 78
Bunevicius, R.
Social Readjustment Rating Scale, 342
Bunkers, S. S.
humanbecoming paradigm, 205
Burchinal, M. R.
Maternal Role Attainment/Becoming a Mother, 252
Burke, L.
evidence-based practice, 259
Burke, M. L.
Theory of Chronic Sorrow, 109–112, 218, 248, 249–250
Burke, R.
shared governance, 456, 457, 458
Burkett, M.
allostasis, 340
Burkhart, L.
Nightingale, 136
nursing curriculum, 487
Burnes-Bolton, L.
California Safe Staffing Law, 464
Burns, D.
symptom-focused diabetes care, 420t
Burns, J. M.
leadership, 362–363
Burns, K.
Health Promotion Model, 236
Burns, N.
nursing research, 432, 433b
Burroughs, E. L.
Bandura's social learning theory, 400
Busby, S.
descriptive theories, 39
Butcher, H. K.
Nursing Intervention Classification system, 422–423, 423t, 424t
prescriptive theories, 78
Butler, M. K.
disease management, 469
Butts, J. B.
grand theories, 117
nursing as discipline, 4
nursing theory, 24
science and philosophy, 5
Buxton, J. A.
Theory of Reasoned Action/Planned Behavior, 326
Byars, L.
Achievement–Motivation Theory, 367
Byrnes, J. P.
cognitive development and learning, 394–395, 402, 404

C

Cahill, J.
Theory of Unpleasant Symptoms, 443
Caldwell, C.
stress theories, 321
Call, V. R. A.
chaos theory, 297
Callister, L. C.
Postpartum Depression Theory, 251
Calvillo, E.
perceived view of science, 9
Calzone, K. A.
genomics in nursing practice, 344–345
Camp, R. C.
benchmarking, 472
Campesino, M.
cultural care diversity and universality theory, 234
Canam, C.
caring as central construct, 45
metaparadigm, 42
Candela, L.
learning theory, 387, 388, 389, 392, 394, 398
Cannella, B.
Piaget's cognitive development theory, 397
Cannon, S.
nursing curriculum, 487
technology in nursing education, 491, 492
Canon, W.
fight or flight, 340
homeostasis, 340
Caplan, E.
Theory X and Theory Y, 359
Caramanica
Model of Evidence-Based Practice, 270
Carbonu, D. M.
chaos theory, 298
Carlson, B.
Theory of Unpleasant Symptoms, 247
Carlson, J.
symptom-focused diabetes care, 420t
Carlson, K. L.
technology in nursing education, 493
Carlson-Sabelli, L. L.
nursing education, 480
Carlsson, M.
psychosocial developmental theory, 310
Carobene, M.
cultural care diversity and universality theory, 234
nursing strategies to reduce caries, 427t

Carpenter, D. R.
epistemology, 12
nursing theory, 25, 72
perceived view of science, 9
research methodology, 17
science, overview, 5
Carpenter, J.
immune function, 343
Carper, B. A.
nursing epistemology, 13–15
Carroll, E. W.
Human Genome Project, 343
Carruth, A.
social exchange theory, 282
Carson, K. D.
power bases, 368
Carson, P. P.
power bases, 368
Carter, L. M.
cognitive-field (gestalt) theory, 394
Carter, S.
nursing epistemology, 19–20
Cartwright, J.
explanatory theories, 76
research to theory approach, 85
Cartwright, S.
transformational leadership, 363
Carver, N.
problem-based learning, 489
Cashman, J.
Leader–Member Exchange Theory, 358
Cason, C.
Artinian Intersystem Model, 168
Castro, S. L.
Path–Goal Theory, 362
Cathcart, D.
span of control, 454
Cathcart, E. B.
model of skill acquisition in nursing, 232
Catlin, A.
Nightingale, 136
Causey, C.
cancer theories, 348
Cesario, S.
theory development, 73
Cha, S. E.
transformational leadership, 363
Chabeli, M. M.
information-processing model, 395
Chaboyer, W.
explanatory theories, 76
Chan, A.
problem-based learning, 489
student-centered teaching, 401
Chan, A. Y.
authentic leadership, 364
Chan, K.
problem-based learning, 489
student-centered teaching, 401
Chan, L. S.
general systems theory, 283
Chan, S.
social networks, 284
Chan, T. S.
cancer theories, 348
Chan, Y. U.
infection prevention, 334
Chan, Z. C. Y.
cancer theories, 348
problem-based learning, 490
Chando, S.
Magnet Recognition Program, 466
Chang, S. H.
predictive theories, 39
Chang, S. J.
practice theories, 418, 502
Chappell, K.
nursing curriculum, 487
Charns, M.
Stetler Model of Evidence-Based Practice, 270
Chase, C.
Health Promotion Model, 236
Chase, S. K.
sustaining health in faith community, 218, 438
Chassin, M.
quality improvement, 375, 376t
Chemers, M.
Contingency Theory of Leadership, 360–361, 361
Chen, M. C.
role theory, 288
Chen, S.
Health as Expanding Consciousness, 201
Self-Transcendence Theory, 248
Chen, Y. C.
infection prevention, 334
Chen, Y. Y.
infection prevention, 334
Chen, Z. X.
Leader–Member Exchange Theory, 358
Cheney, T.
nurse staffing and patient outcomes, 464–465
Chenot, T. M.
nursing curriculum, 487
Chesla, C.
model of skill acquisition in nursing, 232
Cheung, S.
problem-based learning, 489
student-centered teaching, 401
Chi, M. M.
infection prevention, 334
Chin, E.
information-processing model, 395
Chinn, P. L.
assumptions, 81
concept development, 51, 87
evidence-based practice, 261, 263, 264, 502, 504
feminist theory, 292
future issues in nursing, 500
knowledge development, 500
metatheory, 37
middle range theories, 38, 501
middle range theory, 214
nursing epistemology, 15
nursing theory, 25, 26, 27t–28t
nursing theory development, 29, 31, 32, 34t–36t
postmodernism, 10
practice-based evidence, 262
practice theories, 418, 421t, 502
theory and research, 431–432
theory-based nursing practice, 415, 415t
theory components, 79
theory concepts, 79
theory construction, 88
theory description and critique, 97, 98t, 101–102, 102t, 106, 107t
theory development, 73, 437
theory development process, 86
theory purpose, 79
theory structure and linkages, 81
theory testing in research, 88
theory validation and application in practice, 88
Chiu, M.
logistic teaching, 490
Chmielewski, L.
shared governance, 456, 457, 458
Cho, M.
disease management, 468
Cho, M. O.
health-promoting behaviors, 437
Cho, S. H.
nurse staffing and patient outcomes, 464
Chodorow, N.
psychoanalytic feminism, 291–292
Chou, S. S.
infection prevention, 334
Chrisman, M.
systems model, 164
Christman, L.
shared governance, 456
Christopher, K. A.
descriptive theories, 76
Chung, L.
problem-based learning, 489
student-centered teaching, 401
Ciliska, D.
evidence-based practice, 259, 261
Cimiotti, J. P.
California Safe Staffing Law, 464
nurse staffing and patient outcomes, 464, 465
Clancy, T. R.
chaos theory, 298
Clapper, T. C.
adult learning, 404
Clark, E. G.
natural history of disease, 337, 338f
Clark, M.
postmodern social theory, 300
Clarke, J.
Theory of Goal Attainment, 176
Clarke, P. N.
Roy Adaptation Model, 181
Clarke, S. P.
California Safe Staffing Law, 464
nurse staffing and patient outcomes, 464–465

Clavelle, J. T.
transformational leadership, 458
Clayton, M. F.
Uncertainty in Illness Theory, 222
Cleaves, J.
model of skill acquisition in nursing, 233
Cleland, V. S.
shared governance, 456
Clemmens, D.
Postpartum Depression Theory, 251
Cleveland, L. M.
lead exposure screening and strategies, 424
Clingerman, E.
migration transition model, 420t
Clochesy, J. M.
technology in nursing education, 491
Clouten, K.
patient-focused care, 462
Cloutier, J. D.
comparison of concept development models, 67
concept development, 51
Cobb, K. A.
lead exposure screening and strategies, 424
Cobb, R. K.
predictive theories, 39
Cochrane, A.
evidence-based practice, 258–259
Cochrane, D.
psychoanalytic theory, 309
Cody, W. K.
evidence-based practice, 118, 131
humanbecoming paradigm, 205
middle range theory, 214, 215
nursing as human science, 16, 17
parsimony of theory, 127
Rogerian theory, 196
theory-based nursing practice, 415
Coggin, C.
Artinian Intersystem Model, 168
Cohen, B.
infection prevention, 334
Cohen, S. R.
general systems theory, 283
Coke, L.
cultural care diversity and universality theory, 233–234
Coleman, C.
Six Sigma, 381
Coleman, J.
rational choice theory, 281
Cone, P. H.
Artinian Intersystem Model, 168
Conger, J. A.
charismatic leadership, 364
Conley, Y. P.
nursing curriculum, 487
Connors, R.
stress theories, 321
Conway, J.
patient-focused care, 462
Cook, D. J.
disease management, 468
Cooley, C. H.
concept of self, 285
Cooper, C.
problem-based learning, 489
Cope, V. C.
generational differences, 287
Corbin, J. M.
chronic illness trajectory framework, 242t
Corcoran, P.
social networks, 284
Corcoran-Perry, S. A.
caring as central construct, 45
nursing as discipline, 4
Cormier, E.
generational differences, 287
Cornally, N.
research-based concepts, 54
Corrigan, J. M.
quality improvement, 470
Coser, L.
conflict theories, 290
Costigan, S. A.
social cognitive theories, 322
Cottingham, C.
transformational leadership, 458
Coulter, M.
Kotter's Eight Step Plan for Implementing Change, 371
Path–Goal Theory, 362
transactional and transformational leadership, 363
Courneya, K. S.
Bandura's social learning theory, 400
Covell, C. L.
nursing intellectual capital, 218
Coward, D. D.
Self-Transcendence Theory, 248
Cowles, K. V.
sources of concepts, 54t
Cox, C.
motivation in health behavior, 242t
Coyle, J. S.
model of skill acquisition in nursing, 232
Craig, G. P.
adult learning, 404
Crandell, J.
Uncertainty of Illness Theory, 244
Cranley, L. A.
Theory of Nurses' Recognizing and Responding to Uncertainty, 435
Crede, M.
transformational leadership, 363
Cristancho, S.
operational teaching, 490
Critchley, S.
Artinian Intersystem Model, 168
Crogan, N. L.
predictive theories, 39
Cromwell, J. L.
Nightingale, 133, 134, 135, 136
Cronenwett, L.
nursing curriculum, 487
Cronin, P.
philosophy, overview, 6
Cropley, S.
patient-focused care, 463
Crosby, F. E.
Gagne's learning principles, 398
Crosby, P. B.
quality improvement, 377–378
Crowley, D. M.
metaparadigm, 42–44
nursing as discipline, 4
Crowther, S.
Lean Thinking, 379
Cull-Willby, B. L.
empiricism, 8
Cunningham, D. J.
constructivism, 402
Curley, M. A. Q.
Synergy Model for Patient Care, 96
Transitions Theory, 239, 240
Curry, D. M.
gate control theory, 350
Curtis, A. B.
cultural care diversity and universality theory, 233
Cusack, G.
genomics in nursing practice, 344–345
Cutcliff, J. R.
concept development, 50

D

Daack-Hirsch, S.
nursing curriculum, 487
Daft, R. L.
conflict mode model, 374
empowerment, 369
quality improvement, 378
Theory X and Theory Y, 359
Dahinten, S.
caring as central construct, 45
metaparadigm, 42
Dahnke, M. D.
empiricism, 8
future issues in nursing education, 507
perceived view of science, 9
philosophy, overview, 6
science, overview, 6
Dahrendorf, R.
conflict theory, 290
Dale, A. E.
theory application in practice, 413
D'Alonzo, K. T.
web of causation, 337
Daly, J.
humanbecoming paradigm, 205
maintaining hope in transition theory, 420t
Damgaard, G.
humanbecoming paradigm, 205
Damus, K.
Johnson model, 149
Danford, C. A.
social justice, 44
Daniel, L.
technology in nursing education, 493
Daniel, L. G.
nursing curriculum, 487

da Silva, L. de F.
Theory of Goal Attainment, 177
Daubenmire, M. J.
King's conceptual framework, 176
Davidow, S. L.
nurse staffing and patient outcomes, 464
quality improvement, 375, 377
Davidson, J. E.
descriptive theories, 76
Facilitated Sensemaking, 218
theory to practice to theory approach, 84
Davidson, P. M.
maintaining hope in transition theory, 420t
Davies, A.
Leader–Member Exchange Theory, 370
Davis, A. L.
Theory X and Theory Y, 359
Davis, D. M.
nursing as profession, 3
Davis, J.
Health Belief Model, 326
Davis, J. E.
Nurse Practitioner Practice Model, 231t
Davis, S.
predictive theories, 77
Day, L.
nursing curriculum, 508
Dearholt, S.
Johns Hopkins Nursing Evidence-Based Practice Model, 264, 267–270, 269b
DeChurch, L.
Path–Goal Theory, 362
Dee, V.
Johnson model, 149
Deering, C. G.
Piaget's cognitive development theory, 397
Defloor, T.
general systems theory, 283
de Freitas, M. C.
Theory of Goal Attainment, 177
Degner, L. F.
theory of keeping the spirit alive, 249t
DeJoseph, J.
cultural diversity and cultural bias, 295
de Koning, H.
quality improvement, 379–380
Delac, K.
technology in nursing education, 493
Delaney, A.
logistic teaching, 490
Delgado, M.
mobile device for nursing, 139
Dellinger, A.
Health Belief Model, 326
DeLuca, J.
natural history of disease, 339
Demark-Wahnefried, W.
cancer theories, 348
Deming, W. E.
quality improvement, 375, 377, 377t
Demiralp, M.
Postpartum Depression Theory, 251
Denholm, C.
model of skill acquisition in nursing, 232
Derdiarian, A. K.
Johnson model, 149
DeSanto-Madeya, S.
grand theories, 37
metaparadigm, 44
middle range theories, 38
middle range theory, 214, 215, 217
nursing theory development, 41
nursing theory in nursing research, 444
theory analysis and evaluation, 97, 100–101
theory and research, 432
theory as conceptual framework, 442–443
Descartes, R.
philosophy, overview, 7
de Slavy, J. R.
technology in nursing education, 493
Dever, M.
Conservation Model, 163
Devran, A.
Postpartum Depression Theory, 251
DeVries, A.
disease management, 470
Dewey, D.
concept of mind, 285
DeYoung, A.
Health Promotion Model, 236
DeYoung, S.
learning theories, 407
DiBartolo, M. C.
empiricism, 8
operational teaching, 490
perceived view of science, 9, 10
philosophy, overview, 6
postpositivism, 8
Dibble, S.
cultural diversity and cultural bias, 295
DiCenso, A.
evidence-based practice, 259, 261
Dickey, S. B.
Piaget's cognitive development theory, 396–397
Dickinson, J.
critical social theory, 293
Dickoff, J.
explanatory theories, 76
nursing theory, 25, 38, 72, 132
nursing theory development, 30
predictive theories, 76
prescriptive theories, 77, 434
theory categorization, 75
Diedrick, L.
ACE Star Model, 266
evidence-based practice, 270–271
Diekelmann, N.
nursing curriculum, 482
Dieter, C.
nursing curriculum, 487
Dijkstra, A.
Care Dependency Scale, 139
Dillard, N.
nursing curriculum, 481, 481b, 484
Dilthey, W.
nursing as human science, 16
Disch, J.
future issues in nursing, 499
nursing curriculum, 487
Dluhy, N. M.
information-processing model, 395
Doane, G. H.
theory–practice gap, 416
Dobbins, J. A.
learning styles, 405
Dobratz, M. C.
middle range theory of adaptation in death and dying, 220, 439
Dochterman, G. M.
prescriptive theories, 78
Dochterman, J. M.
Nursing Intervention Classification system, 422–423, 423t, 424t
Dodge, T.
Theory of Reasoned Action/Planned Behavior, 326
Doering, J.
explanatory theories, 76
normalcy after childbirth, 419
Does, R. J. M. M.
quality improvement, 379–380
Dokken, D.
patient-focused care, 463
Dolansky, M. A.
nursing curriculum, 487
Dole, D.
critical social theory, 293
Dombrowsky, T. A.
descriptive theories, 38–39
Donahue, M. P.
Harvey's study of circulation, 333
nursing theory development, 29, 30, 33t
Donald, A.
evidence-based practice, 381
Donaldson, M. S.
quality improvement, 470
Donaldson, N.
California Safe Staffing Law, 464
Donaldson, S. K.
metaparadigm, 42–43
nursing as discipline, 4
Donnelly, T. T.
postmodern social theory, 300
Doolin, C. T.
Theory of Comfort, 246
Doornbos, M. M.
Theory of Goal Attainment, 177
Doran, D. M.
Theory of Nurses' Recognizing and Responding to Uncertainty, 435
Dossa, A.
Transitions Theory, 239
Dossey, B. M.
Nightingale, 132, 133, 134, 135, 136

Dougherty, C. M.
study of implantable cardioverter defibrillator, 436–437, 443
Dover, L.
Artinian Intersystem Model, 168
Dow, K. H.
technology in nursing education, 491
Doyle, C.
cancer theories, 348
Dracup, K.
maintaining hope in transition theory, 420t
Drafke, M.
Achievement–Motivation Theory, 366
leadership traits, 356
Drake, D. A.
practice to theory approach, 85
Draucker, C. B.
symbolic interactionism, 286
Dreher, H. M.
empiricism, 8
future issues in nursing education, 507
perceived view of science, 9
philosophy, overview, 6
science, overview, 6
Dreifuerst, K. T.
dialectic learning, 489
Drenkard, K.
transformational leadership, 458
Drenning, C.
evidence-based practice, 474
Dreyfus, H. L.
theory-based nursing practice, 415
Dreyfus, S. E.
theory-based nursing practice, 415
Driscoll, J. W.
Postpartum Depression Theory, 251
Driver, E.
Transitions Theory, 241
Droes, N. S.
Theory of Chronic Sorrow, 110
Dubin, R.
concepts, types of, 51, 51t
DuBrin, A. J.
administration and management, 366
decision-making process, 373–374
emotional intelligence, 356, 357
leadership, 355, 356, 357, 362
Dubrowski, A.
operational teaching, 490
Ducharme, F.
Roy Adaptation Model, 181
Dudley-Brown, S. L.
theory evaluation, 98t, 104–105, 106, 107t
Duffey, M.
theory analysis and evaluation, 97, 98t, 99, 99b, 106
Duffy, T. M.
constructivism, 402
Duke, G.
cancer theories, 348
evidence-based practice, 259, 261, 504
Dumchin, M.
model of skill acquisition in nursing, 232
Dunbar, S. B.
postmodernism, 10
research methodology, 18
Duncan, C.
comparison of concept development models, 67
concept development, 51
Duncan, M.
human needs theory, 317
Dunn, D. G.
Roy Adaptation Model, 181
Dunn, H. C.
Roy Adaptation Model, 181
Dunn, K.
learning styles, 405
Dunn, K. S.
model of skill acquisition in nursing, 232
Theory of Adaptation to Chronic Pain, 86, 221, 249t
Dunn, R.
learning styles, 405
Dunne, P. J.
logistic teaching, 490
Duquette, A.
Roy Adaptation Model, 181
Durfor, S. L.
explanatory theories, 76
normalcy after childbirth, 419
Durney-Crowley, J.
nursing curriculum, 487, 487t
Du Thoit, G.
Health Belief Model, 326
Dworkin, S. L.
symbolic interactionism, 286
Dyess, S. M.
sustaining health in faith community, 218, 438

E

Eakes, G.
Theory of Chronic Sorrow, 109–112, 218, 248, 249–250
Early, T. J.
psychosocial developmental theory, 310
Edmonds, M. L.
operational teaching, 490
Edwards, A.
Health Belief Model, 326
Edwards, Q. I.
genomics in cancer care, 346
Edwards, S. B.
symbolic interactionism, 286
Eggert, J.
nursing curriculum, 487
Ehlers, V.
human needs theory, 317
Ehlman, K.
psychosocial developmental theory, 310
Eichelberger, L. W.
nursing theory, 25
Eilam, G.
authentic leadership, 364
Einstein, A.
paradigm shift, 120
parsimony of theory, 127
Eitzen, D. S.
conflict theories, 289, 289b, 290
feminist theory, 290
Eliason, M. J.
cultural diversity and cultural bias, 295
Ellefsen, B.
research methodology, 18
Ellington, L.
interpersonal theory, 312
Elliot, N. L.
future issues in nursing, 507
Elliott, J. E.
experimental research on cancer pain, 434t
Ellis, A.
Rational Emotive Theory, 314–315, 327t
Ellis, J. R.
administration and management, 506
nursing as profession, 2
Ellis, R.
characteristics of significant theories, 98, 98t, 106, 107t, 124
Ellrodt, G.
disease management, 468
Elsahoff, J.
California Safe Staffing Law, 464
Elsayed, N. G.
perceived view of science, 9
Emerson, R.
social exchange theory, 280
social networks, 284
Emerson, R. J.
allostasis, 340
fight or flight, 340
Endo, E.
Health as Expanding Consciousness, 201
Engebretson, J.
cultural diversity and cultural bias, 295
Erci, B.
interpersonal theory, 312
Erdley, W. S.
disease management, 469
Erdmann
Artinian Intersystem Model, 165t
Erickson, H.
assumptions, concepts, and relationships, 170–172, 171t
background, 169
caring as central construct, 45
interactive–integrative paradigm, 122
middle range theory, 214
Modeling and Role-Modeling, 160
nursing theory, 36t, 119, 169–173
parsimony of theory, 173
philosophical underpinnings of theory, 170
testability of theory, 172
usefulness of theory, 172
value in extending nursing science, 173
Erikson, E. H.
psychosocial developmental theory, 307, 307t, 310–311, 327t, 401

Eriksson, K.
nursing theory, 119
Esposito, E. M.
correlational study of exercise, 436
Health Promotion Model, 236
Esposito-Smythers, C.
cognitive behavioral therapies, 315
Ethridge, P.
Health as Expanding Consciousness, 201
Evans, K. C.
philosophy, overview, 6, 7
Everett, L. Q.
Iowa Model, of evidence-based practice, 264

F

Fahey, K. F.
experimental research on cancer pain, 434t
Fairbanks, E.
evidence-based practice, 266
Falk-Rafael, A.
practice to theory approach, 85
Fallarco, M. D.
Gagne's learning principles, 398
Fanfan, D.
web of causation, 337
Fang, Y.
Health Belief Model, 326
Farrell, D.
Theory of Unpleasant Symptoms, 247
Fasnacht, P. H.
concept analysis, 66
Conservation Model, 163
Fawcett, J.
background, 125
California Safe Staffing Law, 464
caring as central construct, 45
concept development, 50
descriptive theories, 76
evidence-based practice, 259, 261, 264
grand theories, 37, 117, 127
health-related behaviors of Korean Americans, 420t
King, 173
metaparadigm, 41, 44
middle range theories, 38
middle range theory, 214, 215, 217
Neuman Systems Model, 131, 149–154
nursing as discipline, 4
nursing epistemology, 14
nursing theory, 24, 25, 41
paradigm categorization of theories, 122–123, 123t, 124, 126
predictive theories, 77
research on cesarean birth, 434t, 441
science and philosophy, 5
social networks, 284
theory analysis and evaluation, 97, 98t, 100–101, 106, 107t, 124, 126
theory and research, 432, 434, 444
theory application in practice, 414b
Fayol, H.
chain of command, 454
classic management theory, 366, 366b
Feinstein, N. F.
evidence-based practice, 266
Ferguson-Pare, M.
humanbecoming paradigm, 205
Fernandez, J.
cultural care diversity and universality theory, 234
nursing strategies to reduce caries, 427t
Ferrans, C. E.
prescriptive theories, 78
Ferrante, J.
cultural diversity and cultural bias, 294, 294b
Fetter, N. S.
technology in nursing education, 493
Fiedler, F.
Contingency Theory of Leadership, 360–361
Fielder, R. A.
nursing education, 480
Fields, B.
critical social theory, 293
principle-based concept analysis, 66
Fike, A.
Magnet Recognition Program, 466
Finegan, J.
shared governance, 456
Fineout-Overholt, E.
ARCC Model, 264, 266
evidence-based practice, 32, 258–261, 263–264, 266–267, 270, 380–382, 421t, 474
Johns Hopkins Nursing Evidence-Based Practice Model, 267
Stetler Model of Evidence-Based Practice, 270
Finke, L. M.
nursing curriculum, 482, 486, 487
Finkelman, A.
evidence-based practice, 261, 263
nursing as profession, 2, 3
Finnegan, L.
prescriptive theories, 78
Finney, K.
operational teaching, 490
Firestone, S.
radical feminism, 291
Fishbein, M.
Theory of Reasoned Action/Planned Behavior, 222–223, 322–326, 325f, 327t
Fisher, A.
theory–practice gap, 416
Fitzgerald, K.
learning theories, 407
Fitzpatrick, J.
background, 125
evidence-based practice, 261, 264
middle range theory, 214
nursing epistemology, 14
nursing theory, 36t
theory evaluation, 98t
theory in research, 433
Fitzpatrick, J. J.
correlational study of exercise, 436
cultural diversity and cultural bias, 295
Health Promotion Model, 236
Rogerian theory, 196
Self-Transcendence Theory, 248
transformational leadership, 458
Flaskerud, J. H.
theory-research-practice relationship, 82
Fletcher, B. J.
natural history of disease, 339
Flood, M. E.
nursing curriculum, 482
Floria-Santos, M.
genomics in cancer care, 346
Floyd, J. M.
Magnet Recognition Program, 466
Flynn, L.
California Safe Staffing Law, 464
nurse staffing and patient outcomes, 465
patient care delivery models, 463
Fogarty, K. J.
cultural care diversity and universality theory, 233
Fogg, L.
cultural care diversity and universality theory, 233–234
nursing education, 480
Foley, G. V.
patient-focused care, 463
Folkman, S.
stress coping adaptation theory, 221, 320
Folta, J. R.
pure *vs.* applied science, 306
Ford, D.
Theory of Reasoned Action/Planned Behavior, 326
Ford, H.
Lean Thinking, 379
Ford-Gilboe, M.
descriptive research on abused women, 434t
Foreman, M. D.
Conservation Model, 163
Forrest, S.
learning, 387
Foss, C.
research methodology, 18
Fouquier, K. F.
feminist theory, 292
Fowles, E. R.
Maternal Role Attainment/Becoming a Mother, 252
Frazier, L.
genetics of cardiovascular disease, 346
Fredericks, S.
critical social theory, 293
Frederickson, K.
Roy Adaptation Model, 181
Frederiksen, K.
principle-based concept analysis, 66
Fredland, N.
Transitions Theory, 238
Freeman, L. C.
infection prevention, 334

Freiberg, H. J.
cognitive development/interaction theories, 396
French, J.
concept of power, 368
Freud, S.
paradigm shift, 306–307
psychoanalytic theory, 307–309, 307t, 327t, 400
Frew, A.
Health Belief Model, 326
Frey, M. A.
King's conceptual framework, 176
Fridman, M.
California Safe Staffing Law, 464
Friedan, B.
liberal feminism, 291
Friesner, S. T.
gate control theory, 350
Friesth, B. M.
technology in nursing education, 492
Fruewirth, S. E. S.
Johnson model, 149
Fujino, N.
general systems theory, 283
Fuller, B.
technology in nursing education, 493
Fung, S. C.
logistic teaching, 490
Funnell, M. M.
technology in nursing education, 493

G

Gable, R. K.
Postpartum Depression Theory, 251
Gaffney, K. F.
Maternal Role Attainment/Becoming a Mother, 252
Gagne, R. M.
learning theory, 396, 397–398, 397b
Gallagher, P.
practice to theory approach, 85
Gallagher-Ford, L.
evidence-based practice, 381–382
Galvao, C. M.
Conservation Model, 163
Ganz, F. D.
general adaptation syndrome, 342
Garcia, S. P. Q.
genomics in education, 345
Gardner, H.
multiple intelligences, 404–405
Gardner, W. L.
authentic leadership, 364
Garity, J.
evidence-based practice, 259
Garmon, S. C.
theory of perceived access to breast health care, 90–91
Gassaway, J.
practice-based evidence, 261, 262
Gauvreau, K.
California Safe Staffing Law, 464
Gavriloff, C.
quality improvement to promote safety, 473
Geary, C. R.
research-based concepts, 54
Transitions Theory, 239
Gedaly-Duff, V.
cancer theories, 348
Geden, E.
Orem, 142
Gelmon, S. B.
quality improvement, 470
Gemmill, R.
Theory of Goal Attainment, 176
George, J. B.
evidence-based practice, 264
Health as Expanding Consciousness, 202
theory evaluation, 106
Transitions Theory, 237, 238
Georges, J. M.
critical social theory, 293
practice to theory approach, 85
research-based concepts, 54
Shared Presence: Caring for a Dying Spouse, 39, 435
Georgopoulos, B.
Path–Goal Theory, 361
German, V. F.
lead exposure screening and strategies, 424
Germino, B. B.
Uncertainty of Illness Theory, 244
Gharaibeh, H.
cultural diversity and cultural bias, 295
Gharaibeh, M.
cultural diversity and cultural bias, 295
Giarelli, E.
nursing curriculum, 487
web of causation, 337
Giblin, J. C.
psychosocial developmental theory, 310
Giddens, J. F.
nursing education, 480
Gift, A.
Theory of Unpleasant Symptoms, 218, 241, 246–247
Gigliotti, E.
theory-testing research, 441
Gillem, T.
quality improvement, 377t
Gillespie, B. M.
explanatory theories, 76
Gilligan, D.
psychoanalytic feminism, 292
Gillum, D. R.
cultural care diversity and universality theory, 233–234
Gilmour, J.
postmodern social theory, 300
Giordano, J.
therapeutic milieu, 313
Giske, T.
Artinian Intersystem Model, 168
Giuliano, K. K.
nursing philosophy, 11
Glanville, I.
evidence-based practice, 474
Glanz, K.
social psychology theories, 325
Glaser, D.
Perry's theory of intellectual and ethical development, 399
Gleason-Wynn, P.
Artinian Intersystem Model, 168
GlenMaye, L. F.
psychosocial developmental theory, 310
Gobert, M.
general systems theory, 283
Goldenberg, D.
nursing education, 480
Goldman, B. D.
Maternal Role Attainment/Becoming a Mother, 252
Goleman, D.
emotional intelligence, 356–357
Gonzalez, S. A.
cancer theories, 348
natural history of disease, 339
Good, M.
acute pain management, 224, 249t
Goodfellow, L. M.
Theory of Goal Attainment, 176–177
Goodman, D.
postmodern social theory, 299–300, 299t
Goran, S. F.
Synergy Model, 443
Gordon, J.
Theory of Chronic Sorrow, 109, 250, 425–426
Gortner, S. R.
empiricism, 8
metaparadigm, 42–44
nursing philosophy, 11
research methodology, 17
science, overview, 5, 6
Gottman, J. M.
chaos theory, 297
Goubergen, D. V.
general systems theory, 283
Grace, P. J.
boys' healing from being bullied, 427t
Graen, G.
Leader–Member Exchange Theory, 358
Graicunas, A.
span of control, 455
Granner, M. L.
Bandura's social learning theory, 400
Grant, M.
Theory of Goal Attainment, 176
Grant, M. L.
Theory of Chronic Sorrow, 109
Grassley, J.
research to theory approach, 85
Graungaard, A.
stress theories, 321
Gray, E. R.
Theory X and Theory Y, 359
Gray, I.
nursing education, 480
Gray, J.
Client Experience Model, 218
descriptive theories, 38–39

Gray, J. R.
nursing research, 432, 433b
Greco, K. E.
explanatory theories, 76
genomics in education, 345
research to theory approach, 85
Green, A.
predictive theories, 77
Green, B.
Health Belief Model, 326
Green, J. P.
Theory X and Theory Y, 359
Greenwald, B.
cancer theories, 348
Gregory, J. W.
Theory of Chronic Sorrow, 109, 250
Griffith, M. B.
principle-based concept analysis, 66
Griggs, S. A.
learning styles, 405
Grimbeck, P.
explanatory theories, 76
Grindley, J.
Conservation Model, 163
Gross, D.
correlational research, 434t
Grove, S. K.
nursing research, 432, 433b
Grubbs, J.
Johnson, 147, 148t, 149
Grupp, K.
natural history of disease, 339
Guarnero, P.
symbolic interactionism, 286
Gudmundsdottir, M.
postmodern social theory, 300
Guedes, M. V. C.
Theory of Goal Attainment, 177
Guhde, J.
dialectic learning, 489
Gunther, M. E.
Rogers, 193
Gustafsson, B.
empiricism, 8
science and philosophy, 5
Guvenc, G.
cancer theories, 348
Guyatt, G.
evidence-based practice, 259, 261
Guyton, A. C.
concepts of physiology, 54

H

Haag-Heitman, B.
model of skill acquisition in nursing, 233
Haas, B.
evidence-based practice, 259, 261, 504
Haber, J.
correlational research, 436
evidence-based practice, 31, 259, 419, 421t
experimental research, 436
research framework, 433–434
research process, 433b
theory-testing research, 439
Habermas, J.
critical social theory, 292
Hacker, M.
Self-Transcendence Theory, 248
Hackett, R. D.
Leader–Member Exchange Theory, 358
Haddad, V. C. N.
Nightingale, 135
Haefner, D. P.
Health Belief Model, 323f
Haggstrom, M.
theory of ICU transitional care, 435
Transitions Theory, 238
Hainsworth, M. A.
Theory of Chronic Sorrow, 109–112, 218, 248, 249–250
Halding, A. G.
Transitions Theory, 238
Hall, C. S.
defense mechanisms, 308
Hall, E. O. C.
model of skill acquisition in nursing, 232
Hall, J.
critical social theory, 293
Hall, J. E.
concepts of physiology, 54
Hall, J. L.
research on cesarean birth, 434t, 441
Hall, J. M.
principle-based concept analysis, 66
Hall, L. E.
nursing theory, 31, 34t, 119
Hall, L. M.
natural history of disease, 339
Hall, S.
Conservation Model, 163
Hall, W.
caring as central construct, 45
metaparadigm, 42
Hallas, D.
cultural care diversity and universality theory, 234
nursing strategies to reduce caries, 427t
Halliday, L. E.
Uncertainty of Illness Theory, 244
Halperin, B.
Theory of Reasoned Action/Planned Behavior, 326
Halstead, J. A.
future issues in nursing education, 507
technology in nursing education, 492
Hamilton, R. J.
Theory of Genetic Vulnerability, 220
theory to research to theory approach, 86
Hammer, V. R.
adult learning, 404
Hamrin, V.
social exchange theory, 281
Hanchett, E.
nurse-expressed empathy, 219
Handley, S. M.
psychosocial developmental theory, 310
Hann, H. W.
health-related behaviors of Korean Americans, 420t
social networks, 284
Hanna, D.
Roy Adaptation Model, 181
Hannah, D.
Transitions Theory, 238
Hannon-Engel, S. L.
practice theory derived from Roy Adaptation Model, 419
Hansen, L.
role theory, 288
Hanson, K. J.
cognitive-field (gestalt) theory, 394
Hardin, P. K.
nursing education/curriculum, 480, 487
Hardin, S. R.
nursing theory development, 33t
Synergy Model application, 426, 427t
theoretical statements, 79
theory and research, 431
theory components, 79
theory concepts, 79
theory structure and linkages, 81
Transitions Theory, 239, 240, 241
variable *vs.* nonvariable concepts, 52
Hardy, M.
concept development, 51
concepts, type of, 52
theoretically *vs.* operationally defined concepts, 53
theoretical statements, 80t
theory evaluation, 97, 98–99, 98t, 106, 107t, 124
variable *vs.* nonvariable concepts, 52
Harms, P. D.
transformational leadership, 363
Harp, R.
Contingency Theory of Leadership, 361
Hartley, C. L.
nursing as profession, 2
Hartley, L.
administration and management, 506
Harvey, G.
context analysis, 66
Harvey, W.
blood circulation, 333
Harwood, L.
model of skill acquisition in nursing, 232
Hasbargen, B.
dialectic learning, 489
Hastings-Tolsma, M.
Theory of Diversity of Human Field Pattern, 219
theory to research to theory approach, 86
Hatfield, B.
model of skill acquisition in nursing, 232

Hatfield, L. A.
gate control theory, 350
Hatlevik, I. K. R.
theory–practice gap, 416
Haussler, S.
research on cesarean birth, 434t, 441
Havens, D. S.
Magnet Recognition Program, 466
Havighurst, R.
readiness to learn, 401
Hawkins, M.
shared governance, 456
Hawks, J. H.
germ theory, 333
immune system, 342
Hawver, T. H.
emotional intelligence, 363
Hayat, M. J.
correlational research, 434t
Hayles, N. K.
chaos theory, 296
Hayman, L.
California Safe Staffing Law, 464
Hayman, L. L.
Health Promotion Model, 236
Haynes, R. B.
evidence-based practice, 259
Hayward, R. D.
predictive theories, 77
Heater, B. S.
Theory of Chronic Sorrow, 110
Heaton, T. B.
chaos theory, 297
Hechter, M.
rational choice theory, 281
Hecke, A. V.
general systems theory, 283
Heggdal, K.
Transitions Theory, 238
Heifner, C.
Health Promotion Model, 236
Heineken, J.
power concepts, 368
Heinitz, K.
charismatic leadership, 364
Heino, E.
model of skill acquisition in nursing, 233
Heise, B.
dialectic learning, 489
Heitkemper, M.
health-promoting behaviors, 437
Hektor, L. M.
Rogers and Rogerian theory, 193, 196
Heller, B. R.
nursing curriculum, 487, 487t
Hellriegel, D.
leadership, 355
Helms, J. E.
gate control theory, 349
Henderson, A.
caring as central construct, 45
parsimony of theory, 138
value in extending nursing science, 138–139
Henderson, J.
cognitive behavioral therapies, 315
Henderson, V.
activities for client assistance, 137–138, 138t
assumptions, concepts, and relationships, 137
background, 136–137
metaparadigm, 42, 132
nursing theory, 34t, 119, 124, 124t, 136–139
philosophical underpinnings of theory, 137
testability of theory, 138
usefulness of theory, 138
Hendricks, J. M.
generational differences, 287
Hennig, L. M.
technology in nursing education, 491
Hergenhahn, B. R.
definition of learning, 387
learning theory, 389, 390, 392
Herring, P.
Shared Presence: Caring for a Dying Spouse, 39, 435
Herrman, J. W.
operational teaching, 490
Herrmann, E. K.
Henderson, 137
Hersey, P.
situational leadership theory, 362
Herting, J. R.
natural history of disease, 339
Hervé, R.
causative agent in disease, 334
Herzberg, F.
motivation–hygiene (two-factor) theory, 359–360, 366
Hess, R. G.
shared governance, 458
Hickey, P. A.
California Safe Staffing Law, 464
Hickman, J. S.
concept development and research, 57
grand theories, 74
metatheory, 37, 74
nursing theory development, 34t–36t
received and perceived views of science, 7
research-practice relationship, 83
theory description, 97
theory evaluation, 97
theory-research-practice relationship, 82
Transitions Theory, 237, 238
Higgins, P. A.
explanatory theories, 39
grand theories, 37, 74, 117
middle range theories, 38, 74
middle range theory, 215
nursing theory, 37
practice theories, 38, 75
relationship among levels of theory, 75
theory of music, mood, and movement, 218
Hill, K.
Caring Science as Sacred Science, 186
Hill, T. L.
logistic teaching, 490
Hills, M.
Caring Science as Sacred Science, 186
Hilton, P. A.
Nightingale, 26
nursing theory development, 34t–36t
Himes, D.
dialectic learning, 489
Himmelfarb, C. D.
natural history of disease, 339
Hinshaw, A. S.
areas of evolving nursing science, 446–448, 447t
Magnet Recognition Program, 466
Hitt, M. A.
behavioral theories of leadership, 357
Contingency Theory of Leadership, 361
Hobdell, E. F.
Theory of Chronic Sorrow, 109
Hodges, H. F.
career persistence in acute care, 218
Hodges, T. D.
authentic leadership, 364
Hodgins, M. J.
testing of caregiving theory, 441
Hodson-Carlton, K. E.
technology in nursing education, 491
Hoenig, H.
Transitions Theory, 239
Hoerl, R. W.
quality improvement, 379
Hogan, M.
operational teaching, 490
Hogan, N.
Nightingale, 136
Hohman, M.
humanbecoming paradigm, 205
Hoke, M. M.
Health Promotion Model, 236, 443
Holaday, B.
Johnson model, 149
Holden, J. E.
gate control theory, 350
Holditch-Davis, D.
Maternal Role Attainment/Becoming a Mother, 252
Holland, B. E.
Client Experience Model, 218
Hollander, M.
nurse staffing and patient outcomes, 464
quality improvement, 375, 377
Hollenbeck, J. R.
behavioral theories of leadership, 357
Rational Decision-Making Model, 372
Holmes, C.
critical social theory, 293
Holmes, D.
postmodernism, 10

Holmes, T.
general adaptation syndrome, 341–342
Holton, E. F.
adult learning, 402–404, 403b
cognitive-field (gestalt) theory, 393
psychodynamic learning theory, 400
Holtz, C.
cultural care diversity and universality theory, 233
Holzemer, W. L.
nursing science, 12
research methodology, 16
science, overview, 6
Homans, G.
social exchange theory, 280, 281
Hood, L. J.
nursing as profession, 3
postmodernism, 10
Hopkin, R. J.
genetic counseling, 345
Hopkins, B. A.
theory-testing research, 439
Horn, S. D.
practice-based evidence, 261, 262
Horswell, R.
disease management, 469
Horton, K. L.
symbolic interactionism, 286
Houldin, A. D.
Theory of Reasoned Action/Planned Behavior, 326, 443
House, R. J.
charismatic leadership, 364
Path–Goal Theory, 361–362
Houston, S.
Magnet Recognition Program, 466
Howie, L.
cognitive-field (gestalt) theory, 393–394
Hoyt, S.
Nightingale, 135
Hsieh, S. I.
logistic teaching, 490
Hsu, L. L.
logistic teaching, 490
Hudepol, J. H.
humanbecoming paradigm, 205
Hudson, K.
evidence-based practice, 259, 261, 504
Hughes, I.
grand theories, 118
Hughes, R.
Theory of Goal Attainment, 176
Hughes, T.
immune function, 343
Hull, C. L.
reinforcement, 389, 389t, 390
Hume, D.
empiricism, 8
Hummel, J. R.
disease management, 470
Humphrey, R. H.
emotional intelligence, 363
Humphreys, A.
nurses' competence in genetics, 345
Hunker, D. F.
Postpartum Depression Theory, 251
Hunnibell, L. S.
Self-Transcendence Theory, 248
Hunt, D.
disease management, 468
Hunter, J.
infection prevention, 334
Huntington, A.
postmodern social theory, 300
Hupcey, J. E.
comparison of concept development models, 67
concept development, 50, 55, 67, 68t
principle-based concept analysis, 66, 67b
Hurlbut, J. M.
Health Promotion Model, 236, 443
Huseby-Moore, K.
Rogerian theory, 196
Huston, C. J.
administration and management, 506
evidence-based practice, 263
practice-based evidence, 262
Hutchinson, S. W.
Health Belief Model, 326
Huth, M. M.
theory of acute pain management, 224
Hutto, B. E.
Bandura's social learning theory, 400
Hynes, C.
psychoanalytic theory, 309

I

Icaboni, J.
infection prevention, 334
Ihlenfed, J.
social exchange theory, 282
Im, E. O.
Asian Immigrant Women's Menopausal Symptom Experience, 420t
explanatory theories, 76
midlife women's attitudes toward physical activity, 420t
practice theories, 418, 421t, 502
practice to theory approach, 85
Transitions Theory, 237
Ingersoll, G. L.
evidence-based practice, 259, 260, 261
Irvin, B. L.
theory-testing research, 439
Isaksson, A.
Theory of Chronic Sorrow, 109, 250
Isaramalai, S.
Orem, 142
Isbir, G. G.
adaptation in pregnancy, 426
Isenberg, M.
Roy Adaptation Model, 181
Ishikawa, J.
Caring Science as Sacred Science, 186
Iwasiw, C. L.
nursing education, 480

J

Jaarsma, T.
middle range theory of self-care, 219, 439
Jablonski, K.
cancer theories, 348
Jackson, S. E.
leadership, 355
Jacobs, B. B.
Nightingale, 135, 136
Jacobson, J.
cancer theories, 348
Jacobson, L.
nursing education, 480, 507
Jacox, A.
abstract *vs.* concrete concepts, 52
assumptions, 81
concept development, 86
concepts, types of, 51
empiricism, 8
postpositivism, 8
theoretical statements, 80t
theory development process, 86
Jago, A. G.
decision making, 372
leadership theories, 362
James, P.
explanatory theories, 76
nursing theory, 25, 38, 72, 132
nursing theory development, 30
predictive theories, 76
prescriptive theories, 77, 434
theory categorization, 75
James, W.
concept of self, 285
Jampol, M. L.
Theory of Normalizing Risky Sexual Behaviors, 218
Jankowski, S. M.
Health as Expanding Consciousness, 201
Janzen, S. K.
Magnet Recognition Program, 466
Jarrell, A.
interpersonal theory, 313
Jeanerette, C.
Uncertainty of Illness Theory, 244
Jeffries, P. R.
nursing education, 480, 491, 492
Jenkins, B.
research-based concepts, 54
Jenkins, J.
genomics in nursing practice, 344–345
Roy Adaptation Model, 181
Jenkins, K.
California Safe Staffing Law, 464
Jennings, B. M.
evidence-based practice, 259, 261
Jens, R.
charismatic leadership, 364

Jensen, E.
evidence-based practice, 504
Jensen, L.
Conservation Model, 163
Jirovec, M. M.
Roy Adaptation Model, 181
Johnson, A.
logistic teaching, 490
Johnson, A. P.
Magnet Recognition Program, 465
Johnson, B.
patient-focused care, 462
Johnson, B. M.
chaos theory, 296
general systems theory, 282
theory–practice gap, 417
Johnson, D.
assumptions, concepts, and relationships, 147–148, 147t
background, 147
Behavioral System Model, 146–149
metaparadigm, 43t, 147
nursing theory, 34t, 119, 124, 124t, 146–149
parsimony of theory, 149
philosophical underpinnings of theory, 147
testability of theory, 149
totality paradigm, 121
usefulness of theory, 149
value in extending nursing science, 149
writings, 146, 146b
Johnson, D. E.
borrowed theories, 306
Johnson, J.
nursing curriculum, 487
Johnson, N. L.
web of causation, 337
Johnson, R. L.
genetics of cardiovascular disease, 346
Johnson, S.
web of causation, 337
Jonas, C.
humanbecoming paradigm, 205
Jones, C.
grand theories, 118
Health Belief Model, 326
Jones, D.
Health as Expanding Consciousness, 202
Newman and Newman theory, 198
Jones, D. A.
Health as Expanding Consciousness, 201
Jones, N.
Path–Goal Theory, 361
Jones-Parker, H.
natural history of disease, 339
Jonsdottir, H.
nursing as discipline, 4
theory application in practice, 413
Jordan, M.
general systems theory, 283
Joseph, H. A.
Theory of Chronic Sorrow, 250
Joseph, L. M.
Theory of Goal Attainment, 176
Judd, D.
nursing as profession, 3
Judge, C. A.
interpersonal theory, 313
Judge, T. A.
Achievement–Motivation Theory, 366, 367
departmentalization, 456
Equity Theory, 368
organizational design, 453
transactional and transformational leadership, 363
visionary leadership, 364
Junda, T.
social networks, 284
Jung, D. D.
charismatic leadership, 364
Jung, D. I.
transformational leadership, 363
Juran, J. M.
quality improvement, 377–378
Jurgens, C. Y.
Theory of Unpleasant Symptoms, 247
Justin, J. E.
Path–Goal Theory, 362

K

Kacmaz, Z.
interpersonal theory, 312
Kahn, D. L.
Self-Transcendence Theory, 248
Kaiser, M.
disease management, 469
Kalisch, B. J.
Nightingale, 26, 431
nursing theory development, 28, 30, 33t
Pasteur's germ theory, 333
Kalisch, P. A.
Nightingale, 26, 431
nursing theory development, 28, 30, 33t
Pasteur's germ theory, 333
Kameoka, T.
King's conceptual framework, 176
Kanacki, L. S.
research-based concepts, 54
Shared Presence: Caring for a Dying Spouse, 39, 435
Kane, V.
problem-based learning, 489
Kang, D. H.
immune function, 343
Kang, Y.
health-promoting behaviors, 437
predictive theories, 77
Kangas, S.
patient care delivery models, 463
Kant, I.
philosophy, overview, 7
Kanter, R.
Theory of Structural Empowerment, 370
Kanungo, R. N.
charismatic leadership, 364
Kao, C. H.
social networks, 284
Kao, H. F. S.
social networks, 284
Kaplan, L.
evidence-based practice, 381–382
Kapralos, B.
operational teaching, 490
Karian, V. E.
Health as Expanding Consciousness, 201
Karpf, T.
Nightingale, 135
Karunamuni, N.
social cognitive theories, 322
Kaskel, B. L.
nursing curriculum, 484
Kasl, S. V.
Health Belief Model, 323f
Kasper, C. E.
nursing theory, 25
Kasprzyk, D.
Theory of Reasoned Action/Planned Behavior, 323
Katz, N. H.
conflict management, 374
Kaur, R.
infection prevention, 334
Kawano, M.
Caring Science as Sacred Science, 186
Kay, A.
Theory X and Theory Y, 359
Keating, S. B.
nursing education/curriculum, 480, 481, 483, 484–485
Kedziora-Kornatowsa, K.
Care Dependency Scale, 139
Kee, S.
patient care delivery models, 463
Keeley, A. C.
career persistence in acute care, 218
Keene, A.
pain management, 349
Keevil, C.
causative agent in disease, 334
Keilman, L. J.
model of skill acquisition in nursing, 232
Keithley, J. K.
logistic teaching, 490
Keller, C.
experimental study of "sign chi do" exercises, 437
Kelley, H. M.
social exchange theory, 280
Kelley, J.
nursing curriculum, 482
Kelley, L. S.
humanbecoming paradigm, 205
Kelly, C. W.
commitment to health theory, 439
Kelly, K.
immune function, 343
Kelly, M.
patient-focused care, 463
Kelly, T.
cognitive-field (gestalt) theory, 393–394

Kemp, V.
model for smoking prevention, 222–223
Kemper, A. R.
natural history of disease, 339
Kendall, J.
explanatory theories, 76
research to theory approach, 85
Kendall, L. C.
Theory of Chronic Sorrow, 110
Kennedy, H. P.
postmodern social theory, 300
Kenner, C.
evidence-based practice, 261, 263
nursing as profession, 2, 3
Kennerly, S. M.
transformational leadership, 459
Kenney, J. W.
general systems theory, 282
theory application in practice, 413, 414b
theory-based nursing practice, 414
Kerlinger, F. N.
concept development, 50
concept development and research, 57
Ketefian, S.
middle range theories, 38
nurse staffing and patient outcomes, 464
Khoueiry, G.
Six Sigma, 381
Khurana, D. S.
Theory of Chronic Sorrow, 109
Kidd, P.
nursing theory development, 29t, 47
research methodology, 18
Kiefner, J.
Piaget's cognitive development theory, 396–397
Kiesel, M.
homeostasis, 340
Kikuchi, J. F.
theory-based nursing practice, 415
Kilmann, R. H.
conflict mode model, 374
Kim, H. S.
concept development, 50, 61–63, 62t, 64t, 67, 68t
metaparadigm, 41, 44
middle range theory, 214, 501
practice theories, 418t
testability of theories, 127
Kim, S.
cultural diversity and cultural bias, 295
predictive theories, 77
King, I. M.
assumptions, concepts, and relationships, 174–176, 175t
background, 173
nursing theory, 34t, 119, 124, 124t, 173–177
philosophical underpinnings of theory, 174
Systems Framework, 160, 173–177
testability of theory, 176–177
Theory of Goal Attainment, 160, 173–177, 174t
transactional process, 173–177
usefulness of theory, 176
King, J.
parish nursing model, 231t
Kipnis, D.
coercion power, 369
Kirk, M.
genomic health care, 345
nursing curriculum, 487
Kirkham, S. R.
caring as central construct, 45
metaparadigm, 42
postmodern social theory, 300
Kirkley, D.
Magnet Recognition Program, 465
Kitson, A.
context analysis, 66
Kitson, A. L.
general systems theory, 283
Kiviniemi, M. T.
correlational study of mammography, 436
social psychology theories, 326
theories as conceptual framework, 443
Kleiber, C.
Iowa Model, of evidence-based practice, 264, 267
Kleinbeck, S. V. M.
caregiver effectiveness model, 220, 249t
Caregiving Effectiveness Model, 39
Kleinpell, R. M.
Theory of Comfort, 246
Kline, N.
infection prevention, 334
Knafl, K. A.
concept development, 51
Knapp, T. R.
assumptions, 81
empiricism, 8, 9
metaparadigm, 41
metatheory, 37
methodology, 12
nursing philosophy, 11
nursing theory, 27t–28t, 40
science, overview, 5
theory components, 79
theory development, 73
translational research, 32
Kneisl, C. R.
general adaptation syndrome, 319–320
Knowles, M.
adult learning, 402–404, 403b, 492
cognitive-field (gestalt) theory, 393
role of teachers, 391
Knox, A. B.
proficiency, 405
Koch, T.
psychoanalytic theory, 309
Kochinda, C.
caregiver effectiveness model, 220, 249t
Caregiving Effectiveness Model, 39
Koehler, J.
caregiver effectiveness model, 220, 249t
Koenig, H. G.
predictive theories, 77
Koh, W.
transformational leadership, 363
Kohn, L. T.
quality improvement, 470
Kolb, D. A.
cognitive development/interaction theories, 395
learning styles, 405
Kolcaba, K.
Theory of Comfort, 222, 229, 241, 244–246
Kongstvedt, P. R.
disease management, 468
Koop, P. M.
symbolic interactionism, 286
Kopelman, R. E.
Theory X and Theory Y, 359
Koponen, L.
model of skill acquisition in nursing, 232
Koren, M. E.
spirituality of staff nurses, 427t
Korhan, E. A.
Care Dependency Scale, 139
Kothare, S. V.
Theory of Chronic Sorrow, 109
Kotter, J. P.
Eight Step Plan for Implementing Change, 370, 371
Kouzes, J.
transformational leadership, 459
Kowlaski, K.
technology in nursing education, 493
theory-based nursing practice, 414
theory–practice gap, 416
Kralik, D.
psychoanalytic theory, 309
Kramer, M. K.
assumptions, 81
concept development, 51, 87
evidence-based practice, 261, 263, 264, 502, 504
future issues in nursing, 500
knowledge development, 500
metatheory, 37
middle range theories, 38, 501
middle range theory, 214
nursing epistemology, 15
nursing theory, 25, 26, 27t–28t
nursing theory development, 29, 31, 32, 34t–36t
philosophy, overview, 6
postmodernism, 10
practice-based evidence, 262
practice theories, 418, 421t, 502
shared governance, 456, 457, 458
theory and research, 431–432
theory-based nursing practice, 415, 415t
theory components, 79
theory concepts, 79
theory construction, 88

Kramer, M. K. (*continued*)
theory description and critique, 97, 98t, 101–102, 102t, 106, 107t
theory development, 73, 437
theory development process, 86
theory purpose, 79
theory structure and linkages, 81
theory testing in research, 88
theory validation and application in practice, 88
Kraus, R.
evidence-based practice, 266
Kravits, K.
Theory of Goal Attainment, 176
Kristiansen, L.
theory of ICU transitional care, 435
Transitions Theory, 238
Kudenchuk, P. J.
study of implantable cardioverter defibrillator, 436–437, 443
Kuennen, J. K.
dialectic learning, 489
Kuhn, J.
dialectic learning, 489
Kuhn, T. S.
metaparadigm, 41
paradigm shift, 119–120, 203
theory evaluation, 104
KuKanich, K. S.
infection prevention, 334
Kunert, M. P.
homeostasis, 340
Kunkler, K.
allostasis, 340
Kuo, E. S.
natural history of disease, 339
Kurfiss, J. G.
Perry's theory of intellectual and ethical development, 398–399
Kushi, L. H.
cancer theories, 348
Kushniruk, A.
Theory of Nurses' Recognizing and Responding to Uncertainty, 435
Kwekkeboom, K.
Rogerian theory, 196

L

Lachance, L.
Roy Adaptation Model, 181
Ladas, E. L.
immune function, 343
Laffrey, S. C.
predictive theories, 77
LaFleur, C. J.
Piaget's cognitive development theory, 397
Lai, L.
Theory of Goal Attainment, 176
Lake, E. T.
Magnet Recognition Program, 466
nurse staffing and patient outcomes, 464–465
shared governance, 457
Lally, R. M.
correlational study of mammography, 436
social psychology theories, 326
theories as conceptual framework, 443
Lam, S. K.
transformational leadership, 363
Lamb, G. S.
Health as Expanding Consciousness, 201
Lancellotti, K.
cultural care diversity and universality theory, 234
Lane, E.
gate control theory, 350
Lanham, H. J.
general systems theory, 283
LaPlant, M.
Nightingale, 136
Lapum, J.
critical social theory, 293
Larkey, L. K.
experimental study of "sign chi do" exercises, 437
Laroussini, J.
Caring Science as Sacred Science, 186
Larsen, K.
theory–practice gap, 416
Larson, E. L.
infection prevention, 334
Laschinger, H.
Leader–Member Exchange Theory, 370
Laschinger, H. K.
shared governance, 456
Lasiter, S.
descriptive research, 434t
Latham, T.
gate control theory, 350
Latimer, K.
operational teaching, 490
Lau, Y.
social networks, 284
Laughton, D.
Theory of Goal Attainment, 176
Lauver, D.
theory of care-seeking behavior, 242t
Law, K. S.
Leader–Member Exchange Theory, 358
Law, R.
Bridging Worlds theory, 419
practice to theory approach, 85
Lawyer, J. W.
conflict management, 374
Lazarus, R. S.
stress coping adaptation theory, 221, 320, 327t
Le, H. N.
Postpartum Depression Theory, 251
Lea, D.
genomic health care, 345
Leach, M. J.
Conservation Model, 163
Leahy-Warren, P.
social networks, 284
Leavell, H. R.
natural history of disease, 337, 338f
Lee, H.
health-related behaviors of Korean Americans, 420t
social networks, 284
Lee, H. O.
cultural diversity and cultural bias, 295
Lee, J.
disease management, 468
Lee, J. S.
cultural diversity and cultural bias, 295
Lee, P.
perceived view of science, 9
Lee, R. C.
cultural care diversity and universality theory, 234
Lee, T. Y.
social networks, 284
Lee, Y. S.
predictive theories, 77
Lee-Lin, F.
cancer theories, 348
Leeman, J.
symptom-focused diabetes care, 420t
Lefrancois, G. R.
learning theory, 390
Legault, F.
humanbecoming paradigm, 205
Legido, A.
Theory of Chronic Sorrow, 109
Leigh, G. T.
cognitive-field (gestalt) theory, 394
Leininger, M.
caring as central construct, 45
Caring Science as Sacred Science, 186
cultural care diversity and universality theory, 233–234, 497
metaparadigm, 43t
middle range theory, 214, 230
nursing theory, 35t, 119, 230
Lemieux, M. L.
nursing curriculum, 487
Lenz, E. R.
comparison of concept development models, 67
concept development, 55
middle range theory, 215, 225
self-efficacy theory, 242t
Theory of Unpleasant Symptoms, 218, 241, 246–247
Leonard, V.
nursing curriculum, 508
Levelle, M.
Magnet Recognition Program, 466
Levesque, L.
Roy Adaptation Model, 181
Levine, M. E.
assumptions, concepts, and relationships, 161–162, 162t
background, 160
Conservation Model, 160–164, 220, 419, 440–441
middle range theory derived from work, 220, 419, 440–441
nursing theory, 24, 25, 31, 34t, 40, 119, 160–164

parsimony of theory, 163–164
patient-centered approach, 139, 141
philosophical underpinnings of theory, 160–161
testability of theory, 163
usefulness of theory, 163
Levi-Strauss, C.
social exchange theory, 280
Levitan, S. E.
patient-focused care, 462
Lewandowski, W. A.
Rogerian theory, 196
Lewin, K.
adage on theory, 388–389
gestalt theory, 393
leadership behavior, 357
planned change theory, 370–372
Lewis, C.
web of causation, 337
Lewis, D. Y.
nursing curriculum, 487, 487t
Lewis, F. M.
social psychology theories, 325
Lewis, S.
Caring Science as Sacred Science, 186
Li, C.-H.
disease management, 470
Li, H.
evidence-based practice, 266
Li, J.
natural history of disease, 339
Li, R.
information-processing model, 395
Liang, S. Y.
social networks, 284
Liaschendo, J.
theory–practice gap, 416
Liehr, P. R.
middle range theory, 217, 225, 226, 230, 501
practice theories, 421t
theory evaluation, 106
Lievano, J. A.
Theory of Normalizing Risky Sexual Behaviors, 218
Liewehr, D. J.
genomics in nursing practice, 344–345
Ligon, M.
psychosocial developmental theory, 310
Lim, L.
cultural care diversity and universality theory, 234
nursing strategies to reduce caries, 427t
Lin, C.
Bandura's social learning theory, 399–400
Lin, K. C.
social networks, 284
Lin, L.
Uncertainty of Illness Theory, 244
Lin, M.
Health Belief Model, 326
Lindberg, C. E.
gate control theory, 350
Lindebaum, D.
transformational leadership, 363
Lindesmith, A.
role theory, 286
symbolic interactionism, 285t
Lindzey, G.
defense mechanisms, 308
Lippett, R.
leadership behavior, 357
Lipsitz, L. A.
homeostasis, 340
Lira, M. T.
natural history of disease, 339
Litchfield, M. C.
nursing as discipline, 4
theory application in practice, 413
Litt, D.
Theory of Reasoned Action/Planned Behavior, 326
Litwack, K.
gate control theory, 349
pain management, 349
Liu, K. P. Y.
information-processing model, 395
Llewellyn, C.
Health Belief Model, 326
Lloyd, D.
Theory of Goal Attainment, 176
Loan, L. A.
evidence-based practice, 259, 261
LoBiondo-Wood, G.
correlational research, 436
evidence-based practice, 31, 259, 419, 421t
experimental research, 436
research framework, 433–434
research process, 433b
Theory of Unpleasant Symptoms, 443
theory-testing research, 439
Uncertainty of Illness Theory, 244
Lobo, M. L.
concept analysis, 57
Locke, J.
empiricism, 8
Lockhart, J. S.
Theory of Goal Attainment, 176–177
Loeb, J. M.
quality improvement, 375, 376t
Loehler, J.
Caregiving Effectiveness Model, 39
Loescher, L. J.
genomics in education, 345
Logan, J. R.
social networks, 283
Logan, W.
nursing theory, 36t, 118, 119
Logsdon, M. C.
Maternal Role Attainment/Becoming a Mother, 252
Lokken, L.
study of postpartum hospital discharge, 436
Long, A.
nursing care for patients at risk for suicide, 218
Long, J. M.
cultural care diversity and universality theory, 233
Long, K. A.
rural nursing model, 231t
Lopez, M.
Artinian Intersystem Model, 168
Lopez, R. P.
nursing philosophy, 11
Lorenz, E. N.
chaos theory, 298
Lorsch, J.
Theory X and Theory Y, 359
Lottko, B.
web of causation, 335
Loughrey, A.
infection prevention, 334
Lowes, L.
Theory of Chronic Sorrow, 109, 250
Lowry, L. W.
theory application in practice, 413
theory-based nursing practice, 414
theory-research-practice relationship, 82
Lu, J. H.
genetics of addiction, 346
Lubans, D. R.
social cognitive theories, 322
Lucas, R.
principle-based concept analysis, 66
Lucero, N. B.
Postpartum Depression Theory, 251
Lucey, C.
case management, 466–467
Lukose, A.
Caring Science as Sacred Science, 186
Luna, M.
practice to theory approach, 85
Luquire, R.
Magnet Recognition Program, 466
Luthans, F.
authentic leadership, 364
Lyneham, J.
model of skill acquisition in nursing, 232
Lynn, M. R.
Uncertainty of Illness Theory, 244
Lyon, D.
critical social theory, 293
Lyons, A. A.
Theory of Comfort, 246

M

Maaitah, R.
cultural diversity and cultural bias, 295
MacDonald, D. J.
genomics in cancer care, 346
Machin, T.
role theory, 288
Maciag, T.
logistic teaching, 490
Mackay, M.
postmodernism, 10
Mackenzie, S. B.
Path–Goal Theory, 361
Mackey, M. C.
feminist theory, 292

MacLaren, C.
Rational Emotive Theory, 314
MacMahon, B.
web of causation, 335
MacPhail, L. H.
disease management, 470
Madrid, M.
Rogerian theory, 196, 197
Madsen, J. K.
theory–practice gap, 416
Maeve, M. K.
Postpartum Depression Theory, 251
Mager, R. F.
nursing curriculum, 481–482
Magill-Evans, J.
Parenting Under Pressure, 439
Maglione, J. L.
Health Promotion Model, 236
Maguire, P.
shared governance, 456, 457, 458
Mahar, L.
Contingency Theory of Leadership, 360–361
Mahat, G.
Piaget's cognitive development theory, 397
Mahon, S. M.
model of skill acquisition in nursing, 232
natural history of disease, 339
Mahoney, G.
Path–Goal Theory, 361
Mahoney, J. S.
therapeutic milieu, 313
Maier, I.
web of causation, 335
Maiman, L. A.
Health Belief Model, 222
Makaroff, K. L. S.
nursing as discipline, 4
philosophy, overview, 6
Malcolm, J.
testing of caregiving theory, 441
Malinski, V. M.
caring as central construct, 45
metaparadigm, 41
Rogerian theory, 196
Malloch, K.
evidence-based practice, 421t
future issues in nursing, 499, 502, 506, 507
Malone, E.
Theory X and Theory Y, 359
Mang, A. L.
patient-focused care, 461, 462
Manojlovich, M.
future issues in nursing, 499
March, A.
Theory of Comfort, 246
Marchione, J.
Health as Expanding Consciousness, 200t
Marcic, D.
conflict mode model, 374
empowerment, 369
quality improvement, 378
Theory X and Theory Y, 359
Mare, J.
Theory of Chronic Sorrow, 109
Marine, M.
infection prevention, 334
Mark, B.
grand theories, 118
Mark, B. A.
chaos theory, 296, 297–298
Marriage, D.
cognitive behavioral therapies, 315
Marriner-Tomey, A.
total patient care (functional nursing), 460
Marrs, J.
research-practice relationship, 83
theory application in practice, 413
theory-based nursing practice, 414
theory-research-practice relationship, 82
Marsons, L.
homeostasis, 340
Martin, A.
patient-centered approach, 139–142
Martin, K. S.
Omaha System, 218, 231t
Martins, D. C.
critical social theory, 292
Martsolf, D.
symbolic interactionism, 286
Marui, E.
cultural diversity and cultural bias, 295
Marx, K.
conflict theory, 289–290
critical social theory, 292
social exchange theory, 281
Maslow, A.
human needs theory, 54, 131, 315–317, 327t, 359, 363–364, 366, 401
Mason, G.
general systems theory, 282
Masters, K.
theory application in practice, 413
theory evaluation, 106
Masters, M. L.
quality improvement, 377t
Masters, R. J.
quality improvement, 377t
Matheney, R. V.
patient-centered approach, 139–142
Mathews, H. L.
immune function, 343
Matthews, R.
web of causation, 337
Matutina, R. E.
concept analysis, 57
Mauritz, M.
symbolic interactionism, 286
Maxfield, D. G.
whole brain learning, 405
May, B. A.
Theory of Goal Attainment, 177
May, D. R.
authentic leadership, 364
McArdle, T.
immune function, 343
McAuley, E.
Theory of Unpleasant Symptoms, 247
McCallin, A. M.
Artinian Intersystem Model, 168
McCance, T.
nursing theory, 36t
McCarter, B.
patient-focused care, 462
McCarthy, E. M.
social exchange theory, 281
McCarthy, G.
research-based concepts, 54
social networks, 284
McCarty, K.
evidence-based practice, 474
McCauley, E.
natural history of disease, 339
McCay, E.
critical social theory, 293
McClelland, D. C.
power strategy, 369
McCloskey, J.
power concepts, 368
McClure, M. L.
Magnet Recognition Program, 465, 466
McCormack, B.
context analysis, 66
nursing theory, 36t
McCormack, D.
Theory of Comfort, 246
McCormick, M. J.
technology in nursing education, 493
McCoy, T. P.
interpersonal theory, 313
McCreaddie, M.
humor use in nurse–patient interactions, 218
McCullough, M.
cancer theories, 348
McDaniel, R. R., Jr.
general systems theory, 283
McDonald, L.
Nightingale, 136
McElligott, D.
Nightingale, 135
McEwen, M.
epidemiologic triangle, 335
nursing curriculum, 484
theoretical knowledge and skills, 501
theory as conceptual framework in research, 437, 442
McFarland, M.
cultural care diversity and universality theory, 233
McGahee, T. W.
model for smoking prevention, 222–223
McGhee, M. N.
cultural care diversity and universality theory, 234
McGregor, D.
Theory X and Theory Y, 359, 366
McGuinn, K.
nursing curriculum, 487

McGuire, E.
transformational leadership, 459
McIntyre, C.
Theory of Reasoned Action/Planned Behavior, 326
McKee, A.
emotional intelligence, 356–357
McKee-Waddle, R.
patient care delivery models, 463
McKenna, G.
practice theories, 38
McKenna, H. P.
assumptions, 81
concept development, 50
descriptive research, 435
evidence-based practice, 261
McKenna, L.
Perry's theory of intellectual and ethical development, 399
McMahon, M. A.
descriptive theories, 76
McMenamin, E. M.
pain management, 349
McNabb, S.
disease management, 469
McNett, M.
infection prevention, 334
Mead, K.
symbolic interactionism, 285–286
Meadows, R.
caring as central construct, 45
Meadows-Oliver, M.
natural history of disease, 339
Medina, J.
mobile device for nursing, 139
Mefford, L. C.
Conservation Model, 163
Theory of Health Promotion for Preterm Infants, 220, 419, 440–441
Mehta, A.
general systems theory, 283
Meighan, M.
Maternal Role Attainment/Becoming a Mother, 252
Meininger, J. C.
natural history of disease, 339
Meleis, A. I.
abstract *vs.* concrete concepts, 52
concept analysis, 64–65
concept clarification, 64, 64b
concept development, 63–65, 65t, 67, 68t
concept exploration, 63
descriptive theory, 434
epistemology, 12, 13
grand theory categorization, 119, 120t, 123t
metaparadigm, 44
middle range theory, 214, 215, 216, 230, 501
nursing curriculum, 482
nursing epistemology, 15
nursing theory, 119, 230, 236–239
nursing theory development, 33t
postmodernism, 7, 10
practice theories, 418, 502
prescriptive theories, 40, 77, 434
received and perceived views of science, 7
science, views of, 11t
theory description, analysis, and critique, 97, 98t, 102–103, 106, 107t
theory development approaches, 83–86, 84t
theory-practice relationship, 83
theory-research relationship, 82
Transitions Theory, 236–239
Melnyk, B. M.
ARCC Model, 264, 266
evidence-based practice, 32, 258–261, 263–264, 266–267, 270, 380–382, 421t, 474
Johns Hopkins Nursing Evidence-Based Practice Model, 267
Stetler Model of Evidence-Based Practice, 270
Melvin, C. S.
Theory of Chronic Sorrow, 110
Melzack, R.
gate control theory, 349
Melzak, R.
gate control theory of pain, 221
Mendel, G.
theory of genetics, 343
Mensik, J.
King, 173
Mercer, R. T.
Maternal Role Attainment/Becoming a Mother, 222, 248, 251–252
Meretoja, R.
model of skill acquisition in nursing, 232, 233
Merkle, C. J.
cancer theories, 346
Merritt, S.
Caring Science as Sacred Science, 186
Merritt-Gray, M.
descriptive research on abused women, 434t
feminist theory, 292
Messecar, D. C.
explanatory theories, 76
research to theory approach, 85
Messmer, P. R.
King, 173
King's conceptual framework, 176
Mete, S.
adaptation in pregnancy, 426
Meyer, R. M.
general systems theory, 283
Meyers, S. T.
research on cesarean birth, 434t, 441
Mezirow, J.
transformational learning, 405
Miaskowski, C.
experimental research on cancer pain, 434t
Michaels, C.
Health as Expanding Consciousness, 201
Michelow, M. D.
disease management, 470
Mick, J.
evidence-based practice, 475
Mikkelsen, G.
principle-based concept analysis, 66
Miles, M. S.
Maternal Role Attainment/Becoming a Mother, 252
Millar, B.
humanbecoming paradigm, 205
Millar, B. C.
infection prevention, 334
Millet, K.
socialist feminism, 291
Milligan, R. A.
Theory of Unpleasant Symptoms, 218, 241, 246–247
Mills, C. W.
sociological imagination, 279
Milton, C. L.
humanbecoming paradigm, 205
Minor, J.
Contingency Theory of Leadership, 361
Minter, M. L.
lead exposure screening and strategies, 424
Mion, L.
risk factors for pressure ulcers, 218
Mishel, M. H.
Uncertainty in Illness Theory, 222, 241–244
Mitcham, C.
comparison of concept development models, 67
concept analysis, 55, 66
Mitchell, C.
Health as Expanding Consciousness, 201
Mitchell, D.
learning styles, 405
postmodern social theory, 300
Mitchell, G.
theory to implement change, 427t
Mitchell, G. J.
evidence-based practice, 261
nursing as human science, 16, 17
Mitchell, P. H.
King, 173
Miyahara, T.
Health as Expanding Consciousness, 201
Miziniak, H.
dialectic learning, 489
Mock, V.
Conservation Model, 163
Moddeman, G. R.
gate control theory, 350
Moe, K.
Caring Science as Sacred Science, 186
Mokoka, K.
human needs theory, 317
Moloney, M. F.
postmodernism, 10
research methodology, 18
Molzahn, A. E.
metaparadigm, 42

Montalvo-Liendo, N.
cultural diversity and cultural bias, 295
Montano, D. E.
Theory of Reasoned Action/ Planned Behavior, 323
Montgomery, K. S.
Bandura's social learning theory, 399
Monti, E. J.
perceived view of science, 9
research methodology, 17, 18
Moody, L. E.
grand theories, 74
knowledge development, 432
nursing as practice science, 16
nursing theory development, 33t
science, views of, 11t
theory as conceptual framework, 443
theory evaluation, 97, 106
theory-research-practice relationship, 82
Moody-Thomas, S.
disease management, 469
Moore, A.
web of causation, 337
Moore, J. E.
infection prevention, 334
Moore, K.
interpersonal theory, 313
Moore, S. M.
acute pain management, 224, 249t
explanatory theories, 39
flight nursing expertise, 439
grand theories, 37, 74, 117
middle range theory, 38, 74, 215
nursing theory, 37
practice theories, 38, 75
relationship among levels of theory, 75
Theory of the Peaceful End of Life, 224, 224f, 249t
Moreland, S. S.
nursing curriculum, 487
Moreno, D. A.
nurse staffing and patient outcomes, 464
quality improvement, 375, 377
Moreno, J.
sociograms, 283–284
Moreno-Ferguson, M. E.
Roy Adaptation Model, 181
Moretz, J.
patient-focused care, 463
Morinec, J.
infection prevention, 334
Morris, D. L.
middle range theory, 214
Morris, P.
Health Belief Model, 326
Morrison, E. F.
nursing theory development, 29t, 47
research methodology, 18
Morse, J.
theory of suffering, 249t
Theory X and Theory Y, 359
Morse, J. M.
comparison of concept development models, 67
concept clarification, 66
concept comparison, 66
concept delineation, 65
concept development, 55, 65–66, 67, 68t
Morse, J. S.
learning styles, 405
Morton, J. L.
Health Belief Model, 424–425
Moser, D. K.
Theory of Unpleasant Symptoms, 247
Motl, R. W.
Theory of Unpleasant Symptoms, 247
Mott, S.
cultural diversity and cultural bias, 295
Muehlenkord, A.
technology in nursing education, 491
Muething, S.
patient-focused care, 463
Muhlenkamp, A. F.
theory analysis and evaluation, 97, 98t, 99, 99b
Mukhopadhyay, S.
Health Belief Model, 326
Mulvihill, D.
Social Readjustment Rating Scale, 342
Munhall, P. L.
research methodology, 18
Murdaugh, C. L.
Health Promotion Model, 95, 234–236, 235f
Murphy, J.
postmodern social theory, 299
Murphy, R. J.
natural history of disease, 339
Murray, C.
chaos theory, 296
Murray, P. J.
Neuman, 149
Murray, R. P.
Theory of Comfort, 246
Murrock, C. J.
explanatory theories, 39
Health Promotion Model, 236
theory of music, mood, and movement, 218
Musker, K. M.
Health as Expanding Consciousness, 201
Muszalik, M.
Care Dependency Scale, 139
Muurinen, E.
humanbecoming paradigm, 205
Myers, A.
nursing curriculum, 487
Myers, S.
patient-focused care, 461
Myny, D.
general systems theory, 283

N

Nagle, L.
Theory of Nurses' Recognizing and Responding to Uncertainty, 435
Nail, L. M.
explanatory theories, 76
research to theory approach, 85
Nanus, B.
transformational leadership, 458
Napier, G.
therapeutic milieu, 313
Nardi, D.
Theory of Spirituality-Based Nursing Practice, 39
Neal, L. J.
theory of home health nursing, 231t
Neff, D. M.
nurse staffing and patient outcomes, 465
Neill, J.
Health as Expanding Consciousness, 201
Neill, R. M.
Watson, 183
Neils, P. F.
Nightingale, 135
Nelson, A. M.
theory to practice to theory approach, 84
Neswick, R. S.
Conservation Model, 163
Neuhaeuser, M.
web of causation, 335
Neuman, B.
assumptions, concepts, and relationships, 150–152, 151t, 152*f*
background, 150
evidence-based practice, 261, 264
human needs theory, 124t
Johnson model, 149
metaparadigm, 43t, 150
middle range theories derived from work, 219
nursing epistemology, 14
nursing theory, 35t, 119, 132, 149–154
parsimony of theory, 154
philosophical underpinnings of theory, 150
Systems Model, 131, 149–154, 320–321, 441
testability of theory, 153–154
usefulness of theory, 152–153
value in extending nursing science, 154
Newell, A.
problem solving, 405
Newhouse, R. P.
Johns Hopkins Nursing Evidence-Based Practice Model, 264, 267–270, 269b
Newman, M. A.
assumptions, concepts, and relationships, 198–201, 200t
background, 125, 198
caring as central construct, 45

Health as Expanding Consciousness, 192, 198–202, 208, 209t
metaparadigm, 43t
middle range theories derived from work, 219
middle range theory, 214
nursing as discipline, 4
nursing theory, 35t, 119, 124, 124t, 192, 198–202
paradigm categorization of theories, 122, 123t, 124
philosophical underpinnings of theory, 198
Rogerian theory, 196
simultaneity paradigm, 121
simultaneous action paradigm, 126
testability of theory, 201–202
usefulness of theory, 201, 202b
Ng, K. K.
cancer theories, 348
Ngai, F.
social networks, 284
Ngamkham, S.
gate control theory, 350
Nguyen-Truong, C. K. Y.
cancer theories, 348
Nichols, F.
nursing curriculum, 487
Nightingale, F.
application of theory to research, 431
assumptions, concepts, and relationships, 134–135
background, 133–134
feminism, 292
nursing theory, 26, 30, 34t, 119, 124, 124t, 132–136
parsimony of theory, 136
particulate–deterministic paradigm, 122
philosophical underpinnings of theory, 134
quality improvement, 375
testability of theory, 135–136
usefulness of theory, 135
value in extending nursing science, 136
Noel, D. L.
Caring Science as Sacred Science, 186
Noh, C. H.
humanbecoming paradigm, 205–207
Nonnemacher, M.
web of causation, 335
Noonan, D. A.
Theory of Reasoned Action/Planned Behavior, 326
Noor, A. B.
cancer theories, 348
natural history of disease, 339
Norbeck, J. S.
model for social support, 242t
Northcott, H. C.
symbolic interactionism, 286
Northrup, D. T.
nursing as discipline, 4
philosophy, overview, 6
Norwood, S. L.
descriptive theory, 434
explanatory theory, 435
future issues in nursing, 500
methodological triangulation, 500
research report, 445, 446b
theory as conceptual framework in research, 442, 442b
theory-generating research, 438–439
theory-testing research, 439
Nosek, M.
postmodern social theory, 300
Nyatanga, L.
philosophy of science in nursing, 12
Nye, F. I.
social exchange theory, 280

O

Obeisat, S.
cultural diversity and cultural bias, 295
Oberer, J.
learning styles, 405
Oberle, K.
Conservation Model, 163
O'Boyle, E. H.
emotional intelligence, 363
O'Brien-Pallas, L. L.
general systems theory, 283
O'Connor, A.
nurses' competence in genetics, 345
O'Connor, J. J.
Nightingale, 133, 134
Ogola, G. O.
Magnet Recognition Program, 466
Ohmasa, T.
Health as Expanding Consciousness, 201
Okamura, H.
general systems theory, 283
Okonta, N. R.
yoga and stress, 342
Oldnall, A. S.
nursing as discipline, 4
Olson, J.
nurse-expressed empathy, 219
Olson, K.
concept analysis, 66
symbolic interactionism, 286
Olson, M. W.
definition of learning, 387
learning theory, 389, 390, 392
Olynyk, V. G.
nursing as discipline, 4
philosophy, overview, 6
O'Mahony, J. M.
postmodern social theory, 300
O'Malley, J.
Henderson, 136, 138
Omery, A.
perceived view of science, 9
Omrey, A.
nursing theory, 25
O'Neill, E. S.
information-processing model, 395
O'Neill, M.
interpersonal theory, 313
Onyango, M. A.
cultural diversity and cultural bias, 295
Oosthuizen, M.
human needs theory, 317
Orem, D. E.
assumptions, concepts, and relationships, 142–144, 144t
background, 142
human needs theory, 124t
metaparadigm, 43t, 143–144
middle range theories derived from work, 219, 439
nursing theory, 34t, 119, 132, 142–146
parsimony of theory, 146
particulate–deterministic paradigm, 122
philosophical underpinnings of theory, 142
Self-Care Deficit Nursing Theory, 142–146, 425, 484
testability of theory, 145, 145b
totality paradigm, 121
usefulness of theory, 144–145, 145b
value in extending nursing science, 146
Oritz, M.
Theory of Goal Attainment, 176
Orlando, I. J.
background, 125
client participation, 312
interaction theory, 119
middle range theory, 214
nursing theory, 31, 34t, 119, 312
particulate–deterministic paradigm, 122
Ormrod, J. E.
behavioral learning theory, 390, 391
constructivism, 402
information-processing models, 394–395
Piaget's cognitive development theory, 396
Watson's behaviorism, 390
Oros, M. T.
nursing curriculum, 487, 487t
Osmond, M. W.
feminist theory, 290, 291b, 292
Othman, A. K.
correlational study of mammography, 436
social psychology theories, 326
theories as conceptual framework, 443
Oudshoorn, A.
model of skill acquisition in nursing, 232
Ours, C.
Conservation Model, 163
Outland, L.
homeostasis, 340
Oweis, A.
cultural diversity and cultural bias, 295

Owens, A. L.
model of skill acquisition in nursing, 233
Oyetunde, M. O.
role theory, 288
Ozmon, H.
behavioral learning theory, 391

P
Pace, K.
caregiver effectiveness model, 220, 249t
Caregiving Effectiveness Model, 39
Packa, D. R.
case management, 467
Padden, O.
stress theories, 321
Padilla, G.
maintaining hope in transition theory, 420t
Page, G. G.
nursing theory, 25
Paley, J.
postmodernism, 10
Palfreyman, S.
evidence-based practice, 259
Palmer, B.
Self-Transcendence Theory, 248
Palyo, N.
therapeutic milieu, 313
Papamiditriou, C.
spirituality of staff nurses, 427t
Pappas, S. H.
quality improvement, 472
Paradowski, M. B.
Conservation Model, 163
Park, H. J.
health-promoting behaviors, 437
Parker, M.
shared governance, 456
Parker, M. E.
middle range theory, 214
theory application in practice, 413, 414b
theory evaluation, 106
theory–practice gap, 416
Parkinson, C.
model of skill acquisition in nursing, 232
Parks, S. M.
Theory of Reasoned Action/Planned Behavior, 326, 443
Parse, R. R.
assumptions, concepts, and relationships, 203–204, 204b
background, 125, 203
caring/becoming theory, 119
concept development, 51
definition of science, 5
humanbecoming paradigm, 193, 202–208, 209t
middle range theory, 214
nursing as discipline, 4
nursing theory, 36t, 119, 124, 124t, 182–183, 192, 202–208
paradigm categorization of theories, 121, 121f, 123t
parsimony of theory, 207
philosophical underpinnings of theory, 203
research-based concepts, 54
Rogerian theory, 196, 197
simultaneity paradigm, 121
simultaneous action paradigm, 126
testability of theory, 205–207
true presence concept, 192
unitary–transformative paradigm, 122
usefulness of theory, 204–205, 208b
value in extending nursing science, 208
Parsons, M. H.
Health Promotion Model, 95, 234–236, 235f
Pasteur, L.
germ theory, 333
Paterson, J.
interaction theory, 119
nursing theory, 35t
Patrician, P. A.
Health Belief Model, 326
Nursing Work Index-Revised, 463
Patrick, T. E.
Postpartum Depression Theory, 251
Paul, S. M.
experimental research on cancer pain, 434t
Pavlov, I.
classical conditioning, 389, 389t, 390
Pearce, C. L.
Path–Goal Theory, 362
Penberthy, L.
disease management, 468
Pender, N. J.
Health Promotion Model, 95, 234–236, 235f
middle range theory, 214, 230
nursing theory, 119, 230
theory as conceptual framework, 443
Penrod, J.
concept development, 50, 67, 68t
principle-based concept analysis, 66, 67b
Pepin, J. I.
empiricism, 8
Peplau, H.
background, 125
levels of anxiety, 312, 318–320, 319t
middle range theory, 214
nursing theory, 30, 34t, 119, 312
participant–observer, 312
particulate–deterministic paradigm, 122
Perron, A.
postmodernism, 10
Perry, D. F.
Postpartum Depression Theory, 251
Perry, R. N. B.
Caring Science as Sacred Science, 186
Perry, W. G.
intellectual and ethical development, 396, 398–399
Peters, T.
leadership, 355
Peterson, J. Z.
technology in nursing education, 491
Peterson, S. J.
grand theories, 74
middle range theory, 38, 74, 214, 215, 216, 217
nursing theory, 25
practice theories, 38, 75
theory development, 73
theory evaluation, 106
Pfettscher, S. A.
feminist theory, 292
Nightingale, 135
Pfieffer, J. B.
Artinian Intersystem Model, 168
Pharris, M. D.
Health as Expanding Consciousness, 201
Phillips, A.
smoking cessation theories, 425
Phillips, J.
maintaining hope in transition theory, 420t
Phillips, J. R.
Rogers and Rogerian theory, 193, 196, 197
Phillips, K. D.
Roy and Roy Adaptation Model, 178, 181
Piaget, J.
cognitive development theory, 396–397
Piccoli, M.
Conservation Model, 163
Piccoli, R. F.
transactional and transformational leadership, 363
Pickard, C.
Health as Expanding Consciousness, 201
Picot, S.
social exchange theory, 281–282
Pielak, K. L.
Theory of Reasoned Action/Planned Behavior, 326
Pierce, S. T.
evidence-based practice, 381
Pierce, T. B.
Client Experience Model, 218
Pilkington, F. B.
humanbecoming paradigm, 205
Pizzo, J.
learning styles, 405
Plotnikoff, R. C.
social cognitive theories, 322
Plummer, M.
metaparadigm, 42
Podsakoff, N. P.
Path–Goal Theory, 361
Podsakoff, P. M.
Path–Goal Theory, 361
Poe, S.
Johns Hopkins Nursing Evidence-Based Practice Model, 264, 267–270, 269b

Pokorny, M. F.
grand theory categorization, 119
Polifroni, E. C.
logical positivism, 8
philosophy of science in nursing, 12
Polit, D. F.
research defined, 432
research process, 433b
Polivka, B. J.
logistic teaching, 490
Polk, L. V.
theory of resilience, 219, 242t
Pollack, J. M.
emotional intelligence, 363
Polomano, R. C.
pain management, 349
Pond, J. B.
Conservation Model, 163
Ponte, P. R.
Magnet Recognition Program, 465, 466
Pope, D. S.
Nightingale, 136
Pope, R. K.
disease management, 469
Popkess-Vawter, S.
caregiver effectiveness model, 220, 249t
Caregiving Effectiveness Model, 39
Port, O.
quality improvement, 377
Porter, L.
Uncertainty of Illness Theory, 244
Porter, L. W.
behavioral theories of leadership, 357
Contingency Theory of Leadership, 361
Porter-O'Grady, T.
evidence-based practice, 421t
future issues in nursing, 499, 502, 506, 507
shared governance, 456–457
transformational leadership, 458
Porth, C. M.
genetics, 344
Posner, B.
transformational leadership, 459
Poss, J. E.
Theory of Reasoned Action/Planned Behavior, 323
Poster, E. C.
Johnson model, 149
Potylycki, M. J. S.
Conservation Model, 163
Poulin, M. A.
Magnet Recognition Program, 465
Powell, D. A.
infection prevention, 334
Powell, F. A.
technology in nursing education, 493
Powers, B. A.
assumptions, 81
empiricism, 8, 9
metaparadigm, 41
metatheory, 37
methodology, 12
nursing philosophy, 11
nursing theory, 27t–28t, 37, 40
science, overview, 5
theory components, 79
theory development, 73
translational research, 32
Pradhan, S. R.
natural history of disease, 339
Pravikoff, D. S.
evidence-based practice, 381
Press, M. J.
disease management, 470
Prigogine, I.
chaos theory, 297
Prottas, D. J.
Theory X and Theory Y, 359
Province, A.
Health as Expanding Consciousness, 201
Prows, C. A.
genetic counseling, 345
nursing curriculum, 487
Pruthi, R. S.
Uncertainty of Illness Theory, 244
Pryjmachuk, S.
research-practice relationship, 83
theory-research-practice relationship, 82
Pugh, L. C.
Johns Hopkins Nursing Evidence-Based Practice Model, 264, 267–270, 269b
Theory of Unpleasant Symptoms, 218, 241, 246–247
Pugh, T. F.
web of causation, 335
Puja, B.
transformational leadership, 363
Pullis, B.
epidemiologic triangle, 335
Purnell, L.
Model for Cultural Competence, 219
Purtzer, M. A.
Health Belief Model, 326

Q

Quinless, F. W.
future issues in nursing, 507
Quinn, L. D.
Theory of Comfort, 246
Quinn-Griffin, M.
nursing curriculum, 487
Self-Transcendence Theory, 248

R

Racine, L.
postmodernism, 10
Rafeh, N. A.
Six Sigma, 381
Rahe, E.
general adaptation syndrome, 341–342
Rakel, B. A.
Iowa Model, of evidence-based practice, 264
Rami, J. S.
Health Belief Model, 326
Randell, B. P.
Johnson model, 149
Rankin, S. H.
psychomotor learning, 388
Rao, S. M.
experimental research on cancer pain, 434t
Rapps, J.
Perry's theory of intellectual and ethical development, 399
Raven, B. H.
power and power strategy, 368, 369
Ravindran, V.
Parenting Under Pressure, 439
Raway, B.
Piaget's cognitive development theory, 397
Ray, M. A.
chaos theory, 298
Records, K.
Postpartum Depression Theory, 251
Redican, K. J.
Theory of Comfort, 246
Redman, R. W.
middle range theories, 38
Reed, P.
Rogerian theory, 196
Reed, P. G.
empiricism, 9
Nightingale, 133
nursing philosophy, 11
postmodernism, 7, 10
predictive theories, 77
psychosocial developmental theory, 310
Self-Transcendence Theory, 221, 241, 247–248
Reed, T. L.
case management, 467
Reedy, S.
Transitions Theory, 238, 425
Reiff, M.
nursing curriculum, 487
Reiley, P.
patient-focused care, 462
Reiling, D.
cultural care diversity and universality theory, 233–234
Reimer, A. P.
explanatory theories, 39
flight nursing expertise, 439
Reininger, B. M.
cultural diversity and cultural bias, 295
Reller, M. K.
quality improvement, 378, 471, 472
Rempel, G. R.
Parenting Under Pressure, 439
Remple, V. P.
Theory of Reasoned Action/Planned Behavior, 326
Renpenning, K. M.
descriptive theories, 38
nursing theory, 25, 26
Orem, 142, 145
research methodology, 18

Rentschler, D. D.
nursing curriculum, 482
Rentz, C.
infection prevention, 334
Resar, R. K.
quality improvement, 378, 471, 472
Revell, M. A.
cultural care diversity and universality theory, 234
Rew, L.
middle range theory of self-care, 219
Nightingale, 135, 136
Transitions Theory, 238
Reynolds, M. A.
Postpartum Depression Theory, 250–251
Reynolds, P. D.
theoretical statements, 79, 80, 80t
theory development, 73
Rhodewalt, F.
Contingency Theory of Leadership, 361
Ricard, N.
Roy Adaptation Model, 181
Rice, C. E.
web of causation, 337
Rice, M.
Postpartum Depression Theory, 251
Rich, K. L.
nursing as discipline, 4
nursing theory, 24
science and philosophy, 5
Richardson, S. J.
nursing education/curriculum, 480
Richardson, W. S.
evidence-based practice, 259
Riebling, N.
Six Sigma, 381
Riegel, B.
middle range theory of self-care, 219, 439
perceived view of science, 9
Perry's theory of intellectual and ethical development, 399
Riehl, J.
systems model, 164
Rigel, B.
Theory of Unpleasant Symptoms, 247
Riker, G. I.
natural history of disease, 339
Rimer, B. K.
social psychology theories, 325
Risjord, M.
comparison of concept development models, 67
empiricism, 8, 9
future issues in nursing, 500, 502
logical positivism, 8
nursing as discipline, 4
nursing theory development, 32, 40, 118
philosophy, overview, 6
postmodernism, 10
research methodology, 17, 18
science, overview, 6
theory application in practice, 413
theory-based nursing practice, 414
theory–practice gap, 416, 417
Ritchie, J.
Stetler Model of Evidence-Based Practice, 270
Ritzer, G.
postmodern social theory, 298, 299–300, 299t
Riza, L.
logistic teaching, 490
Robb, M. K.
operational teaching, 490
Robbins, L. K.
Health Promotion Model, 236, 443
Robbins, S. P.
Achievement–Motivation Theory, 366, 367
departmentalization, 456
Equity Theory, 368
Kotter's Eight Step Plan for Implementing Change, 371
organizational design, 453
Path–Goal Theory, 362
transactional and transformational leadership, 363
visionary leadership, 364
Roberts, K. L.
nursing theory in nursing research, 444
Roberts, S.
theory to practice to theory approach, 84
Roberts, T. B.
humanistic learning theory, 401
psychodynamic learning theory, 400
reinforcement, 390
Robertson, E. F.
Nightingale, 133, 134
Robinson
chaos theory, 296
Robles-Silva, L.
descriptive theories, 39, 76
Rock, C. L.
cancer theories, 348
Rodgers, B. L.
concept development, 51, 59–61, 60b, 62t, 67, 68t, 69–70
research-based concepts, 54
sources of concepts, 54t
Roe, C. W.
power bases, 368
Rogatto, S. R.
genomics in cancer care, 346
Rogers, B.
occupational health nursing, 218–219, 231t
Rogers, C. E.
experimental study of "sign chi do" exercises, 437
Rogers, C. R.
cognitive development/interaction theories, 396
person-centered theory, 317–318, 327t, 363, 401
student-centered teaching, 401
Rogers, J.
evidence-based practice, 474
Rogers, L. G.
Parenting Under Pressure, 439
Rogers, L. Q.
Bandura's social learning theory, 400
Rogers, M.
assumptions, concepts, and relationships, 194–195, 194b, 195t
background, 125, 193
homeodynamics, 194–195, 194b
metaparadigm, 43t
middle range theories derived from work, 219
nursing theory, 31, 34t, 119, 124, 124t, 193–197
outcome theory, 119
philosophical underpinnings of theory, 193–194
Science of Unitary and Irreducible Human Beings, 193–197, 208, 209t
simultaneity paradigm, 121
simultaneous action paradigm, 126
testability of theory, 196–197
unitary–transformative paradigm, 122
usefulness of theory, 196, 197b
Romaniuk, D.
critical social theory, 293
Rooda, L.
Theory of Spirituality-Based Nursing Practice, 39
Rooke, L.
King's conceptual framework, 176
Rooney, D.
immune function, 343
Roper, N.
nursing theory, 36t, 118, 119
Rosenberg, S.
cancer theories, 348
Rosenberg, W.
evidence-based practice, 259
Rosenstock, I.
Health Belief Model, 222, 321–322, 327t
Rossiter, L. F.
disease management, 468
Roth, P.
research-based concepts, 54
Shared Presence: Caring for a Dying Spouse, 39, 435
Rothbert, D.
science and philosophy, 5
Rowles, C. J.
teaching strategies, 489, 490
Roy, B.
postmodernism, 10
Roy, C.
administration and management, 506b
assumptions, concepts, and relationships, 178–180, 179t, 180f
background, 177–178
interactive–integrative paradigm, 122
Johnson model, 149
metaparadigm, 43t

middle range theories derived from work, 220, 439
middle range theory of adaptation to diabetes, 220
nursing theory, 35t, 119, 124, 124t, 177–181
parsimony of theory, 181
philosophical underpinnings of theory, 178
practice theory derived from work, 419
Roy Adaptation Model, 159, 160, 177–181, 320–321, 419
testability of theory, 181
theory as conceptual framework, 442–443
theory-testing research, 441
theory to practice to theory approach, 84
totality paradigm, 121
usefulness of theory, 180–181, 182t
value in extending nursing science, 181
Royal, P. A.
dialectic learning, 489
Ruchala, P. L.
nursing curriculum, 481
Rue, L. W.
Achievement–Motivation Theory, 367
Ruiz, R. J.
immune function, 343
Ruiz-Lozano, M. D.
mobile device for nursing, 139
Rukholm, E.
cognitive-field (gestalt) theory, 394
Ruland, C. M.
Theory of the Peaceful End of Life, 224, 224f
Rutherford, M. M.
future issues in nursing, 499, 507
Rutland, C. M.
Theory of the Peaceful End of Life, 249t
Rutowski, P.
Postpartum Depression Theory, 250–251
Rutty, J. E.
empiricism, 8
nursing as profession, 2
nursing theory, 24
perceived view of science, 9
philosophy, overview, 7
positivism, 8
research methodology, 16
Ryan, A.
interpersonal theory, 313
Ryan, W.
conflict theories, 289
Rycroft-Malone, J.
context analysis, 66
evidence-based practice, 259, 261
Stetler Model of Evidence-Based Practice, 270
Rydahl-Hansen, S.
stress theories, 321

S

Sackett, D. L.
evidence-based practice, 259
Sackett, K.
disease management, 469
Sadock, B.
projection, 315
Saiki, L. S.
concept analysis, 57
Saint, S.
future issues in nursing, 499
Sakunhongsophon, S.
social networks, 284
Sanchez-Brikhead, A. C.
Postpartum Depression Theory, 251
Sandau, K. E.
ACE Star Model, 266
evidence-based practice, 270–271
Sandelowski, M.
research methodology, 18
Sandhu, M.
California Safe Staffing Law, 464
Sands, D.
Nightingale, 135, 136
Santos, E. M. M.
genomics in cancer care, 346
Santos, T. C. F.
Nightingale, 135
Sauls, D. J.
research to theory approach, 85
Sauter, C.
technology in nursing education, 493
Savage, E.
Theory of Unpleasant Symptoms, 247
Scales, F. S.
nursing curriculum, 483, 485–486, 486t
Schaefer, K. M.
Conservation Model, 163
Levine, 160, 163
Schaffer, M. A.
ACE Star Model, 266
evidence-based practice, 270–271
Schams, K. A.
dialectic learning, 489
Schaubroeck, J.
transformational leadership, 363
Scherer, E. M.
Magnet Recognition Program, 466
Schim, S. M.
social justice, 44
Schirm, V.
evidence-based practice, 474
Schlotfeldt, R. M.
nursing as profession, 3
Schmalenberg, C. E.
shared governance, 456, 457, 458
Schmidt, N. A.
evidence-based practice, 32, 259, 260, 421t
Schmidt, W.
nursing curriculum, 487
Schmidt, W. H.
continuum of leader behavior, 357–358
Schmitt, T. L.
nursing education, 480
Schobel, D.
Johnson model, 149
Schoenhofer, S.
nursing theory, 36t, 118, 119
Schreiber, J.
Caring Science as Sacred Science, 186
Schreier, A. M.
Theory of Chronic Sorrow, 110
Schriesheim, C. A.
Path–Goal Theory, 362
Schuler, P. A.
Nurse Practitioner Practice Model, 231t
Schultz, A.
Stetler Model of Evidence-Based Practice, 270
Schultz, P. R.
empiricism, 8
epistemology, 12, 13
nursing epistemology, 15
research methodology, 17
science, overview, 5, 6
Schumacher, K. L.
research-based concepts, 54
Transitions Theory, 237, 239
Schwartz, K. S.
cultural care diversity and universality theory, 233–234
Schwartz-Barcott, D.
concept development, 61–63, 62t, 64t, 67, 68t
sources of concepts, 54t
Schwind, J.
critical social theory, 293
Scoloveno, M. A.
Piaget's cognitive development theory, 397
Scope, A.
cognitive behavioral therapies, 315
Scott, A.
critical social theory, 293
Scott, A. A.
lead exposure screening and strategies, 424
Scott, L. K.
natural history of disease, 339
Scully, F.
infection prevention, 334
Seago, J. A.
California Safe Staffing Law, 464
Seal, J.
psychosocial developmental theory, 310
Seal, N.
psychosocial developmental theory, 310
Seckel, M. A.
infection prevention, 334
Secker, T.
causative agent in disease, 334
Secomb, J.
Perry's theory of intellectual and ethical development, 399
Secrest, J.
nursing curriculum, 484, 487

Seers, K.
context analysis, 66
Selanders, L. C.
Nightingale, 132, 133, 134, 135
Seldomridge, L. A.
operational teaching, 490
Selye, H.
concept of stress, 54
general adaptation syndrome, 318–320, 327t, 340–342
stages of stress, 318–320, 319t, 341, 341t
Semmelweis, I. P.
quality improvement, 375
Senesac, P. M.
Roy Adaptation Model, 181
Senn, J. F.
interpersonal theory, 312, 427t
Sethares, K.
Theory of Unpleasant Symptoms, 247
Setter, S. M.
natural history of disease, 339
Severn, M.
Postpartum Depression Theory, 251
Sezgin, S.
interpersonal theory, 312
Shambley-Ebron, D.
critical social theory, 293
Shamir, B.
authentic leadership, 364
Sharpe, P. A.
Bandura's social learning theory, 400
Sharps, P. W.
correlational research, 434t
Shasky, C.
disease management, 468
Shattell, M. M.
interpersonal theory, 313
Shaver, J. L.
prescriptive theories, 78
Shaw, P.
cognitive behavioral therapies, 315
Shawler, C.
Gagne's learning principles, 397–398
Sheldon, L. K.
interpersonal theory, 312
Shelley, R. K.
chaos theory, 296, 297
Sheng, X.
Postpartum Depression Theory, 251
Sherman, D. W.
Transitions Theory, 238–239
Shermis, S. S.
learning theory, 389
Sherrod, R. A.
case management, 467
Shi, L.
causative agent of HIV, 333
Shieh, S. C.
social networks, 284
Shiffrin, R. M.
memory, 405
Shin, K. R.
health-promoting behaviors, 437
Shirey, M.
resilience, 372
Shortridge-Baggett, L. M.
self-efficacy theory, 242t
Shu, Y. I. L.
role theory, 288
Shuler, P.
perceived view of science, 9
Shuttleworth, M.
testability of theories, 126
Siegal, B. E.
perceived view of science, 9
Siegel, J. H.
web of causation, 337
Sieloff, C. L.
King, 173, 177
King's conceptual framework, 176
Sikkema, J.
natural history of disease, 339
Siktberg, L.
nursing curriculum, 481, 481b, 484
Silber, E.
cognitive behavioral therapies, 315
Silich, S. J.
Six Sigma, 381
Silva, M. C.
characteristics of science, 5
nursing epistemology, 14
science and philosophy, 5
theory-testing research, 439
Sime, A. M.
caring as central construct, 45
nursing as discipline, 4
Simmel, G.
conflict theory, 289–290
Simmons, L.
patient-focused care, 462
Simon, H. A.
decision making and rationality, 373
problem solving, 405
Simpser, E.
infection prevention, 334
Sims-Giddens, S. S.
nursing education, 480
Singh, D. A.
causative agent of HIV, 333
Singleton, E. K.
Health Belief Model, 326
Sirapo-ngam, Y.
social networks, 284
Sisca, J. R.
nursing theory, 35t
Sitzman, K.
nursing as profession, 3
nursing theory, 25
Skelly, A. H.
symptom-focused diabetes care, 420t
Skiba, D. J.
nursing curriculum, 487
Skinner, B. F.
operant conditioning, 313–314, 327t, 389, 389t, 390
Skirton, H.
genomic health care, 345
nurses' competence in genetics, 345
Skov, L.
stress theories, 321
Slevin, O. D.
assumptions, 81
descriptive research, 435
evidence-based practice, 261
Sloane, D. M.
California Safe Staffing Law, 464
Magnet Recognition Program, 466
nurse staffing and patient outcomes, 464–465
Slocum, J. W.
leadership, 355
Small, H.
Nightingale, 132, 133, 135, 136
Small, L.
evidence-based practice, 266
Small, R. E.
disease management, 468
Smith,
middle range theory, 216
Smith, B.
immune function, 343
Smith, C.
Perry's theory of intellectual and ethical development, 399
Smith, C. E.
caregiver effectiveness model, 220, 249t
Caregiving Effectiveness Model, 39
Smith, C. S.
Theory of Chronic Sorrow, 110, 250
Smith, D. G.
nurse staffing and patient outcomes, 464
Smith, H.
Health Belief Model, 326
Smith, H. L.
Magnet Recognition Program, 466
nurse staffing and patient outcomes, 465
Smith, K.
Public Health Nursing Practice Model, 224, 231t
Smith, K. E.
conflict theories, 289, 289b, 290
feminist theory, 290
Smith, M.
King, 173
Smith, M. C.
Caring Science as Sacred Science, 186
middle range theory, 214, 501
theory application in practice, 413, 414b
theory evaluation, 106, 225–226
theory–practice gap, 416
Smith, M. J.
middle range theory, 217, 225, 226, 230
practice theories, 421t
theory evaluation, 106
Smith, P.
cultural diversity and cultural bias, 293
Smith, S. J.
technology in nursing education, 493
Smith, S. M.
Parse and humanbecoming paradigm, 203, 204, 207
Theory of Normalizing Risky Sexual Behaviors, 218

Smolowitz, J.
infection prevention, 334
Snee, R. D.
quality improvement, 379
Snow, D.
genetics of addiction, 346
Sochalski, J.
Magnet Recognition Program, 466
Sodomka, P.
patient-focused care, 462
Sole, M. L.
technology in nursing education, 491
Song, M. K.
self-care in diabetes mellitus, 420t
Sorrell, C. D.
nursing epistemology, 14
Sorrell, J. M.
nursing epistemology, 14
Sosik, J. J.
charismatic leadership, 364
Sousa, V. D.
middle range theory of diabetes self-care, 221
Southard, K.
interpersonal theory, 313
Sovie, M. D.
Magnet Recognition Program, 465
Soward, A. C. M.
symptom-focused diabetes care, 420t
Sowell, R.
cultural care diversity and universality theory, 233
Sparks, A. M.
generational differences, 287
Sparks, E.
genetics of cardiovascular disease, 346
Spegman, A. M.
nursing curriculum, 482
Spetz, J.
California Safe Staffing Law, 464
Speziale, H. J. S.
nursing education, 480, 507
Spinoza, B.
philosophy, overview, 7
Spirito, A.
cognitive behavioral therapies, 315
Spitze, G.
social networks, 283
Springer, D. L.
cancer theories, 348
natural history of disease, 339
Sridhar, G.
disease management, 470
Stacy, K. M.
Transitions Theory, 241
Staffileno, B. A.
cultural care diversity and universality theory, 233–234
Stallings, K. D.
psychomotor learning, 388
Standard, P. L.
postmodern social theory, 300
Staniute, M.
Social Readjustment Rating Scale, 342
Stanley, D.
operational teaching, 490
Stanley, S. A. R.
logistic teaching, 490
Stanton, M. P.
case management, 467
Stapleton, V.
nursing curriculum, 487
Stark, M. A.
Health Promotion Model, 236
Stark, S.
natural history of disease, 339
Starkweather, A.
immune function, 343
Statham, A.
symbolic interactionism, 285
Steege, L. M. B.
practice to theory approach, 85
Steele-Moses, S.
Theory of Reasoned Action/Planned Behavior, 326
Steelman, V. J.
Iowa Model, of evidence-based practice, 264
Stein, J.
technology, 200
Steinberg, P.
psychoanalytic theory, 309
Steis, M. R.
principle-based concept analysis, 66
Stengers, I.
chaos theory, 297
Stenvig, T. E.
cognitive-field (gestalt) theory, 394
Stetler, C. B.
Model of Evidence-Based Practice, 264, 270, 271t, 272t
Stevens, K. R.
ACE Star Model, 264–266, 265t
evidence-based practice, 261, 264–266
King, 173
Stevenson, C.
role theory, 288
Stewart, B.
role theory, 288
Stewart, J. L.
Uncertainty of Illness Theory, 241, 244
Stock, M.
Theory of Reasoned Action/Planned Behavior, 326
Stoep, A. V.
natural history of disease, 339
Stokowski, L. A.
future issues in nursing, 502, 507, 508
nursing curriculum, 487, 487t, 507, 508
Stoltzfus, J. C.
Theory of Reasoned Action/Planned Behavior, 326, 443
Story, P. A.
emotional intelligence, 363
Stratton, R.
Theory of Comfort, 246
Straus, S. E.
evidence-based practice, 259
Strauss, A.
chronic illness trajectory framework, 242t
role theory, 286
symbolic interactionism, 285t
Streubert, H. J.
epistemology, 12
nursing as human science, 17
nursing theory, 25, 72
perceived view of science, 9
research methodology, 17
science, overview, 5
Stride, P.
infection prevention, 334
Stromberg, A.
middle range theory of self-care, 219, 439
Stryker, S.
symbolic interactionism, 285
Stuifbergen, A. K.
explanatory theories, 76
midlife women's attitudes toward physical activity, 420t
Stusberg, J.
web of causation, 335
Suh, E. E.
breast cancer screening, 419
Suhayda, R.
logistic teaching, 490
Sullivan, H. S.
interpersonal theory, 307, 307t, 311–313, 327t
Sumner, J.
critical social theory, 293
Sun, F. K.
nursing care for patients at risk for suicide, 218
Suppe, F.
empiricism, 8
middle range theory, 214, 215
postpositivism, 8
Theory of Unpleasant Symptoms, 218, 241, 246–247
Sutcliffe, P.
cognitive behavioral therapies, 315
Sutphen, M.
nursing curriculum, 508
Suzuki, M.
Care Dependency Scale, 139
Uncertainty of Illness Theory, 244
Suzuki, S.
Health as Expanding Consciousness, 201
Swain, M. A. P.
assumptions, concepts, and relationships, 170–172, 171t
background, 170
interactive–integrative paradigm, 122
middle range theory, 214
Modeling and Role-Modeling, 169–173
nursing theory, 119, 169–173
parsimony of theory, 173
philosophical underpinnings of theory, 170
testability of theory, 172
usefulness of theory, 172
value in extending nursing science, 173

Swan, B. A.
Theory of Reasoned Action/Planned Behavior, 326, 443
Swanson, B.
logistic teaching, 490
Swanson, K. M.
theory of caring, 219, 242t
Swanson, M.
case management, 467
Swanson, R. A.
adult learning, 402–404, 403b
cognitive-field (gestalt) theory, 393
role of teachers, 391
Swartwout, E.
nursing curriculum, 487
Swatton, A.
psychoanalytic theory, 309
Szabo, J.
nursing as discipline, 4
philosophy, overview, 6

T

Tailor-Ford, R.
Nightingale, 136
Taney, G.
Conservation Model, 163
Tannenbaum, R.
continuum of leader behavior, 357–358
Tanner, A.
evidence-based practice, 381
Tanner, C.
model of skill acquisition in nursing, 232
Tanner, C. A.
nursing curriculum, 482–483, 508
Tansky, C.
gate control theory, 350
Tanyi, R. A.
Nightingale, 136
Tason, M. C.
comparison of concept development models, 67
concept development, 55
Taylor, F. W.
chain of command, 454
scientific management, 365, 365b
Taylor, S. G.
descriptive theories, 38
nursing theory, 25, 26
Orem, 142, 145, 146
research methodology, 18
Teichman, J.
philosophy, definition, 6
Tejero, L. M. S.
Transitions Theory, 241
Telford, K.
psychoanalytic theory, 309
Tellez, M.
California Safe Staffing Law, 464
Thibaut, J. W.
social exchange theory, 280
Thom, B.
infection prevention, 334
Thomas, D. S.
definition of the situation, 285
Thomas, K. W.
conflict mode model, 374–375
Thomas, M.
psychoanalytic theory, 309
Thomas, M. L.
experimental research on cancer pain, 434t
Thomas, W. I.
definition of the situation, 285
Thompson, B.
model of skill acquisition in nursing, 232
Thompson, L.
interpersonal theory, 312
Thomsen, T.
stress theories, 321
Thomson, E. A.
study of implantable cardioverter defibrillator, 436–437, 443
Thorndike, E. L.
behaviorism, 389, 389t, 390
Thorne, B.
feminist theory, 290, 291b
Thorne, S.
caring as central construct, 45
metaparadigm, 42
Thurmond, V. A.
research methodology, 18
Tichen, A.
context analysis, 66
Tierney, A. F.
nursing theory, 25, 36t, 118, 119
Tillery, M.
Conservation Model, 163
Tilley, D. S.
descriptive theories, 76
Timmins, F.
logistic teaching, 490
Tingen, M. S.
model for smoking prevention, 222–223
perceived view of science, 9
research methodology, 17, 18
Tinkle, M. B.
research methodology, 17
Titler, M.
Iowa Model, of evidence-based nursing, 264, 267
To, T.
problem-based learning, 489
student-centered teaching, 401
Tod, A.
evidence-based practice, 259
Todaro-Franceschi, V.
competing paradigms, 128
Rogerian theory, 196
Toikkanen, T.
humanbecoming paradigm, 205
Tomey, A. M.
change, 370
grand theory categorization, 118–119
Nightingale, 134
nursing theory, 27t–28t
theory evaluation, 106, 126
Tomlin, E. M.
assumptions, concepts, and relationships, 170–172, 171t
background, 169–170
interactive–integrative paradigm, 122
middle range theory, 214
Modeling and Role-Modeling, 169–173
nursing theory, 119, 169–173
parsimony of theory, 173
philosophical underpinnings of theory, 170
testability of theory, 172
usefulness of theory, 172
value in extending nursing science, 173
Tough, A.
self-directed learning, 405
Touhy, T. A.
Caring Science as Sacred Science, 186
Tourangeau, A. E.
predictive theories, 77
Theory of Nurses' Recognizing and Responding to Uncertainty, 435
Trangenstein, P. A.
Transitions Theory, 238
Travelbee, L. E.
interaction theory, 119
nursing theory, 34t, 119
Tredway, C. A.
dialectic learning, 489
technology in nursing education, 492
Trevino, E.
Artinian Intersystem Model, 168
Triolo, P. K.
Magnet Recognition Program, 465, 466
Tripp-Reimer, T.
middle range theory, 214, 216
nursing theory–nursing research connection, 431
reliance on nursing models in research, 444–445
social networks, 284
Troutman, M. F.
theory of successful aging, 424
Troyan, P. J.
career persistence in acute care, 218
Tsai, P. F.
caregiver stress theory, 220, 249t
Tsai, W. C.
role theory, 288
Tsao, L. I.
nursing care for patients at risk for suicide, 218
Tschannen, D.
technology in nursing education, 493
Tschanz, C. L.
nursing as discipline, 4
philosophy, overview, 6
Tu, A. W.
Theory of Reasoned Action/Planned Behavior, 326
Tullai-McGuinness, S.
transformational leadership, 458
Tung, H. S.
social networks, 284

Turner, J. H.
process role theory, 288
social exchange theory, 279, 280, 280t
social networks, 283, 284
structural role theory, 288
symbolic interactionism, 285t
Turner-Henson, A.
Johnson model, 149
Tweet, A. G.
benchmarking, 472
Tyer-Viola, L.
nursing philosophy, 11
Tyler, D.
Transitions Theory, 238
Tyler, R.
Theory of Unpleasant Symptoms, 247
Tyson, V.
social exchange theory, 281

U

Uhl, K.
cognitive behavioral therapies, 315
Uhl-Bien, M.
Leader–Member Exchange Theory, 358
Uhrenfeldt, L.
model of skill acquisition in nursing, 232
Ulbrich, S. L.
Theory of Exercise as Self-Care, 221
Upshaw-Owens, M.
infection prevention, 334
Upton, D. J.
evidence-based practice, 261
Utley-Smith, Q.
nursing practice competencies, 503, 503t

V

Vacek, J. E.
student-centered teaching, 401
Valencia, I.
Theory of Chronic Sorrow, 109
van Daalen-Smith, C.
feminist theory, 292
Vandall-Walker, V.
Conservation Model, 163
van den Heuvel, J.
quality improvement, 379–380
Vanderwee, K.
general systems theory, 283
Vander Woude, D.
humanbecoming paradigm, 205
Van Dyke, N. F.
web of causation, 337
van Meijel, B.
symbolic interactionism, 286
Van Riper, M.
genetic counseling, 345
Varcoe, C.
descriptive research on abused women, 434t
theory–practice gap, 416
Varkey, P.
quality improvement, 378, 380, 471, 472
Varnell, G.
evidence-based practice, 259, 261, 504
Vecchio, R. P.
Path–Goal Theory, 362
Verhulst, G.
sources of concepts, 54t
Verver, J. P. S.
quality improvement, 379–380
Vicari, S.
Bandura's social learning theory, 400
Vila, A.
mobile device for nursing, 139
Vogler, J.
cultural care diversity and universality theory, 234
von Bertalanffy, L.
general systems theory, 282
Vroom, V. H.
decision making, 372
Expectancy Theory, 367
leadership theories, 362
Path–Goal Theory, 361
Vukovitch, P. K.
Artinian Intersystem Model, 168
Vuorinen, R.
model of skill acquisition in nursing, 233

W

Wadensten, B.
psychosocial developmental theory, 310
Wagner, C.
Nursing Intervention Classification system, 422–423, 423t, 424t
prescriptive theories, 78
Wagner, D.
chaos theory, 296, 297
Wagner, D. J.
Nightingale, 135
Wagner, J.
metaparadigm, 41–42
Wagner, J. A.
behavioral theories of leadership, 357
Rational Decision-Making Model, 372
Wagner, L.
Caring Science as Sacred Science, 186
stress theories, 321
Wainwright, S. P.
constructionism, 9
Walker, D. K.
natural history of disease, 339
Walker, D. S.
practice-based evidence, 262
social justice, 44
Walker, L.
midlife women's attitudes toward physical activity, 420t
Walker, L. O.
associational statements, 80
concept derivation, 59, 59b
concept development, 58–59, 58b, 60t, 67, 68t
evidence-based practice, 261, 263, 504
explanatory theories, 76
grand theories, 74, 127
Maternal Role Attainment/Becoming a Mother, 252
metatheory, 37, 74
middle range theories, 74
postmodernism, 10
practice theories, 74
relationship among levels of theory, 75
statement development, 87, 87b
theory analysis, 96, 97, 98t, 100, 101t, 106, 107t, 124, 126, 127
theory concepts, 79
theory development, 73
theory development process, 86
theory–practice gap, 417
theory synthesis, 88, 88b
Walker, P. H.
evidence-based practice, 261, 264
nursing epistemology, 14
Wall, P. D.
gate control theory, 349
gate control theory of pain, 221
Wallace, R.
relaxation response, 221
Wallen, E. M.
Uncertainty of Illness Theory, 244
Wallen, G. R.
genomics in nursing practice, 344–345
Walling, A.
prescriptive theories, 40
Wallis, M.
explanatory theories, 76
Walsh, S. M.
Self-Transcendence Theory, 248
Walumbwa, F. O.
transformational leadership, 363
Wandelt, M. A.
Magnet Recognition Program, 465
Wang, C. H.
sources of concepts, 54t
Wang, D.
Leader–Member Exchange Theory, 358
Wang, F. D.
infection prevention, 334
Wang, H.
Leader–Member Exchange Theory, 358
Wang, J.
cancer theories, 348
natural history of disease, 339
Wang, M. M.
social networks, 284
Wang, Y. N.
role theory, 288
Ward, D. J.
Theory of Reasoned Action/Planned Behavior, 326
Ward, M.
chaos theory, 296, 297–298

Ward, S.
Rogerian theory, 196
Wardell, D. W.
cultural diversity and cultural bias, 295
Ward-Smith, P.
psychosocial developmental theory, 310
Warelow, P. J.
critical social theory, 293
Warner, J.
Theory of Chronic Sorrow, 109, 250
Warren, N.
patient-focused care, 462–463
Warren, N. A.
research-based concepts, 54
Washington, R. R.
transactional and transformational leadership, 363
Wassef, M. E.
logistic teaching, 490
Waters, M.
feminist theory, 290, 291
social exchange theory, 281t
Watson, J.
assumptions, concepts, and relationships, 183–185, 184b, 185t
background, 183
caring as central construct, 45
caring/becoming theory, 119
Caring Science as Sacred Science, 160, 182–187, 479–480
evidence-based practice, 261, 264
interactive–integrative paradigm, 122
interactive theory, 124, 124t
metaparadigm, 43t
middle range theories derived from work, 213
nursing epistemology, 14
nursing theory, 35t, 119, 182–187
parsimony of theory, 186
philosophical underpinnings of theory, 183
testability of theory, 186
usefulness of theory, 186, 187b
Watson, J. B.
behaviorism, 389, 389t
Watson, M. J.
theory of transpersonal caring, 490
Weaver, K.
comparison of concept development models, 67
concept analysis, 66
Weaver, M. T.
immune function, 343
Webber, P. B.
chaos theory, 296
general systems theory, 282
theory–practice gap, 417
Weber, A. L.
Magnet Recognition Program, 466
Weber, M.
bureaucracy, 365
chain of command, 454
conflict theory, 289–290
Weber, R.
patient-focused care, 462
Wechter, S. M.
Theory of Comfort, 246
Weick, K. E.
theory to practice to theory approach, 84
Weigarten, S.
disease management, 468
Weigel, D.
chaos theory, 296
Weinert, C.
rural nursing model, 231t
Weinke, C.
Nightingale, 136
Weiss, J. A.
study of postpartum hospital discharge, 436
Theory of Normalizing Risky Sexual Behaviors, 218
Weiss, M.
research on cesarean birth, 434t, 441
Welch, A. J.
humanbecoming paradigm, 205, 206t–207t
unitary process theory, 208
Welch, M.
logical positivism, 8
philosophy of science in nursing, 12
Welsh, D.
Social Readjustment Rating Scale, 342
Werner, J. S.
Nightingale, 136
West, J.
feminist theory, 292
West, K. S.
Artinian Intersystem Model, 168
Westfall, U. B.
role theory, 288
Weston, M. J.
shared governance, 458
Wetz, R. V.
Six Sigma, 381
Weyneth, C. C.
Nightingale, 135
Whaite, B.
Nightingale, 135
Whall, A. L.
middle range theories, 38
practice theories, 38, 434
theory evaluation, 95, 98t, 103–104, 105t, 106, 107t, 225
White, K.
Johns Hopkins Nursing Evidence-Based Practice Model, 264, 267–270, 269b
Whitehead, D.
concept analysis, 66
Whitehead, P. B.
Theory of Comfort, 246
Whitehurst Cook, M. Y.
disease management, 468
White-Traut, R. C.
principle-based concept analysis, 66
Whittemore, R.
middle range theory of adaptation to diabetes, 220
Wicklund-Gustin, L.
Caring Science as Sacred Science, 186
Wiedenbach, E.
explanatory theories, 76
interaction theory, 119
nursing theory, 31, 34t, 72, 119, 132
nursing theory development, 30
predictive theories, 76
prescriptive theories, 77
theory categorization, 75
Wiggins, S.
humor use in nurse–patient interactions, 218
Wikie, D. J.
prescriptive theories, 78
Wilcox, S.
Bandura's social learning theory, 400
Wilfong, D.
technology in nursing education, 493
Wilkie, D. J.
gate control theory, 350
Williams, C. R.
bureaucracy, 365
quality improvement, 378
Williams, J. K.
nursing curriculum, 487
Williams, S.
feminist theory, 292
Willis, D. G.
boys' healing from being bullied, 427t
Wilson, A. F.
relaxation response, 221
Wilson, B.
model of skill acquisition in nursing, 232
Wilson, J.
concept development, 57–58, 67
theory–practice gap, 416
Wineman, N. M.
evidence-based practice, 474
Winstead-Fry, P.
Rogerian theory, 196, 197
Winter, D. G.
power strategy, 369
Wise, N. J.
Health Promotion Model, 236
Wisner, K. L.
Postpartum Depression Theory, 251
Witek-Janusek, L.
immune function, 343
Witucki-Brown, J.
descriptive theories, 39
Wojcik, J.
disease management, 469
Wolf, G.
Magnet Recognition Program, 465, 466
Wolfer, J.
research methodology, 17

Wolff, J.
cognitive behavioral therapies, 315
Wong, C. A.
Leader–Member Exchange Theory, 370
Wong, F. K. Y.
problem-based learning, 489
student-centered teaching, 401
Wong, M. L.
cancer theories, 348
Wongyatunyu, S.
Orem, 142
Wood, M. J.
Artinian, 164
Woodgate, R. L.
theory of keeping the spirit alive, 249t
Woods, A. B.
correlational research, 434t
Worden, C.
logistic teaching, 490
Workman, M. L.
immune system, 342, 343
Wright, B. W.
King, 173
Wright, M.
nursing education, 480
Wrubel, J.
nursing theory, 36t
Wu, E. S.
nurse staffing and patient outcomes, 464
Wu, R. R.
nursing curriculum, 482
Wu, Y. W.
correlational study of mammography, 436
social psychology theories, 326
theories as conceptual framework, 443
Wuest, J.
descriptive research on abused women, 434t
testing of caregiving theory, 441
Wung, S. F.
predictive theories, 39
Wurster, J. L.
Theory of Normalizing Risky Sexual Behaviors, 218
Wysocki, J.
Contingency Theory of Leadership, 361
Wysong, P. R.
Transitions Theory, 241

Y

Yamamoto, L.
case management, 466–467
Yang, J.
social networks, 284
Yang, J. H.
health-related behaviors of Korean Americans, 420t
Yang, P. S.
role theory, 288
Yao, G.
role theory, 288
Yates, E.
homeodynamics, 340
Yates, J.
genomics in nursing practice, 344–345
Yeh, C. H.
Uncertainty of Illness Theory, 244
Yehle, K. S.
dialectic learning, 489
Yenen, M. C.
cancer theories, 348
Yeo, S. A.
homeostasis, 340
Yetton, P. W.
decision making, 372
Yönt, G. H.
Care Dependency Scale, 139
You, K. S.
cultural diversity and cultural bias, 295
Young, A.
descriptive theories, 38
nursing theory, 25, 26
research methodology, 18
Young, T. R.
chaos theory, 296
Youngblut, J.
social exchange theory, 281–282

Z

Zanni, K. L.
natural history of disease, 339
Zarubi, K. L.
patient-focused care, 462
Zauderer, C. R.
descriptive theories, 76
Zauszniewski, J.
methodological triangulation, 500
Zauszniewski, J. A.
middle range theory of diabetes self-care, 221
Zderad, L.
interaction theory, 119
interactive–integrative paradigm, 122
nursing theory, 35t
Zeigler, V. I.
descriptive theories, 76
Zeller, J. M.
logistic teaching, 490
Zeller, R.
social exchange theory, 281–282
Zenk, S. N.
prescriptive theories, 78
Zhao, S.
postmodern social theory, 299
Zhou, G.
Theory of Reasoned Action/Planned Behavior, 326, 443
Zhou, L.
natural history of disease, 339
Zhou, X. T.
Path–Goal Theory, 362
Zhu, W.
transformational leadership, 363
Ziebarth, T. H.
cancer theories, 348
natural history of disease, 339
Ziegler, S. M.
nursing theory, 25
Zimmerman, M.
stress theories, 321
Zoucha, R.
cultural care diversity and universality theory, 234
Zurakowski, T. L.
Nightingale, 133, 134
Zwirn, E. E.
technology in nursing education, 491

SUBJECT INDEX

Note: Page numbers followed by b indicate material in boxes, those followed by f indicate material in figures, and those followed by t indicate material in tables.

A

AACN. *See* American Association of Colleges of Nursing; American Association of Critical Care Nurses
Abstract concepts, 52
Abstraction level, of theories, 36–38, 37f, 73–75
  in categorization of grand theories, 118–119
  in middle range theories, 217, 230
  in theory evaluation, 104, 106, 107t
Academic Center for Evidence-Based Practice Star Model (ACE Star Model), 264–266, 265f, 265t, 272t
Academic discipline. *See* Discipline(s)
Accelerated programs, in nursing education, 480
Accessibility, of theory, 102
Accommodation
  in conflict handling, 374–375
  in learning, 402
Accountability
  in patient care delivery models, 459
  in shared governance, 456–458
Accountable care organizations (ACOs), 470
Accreditation, nursing curriculum and, 482–483
Accuracy, of theory, 104, 106, 107t
ACE Star Model, of evidence-based practice, 264–266, 265f, 265t, 272t
Achievement, need for, 369
Achievement–Motivation Theory, 366–367, 367t
Achievement-oriented leader, 361
Achievement system, 148
ACOs. *See* Accountable care organizations
Active potential assessment model (APAM), 170–172
Activities for client assistance, 137–138, 138b
Actual caring occasion, 185t, 213
Acute pain management, theory of, 224, 249t
Adaptation
  in Conservation Model, 162t
  in Modeling and Role-Modeling, 170
  in Roy Adaptation Model, 179t. *See also* Roy Adaptation Model
  in stress theories, 318–321
  in systems, 282
Adaptation to Chronic Pain, Theory of, 86, 221, 241t, 249t
Adaptive modes, in Roy Adaptation Model, 179–180, 180f
Administration and management, 78t, 354–385
  application of theory in, 452–478
  authority and responsibility in, 455
  bureaucracy/organization theory in, 365
  case management in, 459, 466–468
  centralization *vs.* decentralization in, 455–456
  chain of command in, 454
  change in, 370–372
  classic management theory in, 366
  conflict management in, 374–375
  decision-making processes in, 372–374
  departmentalization in, 456
  disease/chronic illness management in, 468–470, 468b
  empowerment in, 369–370
  evidence-based practice in, 380–382
  Fayol's principles of, 366, 366b
  future issues in, 506–507, 506b
  leadership theories in, 355–364
  Magnet Recognition Program in, 458–459, 465–466, 466b
  motivational theories in, 366–368
  organizational design in, 453–456, 453b
  organizational/management theories in, 365–366
  overview of concepts in, 355
  patient care delivery models in, 459–466
  patient-focused care in, 460, 461–463, 461b
  power in, 368–369
  primary nursing in, 459–460, 461
  problem-solving in, 372–374
  quality improvement/management in, 375–380, 470–475
  scientific management in, 365
  shared governance in, 456–458
  Taylor's principles of, 365, 365b
  team nursing in, 459–461
  total patient care (functional nursing) in, 459–460
  transformational leadership in, 362–363, 458–459
  work specialization in, 453–454
Administrative model, of shared governance, 457
Adolescent Support Model, 85
Adult learning, 402–404, 403b, 405t
Adult Uncertainty in Illness Scale, 243
Advanced practice nurses (APNs), 31–32, 382
  authority and responsibility of, 455
  case management by, 467
  in community-based health care systems, 503
  disease management role of, 470
  in evidence-based practice, 474
  theoretical knowledge and skills of, 500–501, 501b
Advancing Research and Clinical Practice Through Close Collaboration (ARCC) Model, 264, 266, 267b, 272t
Affective learning, 387–388
Affiliated-individuation, 171t
Affiliation, need for, 369
Affiliative subsystem, 148
Ageism, 294
Agency, concept of, 281, 281t
Agency for Healthcare Research and Quality, 259, 260
Agenda for Change (Joint Commission), 375
Aggressive subsystem, 148
Aging, successful, theories of, 424
Aging population, 498b
AIM. *See* Artinian Intersystem Model
Aim of instinct, 308
Alarm, as stage of stress, 318–319, 319t, 341, 341t
Allostasis, 340
AMA. *See* American Medical Association
American Academy of Nursing, 465
American Association of Colleges of Nursing (AACN)
  Commission on Collegiate Nursing Education (CCNE), 483
  competencies and skills needed by generalist nurses, 498–499, 499b
  doctor of nursing practice proposed, 31
  theoretical knowledge and skills, 500–501, 501b
American Association of Critical Care Nurses (AACN), Synergy Model for Patient Care, 96, 230, 239–241. *See also* Synergy Model for Patient Care
American Medical Association (AMA), on nursing education, 28
American Nurses Association (ANA), education initiatives of, 30
  Scope and Standards for Nursing Administrators, 466
  survey on evidence-based practice, 381–382
American Nurses Credentialing Center (ANCC), Magnet Recognition Program, 465–466
ANA. *See* American Nurses Association

Analogizing, in concept development, 65, 65t
Anal stage of development, 307t, 308
Analytical phase, of concept development, 62t, 63
Analytic learners, 406
ANCC. *See* American Nurses Credentialing Center
Andragogy, 402–404, 405t
Antecedents, delineating, 65, 65t
Anthropology
definitions of culture in, 294b
middle range nursing theories derived from, 221–222
Antibody-mediated immunity, 343
Anxiety
in general adaptation syndrome, 318–319, 319t
in interpersonal theory, 311–312
Peplau's levels of, 312, 318–320, 319t
in psychoanalytic theory, 308–309
APAM. *See* Active potential assessment model
APNs. *See* Advanced practice nurses
Application of theory, in nursing administration and management, 452–478
authority and responsibility, 455
case management, 459, 466–468
centralization *vs.* decentralization, 455–456
chain of command, 454
departmentalization, 456
disease/chronic illness management, 468–470, 468b
Magnet Recognition Program, 458–459, 465–466, 466b
organizational design, 453–456, 453b
patient care delivery models, 459–466
patient-focused care, 460, 461–463, 461b
primary nursing, 459–460, 461
quality management, 470–475
shared governance, 456–458
span of control, 454–455
team nursing, 459–461
total patient care (functional nursing), 459–460
transformational leadership, 458–459
work specialization, 453–454
Application of theory, in nursing education, 479–496
curriculum, 481–482
teaching, 488–493
technology, 491–493
Application of theory, in nursing practice, 412–429
borrowed or shared theory, 78t, 424–425
examples from nursing literature, 424–426
grand and middle range theories, 425–426
guidelines for, 415, 415t
health care delivery system and, 417
implied theory, 422, 424–425
in intermittent urinary catheterization, 422–423, 423t
nursing education and, 416–417
in patient contracting, 423, 424t
Roy Adaptation Model, 426
situation-specific (practice) theories in, 418–421
in taxonomy, 422–423
theorist–practitioner disparity and, 417
theory–practice gap in, 416–417
Application of theory, in nursing research, 430–451
borrowed or shared theory, 78t, 424–425
concerns over reliance on nursing models in, 444–445
correlational, 434, 434t, 435–436
description of theory in research report, 445, 446b
descriptive, 434–435, 434t
experimental, 434, 434t, 436–437
framework/process of research, 433–434, 433b
historical overview of, 431–432
Nightingale and, 431
nursing and non-nursing theories, 444–445
purpose of theory in research, 433
rationale for using nursing theories in, 444
theory as conceptual framework, 442–443, 445, 446b
theory fit in research agenda, 445, 446–448, 447b, 448t
theory-generating research, 84t, 85–86, 437–439
theory–research relationship, 432–433
theory-testing research, 437, 439–441, 441b
theory use in, 437–443
types of theories and corresponding research, 434–437, 434t
Application of theory, specific theories
behavioral and cognitive-behavioral theories, 314–315
behavioral learning theories, 391
Benner model of skill acquisition, 232–233, 253
cancer theories, 348
chaos theory, 298
cognitive development/interaction theories, 396–397
cognitive-field (gestalt) theories, 393–394
critical social theory, 293
cultural care diversity and universality theory, 233–234, 253, 497
cultural diversity and cultural bias, 295
feminist theory, 292
Gagne's learning theory, 397–398
gate control theory of pain, 350
general systems theory, 283
genetic principles and theories, 344–346
germ theory and principles of infection, 334
Health Belief Model, 320–321, 424–425, 436, 443, 497
Health Promotion Model, 236, 253, 436, 437, 443
homeostasis, 340
immune system theories, 343
information-processing models, 395
interpersonal theory, 312–313
Knowles' theory of adult learning, 404
learning theories, 391, 397–400, 404, 407–408, 437, 443
Maslow's human needs theory, 316–317
Maternal Role Attainment/Becoming a Mother, 252, 253
multiple middle range theories, 253
natural history of disease, 339
person-centered theory, 318
Piaget's theory of cognitive development, 396–397
postmodern social theory, 300
Postpartum Depression Theory, 251
psychoanalytic theory, 309
psychosocial developmental theory, 310–311
role theory, 288
Roy Adaptation Model, 437
Self-Care Deficit Theory, 425
Self-Transcendence Theory, 248, 253
social exchange theory, 281–282
social learning theory, 399–400, 437, 443
social networks, 284
social psychology theories, 325–326
stress theories, 320–321, 342
symbolic interactionism, 286
Synergy Model for Patient Care, 240–241, 241b, 253, 426, 443
Theory of Chronic Sorrow, 109–110, 250, 253, 425–426
Theory of Comfort, 246, 253
Theory of Reasoned Action/Planned Behavior, 84, 325–326, 436, 443
Theory of Unpleasant Symptoms, 247, 253, 443
Transitions Theory, 238–239, 425, 436
Uncertainty in Illness Theory, 243–244
Applied science, 6, 6t
nursing as, 6, 16, 306
pure science *vs.*, 6, 306
Appraisal, in stress theory, 320
ARCC Model, of evidence-based practice, 264, 266, 267b, 272t
Arizona Social Support Interview Schedule (ASSIS), 282

Artinian Intersystem Model (AIM), 159, 160, 164–169
  assumptions of, 165, 167b
  background of theorist, 164
  concepts of, 165–166, 167t
  parsimony of, 169
  philosophical underpinnings of, 164, 165t, 166f
  relationships in, 166–168
  testability of, 168–169
  value in extending nursing science, 169
Art of nursing, 13, 14t, 19–20
Assertiveness, in conflict handling, 374–375
Assignment systems, 459
Assimilation, 402
ASSIS. *See* Arizona Social Support Interview Schedule
Associational statements, 80–81
Associative concepts, 51t
Assumptions, 27t, 81, 102t
  Abdellah's, 139–141
  Artinian Intersystem Model, 165, 167b
  Caring Science as Sacred Science, 182–187
  Conservation Model, 161
  grand theory, 126
  Health as Expanding Consciousness, 198–199
  Henderson's, 137
  humanbecoming paradigm, 203, 204b
  Johnson's, 147
  Modeling and Role-Modeling, 170
  Neuman Systems Model, 150–152
  Nightingale's, 134–135
  order and conflict synthesis model, 289, 289b
  Orem's, 142–144
  Rational Decision-Making Model, 372–373
  Roy Adaptation Model, 178
  Science of Unitary and Irreducible Human Beings, 194
  social exchange theories, 280b
  symbolic interactionism, 285, 285b
  Theory of Goal Attainment, 174–175
Asthma education, quality improvement in, 474
Asynchronous technology, 491
Attachment subsystem, 148
Attention, and learning, 406
Attitude, in Theory of Reasoned Action/Planned Behavior, 323–324
Attribution theory, 364
Auditory learning style, 405–406
Authentic leadership, 363–364
Authority
  in conflict theories, 289
  definition of, 368
  power *vs.*, 368
Autocratic leadership, 357–358
Automatic thinking scheme, 314
Avoidance, as conflict-handling mode, 374
Axiology, 7, 7t. *See also* Ethics
Axioms, 80t

B

Bandura's social learning theory. *See* Social learning theory
Banner Health, case management venture of, 467–468
Basic duality, 398
Basic or pure sciences, 6, 6t, 306
Basic structure, in Neuman Systems Model, 151t
Behavioral control, perceived, 323–325
Behavioral learning theories, 389–391
  application to nursing, 391
  characteristics of, 391t
  comparison of, 389t
Behavioral sciences, 78t, 305–330
  behavioral and cognitive-behavioral theories in, 313–315, 327t
  comparison of theories, 327t
  humanistic theories in, 315–318, 327t
  middle range nursing theories derived from, 221–222, 222t
  psychodynamic theories in, 306–313, 327t
  social psychology in, 321–326, 327t
  stress theories in, 318–321, 327t
Behavioral system, definition of, 148t
Behavioral System Model, 145–149
  assumptions in, 147
  background of theorist, 147
  concepts in, 147
  philosophical underpinnings of, 147
  relationships in, 148
  testability of, 149
  usefulness of, 149
Behavioral theories, 313–315, 327t
Behavioral theories of leadership, 357–358
Behaviorism, 389–390, 389t
Benchmarking, 472
Benner model of skill acquisition, 230–233
  application in practice, 232–233, 253
  context for use, 232
  evidence of empirical testing, 232–233
  nursing implications of, 232
  purpose and concepts of, 230–232
Best practices guidelines (BPGs), 380
Bias
  cultural, 293–295
  definition of, 294
Bifurcation, 297
Biomedical sciences, 78t, 331–353
  cancer theories, 346–349
  disease causation, 332–339
  genetic principles and theories, 343–346
  pain management, 349–350
  physiology and physical functioning, 339–350
Blocking, in curriculum, 486
Blue Cross Blue Shield of Arizona, case management venture of, 467–468
Borrowed theory, 78–79, 78t. *See also* specific disciplines and theories
  application in nursing practice, 78t, 424–425
  application in nursing research, 78t, 444–445
  definition of, 27t, 306
  vs. unique, 40–41, 306, 431
Boundaries, in Behavioral System Model, 148t
Boundary lines, in Neuman Systems Model, 151t
Bounded rationality, 373
Bovine spongiform encephalopathy (BSE), causative agent of, 334
BPGs. *See* Best practices guidelines
Breast health
  concept development on postmastectomy grief, 49–50, 56, 67
  Perceived Access to Breast Health Care in African American Women Theory, 90–91
BSE. *See* Bovine spongiform encephalopathy
Bureaucracy, theory of, 365
Butterfly effect, 296–297

C

California Safe Staffing Law, 464–465
Canadian Association of Critical Care Nursing, 163
Cancer
  development of, 346–347, 347f, 348t
  lifestyle factors in, 347, 348t
Cancer theories, 346–349
  application to nursing, 348
  goals of, 347–348
Carative factors, 183–184, 184b
Care Dependency Scale, 139
Caregiver Rewards Scale (PCRS), 282
Caregiver roles, 288
Caregiver stress, theory of, 220, 249t
Caregiving Effectiveness Model, 39, 249t
Care-seeking behavior, theory of, 242t
Caring
  as central construct in nursing, 45
  theory of (Swanson), 219, 242t
Caring/becoming theorists, 119, 120t
Caring Science as Sacred Science, 160, 182–187, 479–480
  assumptions of, 183–184
  background of theorist, 183
  carative factors in, 183–184, 184b
  concepts of, 184, 184b, 185t
  middle range theories derived from, 213
  parsimony of, 186
  philosophical underpinnings of, 183
  relationships in, 184–185
  testability of, 186

usefulness of, 186, 187b
value in extending nursing science, 186
Case management, 459, 466–468
coordination of care in, 467–468
definition of, 466
development of, 466
future issues in, 506
high-risk patients in, 467
inpatient ("within the walls"), 467
as nursing competency, 503t
outcomes of, 467
Case Management Society of America (CMSA), 466
Case method model, 459
Causal relationships, 81
Causative agent
in epidemiologic triangle, 334–335, 334f
in germ theory, 333–334
Cause-and-effect diagrams, in quality improvement, 379
CCNE. *See* Commission on Collegiate Nursing Education
Cell-mediated immunity, 343
Centers for Medicare and Medicaid Services (CMS), 377
Centralization *vs.* decentralization, 455–456
Chaining, in Gagne's learning theory, 397b
Chain (web) of causation, 335–337, 336f
Chain of command, 454
Change, 370–372
driving forces for, 371
field of, 371
force of, 371
Kotter's Eight Step Plan for Implementing, 371
planned, theory of, 370–372
restraining forces on, 371
Chaos, definition of, 295–296
Chaos theory, 222, 295–298
application to nursing, 298
concepts from, 296–298
principles of, 296, 296b
Charismatic leadership, 364
Charismatic power, 368
Chief nursing officers (CNOs), 458–459
Chronic conditions, as health care challenge, 498b
Chronic illness management, 468–470
Chronic illness trajectory framework, 242t
Chronic Sorrow, Theory of, 218, 248–250
application in practice and research, 109–110, 250, 253, 425–426
context for use, 250
description of, 110
evaluation of, exemplar of, 109–112
evidence of empirical testing, 250
nursing implications of, 250
purpose and concepts of, 250
Circle of contagiousness, 103
CJD. *See* Creutzfeldt–Jakob disease
Clarity of theory, 102
Classical conditioning, 389–390, 389t
Classification theories, 75–76
Classism, 294
Client. *See also* Person
in nursing metaparadigm, 43t, 44
Client assistance, activities for, 137–138, 138b
Client Experience Model, 218
Client–nurse, in nursing metaparadigm, 44
Client participation, 312
Client problems, Abdellah's steps to identify, 140, 141
Clinical knowledge, 15
Clinical nurse specialists (CNSs), 454, 470
CMS. *See* Centers for Medicare and Medicaid Services
CMSA. *See* Case Management Society of America
CNOs. *See* Chief nursing officers
CNSs. *See* Clinical nurse specialists
Cochrane Collaboration, 259, 260
Cock's Comb model, 133
Coercive power, 368, 369t
Cognator, in Roy Adaptation Model, 179t, 180
Cognition, in interpersonal theory, 312
Cognitive-behavioral theory, 313–315, 327t
Cognitive content, in nursing education, 488
Cognitive development/interaction theories, 395–400, 405t
application to nursing, 396–397
Bandura's social learning theory, 399–400
characteristics of, 396t
Gagne's, 397–398, 397b
Perry's, 398–399
Piaget's, 396–397
Cognitive distortions, 314
Cognitive-field (gestalt) theories, 392–394, 405t
application to nursing, 393–394
characteristics of, 393t
Cognitive learning, 387–388
Cognitive learning theories, 389, 392–404. *See also* specific theories
adult learning, 402–403, 405t
cognitive development/interaction, 395–400, 396t, 405t
cognitive-field (gestalt), 392–394, 393t, 405t
developmental psychology, 401–402, 405t
Gagne's, 397–398, 397b
humanistic, 401, 405t
information-processing models, 394–395, 405t
Perry's, 398–399
Piaget's, 396–397
psychodynamic, 400, 405t
social learning (Bandura), 399–400
summary of, 404–405, 405t
Cognitive theory, 314, 327t
Collaboration, as conflict-handling mode, 374
Collectivism, 280
COM. *See* Commission on Magnet
Comfort, Theory of, 222, 229, 241, 244–246
application in practice, 246, 253
context for use, 244–245
evidence of empirical testing, 246
nursing implications of, 244–245
purpose and concepts of, 244, 245b, 245f
Comfort Behaviors Checklist, 246
Commission on Collegiate Nursing Education (CCNE), 483
Commission on Magnet (COM), 464–465
Commitments, in Perry's development theory, 398–399
Commitment to health theory, 439
Common cause variation, 471
Communication
modes, in Conservation Model, 162t
as nursing competency, 503t
in Theory of Goal Attainment, 175t
Community-based health care systems, 503
Competencies, nurse, 499b
in AACN recommendations, 498–499, 499b
in Synergy Model for Patient Care, 239, 239b
in today's health care system, 503, 503t
Competing, as conflict-handling mode, 374
Complement system, 343
Complex adaptive systems theory, 283
Comprehensibility, in Artinian Intersystem Model, 165t
Compromise, as conflict-handling mode, 374–375
Computer simulation, 480, 491–493
Computer technology, as nursing competency, 503t
Concept(s)
abstract *vs.* concrete, 52
continuous *vs.* discrete, 52
curricular, 485
definitions of, 27t, 50–51
existing, 54, 54t
grand theory, 126
leadership and management, 355
middle range theory, 213, 216–217
naturalistic, 54, 54t
related, 61
research-based, 54, 54t
sources of, 53–54
theoretically *vs.* operationally defined, 53, 53t
as theory component, 79, 102t
types of, 51–53, 51t
variable *vs.* nonvariable, 52

Concept(s), of theorists/theories
Abdellah patient-centered approach, 139–141
Artinian Intersystem Model, 165–166, 167t
Beck's Postpartum Depression Theory, 251
Benner model of skill acquisition, 230–232
chaos theory, 296–298
Eakes, Burke, and Hainsworth's Theory of Chronic Sorrow, 249
Erickson, Tomlin, and Swain's Modeling and Role-Modeling, 170, 171t
Health Belief Model, 322, 323f, 324t
Henderson, 137, 138b
Johnson, 147
King, 175, 175t
Kolcaba's Theory of Comfort, 244, 245b, 245f
Leininger's cultural care diversity and universality theory, 233
Lenz's Theory of Unpleasant Symptoms, 246, 247f
Levine's Conservation Model, 161, 162t
Mercer's Conceptualization of Maternal Role Attainment/Becoming a Mother, 252
Mishel's Uncertainty in Illness Theory, 243, 243f
Neuman Systems Model, 150–152, 151t, 152f
Newman, 199, 200t
Nightingale, 134–135
Orem, 142–144, 143f, 144t
Parse, 203–204
Pender's Health Promotion Model, 234–235
Reed's Self-Transcendence Theory, 248
Rogers, 194, 194b, 195t
Roy Adaptation Model, 179, 179t
social exchange theory, 281, 281t
symbolic interactionism, 285
Synergy Model for Patient Care, 239–240
Transitions Theory, 237, 238f
Watson, 184, 184b, 185t
Concept analysis. *See also* Concept development
exemplar of, 69–70
Meleis' method for, 64–65
Morse's advanced techniques of, 65–66
Penrod and Hupcey's principle-based method for, 66, 67b, 68t
Schwartz-Barcott and Kim's method for, 62t, 63
Walker and Avant's method for, 58, 58b, 68t
Concept-based curriculum, 480
Concept clarification
Meleis' method for, 64, 64b
Morse's method for, 66
Concept comparison, 66
Concept delineation, 65
Concept derivation, 59, 59b
Concept development, 49–71
comparison of methods for, 67, 68t
and conceptual frameworks, 57
context for, 55–56
Meleis' method for, 63–65, 64b, 65t, 68t
Morse's method for, 65–66, 68t
Penrod and Hupcey's method for, 66, 67b, 68t
purposes of, 55
and research, 57
Rodgers' method for, 59–61, 60b, 62t, 68t, 69–70
Schwartz-Barcott and Kim's method for, 61–63, 62t, 64t, 68t
strategies for, 57–67
student-generated examples of, 55, 56
and theory, 57, 86–87, 87t
Walker and Avant's method for, 58–59, 58b, 59b, 60t, 68t
Wilson's method for, 57–58
Concept exploration, 63
Concept synthesis, 58
Conceptual definitions, 79
Conceptual environment, in Conservation Model, 162t
Conceptual framework, 24, 26, 27t
concept development and, 57
in nursing education, 480, 483–487
in research, theory as, 442–443, 445, 446b
Conceptual knowledge, 15
Conceptual meaning, creation of, 86–87
Conceptual model, 24, 26, 27t, 82
relationship with theory and hypotheses, 117, 117f
Concrete concepts, 52
Concrete operational stage, 396
Conditioning
classical, 389–390, 389t
operant, 313–314, 327t, 389–390, 389t
Conflict management, 374–375
Conflict mode model, 374–375
Conflict situation, characteristics of, 374
Conflict theories, 281, 289–295
critical social theory, 292–293
cultural diversity and cultural bias, 293–295
feminist theory, 290–292
Marx's theory of class conflict, 289–290
Congressional model, of shared governance, 457
Congruence, 317
Connecting separating, 204
Connectionism, 389–390, 389t
Consciousness, 200t. *See also* Health as Expanding Consciousness
Consequences, delineating, 65, 65t
Conservation, Levine's definition of, 162t
Conservation Model, 160–164
assumptions about individuals, 161
assumptions about nursing, 161
background of theorist, 160
concepts of, 161, 162t
middle range theory derived from, 220, 220f, 419, 440–441
parsimony of, 163–164
philosophical underpinnings of, 160–161
practice theory derived from, 419
principles of, 161–162
relationships in, 161–162
testability of, 163
usefulness of, 163
value in extending nursing science, 164
Consistency of theory, 102, 104, 106, 107t
Construct
caring as central, in nursing, 45
definition of, 27t
Constructed knowledge stage, of nursing theory, 29t, 31–32
Constructivism, 9–10, 399, 402, 500
Content
curricular. *See* Curriculum, nursing in Neuman Systems Model, 151t
Contextual stimuli, 179t
Contingency theories of leadership, 360–362
Continuous concepts, 52
Continuous quality improvement (CQI), 375
Continuum of leader behavior, 357–358
Control beliefs, 323–325
Control charts, 379
Cooperativeness, in conflict handling, 374–375
Coping, with stress, 320
Correlational research, 76, 434, 434t, 435–436
Correlational statements, 80–81
Cosmology, 7, 7t
Cost
case management and, 466–468
disease management and, 469
evidence-based practice and, 474
nurse staffing levels and, 464
patient-centered medical homes and, 470
patient-focused care and, 461, 462
quality improvement and, 471, 472, 473
shared governance and, 458
total patient care (functional nursing) and, 460
Councilor model, of shared governance, 457
Creative/critical thinking, 507–508
Creutzfeldt–Jakob disease (CJD), 334
Critical caring theory, 85
Critical reflection, 101–102
Critical social theory, 9, 292–293
Critical thinking, 507–508
Cues to action, 322, 324t
Cultural bias, 293–295
in nursing, research on, 295
recommendations for avoidance in research, 295, 295b

Cultural care and universality theory, 233–234
application in practice, 233–234, 253
application in research, 497
context for use, 233
evidence of empirical testing, 233–234, 234b
nursing implications of, 233
purpose and concepts of, 233
Cultural care diversity and universality theory, Leininger's, 233–234
Cultural Competence, Model for, 219
Cultural diversity, 293–295
Cultural feminism, 291
Culture
anthropologic definitions of, 294b
sociologic definitions of, 293–294, 294b
Curriculum, nursing, 481–488
blocking of content in, 486
changes in, 508
components of, 481, 481b
concept-based, 480
concepts of, 485
conceptual/organizational frameworks for, 480, 483–487
components of, 485–486
designing, 484–485
patterns of, 486–487
purposes of, 484
current issues in development of, 487
definition of, 481
design of, 481–482
eclectic approach to, 484–485
enhanced content in, areas of, 487, 487b
and regulatory bodies (accreditation), 482–483
single-theory approach to, 484
structure or sequencing of, 485–486, 486t
threading content in, 487
Tyler model of, 481–482

D

Databases, in evidence-based practice, 262
Data collection, 61
Data management, 61
Death. *See* End-of-life care
Decay theory, of memory, 395
Decentralization
centralization *vs.*, 455–456
shared governance *vs.*, 456–457
support services, in patient-focused care, 462
Decision-making processes, 372–374
evidence-based practice and, 380–382
group, 373
organizational quantitative techniques in, 374
quantitative technology in, 372
Rational Decision-Making Model, 372–373
in shared governance, 457
Defense mechanisms, 308–309, 315, 400
Define, measure, analyze, improve, and control (DMAIC), 380
Defining, in concept development, 65, 65t
Definition of the situation, 285
Definitions, in theories, 102t
Degree of reaction, 151t
Deliberate action, 144t
Delineating antecedents, 65, 65t
Delineating consequences, 65, 65t
Delivery models. *See* Patient care delivery models
Deming Cycle, 473
Democratic leadership, 357–358
Denial, 308, 309
Departmentalization, 456
Dependency subsystem, 148
Descriptive research, 434–435, 434t
Descriptive theories, 38–39, 75–76, 434–435, 434t
Detector, in intrasystem model, 167–168
Developmental psychology. *See also* Development stages; specific theories
learning in, 401–402, 405t
Developmental self-care requisites, 144t
Development stages
in interpersonal theory, 307t, 312
in Perry's intellectual/ethical development theory, 398
in Piaget's cognitive development theory, 396
in psychoanalytic theory, 307t, 308–309
in psychosocial development theory, 307t, 310
Diagnosis-related groups (DRGs), 466
Diagramming, theory, 99, 103
Dialectic learning (teaching), 488–489
The Dialectic of Sex (Firestone), 291
Dialogical engagement, 205
Differentiating, in concept development, 65, 65t
Direct care, as nursing competency, 503t
Directive leader, 361
Discipline(s)
characteristics of, 4
classification of, 4
definition of, 4
multiparadigm, nursing as, 11
nursing as, 4–5, 214
philosophy of, 6
theory classification based on, 78–79, 78t
theory in, 24–25
Discrete concepts, 52
Discrimination learning, 397b
Disease
ancient view of, 332
definition of, 332
empirico-rational approach to, 333
magico-religious approach to, 333
natural history of, 337–339, 338f
Disease causation, theories and models of, 332–339
epidemiologic triangle, 334–335, 334f
evolution of, 332–339
germ theory and principles of infection, 333–334
web of causation, 335–337, 336f
Disease management, 468–470
accountable care organizations in, 470
clinical outcomes of, 469
cost reduction in, potential for, 469
criteria for evaluating services, 468, 468b
definition of, 468
models of, 469
patient-centered medical home models of, 470
return on investment, 469
Disease prevention
levels of, 337–339, 337b
as nursing research priority, 505t
principles of infection in, 334
Dissipative structures, 297–298, 298b
Distance learning/education, 480, 491–493
Diverse population, 498b
Diversity of Human Field Pattern, Theory of, 219
DMAIC steps, in quality improvement, 380
DNA, 344
DNP. *See* Doctor of nursing practice
Doctoral programs
first, 30
growth in, 31–32
Doctor of nursing practice (DNP), 31–32, 501, 501b, 507
Domination/subjugation, 289
Dreyfus model of skill acquisition, 84, 222, 230
DRGs. *See* Diagnosis-related groups
Driving forces, for change, 371
Dualism, 398–399
Dying. *See* End-of-life care
Dynamism, 311

E

EBBS. *See* Exercise Benefits/Barriers Scale
EBP. *See* Evidence-based practice
EBP Beliefs Scale (EBPB), 266
Ecogenetic nursing, 345
Economic class conflict, 289–290
Economic rationality, 372
ECT. *See* Electroshock therapy
Education. *See* Nursing education
Effector, in intrasystem model, 167–168
Ego
in psychoanalytic theory, 307–309, 400
in psychosocial developmental theory, 310

Ego defense mechanisms, 308–309, 315, 400
Ego strength, 310
Eight Step Plan for Implementing Change (Kotter), 371
Electroshock therapy (ECT), feminist theory and, 292
Eliminative subsystem, 148
Emancipatory knowing, 15
Emotion, in learning, 407
Emotional intelligence, of leaders, 356–357, 363
Empathy
  nurse-expressed, middle range theory of, 219
  in symbolic interactionism, 285
Empirical adequacy of theory, 99, 106, 107t
Empirical concepts, 52
Empirical generalizations, 80t
Empirical indicator, 27t, 41
Empirical knowledge
  case study of, 19–20
  definition of, 12
  in nursing, 13, 14t, 15
Empirical models, 82
Empirical testing. *See* Testing, empirical, of theories or models
Empiricism, 7, 8–9, 11t
  contemporary, 8–9
  founding belief of, 8
  future of, 500
  nursing and, 9
  nursing epistemology and, 13, 14t
  quantitative methodology in, 17
Employee variables, in Path–Goal Theory, 361–362
Employment options, for nurses, 502–503
Empowerment, 369–370
Enabling–limiting, 204
End-of-life care
  Dobratz's middle range theory on, 222, 439
  as nursing research priority, 505t
  Psychological Adaptation in Death and Dying, 439
  Shared Presence: Caring for a Dying Spouse, 39, 435
  Theory of the Peaceful End of Life, 224–225, 224f, 249t
Energy conservation, 161, 162t
Energy field, 194–195, 195t
Energy systems, 198
English proficiency, limited, 498b
Entropy, 151t
Enumerative concepts, 51t
Environment
  in Artinian Intersystem Model, 165, 167t
  definition of, 42, 43t
  in epidemiologic triangle, 334–335, 334f
  in Health as Expanding Consciousness, 209t
  in humanbecoming paradigm, 209t
  in interpersonal theory, 312–313
  in Johnson's theory, 147
  in Levine's Conservation Model, 162t
  in Neuman Systems Model, 150
  in Newman's theory, 199
  in Nightingale's theory, 134–135
  in nursing metaparadigm, 41–44, 43t
  in Orem's theory, 143
  in psychoanalytic theory, 308
  in psychosocial developmental theory, 310
  in Roy Adaptation Model, 179t
  in Science of Unitary and Irreducible Human Beings, 194–195, 209t
  in stress theory, 320
  in Theory of Goal Attainment, 175t
  in unitary process theories, 192, 209t
Environmental field, 195t
Environmental variables, in Path–Goal Theory, 361
Epidemiologic triangle, 334–335, 334f
Epistemologic principle, in concept analysis, 66, 67b
Epistemology, 7, 7t, 12–15
  case study of, 19–20
  definition of, 12, 27t
  nursing, 13–15, 14t, 19–20
Equilibrium, in systems, 282
Equity Theory, 368
Erikson's developmental theory. *See* Psychosocial developmental theory
Errors, medical, IOM report on, 470
Essentialism, 59
Esthetic knowledge, 7, 7t, 13, 14t, 19–20
Ethical development, Perry's theory of, 398–399
Ethics
  as branch of philosophy, 7, 7t
  definition of, 13
  in nursing, 14, 14t, 19–20
Evidence-based practice (EBP), 16, 31, 32, 258–275
  ACE Star Model of, 264–266, 265f, 265t, 272t
  advanced practice nurse's role in, 382
  ARCC Model of, 264, 266, 267b, 272t
  barriers to, 263, 263b
  comparison of models, 270–271, 272t
  concerns related to, 261
  definition and characteristics of, 259–260
  developing, process for, 419
  future issues in, 501–502, 504
  grand theory and, 118, 131
  Iowa Model of, 264, 267, 268f, 269b, 272t
  Johns Hopkins model of, 264, 267–270, 269b, 272t
  key resources for, 260
  limitations of, 381
  nurse empowerment in, 370
  nurses' readiness to implement, 381–382
  overview of, 259
  practice-based evidence in, 261–262, 262f
  practice theories and, 419–421, 421t
  prescriptive theory in, 77
  promotion of, 263, 475
  quality improvement in, 380–382, 474–475
  research *vs.*, 259
  role of advanced practice nurses in, 474
  steps in method, 381
  Stetler Model of, 264, 270, 271t, 272t
  support for and commitment to, 474
  theoretical models of, 264–271
  theory and, 263–264, 419
Evolutionary method of concept development, 59–61, 60b, 62t, 68t, 69–70
Exchange theories, 279–284
  general systems theory, 282–283, 283b
  modern social exchange theories, 279–282
  social networks, 283–284
  theory-testing research, 440–441
Exemplar
  concept analysis, 61, 69–70
  middle range theory combining existing nursing and non-nursing theories, 221
  middle range theory derived from grand theory, 220
  middle range theory derived from non-nursing discipline, 222–223
  middle range theory derived from research/practice, 219
  theory as conceptual framework, 442–443
  theory development, 90–91
  theory evaluation, 109–112
  theory-generating research, 438
  theory-testing research, 440–441
Exercise as Self-Care, Theory of, 221
Exercise Benefits/Barriers Scale (EBBS), 436
Exhaustion, as stage of stress, 318–320, 319t, 341, 341t
Existence statements, 79–80
Existing concepts, 54, 54t
Expanding consciousness, 200t. *See also* Health as Expanding Consciousness
Expectancy, definition of, 367
Expectancy Theory, 367
Expected worth, 372
Experience, of adult learners, 403, 403b
Experiential learning model, 395–396
Experimental research, 434, 434t, 436–437
Expert power, 368, 369t

Explanatory theories, 39, 75, 76, 434, 434t, 435–436
External criticism, 100
Extraction–synthesis, 205
Extreme postmodernists, 299

F
Facilitated Sensemaking, 218
Factor-isolating theories. *See* Descriptive theories
Factor-relating theories. *See* Explanatory theories
Factual assumptions, 81
Family-centered care, 462–463
Family systems theory, 283
Feedback, in learning, 407
Feedback mechanisms, physiologic, 340
Feminine mystique, 291
Feminist theory, 290–292
  application to nursing, 292
  as perceived view, 9
  postcolonial, 300
  postmodern, 300
  as postmodern view, 10
  themes in, 290, 291b
  variations of, 290–292
Field, in planned change theory, 371
Fiedler Contingency Theory of Leadership, 360–361, 360b
Field theory, 392
Fieldwork phase, of concept development, 62t, 63
Fight or flight, 340
First-level managers, 455
Flexible line of defense, 151t
Focal stimuli, 179t
Force, in planned change theory, 371
"Forces of Magnetism," 465
Forcing, as conflict-handling mode, 374
Forgetting, theories of, 395
Formal operational stage, 396
Formative testing, in nursing education, 490
Freud's psychoanalytic theory. *See* Psychoanalytic theory
Fruitfulness, of theory, 104
Function, in Behavioral System Model, 148t
Functionalistic perspective, 289
Functional nursing, 459–460
Functional requirements, of humans, 148, 148t
Functional theory of leadership, 357–358
Future issues, 497–512
  Institute of Medicine on, 3, 417, 498–499, 498b
  in nursing education, 507–508
  in nursing leadership and administration, 506–507, 506b
  in nursing practice, 502–504
  in nursing science, 499–500
  in nursing theory, 500–502
  in theory development, 501–502
The Future of Nursing (IOM), 3, 417, 498–499, 498b

G
Gagne's learning theory, 397–398, 397b
GAS. *See* General adaptation syndrome
Gate control theory of pain, 221, 331–332, 349–350, 350f
GCQ. *See* General Comfort Questionnaire
Gender
  in feminist theory, 290–292
  and learning style, 406
Gene(s), 344
General adaptation syndrome (GAS), 318–320, 327t, 340–342
General Comfort Questionnaire (GCQ), 246
Generality of theory, 99, 101t, 102, 106, 107t
Generalized other, 285
General systems theory (GST), 282–283, 283b
  application to nursing, 283
  basic tenets of, 282
Genetics, 343–346
  application to nursing, 344–346
  in cancer theories, 346–347, 347f
  counseling on, nurses' role in, 345–346
  ethics and confidentiality in testing, 345
  in health care, nursing model for, 345t
Genetic Vulnerability, Theory of, 220
Genital stage of development, 307t, 308
Genome, human, 343
Germ theory, 333–334
Gestalt (cognitive-field) theories, 392–394, 405t
  application to nursing, 393–394
  characteristics of, 393t
Glaserian grounded theory, 168
Global learners, 406
Goal
  in Neuman Systems Model, 151t
  of nursing, in Roy Adaptation Model, 179t
Goal Attainment, Theory of, 160, 173–177, 174f
  assumptions of, 174–175
  background of theorist, 173
  concepts of, 175, 175t
  parsimony of, 177
  philosophical underpinnings of, 174
  relationships in, 176
  testability of, 176–177
  usefulness of, 176
  value in extending nursing science, 177
Governance, shared, 456–458
Grand theories, 37, 73, 74. *See also* specific theories
  analysis/evaluation of, 106, 124–128, 125b
  application in practice, 425–426
  background of theorists and, 125
  categorization of, 118–123
  combining, competing paradigms and, 128
  conceptual model *vs.*, 117
  in evidence-based practice, 118
  extending nursing science through, 127
  Fawcett's categorization of, 122–123, 123t
  human needs–based, 131–158. *See also* Human needs theories
  interactive process-based, 159–191. *See also* Interactive theories
  major assumptions, concepts, and relationships in, 126
  Meleis' categorization of, 119, 120t, 123t
  middle range theories derived from, 219–220, 439
  middle range theories *vs.*, 213, 215, 216t
  need to renew or update, 118
  Newman's categorization of, 122, 123t
  nursing domains of, 119
  overview of, 116–130
  paradigms of, 119–123
  Parse's categorization of, 121, 121f, 123t
  parsimony of, 127
  philosophical underpinnings of, 125–126
  practice theories derived from, 419
  relationship with conceptual model and hypotheses, 117, 117f
  research testing, 441
  scope of, 118–119
  specific categories of, 124, 124t
  testability of, 126–127
  unitary process-based, 192–212. *See also* Unitary process theories
  usefulness of, 126
Great Man Theory, 355
Grounded theory approach
  in Artinian Intersystem Model, 168
  in descriptive research, 435
  in middle range theories, 218
  in practice theories, 85, 418, 419
  in symbolic interactionism, 286
  in theory generation, 437–439
Group decision making, 373
Group practice model, 459
Growth process, in learning, 407
GST. *See* General systems theory
"Guarding against cancer" model, 85
Guided imagery, 196

H
HCAHPS. *See* Hospital Consumer Assessment of Healthcare Providers and Systems
Health
  in Artinian Intersystem Model, 165, 167t
  in Caring Science as Sacred Science, 184, 185t
  definition of, 42, 43t
  in Johnson's theory, 147
  in Levine's Conservation Model, 162t

Health (*continued*)
in Modeling and Role-Modeling, 171t
in Neuman Systems Model, 150
in Newman's theory, 199, 200t
in Nightingale's theory, 134–135
in nursing metaparadigm, 41–44, 43t
in Orem's theory, 143
in Roy Adaptation Model, 179t
in Science of Unitary and Irreducible Human Beings, 195t
in Theory of Goal Attainment, 174, 175t
in unitary process theories, 192, 209t
Health Amendments Act (1956), 30
Health as Expanding Consciousness, 193, 198–202
assumptions of, 198–199
background of theorist, 198
comparison with other unitary process theories, 208, 209t
concepts of, 199, 200t
parsimony of, 202
philosophical underpinnings of, 198
relationships in, 199–201
testability of, 201–202
usefulness of, 201, 202b
value in extending nursing science, 202
Health Belief Model, 72, 222, 321–322
application in research, 436, 443, 497
application to nursing, 325–326, 424–425
comparison with other behavioral theories, 327t
concepts of, 322, 323f, 324t
Health care challenges, 498, 498b
Health care costs. *See* Cost
Health care delivery. *See* Patient care delivery models
Health deviation self-care requisites, 144t
Health disparities, 498b
Health information, 387
Health literacy, 387
Health-Promoting Lifestyles Profiles II (HPLP-II), 436
Health promotion
as nursing competency, 503t
as nursing research priority, 505t
Health Promotion for Preterm Infants, Theory of, 220, 220f, 419
application in practice, 236
research testing, 440–441
Health Promotion Model (HPM), 95, 234–236, 235
application in practice, 236, 253
application in research, 436, 437, 443
context for use, 235–236
evidence of empirical testing, 236, 236b
nursing implications of, 235–236
purpose and concepts of, 234–235
Health-related quality of life, theoretical *vs.* operational definition of, 53t
Health risk behaviors, theoretical *vs.* operational definition of, 53t
Helicy, 194–196, 194b
Helson's Adaptation Theory, 84
Heredity, in development, 312, 313
Herzberg's two-factor theory, 359–360
Hierarchy of learning, 406
Hierarchy of needs (Maslow), 315–317, 359
High-fidelity patient simulator, 491
High middle range theories, 217, 230–241, 231t. *See also* specific theories
Benner model of skill acquisition, 230–233
Leininger's cultural care diversity and universality theory, 233–234
Pender's Health Promotion Model, 95, 234–236, 235t
Synergy Model for Patient Care, 96, 230, 239–241, 241b, 253, 426
Transitions Theory, 236–239
Hill-Burton Act, 30
Historicism, 9–10, 11t
HIV/AIDS, determining cause of, 333
Holism
in Conservation Model, 162t
in Modeling and Role-Modeling, 171t
Holistic nursing
homeostasis in, 340
psychosocial developmental theory in, 310–311
Home health nursing, Neal theory of, 231t
Homeodynamics, 194–195, 194b, 340
Homeostasis, 148t, 162t, 340
Hospice Comfort Questionnaire, 246
Hospital Consumer Assessment of Healthcare Providers and Systems (HCAHPS), 463
Hospital nurse force theory, 85
Hospital Standardization Program, 375
Host, in epidemiologic triangle, 334–335, 334f
HPLP-II. *See* Health-Promoting Lifestyles Profiles II
HPM. *See* Health Promotion Model
Humanbecoming paradigm, 121, 193, 202–208
assumptions of, 203, 204b
background of theorist, 203
comparison with other unitary process theories, 208, 209t
concepts of, 203–204
parsimony of, 207
philosophical underpinnings of, 203
relationships in, 204
testability of, 205–207, 206t–207t
usefulness of, 204–205, 208b
Human being. *See* Person
Human Caring, Theory of. *See* Caring Science as Sacred Science
Human Genome Project, 343
Humanism, 122
Humanistic theories, 315–318
comparison with other behavioral theories, 327t
learning theory, 401, 405t
Maslow's human needs theory, 315–317
person-centered theory, 317–318
Human needs theories, 121f, 124, 124t, 131–158
Abdellah's patient-centered approach, 139–142
Henderson's, 136–139
Johnson's Behavioral System Model, 145–149
learning in, 401–402
Maslow's, 54, 131, 315–317, 327t, 359
Neuman Systems Model, 131, 149–154
Nightingale's, 132–136
Orem's Self-Care Deficit Nursing Theory, 142–146
theorists of, 119, 120t
Human science, 6, 6t
vs. natural science, 6
nursing as, 16–17
perceived view of science, 9–10
Hypotheses
concept development and, 57
definition of, 27t
as relational statement, 80t
relationship with theory and conceptual model, 117, 117f

I

IANP. *See* Inpatient asthma nurse practitioner
ICU transitional care, theory of nursing care in, 435
Id, 307–309, 400
Imaging, in humanbecoming paradigm, 203–204
Immunity and immune function, theories of, 342–343
Impetus of instinct, 308
Implications. *See also* Nursing implications of theory
identifying, 61
Implied theory, 422, 424–425
Individual(s). *See also* Person
in Theory of Goal Attainment, 175t
Individualistic social exchange, 280
Individualization, in learning, 406
Inequality
in conflict theories, 289
in critical social theory, 292–293
in feminist theory, 291–292
in social exchange theory, 281
Infection, principles of, 333–334
Infection prevention, 334
Infection risk, 334
Informational power, 368

Information-processing models, 394–395, 405t
application to nursing, 395
forgetting in, 395
memory in, 394–395
Ingestive subsystem, 148
In-group, in Leader–Member Exchange Theory, 358
Innovator control processes, 179t
Inpatient asthma nurse practitioner (IANP), 474
Input, in Neuman Systems Model, 151t
Instability, in Behavioral System Model, 148t
Instinct, characteristics of, 308
Institute for Family-Centered Care, 462
Institute for Patient- and Family-Centered Care, 462
Institute of Medicine (IOM)
To Err Is Human, 470
evidence-based practice, 259, 380
recommendations for nursing, 3, 417, 498–499, 498b, 509
recommendations for nursing education, 509
Instruction. *See* Teaching
Instrumentality, 367
Integrality, 194–196, 194b
Integrated knowledge stage, of nursing theory, 29t, 32
Integration, in social exchange theory, 280
Integration via movement, 200t
Intelligence, emotional, 356–357, 363
Intention, in Theory of Reasoned Action/Planned Behavior, 322–326
Interaction(s)
in symbolic interactionism, 285
in Theory of Goal Attainment, 175t
Interactionist frameworks, 284–288
role theory, 286–288
symbolic interactionism, 285–286, 285b
Interaction theories, of learning, 395–400, 405t
Bandura's social learning theory, 399–400
characteristics of, 396t
Gagne's, 397–398, 397b
Perry's, 398–399
Interaction theorists, 119, 120t
Interactive–integrative paradigm, 122
Interactive theories, 121f, 124, 124t, 159–191
Artinian Intersystem Model, 159, 160, 164–169
Caring Science as Sacred Science, 160, 182–187
Conservation Model, 160–164
Modeling and Role Modeling, 160, 169–173
Roy Adaptation Model, 86, 160, 177–181
Systems Framework (King), 160, 173–177
Theory of Goal Attainment, 160, 173–177, 174f
Interdependence mode, 180, 180f
Interference theory, of memory, 395
Intermittent urinary catheterization, 422–423, 423t
Internal criticism, 100
International Orem Society, 145
Interpersonal communication, as nursing competency, 503t
Interpersonal Relations in Nursing, 312
Interpersonal theory, 311–313
application to nursing, 312–313
comparison with other behavioral theories, 327t
participant–observer in, 312
stages of development in, 307t, 312
Interpretative (perceived) view, 7, 9–10, 11t
Intersystem Model, Artinian. *See* Artinian Intersystem Model
Intersystem Patient-Care Model, 164
Intrasystem model, 164, 167–168
Introduction to Clinical Nursing (Levine), 160
Intuitive knowledge, 13
IOM. *See* Institute of Medicine
Iowa Model, of evidence-based practice, 264, 267, 268f, 269b, 272t

J

JHNEBP. *See* Johns Hopkins Nursing Evidence-Based Practice Model
Joanna Briggs Institute, 260
Johns Hopkins Nursing Evidence-Based Practice Model (JHNEBP), 264, 267–270, 269b, 272t
Joint Commission, 375
Journals, nursing, 431, 444
Justice, social, 44

K

Keeping the Spirit Alive, Theory of, 249t
Kinesthetic learning style, 405–406
Knowledge
definition of, 27t
development in nursing science, 12–15, 432
development in research, 430, 432
development within discipline, 4
future issues in, 499–500
middle range theory and development of, 215
need for, in adult learning, 402–403, 403b
perceived, 9–10
received, 8–9
specialized, in professions, 2–3
types of, 12–13
Knowledge transformation, ACE Star Model of, 264–266, 265b, 265f

L

Laissez-faire leadership, 357–358
Languaging, 204
Latency stage of development, 307t, 308
Law(s), 27t, 80t
LCUs. *See* Life change units
Leader–Member Exchange (LMX) Theory, 358, 370
Leader–member relations, 360–361, 360b
Leadership
authentic, 363–364
autocratic, democratic, and laissez-faire, 357
charismatic, 364
definition of, 355
emotional intelligence of, 356–357, 363
empowerment in, 369–370
formal *vs.* informal, 355
future issues in nursing, 506–507
overview of concepts in, 355
power strategy in, 369
and quality improvement, 378–379
in quality management, 471
in shared governance, 456–458
in team nursing, 460
transactional, 362–363
transformational, 362–363, 458–459
visionary, 364
Leadership Practices Inventory: Self Instrument, 459
Leadership theories
behavioral or functional, 357–358
contemporary, 362–364
contingency, 360–362
early, 355–362
Fiedler's, 360–361, 360b
Great Man, 355
Leader–Member Exchange, 358, 370
motivational, 359–360
motivation–hygiene (two-factor), 359–360
Path–Goal, 361–362
situational, 362
Theory X and Theory Y, 359
trait, 355–357
Lean process management, 379
Lean Thinking, 379
Learning
affective, 387–388
cognitive, 387–388
definition of, 387
Gagne's types of, 397, 397b
hierarchy in, 406
principles of, 406–407
psychomotor, 387–388
strategies in nursing education, 488–490
Learning styles, 405–406
Learning theories, 78t, 386–410. *See also* specific theories
adult learning in, 402–404, 403b, 405t
application in nursing, 407–408
behavioral, 389–391, 389t, 391t
categorization of, 388–389
cognitive, 389, 392–404

Learning theories (*continued*)
cognitive development/interaction, 395–400, 396t, 405t
cognitive-field (gestalt), 392–394, 393t, 405t
constructivism, 399, 402
developmental psychology, 401–402, 405t
Gagne's, 397–398, 397b
humanistic, 401, 405t
information-processing models, 394–395, 405t
Perry's, 398–399
Piaget's, 396–397
psychodynamic, 400, 405t
social learning (Bandura), 399–400
summary of, 404–405, 405t
Least Preferred Coworker (LPC) Scale, 360–361
Legitimacy, of theory, 101
Legitimate power, 368, 369t
Leininger's cultural care and universality theory. *See* Cultural care and universality theory
Leininger Sunrise Model, 233
Leukocytes, 342
Liberal feminism, 291
Life change units (LCUs), 342
Lifetime growth and development, 171t
Line authority, 455
Lines of resistance, 151t
Linguistic principle, in concept analysis, 66, 67b
Literary synthesis, 58
LMX. *See* Leader–Member Exchange Theory
Logic, 7, 7t
Logical adequacy, of theory, 99, 101t, 106, 107t
Logical positivism, 8, 11t
Logical principle, in concept analysis, 66, 67b
Logistic teaching strategies, 490
Long-term memory, 394–395
Looking glass self, 285
Love and belonging needs, 316
Low middle range theories, 217, 230, 248–252. *See also* specific theories
Conceptualization of Maternal Role Attainment/Becoming a Mother, 222, 248, 251–252
Postpartum Depression Theory, 248, 250–251
Theory of Chronic Sorrow, 109–112, 218, 248–250, 253

M

Mad cow disease, causative agent of, 334
Magnet Recognition Program, 465–466
components of, 466, 466b
COM recommendations for, 464–465
designation process in, 466
development of, 464
scope and standards in, 466
transformational leadership in, 458–459
Manageability, in Artinian Intersystem Model, 165t
Managed care, 459, 466–468, 469
Managed care organizations (MCOs), 469
Management. *See also* Administration and management
definition of, 355
Managers
first-level, 455
middle-level, 455
nurse, in case management, 466–468
top-level, 455
Man-Living-Health (Parse), 202
Marxist feminism, 291
Marxist theory, 289–290
Mastectomy, concept development of grief after, 49–50, 56, 67
Maternal Role Attainment/Becoming a Mother, Conceptualization of, 222, 248, 251–252
application in practice, 252, 253
context for use, 252
evidence of empirical testing, 252
nursing implications of, 252
purpose and concepts of, 252
Maturation, and learning, 401–404
Maturity level, 362
MCOs. *See* Managed care organizations
Meaningfulness, in Artinian Intersystem Model, 165t
Measurement, in concept development, 62
Medical errors, IOM report on, 470
Medication administration, specialization in, 453–454
Memory, in information-processing models, 394–395
Metaparadigm, 41–44
Artinian Intersystem Model on, 165–166
definition of, 27t, 41
Johnson on, 147
Neuman on, 150
Nightingale and, 134–135
Orem on, 143–144
relationships among concepts in, 43–44
requirements for, 41b
Roy on, 179, 179t
social justice in, 44
theoretical definitions of concepts in, 43t
Watson on, 184
Metaphysical knowledge, 13
Metaphysics, 7, 7t
Metatheory, 37, 73, 74
Methodological triangulation, 500
Methodology, 12, 16–18
future issues in, 499–500
pluralism in, 18
quantitative *vs.* qualitative, 17–18, 500
Microtheories. *See* Practice theories
Middle-level managers, 455
Middle middle range theories, 217, 230, 241–248, 242t. *See also* specific theories
multiple, application in practice, 253
Self-Transcendence Theory, 221, 241, 247–248
Theory of Comfort, 222, 229, 241, 244–246
Theory of Unpleasant Symptoms, 218, 241, 246–247
Uncertainty in Illness Theory, 222, 241–244
Middle range theories, 27t, 37–38, 73, 74, 213–228. *See also* specific theories
analysis and evaluation of, 225–226, 501–502
approaches for generating, 217, 218t
Benner model of skill acquisition, 230–233
categorization of, 217
characteristics of, 215, 216b, 216t
combining existing nursing and non-nursing theories, 221
concepts of, 213, 216–217
Conceptualization of Maternal Role Attainment/Becoming a Mother, 222, 248, 251–252
derived from behavioral sciences, 221–222, 222t
derived from grand theories, 219–220, 439
derived from practice guidelines or standard of care, 224–225
derived from research and/or practice, 218–219, 438–439
development of, 217–225, 218b, 501–502
evaluation of, 95, 98t, 103–104, 105t, 106
future issues in, 501–502
grand theories *vs.*, 213, 215, 216t
high, 217, 230–241, 231t
legitimizing nursing discipline with, 214
Leininger's cultural care diversity and universality theory, 233–234
low, 217, 230, 248–252
middle, 217, 230, 241–248, 242t
Pender's Health Promotion Model, 234–236, 235t
Postpartum Depression Theory, 248, 250–251
practice theories *vs.*, 215, 216t, 419
purposes of, 214–215
relationships in, 216–217
Self-Transcendence Theory, 221, 241, 247–248
sources for generating, 217
Synergy Model for Patient Care, 230, 239–241, 241b, 253
testability of, 214
Theory of Chronic Sorrow, 218, 248–250, 253
Theory of Comfort, 222, 229, 241, 244–246

Theory of Unpleasant Symptoms, 218, 241, 246–247, 443
Transitions Theory, 236–239
Uncertainty in Illness Theory, 222, 241–244
user-friendly language and style of, 225
Mind, concept of, 285
Mishel's Uncertainty in Illness Theory. *See* Uncertainty in Illness Theory
Model(s), 82. *See also* specific models
application of. *See* Application of theory
concept development and, 57
definition of, 27t
evaluation of, 98t, 103–104, 105t
Modeling
in concept development, 65, 65t
defined by Erickson, Tomlin, and Swain, 170, 171t
Modeling and Role-Modeling (MRM), 160, 169–173
assumptions of, 170
background of theorists, 169–170
concepts of, 170, 171t
philosophical underpinnings of, 170
relationships in, 170–172
testability of, 172
usefulness of, 172, 172b
value in extending nursing science, 173
Modeling and Role-Modeling: A Theory and Paradigm for Nursing (Erickson), 169
Moderate postmodernists, 299
Modular (team) nursing, 459–461
Moral knowledge, 13. *See also* Ethics
Motivation
in adult learning, 403, 403b
in Maslow's human needs theory, 316
Motivational theories, 366–368
Achievement–Motivation Theory, 366–367, 367t
Equity Theory, 368
Expectancy Theory, 367
Motivational theories of leadership, 359–360
Motivation–hygiene theory, 359–360
Motivation in health behavior, theory of, 242t
Movement, in Health as Expanding Consciousness, 199–201, 200t
MRM. *See* Modeling and Role-Modeling
Multiplicity prelegitimate stage, 398
Multiplicity subordinate stage, 398
Multiskilled workers, 462

N

Naming theories, 75
National Guideline Clearinghouse (NGC), 260
National Institute for Nursing Research (NINR), 446, 447, 504, 505t
National Institutes of Health (NIH), on translational research, 32
National League for Nursing (NLN), 31, 136, 482–483
Natural history of disease, 337–339, 338f
Naturalistic concepts, 54, 54t
Natural sciences, 6, 6t
Needs-based theory. *See* Human needs theories
Negentropy, 151t
Network analysis, 283, 284f
Networks, social, 283–284, 284f
Neuman Systems Model, 131, 149–154
background of theorist, 150
concepts of, 150–152, 151*t*, 152*f*
as curricular framework, 484
middle range theories derived from, 219
parsimony of, 154
philosophical underpinnings of, 150
research testing, 441
stress theory and, 320–321
testability of, 153–154
usefulness of, 152–153, 154b
value in extending nursing science, 154
Neuman Systems Model Trustees Group, Inc., 153
New England Hospital, nursing training at, 28
New York University, nursing doctoral program of, 30
NGC. *See* National Guideline Clearinghouse
NGT. *See* Nominal group technique
NIC. *See* Nursing Intervention Classification system
Nightingale Fund, 134
Nightingale School for Nursing, 133–134, 135
NINR. *See* National Institute for Nursing Research
NLN. *See* National League for Nursing
Nominal group technique (NGT), 373
Non-nursing disciplines, middle range theories derived from, 221–223
Non-nursing theory
combined with existing nursing theory, in middle-range theories, 221
in nursing research, 444–445
Normalizing Risky Sexual Behaviors, Theory of, 218
Normal line of defense, 151t
Normative beliefs, 323–324
Notes on Hospitals (Nightingale), 132–133
Notes on Nursing: What It Is and What It Is Not (Nightingale), 26, 34t, 132–133, 134, 431
Nurse case manager, 467
Nurse Practitioner Practice Model, 231t
Nursing
as academic discipline, 4–5, 214
application of models or theories to. *See* Application of theory
art of, 13, 14t, 19–20
caring as central construct in, 45
common elements of, 31
defined, 43t
defined by Artinian, 165–166, 167t
defined by Erickson, Tomlin, and Swain, 170, 171t
defined by Johnson, 147
defined by King, 175, 175t
defined by Levine, 162t
defined by Newman, 199, 200t, 209t
defined by Orem, 143
defined by Parse, 209t
defined by Rogers, 195t, 209t
defined by Watson, 185t
future of, IOM recommendations on, 3, 417
graduate, ANA promotion of, 30
as human science, 16–17
metaparadigm of, 27t, 41–44, 43t
as multiparadigm discipline, 11
as practice or applied science, 6, 16, 306
praxis of, 15
as profession, 2–3
social justice in, 44
Nursing: Human Science and Human Care: A Theory of Nursing (Watson), 182
Nursing action, 165–166, 167t
Nursing Consortium for Research on Chronic Sorrow, 249
Nursing diagnoses
in Neuman Systems Model, 152
vs. nursing functions, 140–141
Nursing education
advanced practice nurses, 31–32
application of content and skills in, 488
application of theory in, 479–496
buzzwords in, 480
change in, 480
closing theory–practice gap through, 416–417
cognitive content of, 488
curriculum in, 481–488
blocking of content in, 486
changes in, 508
components of, 481, 481b
concept-based, 480
concepts of, 485
conceptual/organizational frameworks for, 480, 483–487
current issues in development of, 487
definition of, 481
design of, 481–482
eclectic approach to, 484–485
enhanced content in, areas of, 487, 487b
and regulatory bodies (accreditation), 482–483
single-theory approach to, 484
structure or sequencing of, 485–486, 486t
threading content in, 487
Tyler model of, 481–482

Nursing education (*continued*)
doctor of nursing practice, 31–32
first autonomous school in, 29–30
first doctoral programs in, 30
first training school in, 28
future issues in, 507–508
growth in doctoral programs, 31–32
growth in master's programs, 31
Henderson and, 136
IOM recommendations for, 509
Nightingale and, 133–134
for nurse case manager, 467
psychomotor tasks in, 488
stages of nursing theory in, 28–36
teaching/instruction in, 488–493
dialectic, 488–489
logistic, 490
operational, 490
problem-based, 489–490
theory-based strategies in, 488–490
technology in, 491–493
Nursing epistemology, 13–15, 27t
case study of, 19–20
definition of, 13
patterns of knowing in, 14t
Nursing for the Future (Brown), 30
Nursing goals, in Neuman Systems Model, 152
Nursing implications of theory
Benner model of skill acquisition, 232
Conceptualization of Maternal Role Attainment/Becoming a Mother, 252
Leininger's cultural care and universality theory, 233–234
Pender's Health Promotion Model, 235–236
Postpartum Depression Theory, 251
Self-Transcendence Theory, 248
Synergy Model for Patient Care, 240
Theory of Chronic Sorrow, 250
Theory of Comfort, 244–245
Theory of Unpleasant Symptoms, 247
Transitions Theory, 238
Uncertainty in Illness Theory, 243
Nursing Intervention Classification (NIC) system, 422–423
Nursing metaparadigm, 27t
Nursing of the Sick (Hampton), 133
Nursing philosophy, 11–12. *See also* Philosophical underpinnings of theory
Nursing problems, Abdellah's list of, 140, 140b, 141
Nursing research. *See also* Research
amount and quality of, 431, 504
application of theory in, 430–451
on areas of evolving nursing science, 446–448, 447b
correlational, 76, 434, 434t, 435–436
corresponding, to types of theories, 434–437, 434t
definition of, 432
descriptive, 434–435, 434t
experimental, 434, 434t, 436–437
future issues in, 499–500, 504, 505t
historical overview of, 431–432
NINR priorities in, 446, 447, 504, 505t
non-nursing theory in, 444–445
nursing theory in, 444–445
concern over reliance on, 444–445
rationale for using, 444
purpose of theory in, 433
recommendations for future, 448, 448t
relationship with theory, 432–433
theory as conceptual framework in, 442–443, 445, 446b
theory description in research report, 445, 446b
theory fit in research agenda, 445, 446–448, 447b, 448t
theory-generating, 439
theory-testing, 441
theory use in, 437–443
Nursing science, 11–12
case study of, 19–20
definition of, 12
development of knowledge in, 12–15, 432
empiricism in, 9
evolving, areas of, 446–448, 447b
future issues in, 499–500
as nursing research priority, 505t
phenomenology/constructivism/historicism, 9
philosophical views in, 7–10, 11t
philosophy of, 11–12
postmodernism in, 10
research methodology in, 12, 16–18
Nursing science, value in extending, 127
Abdellah and, 142
Artinian Intersystem Model and, 169
Caring Science as Sacred Science and, 186
Conservation Model and, 164
Health as Expanding Consciousness and, 202
Henderson and, 138–139
humanbecoming paradigm and, 208
Johnson and, 149
Modeling and Role-Modeling and, 173
Neuman Systems Model and, 154
Nightingale and, 136
Orem and, 146
Roy Adaptation Model and, 181
Science of Unitary and Irreducible Human Beings and, 197
Theory of Goal Attainment and, 177
Nursing Services Delivery Theory, 283
Nursing skills, Abdellah's list of, 140, 141
Nursing system, in Self-Care Deficit Theory, 144t
Nursing theory. *See also* Theory(ies); specific theories
borrowed or shared, 78–79, 78t, 424–425. *See also* specific disciplines
borrowed *vs.* unique, 40–41, 431
categorization of, 118–123
chronology of publications on, 34t–36t
classification of, 36–40
and evidence-based practice, 263–264
future issues in, 500–502
importance of, 23, 25
influence on practice, 25
issues in development of, 40–45
Nightingale and, 26
in nursing research, 444–445
concern over reliance on, 444–445
rationale for using, 444
questions and debates about, 23–24
relationships among levels of, 75, 75f
scope of, 36–38, 37f, 73–75
significant events in development of, 33t
stages of development, 26–36, 29t
theory of *vs.* theory for, 444–445
type or purpose of, 38–40
Nursing therapeutics, 237
Nursing Work Index-Revised, 463

O

Object of instinct, 308
Occupation, nursing as, 2–3
Occupational health nurse practice, Rogers' model for, 218–219, 231t
OCRSIEP. *See* Organizational Culture and Readiness Scale for System-wide Integration of Evidence-based Practice
Omaha System, 218, 231t
Online courses, 480, 491–493
Online discussions, dialectic learning in, 489
Ontology, 7, 7t, 12, 16, 27t
Openness, 194–196, 195t
Open system, in Neuman Systems Model, 151t
Open systems theory (OST), 282–283, 283b
Operant, definition of, 390
Operant conditioning, 313–314, 327t, 389–390, 389t
Operational adequacy of theory, 99
Operationally defined concepts, 53, 53t
Operational teaching strategies, 490
Oral stage of development, 307t, 308
Order and conflict synthesis model, 289, 289b
Organism, in person-centered theory, 317–318

Organizational Culture and Readiness Scale for System-wide Integration of Evidence-based Practice (OCRSIEP), 266
Organizational design, 453–456
  authority and responsibility in, 455
  centralization *vs.* decentralization in, 455–456
  departmentalization in, 456
  elements of, 453, 453b
  span of control in, 454–455
Organizational quantitative decision-making techniques, 374
Organizational theory, 365
Orientation to learning, of adults, 403, 403b
Originating, 204
Origins, of theory, 100, 101t
OST. *See* Open systems theory
Outcomes
  in Neuman Systems Model, 152
  in Synergy Model for Patient Care, 240, 240f
Outcome theorists, 119, 120t
Out-group, in Leader–Member Exchange Theory, 358
Output, in Neuman Systems Model, 151t

P

Pain management, 349–350
  acute, theory of, 224, 249t
  gate control theory of, 221, 331–332, 350f
  theory of adaptation to chronic pain, 86, 221, 241t, 249t
Pandimensionality, 194–196, 195t
Paradigm(s). *See also* Metaparadigm
  categorization of grand theories by, 119–123
  competing, combining theories from, 128
  definition of, 28t, 119
  future issues on, 500
  humanbecoming, 121, 193, 202–208
  interactive–integrative, 122
  particulate–deterministic, 122
  reaction, 122, 123t, 125–126
  reciprocal, 122, 123t, 126
  simultaneity, 121, 121f, 192
  simultaneous action, 122–123, 123t, 126
  totality, 121, 121f
  unitary–transformative, 122
Paradigm shift, 119–120, 203, 308
Parataxic cognition, 312
Parenting Under Pressure, 439
Parents' Perception of Uncertainty in Illness Scale, 243–244
Pareto charts, 379
Parish nursing models, 231t
Parsimony of theory, 101t, 127
  Abdellah's patient-centered approach, 141
  Artinian Intersystem Model, 169
  Caring Science as Sacred Science, 186
  Conservation Model, 163–164
  Health as Expanding Consciousness, 202
  Henderson's, 138
  humanbecoming paradigm, 207
  Johnson's, 149
  Modeling and Role-Modeling, 173
  Neuman Systems Model, 154
  Nightingale's, 136
  Orem's, 146
  Roy Adaptation Model, 181
  Science of Unitary and Irreducible Human Beings, 197
  Theory of Goal Attainment, 177
Participant–observer, 312
Participation, shared governance *vs.*, 456–457
Participative leader, 361
Particulate–deterministic paradigm, 122
Path–Goal Theory, 361–362
Pathogenesis, 337–339
Patient and family-centered care (PFCC), 462
Patient care delivery models, 459–466
  current use of, 463–465
  future issues in, 506–507
  Magnet Recognition Program, 464–465, 466b
  nurse and patient satisfaction in, 463
  nurse staffing levels in, 464–465
  patient-focused care, 460, 461–463, 461b
  primary nursing, 459–460, 461
  team nursing, 459–461
  total patient care (functional nursing), 459–460
Patient-centered approach, 139–142
  assumptions, concepts, and relationships in, 139–141
  background of theorist, 139
  parsimony of, 141
  philosophical underpinnings of, 139
  usefulness of, 141, 141b
Patient-centered care. *See* Patient-focused care
Patient-centered medical homes (PCMHs), 470
Patient characteristics, in Synergy Model for Patient Care, 239, 239b
Patient contracting, 423, 424t
Patient-focused care (PFC), 460, 461–463
  goals of, 462
  multiskilled workers in, 462
  outcomes of, 462
  patient redeployment in, 461–462
  principles of, 461, 461b
  support services decentralization in, 462
  task simplification in, 462
Patient Protection and Affordable Care Act (PPACA), 377, 463, 464, 498, 502, 506
Patient redeployment, 461–462
Patient simulator, high-fidelity, 491
Patient-to-nurse ratios, 464–465
Pattern
  in Health as Expanding Consciousness, 199–201
  in Science of Unitary and Irreducible Human Beings, 194–196, 195t
  in Transitions Theory, 237
Pattern recognition, 200t
PBE. *See* Practice-based evidence
PBL. *See* Problem-based learning
PBM. *See* Pharmacy benefits management
PCMHs. *See* Patient-centered medical homes
PCRS. *See* Caregiver Rewards Scale
PDSA. *See* Plan-do-stay-act cycle
Peaceful End of Life, Theory of, 224–225, 224f, 249t
Pedagogy, 402
Pender's Health Promotion Model. *See* Health Promotion Model
Perceived Access to Breast Health Care in African American Women Theory, 90–91
Perceived barriers, 322, 324t
Perceived behavioral control, 323–325
Perceived benefits, 322, 324t
Perceived severity, 322, 324t
Perceived susceptibility, 322, 324t
Perceived view of science, 7, 9–10, 11t
Perception
  in learning theory, 392
  in Theory of Goal Attainment, 175t
Perry's learning theory, 398–399
Person (human being), 43t
  in Artinian Intersystem Model, 164, 165, 167t
  in Caring Science as Sacred Science, 184, 185t
  in Health as Expanding Consciousness, 198–199, 200t, 209t
  in humanbecoming paradigm, 209t
  in Johnson's theory, 147
  in Levine's Conservation Model, 161, 162t
  in Neuman Systems Model, 150
  in nursing metaparadigm, 41–44, 43t
  in Orem's theory, 143
  in Roy Adaptation Model, 179t
  in Science of Unitary and Irreducible Human Beings, 193–197, 195t, 209t
  in Theory of Goal Attainment, 174, 175t
  in unitary process theories, 192, 209t
Personal integrity, 161–162, 162t
Personality traits, of leaders, 355–356
Personalization, in learning, 406
Personal knowledge, 12, 13–14, 14t, 19–20
Person-centered theory, 317–318, 401
Person–environment relationship, in stress theory, 320

Personification, 311
PES-NWI. *See* Practice Environment Scale of the Nursing Work Index revised
PET. *See* Practice question, evidence, and translation
PFC. *See* Patient-focused care
PFCC. *See* Patient and family-centered care
Phallic stage of development, 307t, 308
Pharmacy benefits management (PBM), 469
Phenomena, definition of, 28t
Phenomenal field, 185t, 317
Phenomenology
  perceived view of science, 7, 9–10, 11t
  qualitative methodology in, 17, 18
Philosophical underpinnings of theory
  Abdellah's, 139
  Artinian Intersystem Model, 164, 165t, 166f
  Caring Science as Sacred Science, 183
  Conservation Model, 160–161
  Health as Expanding Consciousness, 198
  Henderson's, 137
  humanbecoming paradigm, 203
  Johnson's, 147
  Modeling and Role-Modeling, 170
  Neuman Systems Model, 150
  Nightingale's, 134
  Orem's, 142
  Roy Adaptation Model, 178
  Theory of Goal Attainment, 174
Philosophy
  branches of, 7, 7t
  definition of, 5, 6, 28t
  metatheory, 37, 74
  of nursing, 11–12
  overview of, 6–7
  of science, 7–10, 7t, 11t
  of science of nursing, 11–12
The Philosophy and Science of Caring (Watson), 182, 187
Physical functioning, theories and principles related to, 339–350
Physiologic needs, 316
Physiologic–physical mode, 179, 180f
Physiology
  middle range nursing theories derived from, 221–222
  theories and principles related to, 339–350
Piaget's cognitive development theory, 396–397
PICO. *See* Practice question, intervention, comparison, and outcome
PKPIC. *See* Power as Knowing Participation in Change
Plan-do-stay-act (PDSA) cycle, 472
Planetree, Inc., 462
Planned Behavior, Theory of, 321, 322–326
  application in research, 436, 443
  application to practice, 84, 325–326
  comparison with other behavioral theories, 327t
  components of, 325f
  smoking behavior model derived from, 222–223
Planned change theory, 370–372
Pleasure principle, 308
Pluralism, methodologic, 18
Polar area diagram, 133
Political philosophy, 7, 7t
Position power, 360–361, 360b
Positivism, 8–9, 11t, 122
Postcolonialism, 10, 11t, 300
Postmastectomy grief (PMG), 49–50, 56, 67
Postmodernism, 7, 10, 11t
  definition of, 298
  extreme, 299
  moderate, 299
  in theory evaluation, 104
Postmodern social theory, 298–300
  application to nursing, 300
  characteristics of, 299b
  vs. modern theory, 299–300
Postpartum Depression Screening Scale, 251
Postpartum Depression Theory, 248, 250–251
  application in practice, 251
  context for use, 251
  evidence of empirical testing, 251
  nursing implications of, 251
  purpose and concepts of, 251
Postpositivism, 8–9, 122
Poststructuralism, 10, 11t
Power, 368–369
  authority *vs.*, 368
  Barrett's theory of, 196
  bases or sources of, 368, 369t
  charismatic, 368
  coercive, 368, 369t
  in conflict theories, 289
  definition of, 368
  expert, 368, 369t
  informational, 368
  of leaders, 355
  legitimate, 368, 369t
  of managers, 355
  in motivational theory, 367, 367t
  need for, 369
  position, 360–361, 360b
  referent, 368, 369t
  reward, 368, 369t
  selecting strategy of, 369
  in social exchange theory, 281
  transfer or delegation of (empowerment), 369–370
Power as Knowing Participation in Change (PKPIC), 196
Powering, 204
PPACA. *See* Patient Protection and Affordable Care Act
Practice
  application of models or theories to. *See* Application of theory
  future issues in, 502–504
  gap between theory and, 416–417
  IOM recommendations for, 509
  middle range theories derived from, 218–219
  in nursing metaparadigm, 44
  relationship among theory, research, and practice, 82–83, 83f, 502
  theory-based, 414–415, 415t. *See also* Application of theory
  theory development in, 83–85, 84t
  theory relationship with, 413–414, 414b
  transformation in, 502
  validation and application of theory in, 87t, 88–89
Practice-based evidence (PBE), 261–262, 262f
Practice Environment Scale of the Nursing Work Index revised (PES-NWI), 465
Practice guidelines, middle range theories derived from, 224–225
Practice question, evidence, and translation (PET), 266, 269b
Practice question, intervention, comparison, and outcome (PICO), 270
Practice science, 6, 6t, 16
Practice theories, 28t, 37, 38, 73, 74–75, 418–421
  characteristics of, 418
  definition of, 418
  development of, 502
  evaluation of, 98t, 103–104, 105t
  and evidence-based practice, 419–421, 421t
  examples from nursing literature, 419, 420t
  future issues in, 501–502
  grand theory-based, 419
  middle range theories *vs.*, 215, 216t, 419
  types needed, 418t
Pragmatic adequacy of theory, 99
Pragmatic principle, in concept analysis, 66, 67b
Pragmatism, 285
Praxis, definition of, 28t
Praxis of nursing, 15
Predictability of theory, 99
Predictive theories, 39, 75, 76–77, 434, 434t, 436–437
Preoperational stage, 396
Preparing Instructional Objectives (Mager), 481–482
Prepathogenesis, 337
Prescriptive theories, 39–40, 75, 77–78
  components of, 77
  list of survey questions for, 77, 77b
Prevention as intervention, 151t, 152
Primary nursing, 459–460, 461
Primary prevention, 337–339, 337b
Principle-based concept analysis, 66, 67b, 68t
Principle or rule learning, 397b
The Principles of Scientific Management (Taylor), 365
Prion, 334
Private duty nursing, 459
Proactive interference, 395

Problem-based learning (PBL), 489–490
Problem-solving, 372–374
in evidence-based practice, 474
in Gagne's learning theory, 397b
in quality improvement, 471–472
Procedural knowledge stage, of nursing theory, 29t, 31
Process improvement, 471
Process role theory, 288
Product of nursing, 144t
Profession(s)
characteristics of, 2
nursing as, 2–3
theory in, 24–25
Projection, 315
Properties, of transitions, 237
Propositions, 80t
Protection Motivation Theory, 322
Prototaxic cognition, 312
Psychic energy, 308
Psychoanalytic feminism, 291–292
Psychoanalytic theory, 307–309
application to nursing, 309
comparison with other behavioral theories, 327t
learning in, 400
stages of development in, 307t, 308–309
Psychodynamic theories, 306–313
comparison of, 327t
interpersonal, 307t, 311–313, 327t
learning in, 400, 405t
psychoanalytic, 307–309, 307t, 327t
psychosocial developmental, 307t, 310–311, 327t
Psychological Adaptation in Death and Dying, 439
Psychological sciences. *See* Behavioral sciences
Psychomotor learning, 387–388
Psychomotor tasks, in nursing education, 488
Psychosocial developmental theory, 310–311
application to nursing, 310–311
comparison with other behavioral theories, 327t
stages of development in, 307t, 310
Publications, of theorists, 34t–36t
Abdellah's, 141b
Johnson's, 146b
Nightingale's, 26, 34t, 132–133, 134
Publications, on theory analysis and evaluation, 98t
Public Health Nursing Practice Model, 224, 231t
Pure or basic sciences, 6, 6t, 306
Purpose of research, 430
Purpose of theories, 79, 102t, 413
Benner model of skill acquisition, 230–232
Conceptualization of Maternal Role Attainment/Becoming a Mother, 252
Kolcaba's Theory of Comfort, 244
Leininger's cultural care diversity and universality theory, 233
middle range theories, 214–215
Pender's Health Promotion Model, 234–235
Postpartum Depression Theory, 251
in research, 433
Self-Transcendence Theory, 248
Synergy Model for Patient Care, 239–240
Theory of Chronic Sorrow, 250
Theory of Unpleasant Symptoms, 246
Transitions Theory, 237
Uncertainty in Illness Theory, 243

Q

QI. *See* Quality improvement/management
QM. *See* Quality improvement/management
Qualitative methodology, 16, 17–18, 500
Qualitative synthesis, 58
Quality improvement/management, 375–380, 470–475
benchmarking in, 472
Crosby's four absolutes of, 378
Deming's 14 points on, 377, 377b
determining and measuring variation in, 379, 471
To Err Is Human as impetus for, 470
evidence-based practice and, 380–382, 474–475
frameworks for, 377–378
in health care
case for, 375–377
initiatives in nursing, 472–473
timeline of, 376t
Juran's trilogy of, 377–378
leadership in, 471
Lean Thinking in, 379
organizational leadership role and, 378–379
processes and tools in, 379–380
process improvement in, 471
quality defined in, 471
safety promotion in, 473
scientific and statistical methods in, 471–472
Six Sigma in, 379–380, 381
vocabulary in, 375
Quality of life
health-related, theoretical *vs.* operational definition of, 53t
in nursing metaparadigm, 42
as nursing research priority, 505t
Quality report cards, 473
Quality systems improvement (QSI), 375
Quantitative decision-making technologies, 372, 374
Quantitative methodology, 16, 17–18, 500
Quantitative synthesis, 58

R

Racism, 294
Radiation Therapy Comfort Questionnaire, 246
Radical feminism, 291
RAM. *See* Roy Adaptation Model
Randomized control trials (RCTs), 259
Rational choice theory, 281
Rational Decision-Making Model, 372–373
Rational Emotive Theory, 314–315, 327t
Rationalism, 7
Rationality, 281, 281t
bounded, 373
economic, 372
RCTs. *See* Randomized control trials
Reaction paradigm, 122, 123t, 125–126
Readiness to learn, of adults, 403, 403b
Reasoned Action, Theory of, 321, 322–326
application in research, 436, 443
application to practice, 84, 325–326
comparison with other behavioral theories, 327t
components of, 325f
smoking behavior model derived from, 222–223
Received knowledge stage, of nursing theory, 29t, 30
Received view of science, 7, 8–9, 11t
Reciprocal determinism, 399
Reciprocal paradigm, 122, 123t, 126
Reciprocity, 280
Reconstitution, 151t
Reference groups, 288
Referent power, 368, 369t
Refreezing, in planned change theory, 371
Regulator, in Roy Adaptation Model, 179t, 180
Reinforcement
in Hull's learning theory, 389–390, 389t
in operant conditioning, 313–314
Related concepts, 61
Relational concepts, 51t
Relational statements, 28t, 79–81, 80t
associational or correlational, 80–81
causal, 81
formulation and validation of, 87, 87b
Relationship behavior, 362
Relationships, in theories, 102t
Abdellah's patient-centered approach, 139–141
Artinian Intersystem Model, 166–168
Caring Science as Sacred Science, 184–185
Conservation Model, 161–162
Health as Expanding Consciousness, 199–201
Henderson's, 137
humanbecoming paradigm, 204

Relationships, in theories (*continued*)
Johnson's, 148
middle range theories, 216–217
Modeling and Role-Modeling, 170–172
Neuman's, 152
Nightingale's, 134–135
Roy Adaptation Model, 179–180
Theory of Goal Attainment, 176
Relativism, 398–399
Relevance, in learning, 406
"Relevance gap," 32
Research
concept development and, 57
correlational, 76, 434, 434t, 435–436
corresponding, to types of theories, 434–437, 434t
cultural bias in, recommendations for avoiding, 295, 295b
definition of, 432
descriptive, 434–435, 434t
evidence-based practice *vs.*, 259
experimental, 434, 434t, 436–437
framework/process of, 433–434, 433b
future issues in, 499–500, 504, 505t
methodology of, 12, 16–18
middle range theories derived from, 218–219
middle range theory use in, 214
nursing and non-nursing theories in, 444–445
purpose of, 430
purpose of theory in, 433
relationship among theory, research, and practice, 82–83, 83f, 502
relationship with theory, 432–433
testing theoretical relationships in, 87t, 88
theory as conceptual framework in, 442–443, 445, 446b
theory development in, 84t, 85–86, 437–439
theory testing in, 437, 439–441, 441b
theory use in, 437–443
translational, 32
Research agenda, 445, 446–448
areas of evolving nursing science, 446–448, 447b
examples of priorities, 448, 448t
NINR research priorities, 446, 447
Research-based concepts, 54, 54t
Research report, 445, 446b
Research utilization (RU), 270
Residual stimuli, 179t
Resilience, 372
Resilience, theory of, 219, 242t
Resistance, as stage of stress, 318–320, 319t, 341, 341t
Resonancy, 194–196, 194b
Resource flows, in networks, 283–284, 284f
Restraining forces, on change, 371
Result interpretation, in concept development, 61
Retrieval cues, loss of, 395
Retroactive interference, 395
Revealing–concealing, 204
Reward power, 368, 369t
Ring structure, 150
Role
concept of, 286
generational changes in, 287
Role ambiguity, 287
Role conflict, 287
Role function mode, 180, 180f
Role incongruity, 287
Role-modeling. *See also* Modeling and Role-Modeling
defined by Erickson, Tomlin, and Swain, 171t
Role overload, 287
Role strain or stress, 287
Role-taking, 285–286
Role theory, 222, 278, 286–288
application to nursing, 288
process, 288
structural, 288
Roy Adaptation Model (RAM), 86, 160, 177–181
adaptive modes in, 179–180, 180f
application in practice, 426
application in research, 437
background of theorist, 177–178
concepts of, 179, 179t
cultural assumptions of, 178
middle range theories derived from, 220, 439
parsimony of, 181
philosophical assumptions of, 178
philosophical underpinnings of, 178
practice theory derived from, 419
relationships in, 170–180
research testing, 441
scientific assumptions of, 178
stress theory and, 320–321
testability of, 181
usefulness of, 180–181, 182b
value in extending nursing science, 181
RU. *See* Research utilization
Rule or principle learning, 397b
Run charts, 379
Rural nursing model, 231t

S

Sacred science. *See* Caring Science as Sacred Science
Safety needs, 316
Safety promotion, 473
Sample, selecting, 60–61
SAMRM. *See* Society for the Advancement of Modeling and Role-Modeling
Satisficing, 373
SBAR. *See* Situation, background, assessment, recommendation
SCDNT. *See* Self-Care Deficit Nursing Theory
Schemes, in Piaget's development theory, 396
Schuler Nurse Practitioner Practice Model, 231t
Science. *See also* Nursing science
applied *vs.* pure or basic, 6, 306
characteristics of, 5b
classifications of, 6, 6t
definition of, 5
overview of, 5–6
perceived view of, 7, 9–10, 11t
philosophies of, 7–10, 7t, 11t
postmodernist view of, 7, 10
received view of, 7, 8–9, 11t
Science of Unitary and Irreducible Human Beings, 193–197
assumptions of, 194
background of theorist, 193
comparison with other unitary process theories, 208, 209t
concepts of, 194, 194b, 195t
middle range theories derived from, 219, 221
parsimony of, 197
philosophical underpinnings of, 193–194
relationships in, 194–195
testability of, 196–197
usefulness of, 196, 197b
value in extending nursing science, 197
Science of Unitary Human Beings, 86, 193, 194
Scientific management, 365
Scientific method, in quality improvement, 471–472
Scope and Standards for Nursing Administrators (ANA), 466
Scope of theory, 36–38, 37f, 73–75
in categorization of grand theories, 118–119
in middle range theories, 217, 230
in theory evaluation, 104, 106, 107t
Secondary prevention, 337–339, 337b
Selector, in intrasystem model, 167–168
Self
in Caring Science as Sacred Science, 185t
concept of, 285–286
in Maslow's human needs theory, 315
in person-centered theory, 317–318
in psychoanalytic theory, 307–309
Self-actualization, 316, 316b, 363–364, 393
Self-awareness, of leaders, 356–357
Self-care
in Modeling and Role-Modeling, 171t
Orem's definition of, 144t
Self-Care, Dependent Care & Nursing (journal), 145
Self-Care Deficit Nursing Theory (SCDNT), 142–146
application in practice, 425
assumptions, concepts, and relationships in, 142–144, 143f, 144t
background of theorist, 142
as curricular framework, 484

middle range theories derived from, 219, 221, 439
parsimony of, 146
philosophical underpinnings of, 142
testability of, 145, 145b
usefulness of, 144–145, 145b
value in extending nursing science, 146
Self-Care of Chronic Illness, 439
Self-care requisites, 144t
Self-concept, 311, 403, 403b
Self-concept–group identity mode, 180, 180f
Self-efficacy, 322, 324t
Self-efficacy theory, 242t, 322
Self-esteem, and power strategy, 369
Self-esteem needs, 316
Self-help model, 242t
Self-management/self-control, of leaders, 357
Self-Transcendence Theory, 221, 241, 247–248
application in practice, 248, 253
context for use, 248
evidence of empirical testing, 248
nursing implications of, 248
purpose and concepts of, 248
Self-transcendent needs, 316
Semantic clarity, 102
Semantic consistency, 102
Sense of coherence (SOC), 164, 165t, 166f, 168
Sensitive dependence on initial conditions, 296–297
Sensorimotor stage, 396
Sensory memory, 394
Sequencing, of curriculum, 485–486, 486t
Sequential learning, 490
Setting, selecting, 60–61
Sexism, 294
Sexual subsystem, 148
Shared governance, 456–458
administrative model of, 457
congressional model of, 457
councilor model of, 457
criticism of, 458
decentralization *vs.*, 456–457
outcomes of, 458
participation *vs.*, 456–457
principles of, 457
Shared Presence: Caring for a Dying Spouse, 39, 435
Shared theory. *See* Borrowed theory
Short-term memory, 394–395
Sick-Nursing and Health-Nursing (Nightingale), 132, 134, 135
Sigma Theta Tau International, 259
Signal learning, 397b
Silent knowledge stage, of nursing theory, 28–30, 29t
Simplicity/complexity of theory, 102, 104, 106, 107t
Simultaneity paradigm, 121, 121f, 192
Simultaneous action paradigm, 122–123, 123t, 126
Situation, background, assessment, recommendation (SBAR), 470
Situation, definition of the, 285
Situational control, 360
Situational leadership theory, 362
Situational sense of coherence (SSOC), 164, 165, 165t, 166f, 168, 169
Situation-producing theories. *See* Prescriptive theories
Situation-relating theories. *See* Predictive theories
Situation-specific theories. *See* Practice theories
Six Sigma, 379–380, 381
Skill(s). *See also* Competencies
of advanced practice nurses, 500–501, 501b
of generalist nurses, 498–499, 499b
Skill acquisition
Benner model of, 230–233, 430, 439
Dreyfus model of, 84, 222, 230
Skinner's behavioral theory. *See* Operant conditioning
Smoking behaviors, theoretical model of, 222–223, 223f
Smoking cessation, theory application in, 425
SOC. *See* Sense of coherence
Social awareness, of leaders, 357
Social exchange theory, 279–282
application to nursing, 281–282
assumptions of, 280b
central concepts of, 281, 281t
Social integrity, 161–162, 162t
Socialist feminism, 291
Social justice, 44
Social learning theory, 322, 399–400
application in research, 437, 443
application to nursing, 399–400
middle range theory derived from, 222–223
Social networks, 283–284, 284f
Social psychology, 321–326. *See also* specific theories
application to nursing, 325–326
Human Belief Model, 321–322
Theory of Reasoned Action/Planned Behavior, 322–325
Social Readjustment Rating Scale (SRRS), 342
Social sciences, 6, 6t
Social skills/relationship skills, of leaders, 357
Social support, model for, 242t
Social support networks, 283
Society for the Advancement of Modeling and Role-Modeling (SAMRM), 169
Sociocultural utility, of theory, 105
Sociograms, 283–284
Sociological imagination, 279
Sociology, 278–304
chaos theory in, 295–298
conflict theories in, 289–295
exchange theories in, 279–284
interactionist frameworks in, 284–288
middle range theories of, 214
nursing theories derived from, 78t, 221–222
Somatic knowledge, 13
Sorrow. *See* Chronic Sorrow, Theory of
Source of instinct, 308
Space, in Health as Expanding Consciousness, 199–201, 200t
Span of control, 454–455
Special cause variation, 471
Spiritual care, theoretical *vs.* operational definition of, 53t
Spirituality-based nursing practice, 39
Spirituality-based nursing practice theory of, 39
Spiritual knowledge, 13
SRRS. *See* Social Readjustment Rating Scale
SSOC. *See* Situational sense of coherence
Stability
in Behavioral System Model, 148t
in Neuman Systems Model, 151t
Stabilizer control processes, 179t
Staff authority, 455
Staffing levels, 464–465
Standard of care, middle range theories derived from, 224–225
Statement development, 87, 87b, 87t
Statistical concepts, 51t
Status, concept of, 286
Stetler Model of Evidence-Based Practice, 264, 270, 271t, 272t
Stimulus–response learning, 397b
Stimulus–response model of behavior, 313–314, 389–390
Strange attractor, 297
Stress
defined by Selye, 318
stages of, 318–320, 319t, 341, 341t
in Theory of Goal Attainment, 175t
Stressor
in Behavioral System Model, 148t
in Neuman Systems Model, 151t
Stress theories, 318–321
application to nursing, 320–321, 342
caregiver, 220, 249t
comparison with other behavioral theories, 327t
general adaptation syndrome, 318–320, 340–342
stress coping adaptation theory, 221, 319–320
Structural clarity, 102
Structural consistency, 102
Structural Empowerment, Theory of, 370
Structural integrity, 161, 162t
Structural role theory, 288
Structure
in Behavioral System Model, 148t
in Neuman Systems Model, 151t
in social exchange theory, 281, 281t
of theory, 81, 88, 102t
Student-centered teaching, 401

Subjective knowledge stage, of nursing theory, 29t, 30–31
Subjective norms, 323–324
Substantia gelatinosa, 349
Suffering, theory of, 249t
Sullivan's interpersonal theory. *See* Interpersonal theory
Summative concepts, 51t
Sunrise Model, Leininger's, 233
Superego, 307–309, 400
Supervision, as nursing competency, 503t
Supportive leader, 361
Surrogate terms, 61
Symbol(s), 285
Symbolic interactionism, 285–286
  application to nursing, 286
  assumptions of, 285, 285b
Synchronous technology, 491
Synergy Model for Patient Care, 96, 230, 239–241
  application in practice, 240–241, 241b, 253, 426
  application in research, 443
  context for use, 240
  evidence of empirical testing, 240–241, 241b
  nurse competencies in, 239, 239b
  nursing implications of, 240
  outcomes in, 240, 240f
  patient characteristics in, 239, 239b
  purpose and concepts of, 239–240
Syntaxic cognition, 312
Synthesizing, in concept development, 65, 65t
Systems
  in Behavioral System Model, 148t
  elements of, 282, 282f
  equilibrium in, 282
  general, theory of, 282–283
Systems Framework (King), 160, 173–177
Systems Model, Neuman's. *See* Neuman Systems Model

T

Tactile learning style, 405–406
Task behavior, 362
Task simplification, 462
Task structure, 360–361, 360b
Taxonomy, 75–76
  application of theory in, 422–423
  definition of, 28t
Teachers College of Columbia University, nursing doctoral program of, 30
Teaching
  definition of, 388
  Gagne's concept of, 397
  as nurse's role, 387
  in nursing education, 488–493
    dialectic, 488–489
    logistic, 490
    operational, 490
    problem-based, 489–490
    technology-based, 491–493
    theory-based strategies in, 488–490
  student-centered, 401
  tools for. *See* Learning theories
Team nursing, 459–461
Technology
  as nursing competency, 503t
  in nursing education, 491–493
Tension, in Behavioral System Model, 148t
Tertiary prevention, 337–339, 337b
Testability of theory, 99, 101t, 106, 107t, 126–127
  Abdellah's, 141
  Artinian Intersystem Model, 168–169
  Caring Science as Sacred Science, 186
  Conservation Model, 163
  Health as Expanding Consciousness, 201–202
  Henderson's, 138
  humanbecoming paradigm, 205–207, 206t–207t
  Johnson's, 149
  middle range theories, 214
  Modeling and Role-Modeling, 172
  Neuman Systems Model, 153–154
  Nightingale's, 135–136
  Orem's, 145, 145b
  Roy Adaptation Model, 181
  Science of Unitary and Irreducible Human Beings, 196–197
  Theory of Goal Attainment, 176–177
Testing, empirical, of theories or models
  Benner model of skill acquisition, 232
  Conceptualization of Maternal Role Attainment/Becoming a Mother, 252
  Leininger's cultural care diversity and universality theory, 233–234, 234b
  Pender's Health Promotion Model, 236, 236b
  Postpartum Depression Theory, 251
  Self-Transcendence Theory, 248
  Synergy Model for Patient Care, 240–241, 241b
  Theory of Chronic Sorrow, 250
  Theory of Comfort, 246
  Theory of Unpleasant Symptoms, 247
  Transitions Theory, 238–239
  Uncertainty in Illness Theory, 243–244
Theoretically defined concepts, 53, 53t
Theoretical models, 82
Theoretical phase, of concept development, 61–62, 62t
Theoretical statements, 79–81
Theorists, background of, 125
  Abdellah, 139
  Artinian, 164
  Erickson, 169
  Henderson, 136–137
  Johnson, 147
  King, 173
  Levine, 160
  Neuman, 150
  Newman, 198
  Nightingale, 133–134
  Orem, 142
  Parse, 203
  Rogers, 193
  Roy, 177–178
  Swain, 170
  Tomlin, 169–170
  Watson, 183
Theorists, paradigms of, 119, 120t
Theorists, publications of, 34t–36t
  Abdellah's, 141b
  Johnson's, 146b
  Nightingale's, 26, 34t, 132–133, 134
Theory(ies). *See also* specific theories, types of theories, and models
  application of. *See* Application of theory
  assumptions of, 81, 102t. *See also* Assumptions
  borrowed or shared, 40–41, 78–79, 78t, 424–425. *See also* specific disciplines and theories
    application in nursing practice, 78t, 424–425
    application in nursing research, 78t, 444–445
    definition of, 27t, 306
    vs. unique, 40–41, 306, 431
  borrowed *vs.* unique, 431
  characteristics of, 98, 98t
  classification of, 36–40, 73–79
  components of, 79–82, 102t
  concept development and, 57, 86–87
  concepts and conceptual definitions of, 79
  definitions of, 25, 28t
  and evidence-based practice, 263–264, 419
  nursing education on, 416–417
  of nursing *vs.* for nursing, 444–445
  origins of, 100, 101t
  overview of, 24–25
  practice relationship with, 413–414, 414b
  as process and product, 413
  purpose of, 79, 102t, 413
  relationships among levels of, 75, 75f
  research relationship with, 432–433
  scope of, 36–38, 37f, 73–75
  source or discipline of, 78–79, 78t
  structure and linkages of, 81, 88, 102t
  terminology of, 24, 26, 27t–28t
  types or classification by purpose, 38–40, 75–78

Theory analysis and evaluation, 95–113
Barnum's method for, 98t, 100, 100b, 106, 107t
Chinn and Kramer's method for, 97, 98t, 101–102, 102t, 106, 107t
comparison of methods, 106, 107t
criteria for, 96
definition of, 96–97
Dudley-Brown's method for, 98t, 104–105, 106, 107t
Duffey and Muhlenkamp's method for, 97, 98t, 99, 99b, 106
Ellis' method for, 98, 98t, 106, 107t, 124
exemplar of, 109–112
Fawcett's method for, 97, 98t, 100–101, 106, 107t, 124
grand theories, 104, 124–128, 125b
Hardy's method for, 98–99, 98t, 106, 107t, 124
historical overview of, 97–105, 98t
Meleis' method for, 97, 98t, 102–103, 106, 107t
middle range theories, 225–226, 501–502
publications on, 98t
purpose of, 96–97, 127–128
single-phase, 97
synthesized method for, 106, 108b
three-phase, 97
two-phase, 97
Walker and Avant's method for, 97, 98t, 100, 101t, 106, 107t, 124
Whall's method for, 95, 98t, 103–104, 105t, 106, 107t
Theory-based nursing practice, 414–415, 415t. *See also* Application of theory
Theory construction, 73, 87t, 88
Theory description, 97, 102
Theory development, 72–94
approaches to, 83–86, 84t
concept development in, 57, 86–87, 87t
exemplar of, 90–91
future issues in, 501–502
integrated approach in, 86
middle range theories, 217–225, 218b, 501–502
overview of, 73
practice to theory, 84t, 85
process of, 86–89, 87t
relationship among theory, research, and practice, 82–83, 83f, 502
research to theory, 84t, 85, 437–439
stages, in nursing, 26–36, 29t
statement development in, 87, 87b, 87t
testing in research, 87t, 88
theory to practice to theory, 83–84, 84t
theory to research to theory, 84t, 86
validation and application in practice, 87t, 88–89
Theory fitting, 443
Theory-generating research, 84t, 85–86, 437–439
exemplar of, 438
nursing studies, 439
process of, 438–439
Theory–practice gap, 416
closing, 416–417
reasons for, 416
Theory synthesis, 88, 88b
Theory-testing research, 437, 439–441
criteria for evaluating, 439, 441b
exemplar, 440–441
lack of clarity on, 439
nursing studies, 441
process of, 439
Theory X on leadership, 359
Theory Y on leadership, 359
Therapeutic interventions, in Conservation Model, 162t
Therapeutic milieu, 312–313
Therapeutic narratives, 300
Therapeutic self-care demand, 144t
"Third force" psychologists, 401
Threading, in curriculum, 487
Tidal model, 231t
Time, in Health as Expanding Consciousness, 199–201
To Err Is Human (IOM), 470
Top-level managers, 455
Totality paradigm, 121, 121f
Total patient care (functional nursing), 459–460
Total quality (TQ), 375
Total quality management (TQM), 375
Total quality systems (TQS), 375
TPB. *See* Planned Behavior, Theory of
TRA. *See* Reasoned Action, Theory of
Trait theories, of leadership, 355–357
Transactional leadership, 362–363
Transactional process, 173–177, 175t
Transcendence. *See* Self-Transcendence Theory
Transformational leadership, 362–363
in nursing and health care, 458–459
results *vs.* process of, 458
strategies for, 458, 459b
Transforming, 204
Transforming Presence: The Difference Nursing Makes (Newman), 198
Transitions, Meleis' definition of, 237
Transitions Theory, 236–239
application in practice, 238–239, 425
application in research, 436
context for use, 238
evidence of empirical testing, 238–239
nursing implications of, 238
purpose and concepts of, 237, 238f
Translational research, 32
Transpersonal caring, 184–185, 185t, 213
Transtheoretical Model, 322, 439
True presence concept, 192
Two-factor theory, Herzberg's, 359–360
Tyler Curriculum Development Model, 481–482
Typology, 75–76

U

UAP. *See* Unlicensed assistive personnel
Uncertainty, Theory of Nurses' Recognizing and Responding to, 435
Uncertainty in Illness Scale, 241, 243–244
Uncertainty in Illness Theory, 222, 241–244
application in practice, 243–244
context for use, 243
evidence of empirical testing, 243–244
nursing implications of, 243
purpose and concepts of, 243, 243f
Unfreezing, in planned change theory, 371
Unitary Man, Theory of, 193, 194
Unitary man/human beings, Rogers' theories of, 193–197. *See also* Science of Unitary and Irreducible Human Beings
Unitary process theories, 121f, 124, 124t, 126, 192–212. *See also* specific theories
comparison of, 208, 209t
Health as Expanding Consciousness, 193, 198–202
humanbecoming paradigm, 121, 193, 202–208
interactive theories *vs.*, 182–183
Science of Unitary and Irreducible Human Beings, 193–197
Science of Unitary Human Beings, 193
Unitary–transformative category, 122
U.S. Preventative Services Task Force, 259, 260
Universal self-care requisites, 144t
University of Pittsburgh, nursing doctoral program of, 30
University of Texas Health Science Center at San Antonio, evidence-based practice model of, 264–266, 265t
Unlicensed assistive personnel (UAP), 460
Unpleasant Symptoms, Theory of, 218, 241, 246–247
application in practice, 247, 253
application in research, 443
context for use, 247
evidence of empirical testing, 247
nursing implications of, 247
purpose and concepts of, 246, 247f
Urinary catheterization, intermittent, 422–423, 423t
Urinary Incontinence and Frequency Comfort Questionnaire, 246
Urine Control Theory, 181

Use, context for
Benner model of skill acquisition, 232
Conceptualization of Maternal Role Attainment/Becoming a Mother, 252
Leininger's cultural care diversity and universality theory, 233
Pender's Health Promotion Model, 235–236
Postpartum Depression Theory, 251
Self-Transcendence Theory, 248
Synergy Model for Patient Care, 240
Theory of Chronic Sorrow, 250
Theory of Comfort, 244–245
Theory of Unpleasant Symptoms, 247
Transitions Theory, 238
Uncertainty in Illness Theory, 243
Usefulness of theory, 99, 101t, 103, 106, 107t, 126
Abdellah's patient-centered approach, 141, 141b
Artinian Intersystem Model, 168
Caring Science as Sacred Science, 186, 187b
Conservation Model, 163
Health as Expanding Consciousness, 201, 202b
Henderson's, 138
humanbecoming paradigm, 204–205, 208b
Johnson's, 149
Modeling and Role-Modeling, 172, 172b
Neuman Systems Model, 152–153, 154b
Nightingale's, 135
Orem's, 144–145, 145b
Roy Adaptation Model, 180–181, 182b
Science of Unitary and Irreducible Human Beings, 196, 197b
Theory of Goal Attainment, 176
Utilitarianism, 279

V
Valence, 367
Validity of theory, 106, 107t
Value assumptions, 81
Valuing, in humanbecoming paradigm, 203–204
Variable(s), 52, 148t
Verbal association, in Gagne's learning theory, 397b
Verbal Rating Scale Questionnaire, 246
Video conferencing, 491
Virtual communities/classrooms, 480, 491–493
Visionary leadership, 364
Visual learning style, 405–406

W
Watson Caring Science Institute and International Caring Consortium (WCSIICC), 183
WCSIICC. *See* Watson Caring Science Institute and International Caring Consortium
Web-based (online) courses, 480, 491–493
Web of causation, 335–337, 336f
Wellness/illness, in Neuman Systems Model, 151t
Working definition, 62
Working (short-term) memory, 394–395
Work specialization, 453–454
Worldviews
definition of, 28t
grand theories categorized by, 119–123
metatheory, 37, 74
perceived, 7, 9–10, 11t
postmodern, 7
received, 7, 8–9, 11t

X
Xerox Corporation, benchmarking in, 472

Y
Yale University school of nursing, 29–30

CCS1214